Elastance	$E = \dfrac{\Delta P}{\Delta V}$	
Total compliance	$\dfrac{1}{C_{total}} = \dfrac{1}{C_L} + \dfrac{1}{C_{cw}}$	
Total elastance	$E_T = E_L + E_{cw}$	Chapter 2, p.
Po$_2$ torr to vol% (oxygen)	vol% = (Po$_2$ torr)(0.003 vol%/torr)	Chapter 3, p. 163
Total carbon dioxide (mmol-liter)	$[HCO_3^-] + PaCO_2 (0.03) = $ total CO_2	Chapter 3, p. 164
Pco$_2$ torr to vol% (carbon dioxide)	vol% = (Pco$_2$ torr)(0.067 vol%/torr)	Chapter 3, p. 166
vol% to mmol/liter (carbon dioxide)	mmol CO_2/liter = $\dfrac{\text{vol}\%}{2.23 \text{ vol}\%/\text{mmol } CO_2/\text{liter}}$	Chapter 3, p. 165
mmol/liter to vol% (carbon dioxide)	vol% = (mmol/liter)(2.23 vol%/mmol/liter)	Chapter 3, p. 165
torr to mmol/liter (carbon dioxide)	mmol/liter = (Pco$_2$ torr)(0.03 mmol/liter/torr)	Chapter 3, p. 166
Graham's law of diffusion (gases)	$r_1 \sqrt{D_1} = r_2 \sqrt{D_2}$	Chapter 3, p. 169
Graham's law of diffusion (gas-liquid)	$\dfrac{r_1}{r_2} = \dfrac{\sqrt{D_2} \times Cs_1}{\sqrt{D_1} \times Cs_2}$	Chapter 3, p. 170
Molarity	$\dfrac{\text{moles}}{\text{liter}} = M$	Chapter 3, p. 173
Normality	$\dfrac{\text{gram equivalent weights}}{\text{liter}} = N$	Chapter 3, p. 176
Hydrogen ion concentration	$pH = -\log[H^+]$	Chapter 3, pp. 178, 195
Hydrogen ion concentration	$pH = \log\left(\dfrac{1}{[H^+]}\right)$	Chapter 3, pp. 178, 195
nanomoles/liter to pH	$pH = 9 - (\log H^+ \text{ in nmol/liter})$	Chapter 3, pp. 182, 195
pH to moles/liter	moles/liter = antilog $(-pH)$	Chapter 3, p. 182
pH to nanomoles/liter	nmol/liter = antilog $(9 - pH)$	Chapter 3, p. 183
Henderson-Hasselbalch equation (HCO_3^-/H_2CO_3)	$pH = 6.10 + \log\dfrac{[HCO_3^-]}{(Pco_2)(0.03)}$	Chapter 3, pp. 192, 195
Density of solid or liquid	$D = \dfrac{g}{cc}$	Chapter 3, pp. 197, 198
Density of gas	$D = \dfrac{g}{22.4 \text{ liters}}$	Chapter 3, p. 199
°Celsius to Kelvin	$K = °C + 273$	Chapter 3, p. 203
°Celsius to °Fahrenheit	$°F = 1.8 (°C) + 32$	Chapter 3, p. 203
°Fahrenheit to °Celsius	$°C = (°F - 32)\tfrac{5}{9}$	Chapter 3, p. 204
°Fahrenheit to Kelvin	$K = (°F - 32)\tfrac{5}{9} + 273$	Chapter 3, p. 204
Electrochemical cell voltage	$E° = E°_{oxidation} + E°_{reduction}$	Chapter 3, p. 211
Work	$W = F \times d$	Chapter 4, p. 225
Power	$P = W/t$	Chapter 4, p. 231
Kinetic energy	$KE = \dfrac{1}{2}mv^2$	Chapter 4, p. 232
	or	
	$KE = \dfrac{1}{2}Dv^2$	Chapter 4, p. 238
Newton's second law of motion	$F = m \times a$	Chapter 4, p. 233
Acceleration from rest	$a = \dfrac{v}{t}$	Chapter 4, p. 233
Potential energy	$PE = m \times g \times h$	Chapter 4, p. 236
	or	
	$PE = D \times g \times h$	Chapter 4, p. 239
Pressure	$P = F/A$	Chapter 4, p. 241
	or	
	$P = h \times D$	Chapter 4, p. 243
Thoracic gas volume	$P_1V_1 = P_2(V_1 + \Delta V)$	Chapter 4, p. 249
Gay-Lussac's law	$\dfrac{P}{T} = k$	Chapter 4, p. 254
Combined gas law	$\dfrac{PV}{T} = k$	Chapter 4, p. 256
Dalton's law of partial pressure	$P_{total} = P_1 + P_2 + P_3 + \ldots P_n$	Chapter 4, p. 258

RESPIRATORY CARE SCIENCES
An Integrated Approach
Third Edition

William V. Wojciechowski

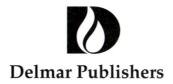

Delmar Publishers

I⟨T⟩P An International Thomson Publishing Company

Albany • Bonn • Boston • Cincinnati • Detroit • London • Madrid • Melbourne
Mexico City • New York • Pacific Grove • Paris • San Francisco • Singapore • Tokyo
Toronto • Washington

Cover Design: TDB Publishing Services

Delmar Staff

Publisher: Susan Simpfenderfer
Acquisitions Editor: Dawn Gerrain
Developmental Editor: Debra Flis
Project Editor: Stacey Prus
Production Coordinator: John Mickelbank

Printed in Canada
3 4 5 6 7 8 9 10 XXX 04 03 02 01 00 99

For more information, contact Delmar, 3 Columbia Circle, PO Box 15015, Albany, NY 12212-0515; or find us on the World Wide Web at http://www.delmar.com

International Division List

Japan:
Thomson Learning
Palaceside Building 5F
1-1-1 Hitotsubashi, Chiyoda-ku
Tokyo 100 0003 Japan
Tel: 813 5218 6544
Fax: 813 5218 6551

Australia/New Zealand:
Nelson/Thomson Learning
102 Dodds Street
South Melbourne, Victoria 3205
Australia
Tel: 61 39 685 4111
Fax: 61 39 685 4199

UK/Europe/Middle East:
Thomson Learning
Berkshire House
168-173 High Holborn
London
WC1V 7AA United Kingdom
Tel: 44 171 497 1422
Fax: 44 171 497 1426

Latin America:
Thomson Learning
Seneca, 53
Colonia Polanco
11560 Mexico D.F. Mexico
Tel: 525-281-2906
Fax: 525-281-2656

Canada:
Nelson/Thomson Learning
1120 Birchmount Road
Scarborough, Ontario
Canada M1K 5G4
Tel: 416-752-9100
Fax: 416-752-8102

Asia:
Thomson Learning
60 Albert Street, #15-01
Albert Complex
Singapore 189969
Tel: 65 336 6411
Fax: 65 336 7411

Spain:
Thomson Learning
Calle Magallanes, 25
28015-MADRID
ESPANA
Tel: 34 91 446 33 50
Fax: 34 91 445 62 18

Library of Congress Cataloging-in-Publication Data:
Wojciechowski, William V.
      Respiratory care sciences : an integrated approach / William
V. Wojciechowski, —3rd ed.
            p.   cm.
      Includes bibliographical references and index.
      ISBN: 0-7668-0780-0
      1. Respiratory therapy. 2. Medical sciences. 3. Respiratory
therapists. I. Title.
      [DNLM: 1. Respiratory Therapy. 2. Physical Sciences. WB 342
W847r 1999]
RC735.I5W65   1999
502'.4616—dc21   99-29382
DNLM/DLC for Library of Congress   CIP

TABLE OF CONTENTS

PREFACE

The content of this text continues to grow. Students and instructors in both technician and therapist programs are discovering that the material in this text fulfills many needs concerning basic science.

Even though this book was initially meant to provide respiratory therapy students with basic science topics skewed toward respiratory care and cardiorespiratory anatomy and physiology, it is finding its way into many programs as a stand-alone text. In many other respiratory therapy programs this book serves as a supplemental text in a number of respiratory therapy courses. I am pleased that the first and second editions were useful to so many students and faculty.

Changes to the Third Edition

The third edition contains changes that are intended to enhance the utility of this book. A list of formulas found in each chapter, along with the page number indicating where each formula is located within the chapter, has added following the chapter objectives. This addition is intended to provide quick reference for students and faculty, and to help make the text even more user friendly.

More practice problems have been added throughout the text. These include:

- calculating airway resistance
- obtaining static and dynamic compliance measurements
- graphing static and dynamic compliance curves
- determining the corrected barometric pressure
- solving problems concerning Dalton's law of partial pressure
- performing air entrainment calculations
- using Staling's law of the capillaries to compute filtration and reabsorption pressures
- computing lung volumes and lung capacities
- calculating shunt problems
- performing calculations concerning carbon dioxide transport

Additional diagrams have been included. These new diagrams reflect an expanded section on graphs, and specifically relate to compliance curves and the oxyhemoglobin dissociation curve. Diagrams in reference to lung volumes and capacities have also been added.

Calculator solutions to numerous sample problems have likewise been included, especially for logarithms, Henderson-Hasselbalch equation problems, and statistics.

The popular detailed solutions to the numerous practice problems (Appendix A) are still present. In fact this section has been expanded to encompass the additional practice problems mentioned in the bulleted list.

Chapter summaries have been added. Page numbers directing the reader to the answers to the practice problems have also been inserted to make locating answers in the Appendix easier and faster.

Again, I would like to extend an open invitation to those of you who use this text to continue providing me with input. I appreciate knowing your impressions and suggestions, favorable or otherwise. The only way this book is going to continually improve is via your critiques. I am grateful for having had the feedback from students and colleagues as this book evolved from the first to third editions. I recognize that there is always room for improvement. Thank you.

W.V.W.

ACKNOWLEDGMENTS

The third edition of this text would not have been possible without the extraordinary effort and perseverance of Deanna Winn who oversaw this project from start to finish. Seemingly endless drafts and rewrites were handled without complaints. Without her, the manuscript would still be in the preparation stages.

The staff at Delmar Publishers is to be thanked for its professional support and adherence to details.

My gratitude also is extended to the contributors who added important, timely content to the text.

I also wish to thank the following colleagues of mine who provided excellent review of the manuscript. Their suggestions proved to be fine additions to the text.

Sharon Baer, MBA, RRT, CPFT, Program Director, Respiratory Care Department, Naugatuck Valley Community-Technical College, Waterbury, Connecticut

Melanie A. Ciesielski, BS, RRT, Faculty, Respiratory Care Program, Forsyth Technical Community College, Winston-Salem, North Carolina

J. Kenneth Le Jeune, MS, RRT, CPFT, Division Chair Allied Health, Program Chair Respiratory Education, University of Arkansas Community College at Hope

Leanna Konechne, Med, RRT, RCP, Respiratory Therapy Program Director, Pima Medical Institute, Tucson, Arizona

Kathy Miller, MA, RRT, Director, Respiratory Care Program, Marygrive College, Detroit, Michigan

I would be remiss if I did not express my appreciation to the fine persons who contributed to the writing of the third edition. They are Ronald Allison, M.D., Kim Cavanagh, M.Ed., R.R.T., Brad Davis, Ph.D., Dean Hess, Ph.D., R.R.T., Alan Jobe, M.D., Ph.D., Pandu Kulkarni, Ph.D., and Larry Sindel, M.D.

Finally, I am grateful for the assistance of my colleague Julio Turrens, Ph.D., who provided valuable insight toward the preparation of the physiologic chemistry chapter.

It is my sincere hope that the efforts of all involved in this writing project benefit the people for whom this book was written—the students.

W.V.W.

DEDICATION

This book is dedicated to: my wife, Leslie; my daughters, Alison and Maria; my son, Matthew; my parents, Joseph and Lorraine.

CONTRIBUTORS

Chapters 1, 2 and 3
William V. Wojciechowski, MS, RRT
Chairman and Associate Professor
Department of Cardiorespiratory Care
University of South Alabama
Mobile, Alabama

Chapter 4
William V. Wojciechowski, MS, RRT

with contributions by:
Kim Cavanagh, MEd, RRT
South Baldwin Hospital
Foley, Alabama

Chapter 5
Pandu M. Kulkarni, PhD
Associate Professor of Statistics
Department of Math and Statistics
University of South Alabama
Mobile, Alabama

Dean Hess, RRT, PhD
Assistant Director of Respiratory Care
Massachusetts General Hospital
Instructor in Anesthesia
Harvard Medical School
Boston, Massachusetts

Chapter 6
William Bradshaw Davis, PhD
Professor of Biomedical Sciences

College of Allied Health Professions
Associate Professor
Department of Microbiology/
    Immunology
College of Medicine
University of South Alabama
Mobile, Alabama

William V. Wojciechowski, MS, RRT

with contributions by:
Ronald C. Allison, MD
Professor of Medicine
Pulmonary and Critical Care Medicine
Department of Medicine
University of South Alabama
Mobile, Alabama

Dean Hess, RRT, PhD

Alan H. Jobe, MD, PhD
Professor of Pediatrics
Harbor-University of California Los
    Angeles Medical Center
Torrance, California

Lawrence Sindel, MD
Associate Clinical Professor
Department of Pediatrics
University of South Alabama
Mobile, Alabama

Chapter 7
William Bradshaw Davis, PhD

CHAPTER ONE

MATHEMATICS

FORMULAS USED IN THIS CHAPTER

$I{:}E = \dfrac{T_I}{T_I} : \dfrac{T_E}{T_I}$ (page 22)

$\dfrac{V_D}{V_T} = \dfrac{PaCO_2 - P\bar{E}CO_2}{PaCO_2}$ (page 26)

$C_1V_1 = C_2V_2$, or $\dfrac{C_1}{C_2} = \dfrac{V_2}{V_1}$ (page 32)

$V/T = k$ (page 35)

$P \times V = k$ (page 35)

$\dfrac{\text{actual } PaCO_2}{\text{desired } PaCO_2} = \dfrac{\text{desired } \dot{V}_A}{\text{actual } \dot{V}_A}$ (page 35)

$\dfrac{\text{content}}{\text{capacity}} \times 100 = \%$ relative humidity   (page 41)

$\dfrac{FEV_T}{FVC} \times 100 = FEV_{T\%}$ (page 42)

$\dfrac{ml\ O_2}{100\ ml\ plasma} = $ volume %   (page 44)

$[Hb] \times 1.34\ ml\ O_2/g\ Hb \times SaO_2 = O_2$ content   (page 45)

$\dfrac{\text{grams of Hb}}{100\ ml\ blood} = [Hb]$ (page 45)

$\dfrac{O_2\ content}{O_2\ capacity} \times 100 = So_2$ (page 45)

$\dfrac{\dot{Q}_s}{\dot{Q}_T} = \dfrac{C\acute{c}O_2 - CaO_2}{C\acute{c}O_2 - C\bar{v}O_2}$ (page 46)

$PAO_2 = FIO_2(PB - PH_2O) - PACO_2\left(FIO_2 + \dfrac{1 - F_IO_2}{R}\right)$ (page 47)

$T_I + T_E = TCT$ (page 51)

slope $= \Delta y/\Delta x$ (page 84)

Respiratory care practitioners and students are frequently confronted with solving mathematical problems. The level of mathematical knowledge required in the area of respiratory care is not overwhelming; however, a fundamental understanding of certain mathematical concepts is necessary. Therefore, the goal of this chapter is to provide the reader the opportunity to become skillful in solving basic mathematical operations and problems encountered in respiratory care.

CHAPTER OBJECTIVES

Upon completing this chapter, the reader will understand the fundamental mathematical skills used in performing calculations associated with respiratory care and will be able to

1-1 SCIENTIFIC NOTATION AND EXPONENTS

- Express in proper scientific notation answers obtained from mathematical calculations.
- Compute basic mathematical problems involving exponents.

1-2 SIGNIFICANT DIGITS

- Differentiate between the precision and accuracy of measurement.
- Discuss the limitations of measuring instruments.
- State the rules that govern the process of determining significant digits.
- Employ the rules governing the use of significant digits when performing calculations.
- Distinguish between random and systematic error.
- Describe how to avoid the problem of parallax.

1-3 RATIOS

- Solve mathematical problems using ratios.
- Compute air/oxygen entrainment ratios.
- Calculate inspiratory/expiratory ratios.
- Solve problems involving solute/solvent ratios.
- Employ the Bohr equation to solve problems concerning the V_D/V_T ratio.

1-4 PROPORTIONS

- Apply proportions to mathematical problems.
- Calculate drug dilution problems (W/W, V/V, and W/V).

- Use Charles' law to understand direct proportions.
- Utilize Boyle's law to conceptualize inverse proportions.
- Determine the ventilatory rate or tidal volume needed to achieve a desired $PaCO_2$ for a patient mechanically ventilated in the control mode.

1-5 PERCENTS

- Calculate percentages.
- Employ concepts of percentage to calculate relative humidity.
- Utilize percent computations to determine $FEV_{T\%}$.
- Distinguish between an actual percent solution (W/W and V/V) and one that is not (W/V).
- Differentiate the term *volumes percent* from an expression that relates to an actual percentage.
- Recognize what is incorporated in the term *grams percent.*
- Apply percent computations to obtain oxygen saturation.
- Solve shunt calculations utilizing the concepts of percentage.

1-6 DIMENSIONAL ANALYSIS

- Apply dimensional analysis to solving mathematical problems.

1-7 UNITS OF MEASUREMENT

- Describe the International System of Units.
- List the seven units that form the basis for the International System of Units.
- Convert various units using the metric system and the International System of Units.
- Convert between the English and metric system, and between the English system and the International System of Units.

1-8 LOGARITHMS

- Determine the logarithm of a number.
- Obtain antilogarithms.
- Perform mathematical operations using logarithms.

1-9 GRAPHS

- Interpret graphic presentation of data.
- Define *independent variable* and *dependent variable.*
- Differentiate among hyperbolic, parabolic, and straight line curves.
- Use basic science and physiologic examples to describe the various curves.

1-1 SCIENTIFIC NOTATION AND EXPONENTS

Some calculations in clinical respiratory care and cardiopulmonary physiology involve using scientific notation and exponents. Although the use of scientific notation and exponents is considered rudimentary mathematics, the principles of their application are presented here essentially as a review. Students enrolled in respiratory care education programs have different backgrounds in mathematics. Therefore, some students may need to spend more time on this subject matter, whereas others may require very little.

To avoid using numbers in a long form, it is useful to be able to express numbers in scientific notation. In addition to allowing easier comprehension of their magnitude, scientific notation provides the additional benefit of expediting mathematical manipulations by simplifying the numbers.

For example, an extremely large number, such as Avogadro's number written in its long form, is rather imposing:

$$602\ 000\ 000\ 000\ 000\ 000\ 000\ 000 \text{ molecules}$$

Similarly, the mass of an electron, represented by an extremely small number, is written in its long form as

$$0.000\ 000\ 000\ 000\ 000\ 000\ 000\ 000\ 000\ 911 \text{ kilogram.}$$

This form of writing numbers makes calculations unwieldy and introduces a source of error.

To facilitate working with these numbers, a shortened form of expressing decimal places as a **power** of ten is available. This method is called exponential or scientific notation. Scientific notation is expressed according to the general format below.

$$M \times 10^m$$

According to this expression, M represents a whole number that must be greater than or equal to ($\geq$) 1 but less than ($<$) 10, and m is a positive or negative **exponent** whose value represents the movement of a decimal point. As an example, Avogadro's number (602 sextillion) is expressed below in scientific notation.

$$6.02 \times 10^{23} \text{ molecules}$$

The decimal point is moved to the left until only one digit to the left of the decimal point remains. That digit must be between 1 and 9, inclusively, as illustrated below.

$$\underset{23\ 22\quad 21\ 20\ 19\quad 18\ 17\ 16\quad 15\ 14\ 13\quad 12\ 11\ 10\quad 9\ 8\ 7\quad 6\ 5\ 4\quad 3\ 2\ 1}{6\ 0\ 2\quad 0\ 0\ 0\quad 0\ 0\ 0\quad 0\ 0\ 0\quad 0\ 0\ 0\quad 0\ 0\ 0\quad 0\ 0\ 0.}\ \text{molecules}$$

or

$$6.02 \times 10^{23} \text{ molecules}$$

In this example, the decimal point was moved 23 places to the left. For large numbers, the rule is to move the decimal point to the left as many times as is necessary until a digit greater than or equal to 1, but less than 10, is encountered. To express the number 8,210 in proper scientific notation, the decimal point must be moved three places to the left to obtain the expression 8.21×10^3. Expressing the number 8,210 as 82.1×10^2 is not correct because the whole, or non-decimal, number (82) is not between 1 and 9, inclusively, as the rule requires.

For values less than 1, a similar rule applies. The difference is the direction in which the decimal point is moved. In this instance, the decimal point is moved to the right until a digit greater than or equal to 1, or less than 10, is obtained. The extremely small number, representing the mass of an electron, is expressed below in scientific notation.

0.0 0 0   0 0 0   0 0 0   0 0 0   0 0 0   0 0 0   0 0 0   0 0 0   0 0 0   0 0 0   9 1 1 kilogram

1 2 3   4 5 6   7 8 9   10 11 12   13 14 15   16 17 18   19 20 21   22 23 24   25 26 27   28 29 30   31

or

$$9.11 \times 10^{-31} \text{ kg}$$

The decimal point has been moved 31 places to the right.

However, in the process of solving mathematical problems, expressing numbers in the form of 82.1×10^2 or 0.749×10^{-1} may be necessary. Placing the decimal point in different locations within the number is sometimes necessary when adding and subtracting numbers expressed in scientific notation. This practice is especially applicable when the exponents are not equal.

When working with numbers that are extremely large and extremely small, knowing the **place value** of each digit is important. Figure 1-1 illustrates the place value for each digit in the number 5,378,214,965.

Similarly, Figure 1-2 represents the place value for each digit in the decimal number 0.5378214965.

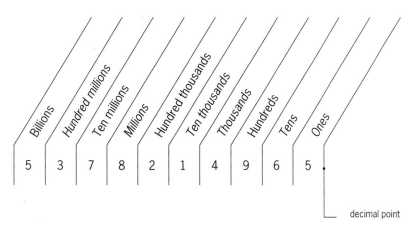

Figure 1-1 *Depiction of the place value of each digit in the number 5,378,214,965. Note the position of the decimal point.*

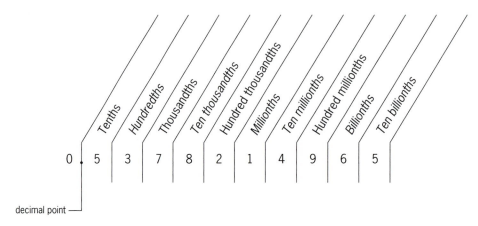

Figure 1-2 *Depiction of the place value of each digit in the decimal number 0.5378214965. Note the location of the decimal point.*

Observe the following examples of various numbers expressed as powers of 10:

Standard Notation	Scientific Notation
1,000	1×10^3
100	1×10^2
10	1×10^1
1	1×10^0
0.1	1×10^{-1}
0.01	1×10^{-2}
0.001	1×10^{-3}
0.0001	1×10^{-4}

Negative powers of 10 are decimals. These numbers can be expressed as a fraction. For example,

$$0.1 \quad = 10^{-1} = \frac{1}{10}$$

$$0.01 \quad = 10^{-2} = \frac{1}{100}$$

$$0.001 = 10^{-3} = \frac{1}{1000}$$

Any number can be expressed exponentially as illustrated by the following examples:

Standard Notation	Scientific Notation
500	5×10^2
93,000,000	9.3×10^7
0.0003	3×10^{-4}
0.000000024	2.4×10^{-8}

Certain rules must be applied when performing calculations involving exponential numbers. The rules governing use of exponential numbers are as follows:

The exponents are algebraically added during multiplication.

$$10^x \cdot 10^y = 10^{x+y}$$

EXAMPLES:

$$10^4 \cdot 10^7 = 10^{4+7} = 10^{11}$$

$$10^4 \cdot 10^{-7} = 10^{4+(-7)} = 10^{-3}$$

$$10^{-4} \cdot 10^7 = 10^{-4+7} = 10^3$$

$$10^{-4} \cdot 10^{-7} = 10^{-4+(-7)} = 10^{-11}$$

The exponents are algebraically subtracted during division.

$$\frac{10^x}{10^y} = 10^x \div 10^y = 10^{x-y}$$

EXAMPLES:

$$\frac{10^4}{10^7} = 10^{4-7} = 10^{-3}$$

$$\frac{10^4}{10^{-7}} = 10^{4-(-7)} = 10^{11}$$

$$\frac{10^{-4}}{10^7} = 10^{-4-7} = 10^{-11}$$

$$\frac{10^{-4}}{10^{-7}} = 10^{-4-(-7)} = 10^3$$

Expressing numbers now as $A \cdot 10^x$ and $B \cdot 10^y$ where A and B are the **coefficients**, and x and y are the exponents, the rules for addition, subtraction, multiplication, and division are as follows:

A. Multiplication

Rule: When multiplying numbers containing exponents, the exponents (powers of 10) are added and the coefficients are multiplied.

$$(A \cdot 10^x) \times (B \cdot 10^y) = (A \cdot B)10^{x+y}$$

$$(A \cdot 10^x) \times (B \cdot 10^{-y}) = (A \cdot B)10^{x+(-y)}$$

EXAMPLE 1:

Multiply $(4.80 \times 10^6) \times (5.30 \times 10^8)$

Step 1: The coefficients, 4.80 and 5.30, are multiplied and the exponents, 10^6 and 10^8, are added.

$$(4.80 \times 5.30)10^{6+8}$$

The product of $4.80 \times 5.30 = 25.44$, and the sum of the exponents is 10^{14}, hence 25.44×10^{14}.

Step 2: Express 25.44×10^{14} in proper scientific notation.

$$(2.544 \times 10^1)(1.0 \times 10^{14}) = 2.54 \times 10^{15}$$

EXAMPLE 2:

Multiply $(4.80 \times 10^6) \times (5.30 \times 10^{-8})$

Step 1: Again, the coefficients, 4.80 and 5.30, are multiplied and the exponents, 10^6 and 10^{-8}, are added.

$$(4.80 \times 5.30)10^{6+(-8)}$$

The product of 4.80 and 5.30 is 25.44, and the sum of the exponents is 10^{-2}, hence 25.44×10^{-2}.

Step 2: Express 25.44×10^{-2} in proper scientific notation.

$$(2.544 \times 10^1)(1.0 \times 10^{-2}) = 2.54 \times 10^{-1}$$

B. Division

Rule: When dividing numbers containing exponents, the exponents are subtracted and the coefficients are divided.

$$(A \cdot 10^x) \div (B \cdot 10^y) = (A \div B)10^{x-y}$$

$$(A \cdot 10^x) \div (B \cdot 10^{-y}) = (A \div B)10^{x-(-y)} = (A \div B)10^{x+y}$$

EXAMPLE 1:

Divide $(4.80 \times 10^6) \div (5.30 \times 10^8)$

Step 1: The coefficient 4.80 is divided by 5.30 and the exponents, 10^6 and 10^8, are subtracted.

$$\left(\frac{4.80}{5.30}\right)10^{6-8}$$

The quotient of $4.80 \div 5.30$ is 0.906 and the remainder of 10^{6-8} is 10^{-2}, hence 0.906×10^{-2}.

Step 2: Express 0.906×10^{-2} in proper scientific notation.

$$(9.06 \times 10^{-1})(1.0 \times 10^{-2}) = 9.06 \times 10^{-3}$$

EXAMPLE 2:

Divide $(4.80 \times 10^6) \div (5.30 \times 10^{-8})$

Step 1: The coefficient 4.80 is divided by 5.30 and the exponents, 10^6 and 10^{-8}, are subtracted.

$$\left(\frac{4.80}{5.30}\right)10^{6-(-8)}$$

The quotient of $4.80 \div 5.30$ is 0.906 and the remainder of $10^{6-(-8)}$ is 10^{14}, hence 0.906×10^{14}.

Step 2:   Express 0.906×10^{14} in proper scientific notation.

$$(9.06 \times 10^{-1})(1.0 \times 10^{14}) = 9.06 \times 10^{13}$$

C. Addition

Rule: When adding numbers containing exponents, the exponents must be equal before the coefficients are added.

$$(A \cdot 10^x) + (B \cdot 10^y) \text{ can only be added if } x = y$$

$$(A \cdot 10^y) + (B \cdot 10^y) = (A + B)10^y$$

The coefficients, A and B, can be added because the exponents are the same (equal).

EXAMPLE 1:

Add $(4.80 \times 10^6) + (5.30 \times 10^6)$

Step 1:   The coefficients, 4.80 and 5.30, can be added because the exponents are equal. The exponents are not involved in any mathematical operation here, hence

$$
\begin{array}{r}
4.80 \times 10^6 \\
+5.30 \times 10^6 \\
\hline
10.10 \times 10^6
\end{array}
$$

Step 2:   Express 10.10×10^6 in proper scientific notation.

$$(1.01 \times 10^1)(1.0 \times 10^6) = 1.01 \times 10^7$$

EXAMPLE 2:

Add $(4.80 \times 10^6) + (5.30 \times 10^7)$

Step 1:   The coefficients, 4.80 and 5.30, cannot be added as shown. However, the addition can be performed after changing 5.30×10^7 to 53.00×10^6, or after changing 4.80×10^6 to 0.48×10^7, hence $(4.80 \times 10^6) + (53.00 \times 10^6)$.

Step 2:   The sum of 4.80 and 53.00 is 57.80. Again, the exponents do not change, hence

$$
\begin{array}{r}
4.80 \times 10^6 \\
+53.00 \times 10^6 \\
\hline
57.80 \times 10^6
\end{array}
$$

Step 3:   Express 57.80×10^6 in proper scientific notation.

$$(5.78 \times 10^1)(1.0 \times 10^6) = 5.78 \times 10^7$$

D. Subtraction

Rule: When subtracting numbers containing exponents, the exponents must be equal before the coefficients are subtracted.

$$(A \cdot 10^x) - (B \cdot 10^y) \text{ can only be subtracted if } x = y$$

$$(A - 10^y) - (B \cdot 10^y) = (A - B)10^y$$

The coefficients, *A* and *B*, can be subtracted because the exponents are the same (equal).

EXAMPLE 1:

Subtract $(5.30 \times 10^6) - (4.80 \times 10^6)$

Step 1: The coefficient 4.80 can be subtracted from 5.30 because the exponents are equal. The exponents are not involved in any mathematical operation here, hence

$$\begin{array}{r} 5.30 \times 10^6 \\ -4.80 \times 10^6 \\ \hline 0.50 \times 10^6 \end{array}$$

Step 2: Express 0.50×10^6 in proper scientific notion.

$$(5.0 \times 10^{-1})(1.0 \times 10^6) = 5.0 \times 10^5$$

EXAMPLE 2:

Subtract $(5.30 \times 10^6) - (4.80 \times 10^5)$

Step 1: The coefficient 4.80 cannot be subtracted from 5.30 as shown. However, the subtraction can be performed after changing 5.30×10^6 to 53.00×10^5, or after changing 4.80×10^5 to 0.48×10^6.

$$(53.00 \times 10^5) - (4.80 \times 10^5)$$

Step 2: The remainder of 53.00 minus 4.80 is 48.20. Again, the exponents do not change, hence

$$\begin{array}{r} 53.00 \times 10^5 \\ -4.80 \times 10^5 \\ \hline 48.20 \times 10^5 \end{array}$$

Step 3: Express 48.20×10^5 in proper scientific notation.

$$(4.82 \times 10^1)(1.0 \times 10^5) = 4.82 \times 10^6$$

PRACTICE PROBLEMS

Refer to Appendix A (pages 548-549) for the solutions and answers to the practice problems.
Express the following numbers in proper scientific notation:

1. $893 \times 10^{-3} =$ _____
2. $67.4 \times 10^9 =$ _____
3. $8,562 \times 10^{10} =$ _____
4. $0.0000732 \times 10^8 =$ _____
5. $4,930,000 \times 10^{-7} =$ _____
6. $54,691 \times 10^{-2} =$ _____
7. $7.03 \times 10^2 =$ _____

8. $0.000509 \times 10^{-9} =$ _____

9. $96.2 \times 10^{-6} =$ _____

10. $321.0 \times 10^{-4} =$ _____

Perform the following calculations:

11. $(9.42 \times 10^{-3}) \div (8.62 \times 10^{9}) =$ _____

12. $(6.40 \times 10^{6}) \div (9.81 \times 10^{5}) =$ _____

13. $(1.41 \times 10^{9}) - (5.61 \times 10^{5}) =$ _____

14. $(8.41 \times 10^{-6})/(7.28 \times 10^{-7}) =$ _____

15. $(7.41 \times 10^{-11}) + (3.65 \times 10^{-9}) =$ _____

16. $(8.15 \times 10^{-6}) - (9.21 \times 10^{-10}) =$ _____

17. $(2.40 \times 10^{-20}) \times (6.67 \times 10^{13}) =$ _____

18. $(5.89 \times 10^{-14}) \cdot (2.22 \times 10^{-7}) =$ _____

19. $(3.59 \times 10^{-8}) \div (3.59 \times 10^{-9}) =$ _____

20. $(1.11 \times 10^{10}) + (3.12 \times 10^{12}) =$ _____

1-2 SIGNIFICANT DIGITS

The respiratory care practitioner and student are frequently confronted with the dilemma of deciding how many digits to retain in an answer to a mathematical problem, or in a measurement. By applying the rules that govern significant digits, the reader will avoid unnecessary work and accurately report measurements and answers to calculations involving measured values. This section will present the rules that apply to significant digits. (Also commonly known as *significant figures*.)

Precision and Accuracy of Measurement

The number of significant digits used for a measurement is imposed by the measuring device itself. Specifically, it is the precision of the measuring instrument that limits the number of significant figures given to a measurement. **Precision** is defined as the degree of exactness to which a measurement can be reproduced. In other words, precision refers to how close successive measurements are to each other.

For example, a respiratory care practitioner obtains three forced vital capacity (FVC) measurements from a patient performing spirometry. The data from the three trials are shown in Table 1-1. These data are closely clustered, as opposed to being dispersed. They represent reproducible data and therefore qualify as being precise.

Accuracy is defined as the extent to which a measurement agrees with a standard, or an accepted value. Accuracy refers to how much the measured (observed) value agrees with the actual (real) value. For instance, immediately after performing the spirometry tests above, the respiratory care practitioner decided to calibrate the spirometer with a standard 3-liter (L) syringe. The following data were obtained from three separate syringe injections. (Table 1-2)

TABLE 1-1 Spirometric Data from Three FVC Maneuvers

Trial	FVC
1	6.50 L
2	6.53 L
3	6.51 L

TABLE 1-2 Calibration Data from 3-liter Syringe*

Trial	Calibration Reading
1	2.85 L
2	2.80 L
3	2.90 L

The three readings obtained here are not accurate because they deviate by more than the acceptable ±3% level from the standard (3.00 L).* The first trial is 5% below the accepted value (2.85 L/3.00 L × 100). Trials 2 and 3 are 7.6% and 4.4% lower than the standard, respectively. Even though the spirometry here is precise, it is not accurate.

Significant Digits and Measurements

The accuracy of a measurement is limited by the precision of the measuring instrument. The precision of an instrument is limited by the finest division on its scale. Note the scale in Figure 1-3. A meter stick is being used to measure a wooden strip. The larger calibrations on the scale indicate centimeters (cm). The smaller calibrations on the scale illustrate millimeters (mm). Therefore, if a linear measurement falls between two millimeter divisions as shown in Figure 1-3, a fraction of a millimeter may be estimated. Therefore, the length of the wooden strip can be expressed as either 9.45 cm, or 94.5 mm. The last digit (5) is an estimate. The number of significant digits in this measurement is three, i.e., 9, 4, and 5.

This measurement is accurate to 0.1 cm, or 1.0 mm because the last digit of this measurement represents an estimate. The estimated digit lies between two of the smallest divisions, or calibrations, on the measuring scale. It would be inappropriate to express the measurement of the wooden strip in Figure 1-3 as 9.450 cm. The implication would be that the measuring instrument was accurate to a hundredth of a centimeter and that

---

*See the following publications for precise information on spirometric deviations.

1. Ferris, B.G., "Epidemiology Standardization Project," *American Review of Respiratory Disease* (1978) 118: Part 2.

2. "American College of Chest Physicians, Scientific Section Recommendations. Statement on Spirometry: A Report of the Section on Respiratory Pathophysiology." *Chest* (1983); 83:547–550.

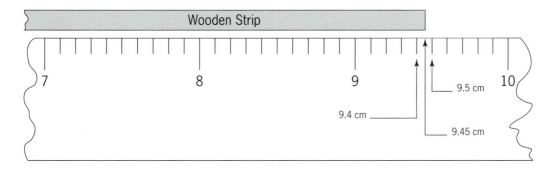

Figure 1-3 *A strip of wood being measured by a meterstick. The edge of the wooden strip extends between the 9.4-cm and 9.5-cm (94-mm and 95-mm) calibrations. The last significant digit of the measurement is an estimation of the smallest unit. Because the edge of the wooden strip appears to be midway between the 9.4-cm and 9.5-cm marks, the measurement is given as 9.45 cm. The estimated value is 5.*

the estimate was zero. Similarly, expressing the length as 94.50 mm is incorrect because that value means that the measuring device was accurate to a tenth of a millimeter and that the zero is the estimate.

If the object measured coincides with a specific calibration, a zero should be added. If the wooden strip in Figure 1-3 measured 9.4 cm, the measurement should be recorded as 9.40 cm, or 94.0 mm. In this situation the zero is considered a significant figure. However, it is an uncertain digit because it is an estimate, as the last digit is for any measurement.

Not all zeros are significant figures. A zero that is used to indicate the location of a decimal point is not significant. For example, the value 0.003 kilogram contains one significant digit, i.e., 3. The zeros are used only to locate the decimal point. If that value were actually 0.003210 kilogram, the number of significant figures would be four (3, 2, 1, and 0). The last zero represents the uncertain digit, or the estimate. It is one of the significant figures.

Consider the value of Avogadro's number. That value is 602,000,000,000,000,000,000,000 molecules. It is difficult to determine the number of zeros that are significant in this number. The digit 2 may be the estimate, or all 21 zeros following the 2 may be significant. Large numbers, such as this one, are expressed in scientific notation to avoid this dilemma. Therefore, with Avogadro's number expressed as 6.02×10^{23}, three significant digits comprise the value (i.e., 6, 0, and 2).

The following rules govern the process of determining significant digits:

- Nonzero digits are always significant (e.g., 486.291 has 6 significant figures).
- All final zeros following the decimal point are significant (e.g., 3.00 has 3 significant figures).
- Zeros between nonzero significant digits are always significant (e.g., 3,010.508 has 7 significant figures).
- Zeros used exclusively for placing the decimal point are not significant (e.g., 0.0009 has 1 significant figure).
- All digits preceding the power of ten in scientific notation are significant (e.g., 2.1500×10^{6} has 5 significant digits).

EXAMPLE 1:

How many significant digits are in the value 8.002010?

Answer: 7

Rationale:
- Nonzero digits are always significant, i.e., 8, 2, and 1.
- All final zeros following the decimal point are significant.
- Zeros between nonzero significant digits are significant.

EXAMPLE 2:

How many significant digits are in the value 0.00009010?

Answer: 4

Rationale:
- Nonzero digits are always significant, i.e., 9 and 1.
- All final zeros following the decimal point are significant.
- Zeros between nonzero significant digits are significant.
- Zeros used exclusively for placing the decimal point are not significant.

Calculations with Significant Digits

Thoughtfulness must be exercised when using significant digits in mathematical operations because the result of any calculation with measurements can never be more precise than the least precise measurement. Consider obtaining the sum of the masses 5.29 grams and 10.0 grams. The least precise of these two measurements is 10.0 grams. Therefore, the result of the addition of these two measurements cannot be more precise than the least precise measurement.

EXAMPLE 1:

Add 5.29 grams and 10.0 grams.

$$\begin{array}{r} 5.29 \text{ g} \\ +10.0 \text{ g} \\ \hline 15.29 \text{ g} \end{array}$$

Answer: 15.3 g

Because 10.0 g is the least precise measurement, the answer must be rounded off to the nearest tenth. However, the answer should be rounded upwards to the nearest tenth of a gram because 9 in the calculated value 15.29 grams 9 is greater than 5. If the calculated value in *Example 1* was 15.24 g, the last digit (4) would be dropped, and the answer would be 15.2 g. The same rules apply to subtraction of measurements.

For multiplication or division of measurements, perform the mathematical operation, then determine the least precise measurement. Finally, round off the product or quotient and express the answer with the same number of decimal places as the least precise measurement.

EXAMPLE 2:

Multiply 3.410 meters by 20.6 meters.

$$3.410 \text{ m}$$
$$\times\ 20.6 \text{ m}$$
$$70.246 \text{ m}^2$$

Answer: 70.2 m²

Because the least precise measurement is 20.6 m, the product is rounded down to the nearest tenth of a meter.

Errors

All measurements contain error. Regardless of the amount of care exercised during a measurement, error still arises. Two types of error enter into a measurement: (1) random error and (2) systematic error.

Consider being assigned the task of measuring the lab floor using a meterstick. Each time the meterstick is placed on the floor, you place a pencil mark at the end of the meterstick. You then place the meterstick again on the floor aligning the other end of the meterstick with the pencil mark you made during the previous measurement. A random error is introduced each time you place the meterstick on the floor.

Random errors are unavoidable. However, they can be minimized. The degree of random error can be reduced by exercising care during the measurement, e.g., making certain that the pencil mark and the end of the meterstick closely align. Also, a number of measurements of the lab floor can be made and the average determined. Again, these practices do not eliminate the random error; they help minimize the random error.

A systematic error is introduced if a faulty measuring device is used or if a procedural flaw is present. In the example discussed here, suppose the meterstick you are using is warped. You are, in essence, using a faulty instrument and are introducing a systematic error. On the other hand, perhaps the mark on the floor is made with a broad magic marker instead of with a finely sharpened pencil. In such a case, the mark will always be made well in front of the meterstick. This procedural flaw contributes to the introduction of systematic error. Systematic errors cannot be minimized by taking repeated measurements and obtaining an average.

Reconsider the spirometric data in Table 1-1. The measuring device (the spirometer) is likely flawed. Therefore, performing repeated volume injections with the 3-L syringe, then averaging the results, will not minimize the systematic error. Even though the measurements may be precise, systematic errors will result if either the measuring instrument or the procedure is flawed.

Another important aspect associated with measurement is parallax error. **Parallax** is the apparent shift in the position of an object when it is viewed from different angles. This problem occurs when a space exists between the calibrated scale and the scale pointer, or indicator.

When viewing the liter flow on a flowmeter (Figure 1-4), the respiratory care practitioner must examine the middle of the flow rate indicator (ball) at eye level to obtain the most accurate reading (Eye B). Viewing the flowmeter ball from above (Eye A) will likely result in a reading greater than that actually indicated, whereas from the perspective below

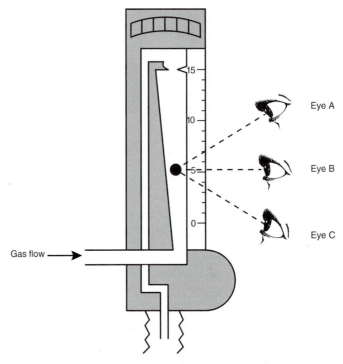

Figure 1-4 *Demonstration of parallax as an oxygen flowmeter is viewed from three perspectives. Eye A views a higher liter flow. Eye B sees the actual flow rate. Eye C perceives a lower liter flow.*

(Eye C), the ball will likely render a reading lower than that actually indicated. Parallax is also a problem associated with reading a pressure gauge. If a circular pressure gauge on a mechanical ventilator indicates a peak inspiratory pressure (PIP) of 20 cm H_2O when viewed at eye level with the line of sight perpendicular to the gauge, it will appear to be delivering a higher PIP when viewed by someone standing to the right of the ventilator. Parallax, of course, is not a problem when digital readouts are provided.

PRACTICE PROBLEMS

Refer to Appendix A (pages 549-550) for the solutions and answers to the practice problems.

List the number of significant figures in the following values:

21. 43 kg _____
22. 0.001 L _____
23. 202.66 kPa _____
24. 7.40×10^{-6} cm _____
25. 2.008010 Å _____
26. 10.00 cm³ _____

Perform the following calculations involving significant figures:

27. Add 3.22 m and 3.414 m. _____
28. Divide 90.0 L/min by 45.000 L/min. _____
29. Divide 63.21 L by 10.000 min. _____
30. Subtract 0.00961 mg from 10.0 mg. _____
31. Multiply 3.140 cm by 30.6 cm. _____
32. Add 16.219 kPa and 101.33 kPa. _____
33. Multiply 0.9900 ml by 0.01 ml. _____
34. Subtract 7.234 m from 12.01 m. _____
35. Multiply 2.32 cm by 20.1 cm. _____

1-3 RATIOS

Basically, a ratio is a fraction of quantities having like units. Therefore, a ratio may be thought of as having a **numerator** and a **denominator.** That is,

$$\frac{\text{numerator}}{\text{denominator}} = \text{fraction, or ratio}$$

If the denominator increases in greater proportion to the numerator, the overall ratio decreases. For example, if we had a ratio of 3 to 5 and the denominator increased to 10 and the numerator increased to 4, the overall ratio decreased. That is,

$$\frac{3}{5} = 0.6 \qquad\qquad \frac{4}{10} = 0.4$$

On the other hand, if the numerator increases in greater proportion to the denominator, the overall ratio increases. For example, if we had a ratio of 2 to 4, and the numerator increased to 4 and the denominator increased to 5, the overal ratio increased. That is,

$$\frac{2}{4} = 0.5 \qquad\qquad \frac{4}{5} = 0.8$$

A **ratio** provides a method of comparing like quantities. It cannot compare unlike quantities. In other words, a ratio must be comprised of quantities having the same **units.**

For example, the measurement compliance (volume/pressure) is not a ratio because the units of the value in the numerator are not the same as the units in the denominator, i.e.,

$$\text{compliance} = \frac{\text{volume}}{\text{pressure}} = \frac{\text{liter}}{\text{cm H}_2\text{O}}$$

The numerical value of compliance retains its units. In a true ratio the units cancel and the numerical result becomes dimensionless. If the units are different, but can be converted to the same unit, a ratio will exist. For example, assuming that the two pressure readings below are being compared,

$$\frac{1{,}034 \text{ cm H}_2\text{O}}{760 \text{ mm Hg}}$$

TABLE 1-3 Respiratory Care Department Staffing Patterns at Two Hospitals

Employee Category	Hospital A	Hospital B
RRTs	18	12
CRTTs	12	6
AS degree therapist graduates	9	10
BS degree therapist graduates	9	2
1 yr. technician graduates	10	6
nontraditional technician graduates	2	0

the comparison cannot be made because the units differ. However, if 1,034 cm H_2O is converted to mm Hg, or if 760 mm Hg is converted to cm H_2O, a comparison can be made. A true ratio will then exist.

Data illustrated in Table 1-3 were compiled to compare respiratory care department staffing patterns between two hospitals. A demonstration of how a ratio can be used to make comparisons will follow.

Answer the following questions using information provided in Table 1-3.

Question 1:

What is the ratio of CRTTs to RRTs employed at Hospital A?

Step 1: Set up the ratio of CRTTs to RRTs at Hospital A.

$$\frac{\text{Hospital A CRTTs}}{\text{Hospital A RRTs}} = \text{Hospital A CRTTs: Hospital A RRTs}$$

Step 2: Insert the appropriate data, and divide by the least common denominator.

$$\frac{12 \text{ CRTTs}}{18 \text{ RRTs}} = \frac{12 \div 6}{18 \div 6} = \frac{2}{3}$$

6 = the least common denominator.

Question 2:

What is the ratio of baccalaureate degree therapist graduates at Hospital A compared with Hospital B?

Step 1: Set up the ratio of baccalaureate degree therapist graduates at Hospital A to Hospital B.

$$\frac{\text{Hospital A BS graduates}}{\text{Hospital B BS graduates}} = \text{Hospital A BS graduates:Hospital B BS graduates}$$

Step 2: Insert the appropriate data, and divide by the least common denominator.

$$\frac{9}{2} = \frac{9 \div 2}{2 \div 2} = \frac{4.5}{1}$$

Air:Oxygen Ratio

In the practice of respiratory therapy, air:oxygen ratios are commonly used. When oxygen therapy devices are used, a certain amount of air and oxygen mix to provide a desired oxygen percentage, or fraction of inspired oxygen, to be delivered to a patient. Through the use of the air:oxygen ratio, you will be able to calculate the flow of air and the flow of oxygen needed to provide a certain percentage of oxygen.

If an air entrainment mask was assembled to deliver 24% oxygen at 4 liters/min (lpm), the air:oxygen ratio would be 25:1. The liter flow of air would be 100 lpm and that of oxygen would be 4 lpm. Consequently,

$$\frac{air}{oxygen} = \frac{100 \; \cancel{lpm}}{4 \; \cancel{lpm}} = \frac{25}{1} = 25:1$$

The colon represents the word *to*. Therefore, the preceding ratio is stated as 25 *to* 1. The symbol also represents division.

Another example of how units may need to be converted to correspond with each other to form a true ratio is that of gas flow rates. The relationship below demonstrates an air:oxygen ratio with units expressed in liters/sec (numerator) and liters/min (denominator).

$$\frac{air}{oxygen} = \frac{80 \; liters/sec}{240 \; liters/min}$$

The calculation of this air:oxygen ratio cannot be performed until either 80 liters/sec is converted to liters/min, or 240 liters/min is converted to liters/sec.

For example, since there are 60 seconds in 1 minute,

$$\frac{240 \; liters/\cancel{min}}{60 \; sec/\cancel{min}} = 4 \; liters/sec$$

Therefore,

$$\frac{air}{oxygen} = \frac{80 \; \cancel{liters/sec}}{4 \; \cancel{liters/sec}} = 20:1$$

Alternatively, convert 80 liters/sec to liters per minute as follows,

$$(80 \; liters/\cancel{sec}) \times (60 \; \cancel{sec}/min) = 4800 \; liters/min$$

Therefore,

$$\frac{air}{oxygen} = \frac{4800 \; \cancel{liters/min}}{240 \; \cancel{liters/min}} = 20:1$$

Knowing both the air and oxygen flow rates, one can ascertain the air:oxygen ratio. Each air:oxygen ratio provides a specific percentage of oxygen. Table 1-4 on the next page outlines air:oxygen ratios and their corresponding oxygen concentrations.

Employing a shortcut method for calculating air:oxygen ratios is demonstrated by the "magic box." One can quickly obtain an estimated air:oxygen ratio for any oxygen concentration using this method. The "magic box" (Figure 1-5) is set up by placing the number 20, or 21, (representing approximate room air O_2%) in the upper left hand corner and

TABLE 1-4 Air:O$_2$ Ratios and Corresponding O$_2$ Concentrations

Air:O$_2$	O$_2$%
0:1	100
0.3:1	80
0.6:1	70
1:1	60
1.7:1	50
2:1	45
3:1	40
5:1	35
8:1	30
10:1	28
25:1	24

100 (indicating 100% O$_2$) in the upper right hand corner. The desired O$_2$% is placed in the center of the box.

The "magic box" is used two ways. First, when the desired O$_2$ concentration is less than 35%, the number in the upper left-hand corner of the box should be 21. Second, when the desired O$_2$ concentration is 35% or greater, then 20 is inserted in the upper left hand corner. The values 20 and 21 represent the O$_2$ concentration in room air.

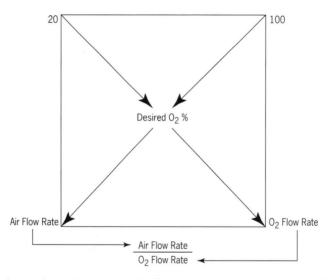

Figure 1-5 *Magic box used to estimate air and O$_2$ flow rates associated with oxygen delivery devices.*

Another way to determine the air:O_2 ratio is to place the "magic box" in formula form. That is,

FOR O₂ CONCENTRATIONS LESS THAN 35%

$$\frac{air}{O_2} = \frac{100 - \text{desired } O_2\%}{\text{desired } O_2\% - 21}$$

FOR O₂ CONCENTRATIONS 35%, OR GREATER

$$\frac{air}{O_2} = \frac{100 - \text{desired } O_2\%}{\text{desired } O_2\% - 20}$$

Let's consider an example for each form of this formula.

EXAMPLE 1:

Calculate the approximate air:O_2 ratio for an air-entrainment mask delivering 28% O_2 to a patient.

Step 1: Use the formula shown below.

$$\frac{air}{O_2} = \frac{100 - \text{desired } O_2\%}{\text{desired } O_2\% - 21}$$

Step 2: Insert the known values.

$$= \frac{100 - 28}{28 - 21}$$

$$= \frac{72}{7}$$

$$\approx \frac{10}{1}, \text{ or } 10{:}1$$

EXAMPLE 2:

Calculate the approximate air:O_2 ratio for an oxygen delivery device providing the patient with 70% O_2.

Step 1: Use the following formula.

$$\frac{air}{O_2} = \frac{100 - \text{desired } O_2\%}{\text{desired } O_2\% - 20}$$

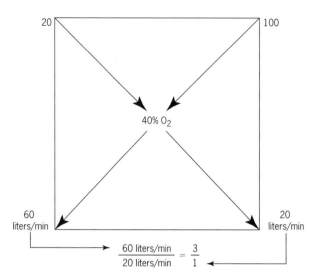

Figure 1-6   *Air:oxygen ratio for 40% oxygen, derived from estimated air and O_2 flow rates.*

Step 2:   Insert the known values.

$$= \frac{100 - 70}{70 - 20}$$

$$= \frac{30}{50}$$

$$= \frac{0.6}{1}$$

The difference between the desired $O_2\%$ and 100 is the air flow rate, and the difference between 20 and the desired $O_2\%$ represents the oxygen flow rate. The ratio of these two flow rates renders the air:oxygen ratio for the oxygen concentration in the middle of the box. Note the example demonstrated in Figure 1-6.

In Section 4-6 of the physics chapter, a discussion of the Venturi Principle will explain how to determine total system flow, as well as how to compute the fraction of inspired oxygen (FiO_2).

Inspiratory:Expiratory Ratio

Applying the rules for ratios and changes with the numerator and the denominator, we examine what happens with changes in either inspiration and expiration. During breathing a certain amount of time is devoted to inspiration and a given amount of time is occupied by exhalation. Placing the inspiratory time (T_I) in the numerator and the expiratory time (T_E) in the denominator establishes the I:E ratio. For example, if T_I is 1 second and T_E is 2 seconds, the I:E ratio is 1:2, that is,

$$\frac{T_I}{T_E} = \frac{1 \text{ sec}}{2 \text{ sec}} = 1:2$$

If expiratory time increases (takes longer), while inspiratory time remains constant, the I:E ratio decreases. Conversely, if inspiratory time increases, while expiratory time remains constant, the I:E ratio increases.

When the expiratory time (T_E) exceeds the inspiratory time (T_I) and when both the T_I and T_E times are known, the relationship for calculating the I:E ratio is

$$\text{I:E} = \frac{T_I}{T_I} : \frac{T_E}{T_I}$$

For example, if T_I = 1.25 sec and T_E = 2.50 sec, then the I:E ratio is

Initial I:E Ratio

$$\text{I:E} = \frac{T_I}{T_I} : \frac{T_E}{T_I}$$

$$\text{I:E} = \frac{1.25 \text{ sec}}{1.25 \text{ sec}} : \frac{2.50 \text{ sec}}{1.25 \text{ sec}} = 1:2$$

If T_E is increased to 3.75 sec while the T_I remains at 1.25 sec, then the I:E ratio becomes

Decreased I:E (Constant T_I, ↑T_E)

$$\text{I:E} = \frac{1.25 \text{ sec}}{1.25 \text{ sec}} : \frac{3.75 \text{ sec}}{1.25 \text{ sec}} = 1:3$$

If T_I is increased to 2.50 sec while the T_E remains at 2.50 sec, then the I:E ratio becomes

Increased I:E (↑T_I, Constant T_E)

$$\text{I:E} = \frac{2.50 \text{ sec}}{2.50 \text{ sec}} : \frac{2.50 \text{ sec}}{2.50 \text{ sec}} = 1:1$$

During positive pressure mechanical ventilation the general principle is to establish an I:E ratio where the inspiratory time is less than the expiratory time. The reason for maintaining the T_E greater than the T_I during positive pressure mechanical ventilation is to minimize the adverse physiologic effects of an increased intrathoracic pressure during inspiration with mechanical ventilation. The graphic below (Figure 1-7) shows the relationship between the T_I and the T_E for an I:E ratio of 1:3 for a total cycle time of 4 seconds.

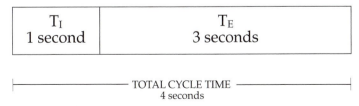

Figure 1-7. *Relationship of T_I to T_E during positive pressure mechanical ventilation. The total cycle time is 4 seconds, i.e., $T_I + T_E$, or 1 sec + 3 sec = 4 sec.*

Inverse ratio ventilation (i.e., T_I greater than T_E) is sometimes used during positive pressure mechanical ventilation. Inverse ratio ventilation is often used with patients who have adult respiratory distress syndrome (ARDS). This technique is essentially applied to improve the oxygenation status of patients who have ARDS. The lungs of ARDS patients are generally stiff (low pulmonary compliance). Therefore, the increased intrathoracic pressure caused by a prolonged T_I ($T_I > T_E$) is not fully transmitted from the lung tissue to the other structures within the thorax. The stiff lungs characteristic of ARDS patients generally allow the increased pressure to be confined to the lungs. The alveoli are forced open more for a longer time during inspiration to attempt to improve gas diffusion at the alveolar-capillary membrane.

The calculation of the I:E ratio changes when inverse ratio ventilation is employed. The relationship then becomes

$$I{:}E = \frac{T_I}{T_E} : \frac{T_E}{T_E}$$

During inverse ratio ventilation, the inspiratory time exceeds the expiratory time. For example, if $T_I = 2.50$ sec and $T_E = 1.25$ sec, then

$$I{:}E = \frac{T_I}{T_E} : \frac{T_E}{T_E}$$

$$I{:}E = \frac{2.50 \text{ sec}}{1.25 \text{ sec}} : \frac{1.25 \text{ sec}}{1.25 \text{ sec}} = 2{:}1$$

Another approach to view the I:E ratio involves dividing the respiratory rate into the number of seconds in a minute, to obtain the total cycle time. The total cycle time (TCT) is defined as the length of the entire ventilatory cycle, i.e., $T_I + T_E$. That is,

$$TCT = \frac{60 \text{ sec/min}}{f \text{ breath/min}}$$

$$TCT = \text{seconds/breath}$$

For example, assume a respiratory rate of 12 breaths/min. Now determine the TCT.

$$TCT = \frac{60 \text{ sec/min}}{12 \text{ breaths/min}}$$

$$TCT = 5 \text{ seconds/breath}$$

This means that the length of the respiratory cycle (inspiration and expiration) is 5 seconds. In other words, the sum of T_I and the T_E would equal 5 seconds.

The T_I and T_E can be determined by dividing the TCT by the sum of the T_I and T_E, or the number of components or parts in the I:E ratio. If the I:E ratio was 2:3, the I:E ratio would have five parts. Then, by dividing the TCT by the number of parts in TCT, the T_I would be obtained. That is,

$$T_I = \frac{TCT}{\# \text{ of parts in TCT}}$$

Using the numbers that we already have,

$$T_I = \frac{TCT}{\# \text{ of parts in TCT}} = \frac{5 \text{ seconds}}{5 \text{ parts}}$$

$$= 1 \text{ second/part}$$

The T_E is determined by subtracting the T_I from the TCT as shown,

$$TCT - T_I = T_E$$

$$5 \text{ seconds} - 1 \text{ second} = 4 \text{ seconds}$$

Insert the T_I and T_E into the formulas previously given for the $T_I{:}T_E$, or I:E, ratio.

Solute:Solvent Ratio

Ratio solutions represent still another example. They express the relationship of the **solute** to the **solvent** as a ratio. More familiarly, they are seen as 1:100, 1:200, 1:1,000, and so on. However, they may be quantitatively represented as 1/100, 1/200, 1/1,000, and so on. Certain drug dilution problems require converting ratio solutions to a percentage. Keep in mind, though, that ratio solutions are true **percent** solutions. (See the topics entitled "Drug Dilution" in the following section and "Drug Concentration" in Section 1-5.)

Dead Space Volume:Tidal Volume Ratio

The Bohr equation provides for the determination of the dead space volume (V_D) to tidal volume (V_T) ratio. The tidal volume is the amount of air a person inspires each breath. The dead space volume is the amount of air that enters the respiratory system each breath not participating in gas exchange. All the air we inspire each breath does not enter the alveoli and participate in gas exchange. Some of the inspired volume remains in the mouth, nose, pharynx, larynx, trachea, bronchi, segmental bronchi, subsegmental bronchi, bronchioles, and terminal bronchioles. These anatomic structures are called the gas-conducting airways, or the anatomic dead space. The air occupied within these structures does not participate in gas exchange. The remainder of the inspired tidal volume enters the alveoli where gas exchange does take place.

In some lung diseases, such as pulmonary embolism, alveoli do not receive normal blood flow through the pulmonary capillaries. In these cases gas exchange in the affected alveoli is either compromised or absent. Such conditions cause the volume of dead space gas to increase. This added dead space differs from the anatomic dead space described above. The dead space that develops from poorly perfused, or non-perfused alveoli receiving ventilation is called **alveolar dead space**. In other words, alveolar dead space units either participate in gas exchange submaximally, or they do not participate in gas exchange at all. The extent to which perfusion is lacking determines the degree to which gas exchange in compromised.

The dead space volume that is represented in the Bohr equation is called **physiologic dead space.** Physiologic dead space volume (V_{Dphys}) is the sum of anatomic dead space volume (V_{Danat}) and alveolar dead space volume (V_{Dalv}). That is,

$$V_{Dphys} = V_{Danat} + V_{Dalv}$$

The Bohr equation reads as follows:

$$\frac{V_D}{V_T} = \frac{PaCO_2 - P\bar{E}CO_2}{PaCO_2}$$

where

V_D = the anatomic dead space volume plus the alveolar dead space volume

V_T = the tidal volume

$PaCO_2$ = the partial pressure of carbon dioxide dissolved in arterial blood

$P\bar{E}CO_2$ = the mean expired carbon dioxide tension

Since there is an insignificant amount of carbon dioxide in normal ambient air, the $P\bar{E}CO_2$ reflects mainly the amount of carbon dioxide entering the alveoli from the pulmonary vasculature, that is, those receiving both perfusion and ventilation.

The mean expired carbon dioxide tension is defined as the average partial pressure of carbon dioxide gas in a volume of gas collected throughout the entire expiratory phase. As the mean expired carbon dioxide tension approaches zero, the quality of ventilation approaches that of dead space ventilation. Dead space ventilation is described as gas entering the lungs but not participating in gas exchange. Assuming a normal $PaCO_2$ of 40 mm Hg, the V_D/V_T ratio would equal unity if the $P\bar{E}CO_2$ were 0 mm Hg. For example,

$$\frac{V_D}{V_T} = \frac{40 \text{ mm Hg} - 0 \text{ mm Hg}}{40 \text{ mm Hg}}$$

$$= \frac{40 \cancel{\text{ mm Hg}}}{40 \cancel{\text{ mm Hg}}}$$

$$= 1$$

On the other hand, if the $P\bar{E}CO_2$ is equal to the $PaCO_2$ (40 mm Hg), no dead space ventilation would exist. This means that all the air inspired into the lungs takes part in gas exchange. For example,

$$\frac{V_D}{V_T} = \frac{40 \text{ mm Hg} - 40 \text{ mm Hg}}{40 \text{ mm Hg}}$$

$$= \frac{0 \cancel{\text{ mm Hg}}}{40 \cancel{\text{ mm Hg}}}$$

$$= 0$$

Neither of these two extreme situations is clinically nor physiologically possible. Each was presented merely to demonstrate how changes in the $\overline{P}ECO_2$ and $PaCO_2$ affected the V_D/V_T ratio.

Knowing a person's V_D and V_T, one can readily determine the V_A (alveolar volume) by rearranging the formula shown below.

$$V_T = V_A + V_D$$

Rearranging to solve for V_A, the formula becomes,

$$V_A = V_T - V_D$$

Let's assume that a person has a V_T of 500 cc and a dead space volume of 150 cc. The V_A would then be obtained as follows.

$$V_A = V_T - V_D$$

$$V_A = 500 \text{ cc} - 150 \text{ cc}$$

$$V_A = 350 \text{ cc}$$

These numbers show that when 500 cc of air are inhaled, 150 cc remain in the conducting airways (anatomic dead space), and 350 cc enter the alveoli for gas exchange. Notice that about 70% of the tidal volume enters the alveoli for gas exchange, i.e.,

$$\frac{350 \text{ cc}}{500 \text{ cc}} \times 100 = 70\%$$

Furthermore, 30% of the tidal volume remains in the anatomic dead space at end-inspiration, i.e.,

$$\frac{150 \text{ cc}}{500 \text{ cc}} \times 100 = 30\%$$

When each of the three volumes given above (V_T, V_A, and V_D) is multiplied by the respiratory rate (f), the rate of ventilation for each volume is obtained.

To determine the minute ventilation ($\dot{V}_E$), multiply the ventilatory rate by the tidal volume,

$$f \times V_T = \dot{V}_E$$

For example, if a person has a 500-cc V_T and a ventilatory rate of 12 breaths/min, the minute ventilation would be

$$12 \text{ breaths/min} \times 500 \text{ cc/breath} = 6{,}000 \text{ cc/min}$$

To calculate the dead space ventilation ($\dot{V}_D$), multiply the ventilatory rate by the dead space volume,

$$f \times V_D = \dot{V}_D$$

For example, a person with an ideal body weight of 150 lbs will have about 150 cc of anatomic dead space. A person's anatomic dead space is estimated to be 1 cc per pound of ideal body weight. If the person had a ventilatory rate of 12 breaths/min, the dead space ventilation would be

$$12 \text{ breaths/min} \times 150 \text{ cc/breath} = 1{,}800 \text{ cc/min}$$

The calculation of the alveolar ventilation ($\dot{V}_A$) is performed by multiplying the ventilatory rate by the alveolar volume. That is,

$$f \times V_A = \dot{V}_A$$

For example, a person with an alveolar volume of 350 cc and a ventilatory rate of 12 breaths/min would have a $\dot{V}_A$ of,

$$12 \text{ breaths/min} \times 350 \text{ cc/breath} = 4{,}200 \text{ cc/min}$$

The following relationship therefore exists.

$$\dot{V}_E = \dot{V}_A + \dot{V}_D$$

Using the value above for the $\dot{V}_A$ and $\dot{V}_D$, the $\dot{V}_E$ can be calculated.

$$\dot{V}_E = 4{,}200 \text{ cc/min} + 1{,}800 \text{ cc/min}$$

$$= 6{,}000 \text{ cc/min}$$

Let's consider a sample problem.

EXAMPLE:

Calculate the tidal volume of a patient weighing 165 lbs (ideal body weight) and a respiratory rate of 14 breaths per minute, along with an alveolar ventilation of 3,990 cc/min.

Step 1: Determine the dead space ventilation.

$$\dot{V}_D = f \times V_D$$

$$= 14 \text{ breaths/min} \times 165 \text{ cc/breath}$$

$$= 2{,}310 \text{ cc/min}$$

Step 2: Obtain the minute ventilation.

$$\dot{V}_E = \dot{V}_A + \dot{V}_D$$

$$= 3{,}990 \text{ cc/min} + 2{,}310 \text{ cc/breath}$$

$$= 6{,}300 \text{ cc/min}$$

Step 3: Calculate the tidal volume.

$$V_T = \frac{\dot{V}_E}{f}$$

$$V_T = \frac{6{,}300 \text{ cc/min}}{14 \text{ breaths/min}}$$

$$V_T = 450 \text{ cc/breath}$$

Let's consider a couple of examples concerning the calculation of the V_D/V_T ratio and the $P\overline{E}CO_2$ using the Bohr equation.

EXAMPLE 1:

Determine the V_D/V_T ratio of a patient who has a $PaCO_2$ of 50 mm Hg and a $P\overline{E}CO_2$ of 35 mm Hg.

V_D/V_T = dead space-tidal volume ratio

$PaCO_2$ = arterial CO_2 tension (50 mm Hg)

$P\overline{E}CO_2$ = mean exhaled CO_2 tension (35 mm Hg)

$$\frac{V_D}{V_T} = \frac{PaCO_2 - P\overline{E}CO_2}{PaCO_2}$$

$$\frac{V_D}{V_T} = \frac{50 \text{ mm Hg} - 35 \text{ mm Hg}}{50 \text{ mm Hg}}$$

$$\frac{V_D}{V_T} = \frac{15 \cancel{\text{ mm Hg}}}{50 \cancel{\text{ mm Hg}}}$$

$$\frac{V_D}{V_T} = 0.3$$

EXAMPLE 2:

Determine the $P\overline{E}CO_2$ of a patient who has an ideal body weight of 150 lbs, has a tidal volume of 500 cc, and a $PaCO_2$ of 40 torr.

V_D = 150 cc

V_T = 500 cc

$PaCO_2$ = 40 torr

$P\overline{E}CO_2 = x$

$$\frac{V_D}{V_T} = \frac{PaCO_2 - P\overline{E}CO_2}{PaCO_2}$$

$$\frac{150 \text{ cc}}{500 \text{ cc}} = \frac{40 \text{ torr} - x}{40 \text{ torr}}$$

$$0.3 = \frac{40 \text{ torr} - x}{40 \text{ torr}}$$

$$(0.3)(40 \text{ torr}) = 40 \text{ torr} - x$$

$$12 \text{ torr} = 40 \text{ torr} - x$$

$$x = 40 \text{ torr} - 12 \text{ torr}$$

$$x = 28 \text{ torr}$$

PRACTICE PROBLEMS

Refer to Appendix A (pages 550-554) for the solutions and answers to the practice problems.

Calculate the following ratios:

36. 10 lpm airflow and 10 lpm O_2 flow _____

37. 43 lpm airflow and 6 lpm O_2 flow _____

38. 32 lpm total flow and 8 lpm O_2 flow _____

39. Calculate the air:O_2 ratio for a 40% air-entrainment mask. _____

40. Determine the air:O_2 ratio for a non-rebreather mask delivering 100% O_2 to a patient. _____

41. Obtain the air:O_2 ratio for a patient breathing 21% O_2. _____

42. Calculate the air:O_2 ratio for an O_2 delivery device delivering 29% O_2. _____

43. Compute the air:O_2 ratio for an air-entrainment mask delivering 50% O_2 to a patient. _____

44. 3 sec inspiratory time and 1.5 sec expiratory time _____

45. 4.5 lpm alveolar ventilation and 5.6 lpm pulmonary perfusion _____

46. 225 ml/min O_2 consumption and 281 ml/min CO_2 production _____

47. 1.75 sec inspiratory time and 3.50 sec expiratory time _____

48. 80 cm H_2O and 10 liters/sec _____

49. Determine the V_D/V_T ratio for an individual who has an arterial CO_2 tension of 35 mm Hg and a mean end-exhaled CO_2 tension of 30 mm Hg. _____

50. Find the $P\bar{E}CO_2$ for a patient who has an ideal body weight of 79.5 kg, a tidal volume of 565 cc, and an arterial CO_2 tension of 33 torr. _____

51. 80 liters/sec airflow and 240 liters/min oxygen flow _____

52. 1,034 cm H_2O and 760 mm Hg _____

53. T_I 1.8 seconds and T_E 0.6 second _____

54. T_I 1.28 seconds and T_E 3.84 seconds _____

55. Determine the air:O_2 ratio for 36% O_2. _____

56. Determine the air:O ratio for 66% O_2. _____

57. Determine the air:O_2 ratio for 54% O_2. _____

1-4 PROPORTIONS

A proportion is a statement indicating that two ratios are equal. Proportions can be written a variety of ways. Examples include

1. $\dfrac{a}{b} = \dfrac{x}{y}$

The ratio *a/b* is equal to the ratio *x/y*, or it can be said that "*a*" divided by "*b*" equals "*x*" divided by "*y*." When a proportion is expressed in this form, the terms "*a*" and "*y*" are called the **extremes,** and the terms "*b*" and "*x*" are called the **means.** This relationship is shown below.

$$\frac{\text{extremes}}{\text{means}} = \frac{\text{means}}{\text{extremes}}$$

2. *a:b = x:y*

   Again, the terms "*a*" and "*y*" are called the *extremes,* and the terms "*b*" and "*x*" are called the *means.*

3. *ay = bx*

   The product of "*a*" times "*y*" equals the product of "*b*" times "*x*." The product of the extremes equals the product of the means.

4. *a:b :: x:y*

   The colon signifies the words *is to,* and the four dots represent the word *as.* The proportion here is therefore verbalized as

   "*a*" is to "*b*" as "*x*" is to "*y*."

Knowing the values of any three of the four terms in a proportion allows for the calculation of the missing quantity. This situation is illustrated in the drug dilution examples that follow.

To show that a proportion does not exist if the products of the means and the extremes are not equal, note the following example:

$$\text{extremes} = 2 \text{ and } 10$$

$$\text{means} = 6 \text{ and } 4$$

$$\frac{2}{4} = \frac{6}{10}$$

The product of the means, i.e., $2 \times 10 = 20$, does not equal the product of the extremes, i.e., $4 \times 6 = 24$. Therefore, a proportion does not exist.

Drug Dilution

Before we actually discuss and present drug dilution problems, it is essential that the respiratory care practitioner understands the three types of solutions. One type is the weight-to-weight (W/W) solution. This preparation involves mixing a certain weight of solute with a certain weight of solvent. For example, a 20% W/W solution might contain 20 g of solute mixed with 80 g of solvent rendering 100 g of solution. Thus, a 20% W/W solution is a true percent solution.

A second type of solution is the volume-to-volume (V/V) solution. This solution is comprised of a certain volume of solute mixed with a certain volume of solvent. A 20% V/V solution might have 20 ml of solute combined with 80 ml of solvent resulting in a total of 100 ml of solution. A V/V solution is also a true percent solution.

The third type of solution is prepared by dissolving a certain mass of solute in a certain volume of solvent. Therefore, for weight-to-volume (W/V) solutions, the concentration (percentage) represents the number of grams of solute per 100 milliliters of solution. For instance, a 5% W/V solution indicates that 5 g of solute is dissolved in 100 ml of solution.

Weight-to-volume solutions are not true percent solutions because the units in the numerator and the denominator of the ratio are not identical. In a W/V solution the solute is expressed in units of weight, whereas the solvent is expressed in units of volume.

Weight-to-volume solutions are nonetheless also represented as ratios. For example, 1:100 solution is one containing 1 g of solute per 100 ml of solvent. A ratio solution of 1:200 represents 1 g of solute dissolved in 200 ml of solvent.

EXAMPLE 1:

How many mg of acetylcysteine are in 4 ml of a 20% W/V Mucomyst solution?

Step 1: Establish the ratio of solute to solvent in the 20% solution.

$$20\% \text{ W/V solution} = 20 \text{ g per 100 ml}$$
$$= 20{,}000 \text{ mg per 100 ml}$$
$$= 200 \text{ mg per ml}$$

Step 2: Set up a proportion comparing ratios of the 20% W/V Mucomyst solution and the unknown amount (x) of mg in 4 ml of that solution.

$$\frac{200 \text{ mg}}{x \text{ mg}} = \frac{1 \text{ ml}}{4 \text{ ml}}$$

$$\frac{800 \text{ mg-ml}}{1 \text{ ml}} = x \text{ mg}$$

$$800 \text{ mg} = x$$

Therefore, 4 ml of a 20% W/V Mucomyst solution contains 800 mg of acetylcysteine.

EXAMPLE 2:

What concentration of racemic epinephrine would result if 0.5 cc of 2.25% W/V racemic epinephrine was diluted with 5 cc of 0.9% W/V NaCl?

Step 1: Disregard the concentration of the **diluent,** i.e., 0.9% W/V NaCl; it will not enter into the calculations.

Step 2: Set up a proportion.

$$\text{(concentration) (volume)} = \text{(concentration) (volume)}$$

$$C_1V_1 = C_2V_2$$

where

C_1 = 2.25% W/V racemic epinephrine
V_1 = 0.5 cc racemic epinephrine
C_2 = unknown or X (final concentration)
V_2 = 5 cc diluent + 0.5 cc racemic epinephrine

$$C_1V_1 = C_2V_2$$

$$(2.25\%)\,(0.5\ cc) = (X)\,(5.5\ cc)$$

$$\frac{C_1}{C_2} = \frac{V_2}{V_1}$$

$$\frac{2.25\%}{X} = \frac{5.5\ cc}{0.5\ cc}$$

$$X = \frac{(2.25\%)\,(0.5\ \cancel{cc})}{5.5\ \cancel{cc}}$$

$$X = 0.205\%\ W/V$$

Answer: A concentration of 0.205% W/V racemic epinephrine will result when 0.5 cc of 2.25% W/V racemic epinephrine is diluted with 5 cc of 0.9% W/V NaCl.

Table 1-5 lists a variety of equivalents of concentration. Notice how the percentage (%) of a solution (column one) relates to the ratio of solute to solvent (column two). For example, along the first row we see that one part of solute divided by the total amount of solution (10) equals 10%. That is,

$$\frac{1}{10} \times 100 = 10\%$$

Column three indicates that a 10% W/V (g/L) solution contains 100 g of solute per liter of solution. Column four shows that a 10% W/V solution has 100 mg per milliliter (ml) of solution, and column five demonstrates that a 10% W/V solution is comprised of 10,000 ml per deciliter (dl) of solution.

TABLE 1-5   Expressions of Equivalents of Concentration

%	Ratio	g/L	mg/ml	mg/dl
10.0	1:10	100	100	10,000
1.0	1:100	10	10	1,000
0.1	1:1,000	1.0	1.0	100
0.01	1:10,000	0.1	0.1	10
0.001	1:100,000	0.01	0.01	1.0
0.0001	1:1,000,000	0.001	0.001	0.1

PRACTICE PROBLEMS

Refer to Appendix A (pages 554-555) for the solutions and answers to the practice problems.

Compute the following drug dilution problems:

58. How many milligrams are there in 4 cc of a 10% W/V Mucomyst solution?
_____

59. If you receive an order to administer 2.5 ml of 10% M/V Mucomyst, but have only 20% W/V Mucomyst available, how much of the 20% W/V solution would you use to give the same dose? _____

60. How many milliliters of a solution containing 100 mg of Demerol per ml are needed if only 50 mg of Demerol was ordered? _____

61. You are requested to prepare 10 cc of 40% ethyl alcohol (ETOH) solution. You have a container of 70% ETOH from the pharmacy. How much 70% ETOH should you draw up from the container? _____

62. A physician presents you with an order to administer 30 ml of 6% W/V NaHCO₃. All that is available to you is 10% W/V NaHCO₃. How much of the 10% W/V NaHCO₃ would you need to make 30 cc of the 6% W/V solution? _____

63. What volume would be needed to administer 5 mg of a 20% W/V Mucomyst solution? _____

Aside from drug dilution problems, a variety of other problems can be solved by the proportion method, e.g., Boyle's law, Charles' law, and Gay-Lussac's law.

Charles' Law

Before proceeding further, it should be noted that two types of proportions should be identified. One type is the direct proportion. For example, assume that two variables are interrelated as follows:

$$A \propto B$$

or

$$\frac{A}{B} = k$$

This first expression reads "*A* is proportional to *B*." The symbol $\propto$ means "is proportional to." In the second expression, the equals sign and constant *k* substitute for the proportionality sign. The variables *A* and *B* are said to be directly proportional. What this relationship means is that as *A* increases, *B* also increases proportionately, maintaining the value of **constant** *k*.

Charles' law, which describes the relationship between volume (*V*) and absolute temperature (*T*) for a gas in which the pressure (*P*) and mass are held constant, will serve as an illustration of a direct proportion. Mathematically, Charles' law can be expressed as

$$\frac{V}{T} = k$$

when P and the amount of gas (number of moles) are constant. Here the variables V and T are directly proportional (related). As the temperature increases, the volume occupied by the gas also increases, thus maintaining a constant pressure. The converse is likewise true. (See Chapter 4, Section 4-5 for more information concerning Charles' law.)

For example, if the temperature of the gas doubles ($2T$), the volume likewise doubles ($2V$). The constant k, of course, would be maintained. Note the equation below:

$$\frac{2V}{2T} = k$$

Boyle's Law

Boyle's law, which states that the pressure (P) and volume (V) of a gas are inversely related when the temperature (T) and mass are held constant, will illustrate the second type of proportion, i.e., an inverse proportion. Boyle's law can be shown as follows:

$$V \propto \frac{1}{P}$$

or

$$P \times V = k$$

If the pressure increases, gas volume will decrease proportionately to maintain the constant k. The converse is also true. (See Chapter 4, Section 4-5, for a more in-depth discussion of Boyle's law.)

For example, if the gas pressure doubles ($2P$), the volume that it occupies will be halved ($V/2$). The value of the constant k would still be maintained. Observe the following relationship:

$$2P \times \frac{V}{2} = k$$

Changing Arterial P_{CO_2}

Controlled mechanical ventilation provides the patient with a preset ventilatory rate, tidal volume, oxygen concentration, inspiratory flow rate, and I:E ratio. By altering certain ventilator settings, the respiratory care practitioner can manipulate the amount of CO_2 dissolved in the patient's arterial blood, i.e., the $PaCO_2$ expressed in torr or mm Hg.

The following proportion can be used to achieve arterial P_{CO_2} changes during volume-controlled mechanical ventilation:

$$(\text{actual } PaCO_2)(\text{actual } \dot{V}_A) = (\text{desired } PaCO_2)(\text{desired } \dot{V}_A)$$

$$\frac{\text{actual } PaCO_2}{\text{desired } PaCO_2} = \frac{\text{desired } \dot{V}_A}{\text{actual } \dot{V}_A}$$

where

actual $PaCO_2$ = most recent $PaCO_2$ (torr)

desired $PaCO_2$ = $PaCO_2$ that is intended to be achieved (torr)

desired $\dot{V}_A$ = alveolar ventilation that would render the desired $PaCO_2$ (liters/min)

actual $\dot{V}_A$ = alveolar ventilation responsible for the actual $PaCO_2$ (liters/min)

Because the patient's anatomic dead space essentially remains constant from breath to breath, either the tidal volume (V_T) or ventilatory rate (f) can substitute for $\dot{V}_A$. The equation will be modified as follows, depending on which factor (V_T or f) substitutes for $\dot{V}_A$:

A. V_T substituting for $\dot{V}_A$, while f remains constant:

$$\frac{actual\ PaCO_2}{desired\ PaCO_2} = \frac{desired\ V_T}{actual\ V_T}$$

B. f substituting for $\dot{V}_A$, while V_T remains constant:

$$\frac{actual\ PaCO_2}{desired\ PaCO_2} = \frac{desired\ f}{actual\ f}$$

The clinical situation will dictate whether the V_T or the f needs to be changed to achieve a particular $PaCO_2$. The following clinical examples illustrate this point:

EXAMPLE 1:

Using the V_T to alter the $PaCO_2$.
A 77-kg patient of ideal body weight (IBW) receiving volume-controlled mechanical ventilation has a V_T of 700 cc. The ventilatory rate is 12 breaths/min and the arterial Pco_2 is 50 torr. The desired arterial Pco_2 is 40 torr. What setting must be changed to achieve the desired $PaCO_2$?

Step 1: Evaluate the appropriateness of the V_T using the general V_T guideline of 10 to 15 ml/kg of ideal body weight (IBW).*

$$\frac{V_T}{IBW} = ml/kg$$

$$\frac{700\ ml}{77\ kg} = 9.0\ ml/kg$$

Based on the fact that the patient is receiving 9 ml/kg of volume, which is below the lower limit of the guideline, the V_T should be increased and the f should remain unchanged.

Step 2: Insert the known values into the appropriate formula to determine the V_T that will achieve the desired $PaCO_2$.

*Please keep in mind that the V_T guideline of 10 to 15 ml/kg (IBW) is not advocated for all mechanically ventilated patients. The V_T for mechanically ventilated COPD, status asthmaticus, and ARDS patients is in the range of 7 to 10 ml/kg (IBW). In those conditions the V_T guideline of 10 to 15 ml/kg (IBW) would not be used.

$$\frac{\text{actual PaCO}_2}{\text{desired PaCO}_2} = \frac{\text{desired V}_T}{\text{actual V}_T}$$

$$\frac{50 \text{ torr}}{40 \text{ torr}} = \frac{\text{desired V}_T}{700 \text{ ml}}$$

Rearrange the formula to solve for the unknown.

$$\text{desired V}_T = \frac{(50 \text{ torr})(700 \text{ ml})}{(40 \text{ torr})}$$

$$= \frac{35{,}000 \text{ torr--ml}}{40 \text{ torr}}$$

$$= 875 \text{ ml}$$

A V_T of 875 ml delivered at a rate of 12 breaths/min will provide a $PaCO_2$ of approximately 40 torr.

EXAMPLE 2:

Using the f to alter the PaCO$_2$.
   A patient weighing 130 lbs (IBW) is receiving volume-controlled mechanical ventilation at a V_T of 900 ml with a ventilatory rate of 8 breaths/min. This patient's $PaCO_2$ is 60 torr. What can be done to achieve a $PaCO_2$ of 40 torr?

Step 1:   Evaluate the appropriateness of the V_T using the general V_T guideline of 10 to 15 ml/kg (IBW).

$$\frac{V_T}{\text{IBW}} = \text{ml/kg}$$

$$\frac{900 \text{ ml}}{130 \text{ lb}/2.2 \text{ lb/kg}} = \frac{900 \text{ ml}}{59.09 \text{ kg}} = 15.2 \text{ ml/kg}$$

A V_T of 900 ml or 15.2 ml/kg for a 130-lb patient is at the upper limit of the guideline, and should not be increased. The ventilatory rate should now be assessed.
   It is prudent to evaluate the V_T first because a 100-ml V_T increase does not impact the mean intrathoracic pressure of the patient as much as a 1- to 2-breath/min increase in ventilatory rate. This statement applies to clinical situations where the patient's V_T resides on the flat portion of the compliance curve. Further V_T increases beyond that point contribute only to hyperinflation, cardiovascular compromise, and barotrauma.

Step 2:   Insert the known values into the appropriate formula to determine the f that will achieve the desired $PaCO_2$.

$$\frac{\text{actual PaCO}_2}{\text{desired PaCO}_2} = \frac{\text{desired f}}{\text{actual f}}$$

$$\frac{60 \text{ torr}}{40 \text{ torr}} = \frac{\text{desired f}}{8 \text{ breaths/min}}$$

Rearrange the formula to solve for the unknown.

$$\text{desired f} = \frac{(60 \text{ torr})(8 \text{ breaths}/\text{min})}{(40 \text{ torr})}$$

$$= \frac{(480 \text{ breaths}/\text{min})}{40}$$

$$= 12 \text{ breaths}/\text{min}$$

PRACTICE PROBLEMS

Refer to Appendix A (pages 555-556) for the solutions and answers to the practice problems.

Calculate the desired arterial P_{CO_2}.

64. A 180-lb (IBW) patient is receiving controlled mechanical ventilation at a V_T of 900 cc. The ventilator rate is 16 breaths/min and the $PaCO_2$ is 25 torr. The desired $PaCO_2$ is 40 torr. To what value must the ventilator setting be changed to achieve the desired $PaCO_2$? _____

65. A 145-lb (IBW), COPD patient, receiving controlled mechanical ventilation, has a V_T of 1,000 cc. The ventilator rate is 12 breaths/min and the $PaCO_2$ is 30 torr. The desired $PaCO_2$ is 50 torr. To what value must the ventilator setting be changed to achieve the desired $PaCO_2$? _____

66. An 80-kg (IBW) patient is receiving controlled mechanical ventilation with a V_T of 600 cc. The ventilatory rate is 12 breaths/min and the $PaCO_2$ is 60 torr. The desired $PaCO_2$ is 40 torr. To what value must the ventilator setting be changed to achieve the desired $PaCO_2$? _____

67. A 165-lb (IBW) patient is receiving controlled mechanical ventilation with a V_T of 900 ml. The ventilatory rate is 8 breaths/min and the $PaCO_2$ is 50 mm Hg. To what value must the ventilator setting be changed to achieve a $PaCO_2$ of 30 mm Hg? _____

1-5 PERCENTS

The term *percent* is derived from the Latin words *per centum,* which mean "by the hundreds." Basically, a percent is a ratio, i.e., some portion of 100 (numerator) over 100 (denominator). For example, 15% represents 15 parts of 100, or 15/100.

Commonly, percents are expressed with the % sign. This sign replaces the fraction line and the denominator 100. Therefore, 15% means 15/100. The decimal equivalent of 15% can be obtained by dropping the % sign and dividing by 100, that is, 15/100 = 0.15.

Graphically, 15/100 or 15% can be illustrated in the grid Figure 1-8 where 15 of the 100 squares are shaded.

1	11	6	16	26	36	46	56	66	76	1
2	12	7	17	27	37	47	57	67	77	2
3	13	8	18	28	38	48	58	68	78	3
4	14	9	19	29	39	49	59	69	79	4
5	15	10	20	30	40	50	60	70	80	5
6	1	11	21	31	41	51	61	71	81	6
7	2	12	22	32	42	52	62	72	82	7
8	3	13	23	33	43	53	63	73	83	8
9	4	14	24	34	44	54	64	74	84	9
10	5	15	25	35	45	55	65	75	85	10
1	2	3	4	5	6	7	8	9	10	

Figure 1-8 *Pictorial representation of percent. A grid of 100 squares showing 15/100 squares (15%) as shaded and 85/100 squares (85%) as unshaded. The numbers 1–10 outside the grid along the right and bottom borders indicate a 10-by-10 grid.*

EXAMPLES:

$$97.5\% = \frac{97.5}{100} = 0.975$$

$$75\% = \frac{75}{100} = 0.75$$

$$2.5\% = \frac{2.5}{100} = 0.025$$

$$0.9\% = \frac{0.9}{100} = 0.009$$

By the same token, multiplying the decimal number by 100 provides the percent. For example,

$$0.15 \times 100 = 15\%$$

There are three types of percent problems: (1) finding the percent of a number, (2) determining what percent one number is of another, and (3) calculating the number when the percent of it is known.

EXAMPLE 1:

Find the percent of a number. What number is 75% of 200?

$$n = \text{the number}$$

$$n = 75\% \text{ of } 200$$

$$n = \frac{75}{100}(200)$$

$$n = 150$$

EXAMPLE 2:

Determine what percent one number is of another. What percent of 3 is 2?

$$\% = \text{the percent}$$

$$2 = \%(3)$$

$$\% = \frac{2}{3}(100)$$

$$\% = 66.67\%$$

EXAMPLE 3:

Calculate the number when the percent of it is known. Twenty-five percent (25%) of what number is 1.5?

$$y = \text{the number}$$

$$1.5 = y(25\%)$$

$$1.5 = y\left(\frac{25}{100}\right)$$

$$y = \frac{1.5}{0.25}$$

$$y = 6$$

Some clinically applicable percent problems follow.

EXAMPLE 1:

Find the percent of a number.

If a mechanically ventilated patient has an inspiratory time percent of 40% and a total cycle time of 3.5 seconds, how long is the inspiratory cycle?

$$n = \text{length of inspiratory cycle}$$

$$n = 40\% \text{ of } 3.5 \text{ seconds}$$

$$n = \left(\frac{40}{100}\right)3.5 \text{ seconds}$$

$$= \frac{140}{100} \text{ seconds}$$

$$= 1.4 \text{ seconds}$$

EXAMPLE 2:

Determine what percent one number is of another.

    Calculate the percent saturation for a patient who has an oxygen content of 18.4 volumes percent and an oxygen capacity of 20.1 volumes percent. (See Chapter 3 Chemistry page 163 for a discussion on volumes percent, or vol%.)

$$\% = \text{the percent}$$

$$\% = \frac{\text{oxygen content}}{\text{oxygen capacity}} \times 100$$

$$\% = \frac{18.4 \text{ vol \%}}{20.1 \text{ vol \%}} \times 100$$

$$\% = 91.5\% \text{ saturation}$$

EXAMPLE 3:

Calculate the number when the percent of it is known.

    If a mechanically ventilated patient has an inspiratory time of 2.5 seconds, which is 30% of the total cycle time, calculate the total cycle time.

$$y = \text{the number}$$

$$2.5 \text{ sec} = y(30\%)$$

$$2.5 \text{ sec} = y\left(\frac{30}{100}\right)$$

$$y = \frac{2.5}{0.3} \text{ seconds}$$

$$y = 8.3 \text{ seconds}$$

Relative Humidity

Relative humidity is derived from a fraction and is expressed as a percentage. The mathematical relationship is

$$\frac{\text{content}}{\text{capacity}} \times 100 = \text{relative humidity}$$

Content is defined as the actual weight of water present in a given volume of air expressed in terms of either grams per cubic meter (g/m^3) or milligrams per liter (mg/l). Capacity describes the maximum amount of water that the air can hold at a given temperature. Capacity is usually expressed in either g/m^3 or mg/l. Both content and capacity can be measured as water vapor pressure and can be expressed as mm Hg or torr.

EXAMPLE 1:

Calculate the relative humidity for a volume of air containing 18 g/m³ of water at 37°C. The capacity for water at this temperature is 43.8 g/m³.

Step 1: Set up the problem.

$$\frac{\text{content}}{\text{capacity}} = \frac{18 \text{ g/m}^3}{43.8/\text{m}^3} \times 100 = \text{relative humidity}$$

Step 2: Solve for relative humidity.

$$\frac{18 \text{ g/m}^3}{43.8 \text{ g/m}^3} \times 100 = 41\%$$

Answer: 41%

EXAMPLE 2:

Air at 25°C can exert a maximum water vapor pressure of 24 torr. Calculate the relative humidity when the water vapor pressure is 17 torr.

Step 1: Set up the problem.

$$\frac{\text{content}}{\text{capacity}} = \frac{17 \text{ torr}}{24 \text{ torr}} \times 100 = \text{relative humidity}$$

Step 2: Solve for relative humidity.

$$\frac{17 \text{ torr}}{24 \text{ torr}} \times 100 = 71\%$$

Answer: 71%

FEV$_{T\%}$

When spirometry is performed to obtain a patient's forced vital capacity (FVC), four timed forced expiratory volumes (FEV$_{TS}$) can be measured. The FEV$_T$ refers to the volume of air exhaled at four different times from the point where the forced exhalation begins. These forced expiratory volumes are the FEV$_{0.5}$, FEV$_1$, FEV$_2$, and FEV$_3$. The subscripts denote the time in seconds from the time the forced expiratory effort began. In other words, the FEV$_{0.5}$ refers to the volume forcefully expired during the first half second of the FVC maneuver. The FEV$_1$ represents the volume forcefully exhaled during the first second of the FVC maneuver, and so on.

Another calculation involving percentages includes the determination of the percent of the forced vital capacity exhaled within a given amount of time. Timed forced expiratory volumes are compared to the FVC and multiplied by 100 to obtain percent of the FVC exhaled within the time (seconds) represented by the FEV$_T$ subscripts. The equation can be written as

$$\frac{\text{FEV}_T}{\text{FVC}} \times 100 = \text{FEV}_{T\%}$$

EXAMPLE 1:

Given the pulmonary function data below, calculate the $FEV_{1\%}$.

	Predicted	*Actual*
FVC	5.43 L	6.44 L
FEV_1	4.43 L	5.02 L

Step 1: Divide the actual FEV_1 by the actual FVC.

$$\frac{5.02 \text{ L}}{6.44 \text{ L}} = 0.779$$

Step 2: Multiply the quotient (0.779) by 100 to obtain the percentage ($FEV_{1\%}$).

$$0.779 \times 100 = 77.9\%$$

EXAMPLE 2:

Calculate the $FEV_{0.5\%}$ from the following pulmonary function data.

	Predicted	*Actual*
FVC	5.54 L	6.79 L
$FEV_{0.5}$	3.00 L	3.91 L
FEV_1	4.24 L	5.22 L

Step 1: Divide the actual $FEV_{0.5}$ by the actual FVC.

$$\frac{3.91 \text{ L}}{6.79 \text{ L}} = 0.576$$

Step 2: Multiply the quotient (0.576) by 100 to obtain the percentage ($FEV_{0.5\%}$).

$$0.576 \times 100 = 57.6\%$$

Drug Concentration

A fraction can be converted to a percent by multiplying it by 100. A ratio solution can be written as a fraction and then converted to a percent. The reader is asked to review the earlier section entitled "Drug Dilution" to ensure a firm understanding of W/W, V/V, and W/V solutions. Be mindful that a ratio solution, although it can be expressed as a percentage, is not a true percent solution. A W/V solution is a ratio solution. Observe this illustration. Given: 1:200 solution of Isuprel. As a fraction, this ratio solution becomes 1/200; to convert to percent: (1/200) × 100 = 0.5% W/V.

Dissolved Oxygen

Dissolved oxygen is ordinarily expressed in terms of partial pressure using either the units *mm Hg* or *torr* (in the United States). Some calculations, though, require the amount of dissolved oxygen to be expressed as **volumes percent.** (See the discussion in Section 3-2 on Henry's law of solubility.) The unit volumes percent (vol%) refers to the amount of gas in milliliters dissolved in 100 ml of plasma. In other words, the average normal adult PaO_2

of 100 torr is equivalent to 0.3 vol%. This means that 0.3 ml of oxygen is dissolved in each 100 ml of plasma. Quantitatively, this can be shown as

$$\frac{0.3 \text{ ml oxygen}}{100 \text{ ml plasma}} = 0.3 \text{ vol}\%$$

The term *volume* is retained in the value in order to identify the quantity as a measurement of volume. Be mindful, however, that this relationship does not represent a true percentage.

Combined Oxygen

Hemoglobin has the ability to chemically and reversibly combine with oxygen. A certain amount of oxygen normally combines with hemoglobin in the arterial blood. Usually, between 19.10 vol% and 19.59 vol% of oxygen is in the combined form in the arterial blood. The quantitative basis for these values is shown below.

$$19.10 \text{ vol}\% = 15 \text{ g}\% \text{ Hb} \times 1.34 \text{ ml } O_2/\text{g Hb} \times 95\%$$

and

$$19.60 \text{ vol}\% = 15 \text{ g}\% \text{ Hb} \times 1.34 \text{ ml } O_2/\text{g Hb} \times 97.5\%$$

In venous blood, the oxygen content likewise represents the amount of oxygen combined with hemoglobin. The normal range for the venous oxygen content ($C\bar{v}O_2$) is 14.07 vol% to 15.08 vol%. The normal $S\bar{v}O_2$ range is between 70% and 75%. The calculations for these values are shown here.

$$14.07 \text{ vol}\% = 15 \text{ g}\% \text{ Hb} \times 1.34 \text{ ml } O_2/\text{g Hb} \times 70\%$$

and

$$15.08 \text{ vol}\% = 15 \text{ g}\% \text{ Hb} \times 1.34 \text{ ml } O_2/\text{g Hb} \times 75\%$$

The unit *vol*% is not a true percent because the units in the numerator and denominator are not the same. The numerator is expressed in *ml* O_2, whereas the denominator is described as *100 ml of blood.*

Hemoglobin Concentration

The concentration of hemoglobin in the blood is expressed as *grams percent*, or *g*%. Similar to the unit volumes percent, or vol%, this expression refers to a certain number of grams of hemoglobin per 100 ml of blood.

The average normal adult has 15 grams of hemoglobin in 100 ml of blood. This value is customarily shown as 15 g%. Quantitatively, this expression appears as

$$\frac{15 \text{ g of hemoglobin}}{100 \text{ ml of blood}} = 15 \text{ g}\%$$

The unit *gram* indicates the weight of hemoglobin contained in 100 ml of blood. As was the situation with the dissolved oxygen, the combined oxygen value is not a true percent.

Oxygen Saturation

Still another example is the concept of oxygen saturation (SO_2). This measurement represents the amount of oxygen combined to hemoglobin compared to the maximum amount of oxygen the hemoglobin is capable of carrying. Essentially, this measurement is mathematically identical to that used for the calculation of relative humidity. It is expressed as a percentage derived from the ratio of content/capacity multiplied by 100, that is

$$\frac{content}{capacity} \times 100 = \% \text{ saturation}$$

This formula applies to both arterial and venous blood. For arterial blood, the arterial oxygen content (the actual amount of oxygen bound to hemoglobin) divided by the capacity of hemoglobin to hold oxygen, multiplied by 100 provides the arterial oxygen saturation (SaO_2). For mixed venous blood, the mixed venous oxygen content (actual amount of oxygen bound to hemoglobin) divided by hemoglobin's capacity to combine with oxygen, multiplied by 100 renders the mixed venous oxygen saturation ($S\bar{v}O_2$). Mixed venous blood is blood obtained from the pulmonary artery via a pulmonary artery catheter.

Assuming normal physiologic and ambient conditions, the denominator (capacity) in the equation is primarily influenced by the hemoglobin concentration. As previously stated, the average amount of hemoglobin in a normal adult is 15 g%. This value is multiplied by the factor 1.34. The factor 1.34 indicates the number of milliliters of oxygen that combine with each gram of hemoglobin. The capacity of hemoglobin for oxygen is obtained as follows:

$$[\text{Hb}] \times 1.34 \text{ ml } O_2/\text{g Hb} = capacity$$

To avoid confusion with terminology, the reader should be aware of the expressions **total arterial oxygen content** and **total mixed venous oxygen content.** These two terms describe the sum of the amount of oxygen combined with hemoglobin (i.e., oxygen content) and the amount of oxygen dissolved in the plasma expressed in volumes percent (vol%). The total arterial oxygen content is symbolized as CaO_2 and that for mixed venous blood is $C\bar{v}O_2$.

EXAMPLE 1:

Calculate the SaO_2 for a patient who has 12 g% Hb and 14.50 vol% oxygen reversibly attached to Hb.

Step 1: Determine the capacity.

$$[\text{Hb}] \times 1.34 \text{ ml } O_2/\text{g Hb} = capacity$$

$$12 \text{ g Hb}/100 \text{ ml blood} \times 1.34 \text{ ml } O_2/\text{g Hb} = 16.08 \text{ vol\%}$$

Step 2: Apply the equation for calculating the SaO_2.

$$\frac{content}{capacity} = \frac{14.50 \text{ vol\%}}{16.08 \text{ vol\%}} \times 100 = 90\%$$

Answer: 90% SaO_2

EXAMPLE 2:

Calculate the quantity of oxygen attached to Hb for a patient who has an SaO_2 of 88% and a hemoglobin concentration of 14 g%.

Step 1: Determine the capacity.

$$[Hb] \times 1.34 \text{ ml } O_2/\text{g Hb} = \text{capacity}$$

$$14 \text{ g Hb}/100 \text{ ml blood} \times 1.34 \text{ ml } O_2/\text{g Hb} = 18.76 \text{ vol}\%$$

Step 2: Rearrange the equation for calculating the SaO_2 to solve for the content.

$$\text{saturation} \times \text{capacity} = \text{content}$$

$$88\% \times 18.76 \text{ vol}\% = 16.51 \text{ vol}\%$$

Answer: 16.51 vol%

Shunts

The term **shunt** refers to blood that flows from the venous side of circulation, past the pulmonary vasculature, and enters the left ventricle without becoming arterialized. In other words, a shunt prevents venous blood from becoming oxygenated and from getting rid of carbon dioxide. Shunted blood tends to lower the oxygen level of arterial blood and to raise the carbon dioxide level of arterial blood. The amount of shunt present in circulation can be quantified via shunt equations.

Two shunt equations will be presented here. They are the physiologic shunt equation and the clinical shunt equation.*

The physiologic shunt equation is certainly a less cumbersome equation and, in the author's opinion, allows for an easier understanding of the concept of shunt as compared to other shunt equations.

Mathematically, it is shown as

$$\frac{\dot{Q}_S}{\dot{Q}_T} = \frac{C\dot{c}O_2 - CaO_2}{C\dot{c}O_2 - C\bar{v}O_2}$$

where

$\dot{Q}_S$ = shunted cardiac output (C.O.)

$\dot{Q}_T$ = total C.O.

$C\dot{c}O_2$ = end-pulmonary capillary oxygen content (vol%)

CaO_2 = arterial oxygen content (vol%)

$C\bar{v}O_2$ = mixed venous oxygen content (vol%)

---

*The derivation of these two equations will not be included here; however, the reader is directed to the following texts for such information.

1. Kacmarek, et al. *The Essentials of Respiratory Therapy*, 3rd ed. (Chicago: Mosby-Year Book, Inc., 1990), pp. 181–184.
2. Shapiro, et al. *Clinical Applications of Blood Gases*, 5th ed. (Chicago: Mosby-Year Book, Inc., 1994), pp. 87–91.

The physiologic shunt equation is a ratio of the shunted cardiac output compared to the total cardiac output. The simplicity of the equation allows one to readily see that, as $\dot{Q}_S$ nears zero, CaO_2 approaches $C\acute{c}O_2$, and that the CaO_2 will always be less than $C\acute{c}O_2$, as long as the shunt exists. Figure 1-9 illustrates the relationships among the factors present in the physiologic shunt equation.

Since end-pulmonary capillary blood is impossible to obtain, the alveolar oxygen tension (PaO_2) is assumed to be equal to the partial pressure of oxygen at the end-pulmonary capillary level. The alveolar oxygen tension can be determined from the alveolar air equation.

$$PaO_2 = FiO_2 (P_B - P_{H2O}) - PaCO_2{}^*\left(FiO_2 + \frac{1 - FiO_2}{R}\right)^{**}$$

EXAMPLE:

Calculate the percent shunt in a patient who, after breathing 100% O_2 for 20 minutes, has a PaO_2 of 525 torr, $PaCO_2$ of 45 torr, and a hemoglobin concentration of 17 g%.

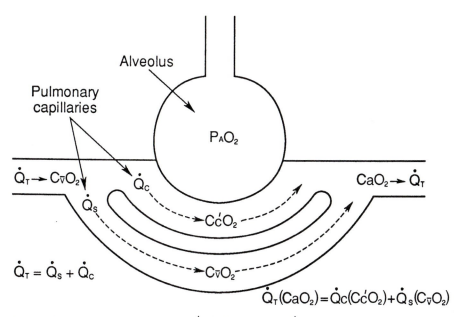

Figure 1-9 *Relationship among total C.O. ($\dot{Q}_T$), shunted C.O. ($\dot{Q}_S$), and pulmonary capillary blood flow ($\dot{Q}_C$). Corresponding oxygen contents are also shown, i.e., (CaO_2) = ($C\overline{V}O_2$) + ($Cc'O_2$).*

---

*The $PaCO_2$ can substitute for the $PaCO_2$ since complete equilibration across the alveolar-capillary membrane is assumed for carbon dioxide.

**R represents the respiratory quotient reflecting internal respiration and is normally 0.8.

†The derivation of the factor 0.003 vol%/torr will be discussed in Chapter 3, Section 3-2, "Henry's law of solubility."

Step 1: Calculate the P_{AO_2}, which represents the end-pulmonary capillary oxygen tension.

$$P_{AO_2} = F_{IO_2}(P_B - P_{H_2O}) - P_{aCO_2}\left(F_{IO_2} + \frac{1 - F_{IO_2}}{R}\right)$$

$$= 1(760 \text{ torr} - 47 \text{ torr}) - 45 \text{ torr}\left(1 + \frac{1 - 1}{0.8}\right)$$

$$= 1(713 \text{ torr}) - 45 \text{ torr}(1)$$

$$= 668 \text{ torr}$$

$$P_{AO_2} = 668 \text{ torr (The end-pulmonary capillary oxygen}$$
$$\text{tension, or } P\acute{c}O_2, \text{ is also assumed to be 668 torr.)}$$

Step 2: Calculate $C\acute{c}O_2$.

$$C\acute{c}O_2 = \text{combined } O_2 \text{ (vol\%)} + \text{dissolved } O_2 \text{ (vol\%)}$$

$$= (17 \text{ g\%} \times 1.34) + (668 \text{ torr} \times 0.003)^\dagger$$

$$= 22.78 \text{ vol\%} + 2.00 \text{ vol\%}$$

$$= 24.78 \text{ vol\%}$$

Step 3: Calculate CaO_2.

$$CaO_2 = \text{combined } O_2 \text{ (vol\%)} + \text{dissolved } O_2 \text{ (vol\%)}$$

$$= (17 \text{ g\%} \times 1.34) + (525 \text{ torr} \times 0.003)$$

$$= 22.78 \text{ vol\%} + 1.58 \text{ vol\%}$$

$$= 24.36 \text{ vol\%}$$

Step 4: Estimate the $C\bar{v}O_2$.

$$C\bar{v}O_2 = CaO_2 - 3.5 \text{ vol\%}$$

If a pulmonary artery sample is not available, assume a normal **a-v difference** of 5 vol%. However, for patients who have a stabilized cardiovascular status while receiving mechanical ventilatory support, an a-v difference of 3.5% can be assumed.

$$C\bar{v}O_2 = 24.36 \text{ vol\%} - 3.5 \text{ vol\%}$$

$$= 20.86 \text{ vol\%}$$

Step 5: Use the physiologic shunt equation.

$$\frac{\dot{Q}_S}{\dot{Q}_T} = \frac{C\acute{c}O_2 - CaO_2}{C\acute{c}O_2 - C\bar{v}O_2}$$

$$= \frac{24.78 \text{ vol\%} - 24.36 \text{ vol\%}}{24.78 \text{ vol\%} - 20.86 \text{ vol\%}} \times 100$$

$$= \frac{0.42 \text{ vol}\%}{3.92 \text{ vol}\%} \times 100$$

$$= 10.71\%$$

Basically, this shunt equation is a ratio converted to a percentage by multiplying the resulting fraction by 100. The factors that are required for the calculation of percent shunt with this equation include:

- $PaCO_2$; used in the alveolar air equation to calculate PAO_2, which substitutes for the end-pulmonary capillary oxygen tension. The PB, PH_2O, and FIO_2 are also used in the alveolar air equation.

- PaO_2; used to determine the dissolved arterial O_2 in terms of vol%.
- [Hb]; used to determine hemoglobin's oxygen-carrying capacity.
- 3.5 vol%; assumed a-v difference used for stabilized ventilator patient. The normal a-v difference (5 vol%) can be used in some situations. Pulmonary artery catheter data make this calculation more accurate because pulmonary artery blood can be directly obtained.

The other shunt equation that will be discussed is the clinical shunt equation. The clinical shunt equation provides a means by which the percent shunt or shunt fraction can be estimated. When access to a mixed venous blood sample is not possible, the arterial-mixed venous oxygen content difference ($CaO_2 - C\bar{v}O_2$) cannot be calculated. The $CaO_2 - C\bar{v}O_2$ is then estimated to be either normal (5.0 volumes %), or reflective of a stable critically ill patient, i.e., 3.5 volumes %.

$$\frac{\dot{Q}_S}{\dot{Q}_T} = \frac{C\acute{c}O_2 - CaO_2}{(CaO_2 - C\bar{v}O_2) + (C\acute{c}O_2 - CaO_2)}$$

The CaO_2 and $C\bar{v}O_2$ are calculated as shown with the physiologic shunt equation. The calculation of the $C\acute{c}O_2$, which represents the end-pulmonary capillary oxygen content, involves assuming that the PAO_2 is equal to the partial pressure of oxygen in the pulmonary capillaries, and that the hemoglobin in the pulmonary capillaries is 100% saturated with oxygen. For example,

$$C\acute{c}O_2 = ([Hb] \times 1.34 \times 1.0) + (PAO_2 \times 0.003)$$

EXAMPLE:

A patient with a pulmonary artery catheter in place has received 100% oxygen for 20 minutes. Calculate the percent shunt given the data below. Assume a normal respiratory quotient and normal ambient conditions.

PaO_2 500 torr
$PaCO_2$ 60 torr
[Hb] 16 g%
SaO_2 100%
$P\bar{v}O_2$ 70 torr
$P\bar{v}CO_2$ 65 torr
$S\bar{v}O_2$ 85%

Step 1: Calculate the P_AO_2 using the alveolar air equation.

$$P_AO_2 = F_IO_2(P_B - P_{H_2O}) - P_aCO_2\left(F_IO_2 + \frac{1 - F_IO_2}{R}\right)$$

$$= 1(760 \text{ torr} - 47 \text{ torr}) - 60 \text{ torr } (1)$$

$$= (1) \, 713 \text{ torr} - 60 \text{ torr}$$

$$= 653 \text{ torr}$$

Step 2: Calculate the $Cc'O_2$ and CaO_2 **gradient.**

A. $Cc'O_2$ = combined O_2 (vol%) + dissolved O_2 (vol%)

$\qquad = ([Hb] \times 1.34 \times 100\%) + (P_AO_2 \times 0.003)$

$\qquad = (16 \text{ g\%} \times 1.34 \times 100\%) + (653 \text{ torr} \times 0.003)$

$\qquad = 21.44 \text{ vol\%} + 1.96 \text{ vol\%}$

$\qquad = 23.4 \text{ vol\%}$

B. CaO_2 = combined O_2 (vol%) + dissolved O_2 (vol%)

$\qquad = ([Hb] \times 1.34 \times SaO_2) + (PaO_2 \times 0.003)$

$\qquad = (16 \text{ g\%} \times 1.34 \times 100\%) + (500 \text{ torr} \times 0.003)$

$\qquad = 21.44 \text{ vol\%} + 1.5 \text{ vol\%}$

$\qquad = 22.94 \text{ vol\%}$

C. $Cc'O_2 - CaO_2 = 23.4 \text{ vol\%} - 22.94 \text{ vol\%}$

$\qquad\qquad\quad\;\; = 0.46 \text{ vol\%}$

Step 3: Calculate the a-v difference. If a pulmonary artery blood sample is unavailable, either a normal a-v difference (5 vol%) or that reflecting a stable critically ill patient (3.5 vol%) may be used, depending on the situation.

A. CaO_2 = combined O_2 (vol%) + dissolved O_2 (vol%)

$\qquad = ([Hb] \times 1.34 \times SaO_2) + (PaO_2)(0.003)$

$\qquad = (16 \text{ g\%} \times 1.34 \times 100\%) + (500 \text{ torr})(0.003)$

$\qquad = 21.44 \text{ vol\%} + 1.50 \text{ vol\%}$

$\qquad = 22.94 \text{ vol\%}$

B. $C\bar{v}O_2$ = combined O_2 (vol%) + dissolved O_2 (vol%)

$\qquad = ([Hb] \times 1.34 \times S\bar{v}O_2) + (P\bar{v}O_2)(0.003)$

$\qquad = (16 \text{ g\%} \times 1.34 \times 85\%) + (70 \text{ torr})(0.003)$

$\qquad = 18.22 \text{ vol\%} + 0.21 \text{ vol\%}$

$\qquad = 18.43 \text{ vol\%}$

C. a-v difference $= CaO_2 - C\bar{v}O_2$

$\qquad = 22.94 \text{ vol\%} - 18.43 \text{ vol\%}$

$\qquad = 4.51 \text{ vol\%}$

Step 4: Set up the shunt equation.

$$\frac{\dot{Q}_S}{\dot{Q}_T} = \frac{C\dot{c}O_2 - CaO_2}{(CaO_2 - C\bar{v}O_2) + (C\dot{c}O_2 - CaO_2)}$$

$$= \frac{0.46 \text{ vol\%}}{4.51 \text{ vol\%} + 0.46 \text{ vol\%}}$$

$$= 0.093, \text{ or } 0.093 \times 100$$

$$= 9.3\%$$

Inspiratory Time Percent

In total cycle time (TCT) of a patient's breath is the sum of the inspiratory time (T_I) and the expiratory time (T_E). Therefore,

$$T_I + T_E = TCT$$

The portion of the total cycle time devoted to inspiration is sometimes expressed as the *inspiratory time percent*, or $T_{I\%}$. The inspiratory time percent can be calculated using the following formula:

$$T_{I\%} = \frac{T_I}{TCT} \times 100$$

For example, if a patient had an inspiratory time of 1.5 seconds and an expiratory time of 3.0 seconds, the $T_{I\%}$ would be determined as follows:

$$T_{I\%} = \frac{1.5 \text{ sec}}{1.5 \text{ sec} + 3.0 \text{ sec}} \times 100$$

$$= \frac{1.5 \text{ sec}}{4.5 \text{ sec}} \times 100$$

$$= 33\%$$

On the Siemens Servo 900C ventilator, the I:E ratio can be established by setting the inspiratory time percent and the pause time percent during control mode ventilation. These two settings establish the length of the inspiratory cycle. For example, if the inspiratory time percent were set at 20% and the inspiratory pause percent at 5%, the length of the inspiratory cycle would be 25% (i.e., 20% + 5% = 25%) of the total cycle time. The remaining 75% of the total cycle time would be devoted to exhalation.

PRACTICE PROBLEMS

Refer to Appendix A (pages 556-559) for the solutions and answers to the practice problems.

Work the following percentage problems:

68. Using Figure 1-10, determine the percentage of the squares that are (a) shaded and (b) unshaded.

    (a) shaded squares: _____   (b) unshaded squares: _____

69. Calculate the inspiratory time for a mechanically ventilated patient with an inspiratory time percent of 30% and a total cycle time of four seconds. _____

70. Calculate the total cycle time of a patient who is receiving mechanical ventilation with a T_I of 3.0 seconds, which is 60% of the total cycle time.

    _____

71. How much water must be added to achieve saturation of 1 liter of air at 37°C with a 75% relative humidity? _____

72. Determine the percentage equivalent of a 1:100 solution of isoproterenol hydrochloride. _____

73. Calculate the percent shunt for a patient being mechanically ventilated on an F_IO_2 of 0.6, and with arterial blood gas values as follows.

    PaO_2 70 torr, $PaCO_2$ 44 torr, pH 7.34, HCO_3^- 23 mEq/L, SaO_2 85%, [Hb] 15g%

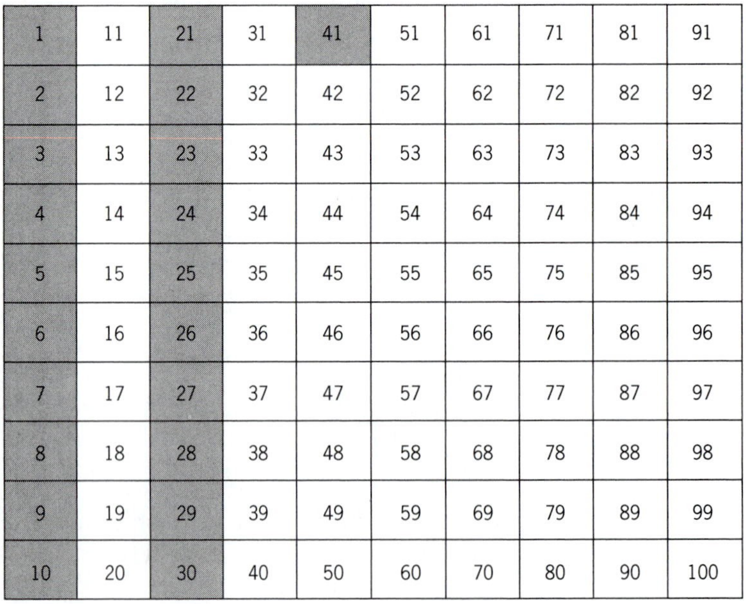

1	11	21	31	41	51	61	71	81	91
2	12	22	32	42	52	62	72	82	92
3	13	23	33	43	53	63	73	83	93
4	14	24	34	44	54	64	74	84	94
5	15	25	35	45	55	65	75	85	95
6	16	26	36	46	56	66	76	86	96
7	17	27	37	47	57	67	77	87	97
8	18	28	38	48	58	68	78	88	98
9	19	29	39	49	59	69	79	89	99
10	20	30	40	50	60	70	80	90	100

Figure 1-10   *100-square grid.*

This patient's mixed venous blood values are:

$$P\bar{v}O_2 \text{ 50 torr, } P\bar{v}CO_2 \text{ 50 torr, } S\bar{v}O_2 \text{ 60\%}$$

The patient is afebrile and has a normal respiratory quotient. _____

74. Calculate the percent shunt for a patient who has the following blood gas tensions after breathing 100% O_2 for 20 min: PaO_2 515 torr, $PaCO_2$ 60 torr. This patient also has a hemoglobin concentration of 13 g%. Assume (a) an arterial-venous oxygen content difference of 3.5 vol%, (b) a body temperature of 37°C, and (c) a normal respiratory quotient. _____

75. A ratio solution of 1:1000 is equivalent to what percentage? _____

76. Calculate the actual $FEV_{1\%}$ and the actual $FEV_{3\%}$ given the following data:

	Predicted	Actual
FVC (liters)	5.38	6.38
FEV_1 (liters)	4.42	5.19
FEV_3 (liters)	5.21	6.35

$FEV_{1\%}$: _____ ; $FEV_{3\%}$: _____

77. Calculate the oxygen content of arterial blood for a patient who has an 18 g% hemoglobin concentration and a 65% SaO_2. _____

78. Calculate the arterial oxygen saturation for someone who has a hemoglobin concentration of 16 g% and an oxygen content of 17.5 vol%. _____

79. Calculate the percent shunt in a patient having a pulmonary artery catheter in place while breathing an FiO_2 of 1.0 for 20 min. The following data were obtained:

$PACO_2$ 55 torr	SaO_2 100%
PaO_2 514 torr	$P\bar{v}O_2$ 80 torr
$PaCO_2$ 55 torr	$P\bar{v}CO_2$ 61 torr
pH 7.32	pH 7.30
[Hb] 13 g%	$S\bar{v}O_2$ 92%

Assume normal ambient conditions and a normal respiratory quotient.

_____

80. If a mechanically ventilated patient has an I:E ratio of 1:2.5, what is the inspiratory time percent? _____

81. Calculate the length of the inspiratory cycle for a mechanically ventilated patient who has an inspiratory time percent of 33% and a total cycle time of 5 seconds.

_____

82. If an inspiratory time of 1.25 seconds is 25% of the ventilatory cycle, calculate the total cycle time. _____

1-6 DIMENSIONAL ANALYSIS

The term **dimension** is synonymous with the term **unit.** Most numbers that a respiratory care student or practitioner encounters consist of both a quantitative value and a dimensional component. For instance, it can be stated that a certain ventilator patient is receiving a tidal volume (V_T) of 800 cc, and has a PaO_2 of 95 torr. Both of these measurements contain two components—a quantitative value and a dimensional (unit) value. Any measurement is meaningless without its appropriate dimension, that is, unless the number is a dimensionless value.

A dimensionless value is a numerical value that has no units. For example, in the section on ratios it was shown that, for a true ratio to exist, like entities must be compared, i.e., sec/sec (I/E); ml/ml (V_D/V_T). The numerical result of such a relationship is termed a *dimensionless* number because the units cancel.

In either case, as the solution of a problem is sought, both the quantitative value and its dimensional component should be considered. Solving a problem using the dimensional aspects of quantities allows the problem-solver to observe how the units will interrelate in a given equation and to determine if the problem is set up correctly.

Using dimensional analysis does not ensure that the quantitative outcome will be correct. It does, however, ensure that the solution to the problem will yield the appropriate units. Therefore, it is prudent to retain the units throughout the calculation, as the units are multiplied, divided, and/or canceled.

An essential aspect associated with dimensional analysis is the use of conversion factors. A conversion factor is a fraction having unlike units in the numerator and denominator, e.g.,

$$\frac{1{,}034 \text{ cm } H_2O}{760 \text{ mm Hg}} = 1.36 \text{ cm } H_2O/\text{mm Hg}$$

Because the unlike units do not cancel when they are divided here, this relationship allows for the conversion of any pressure expressed as mm Hg to be converted to cm H_2O by being multiplied by 1.36 cm H_2O/mm Hg.

$$(100 \text{ mm Hg})(1.36 \text{ cm } H_2O/\text{mm Hg}) = 136 \text{ cm } H_2O$$

Reciprocally expressed, this conversion factor becomes

$$\frac{760 \text{ mm Hg}}{1{,}034 \text{ cm } H_2O} = 0.735 \text{ mm Hg}/\text{cm } H_2O$$

In this instance any pressure expressed in cm H_2O can be converted to mm Hg by being multiplied by 0.735 mm Hg/cm H_2O or divided by 1.36 cm H_2O/mm Hg.

$$(136 \text{ cm } H_2O)(0.735 \text{ mm Hg}/\text{cm } H_2O) = 100 \text{ mm Hg}$$

Note that the position of the units changes when the reciprocal is used.

Again, retaining the units throughout a calculation does not ensure that the correct solution will be obtained, but it certainly increases the likelihood of that outcome when the final units conform with the anticipated dimension. Whenever a calculation is performed, the answer should always be scrutinized from the standpoint of making sense. The cartoon (Figure 1-11) illustrates this point perfectly.

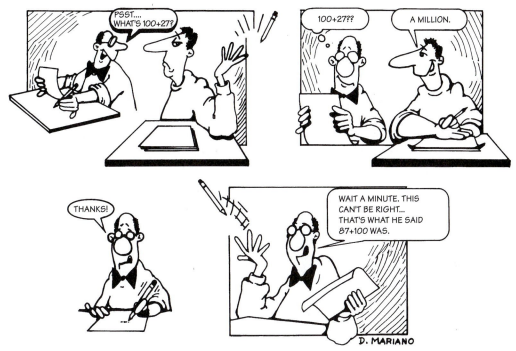

Figure 1-11 *When applying dimensional analysis to calculations, be sure to determine if the numerical value is quantitatively reasonable.*

Dimensions in Addition and Subtraction

To add or subtract numbers, the numbers must have the same dimensions. One could not, for example, add 10 vol% to 15 g%. The result would be meaningless.

Numbers with unlike units may be added or subtracted only if the units can be converted to the same dimension. Consider the following example: Determine the total arterial oxygen content if the amount of oxygen bound to hemoglobin is 19.5 vol% and the dissolved oxygen (PaO_2) is 100 torr. The combined oxygen (19.5 vol%) cannot be added to the dissolved oxygen expressed in torr (PaO_2 100 torr). However, the unit *torr* can be converted to vol% by multiplying the PaO_2 by the factor 0.003 vol%/torr. Therefore,

$$100 \ \text{torr} \times 0.003 \ \text{vol\%/torr} = 0.3 \ \text{vol\%};$$

then

$$\text{total arterial O}_2 \text{ content} = \text{combined O}_2 \ (\text{vol\%}) + \text{dissolved O}_2 \ (\text{vol\%})$$

$$= 19.5 \ \text{vol\%} + 0.3 \ \text{vol\%}$$

$$= 19.8 \ \text{vol\%}$$

Dimensions in Multiplication and Division

Like entities, as well as unlike entities, can be multiplied or divided. The units can also be dealt with mathematically in the same fashion as the quantities. The following examples will illustrate these points.

EXAMPLE 1:

Find the volume of a cube measuring 1 cm high, 3 cm wide, and 4 cm long.

$$\text{length} \times \text{width} \times \text{height} = \text{volume}$$

$$4 \text{ cm} \times 3 \text{ cm} \times 1 \text{ cm} = 12 \text{ cc (or cm}^3)$$

EXAMPLE 2:

Calculate the airway resistance encountered by a 450-cc tidal volume moving through the tracheobronchial tree during a 1-sec inspiration. The intraalveolar pressure is -5 cm H_2O. Assume normal ambient conditions (1,034 cm H_2O = 1 atmosphere).

$$R_{\text{airway}} = \frac{\text{pressure gradient}}{\text{volume/time}} = \frac{\text{pressure}}{\text{flow rate}} = \frac{\text{cm } H_2O}{\text{liter/sec}}$$

$$= \frac{1,034 \text{ cm } H_2O - 1,029 \text{ cm } H_2O}{0.45 \text{ liter/1 sec}}$$

$$= \frac{5 \text{ cm } H_2O}{0.45 \text{ liter/sec}}$$

$$= 11.11 \text{ cm } H_2O/\text{liter/sec}$$

In the first example the like units were mathematically treated like the numbers. Hence, multiplied by itself three times, the dimension (centimeters) becomes cubed (cm³).

Three different units were encountered in the second example. The denominator of the ratio was first simplified by dividing time into volume to obtain the flow rate. Next, the flow rate was divided into the pressure gradient. All the units were ultimately retained to yield the unit denoting resistance (cm H_2O/liter/sec).

Factor-Units Method

In some of the more complicated equations, it is useful to write the units into the formula to determine the remaining dimension(s) after the appropriate cancellations are made. The clinical shunt equation is shown with the units written in to demonstrate the technique.

$$\frac{\dot{Q}_S}{\dot{Q}_T} = \frac{(\text{torr} - \text{torr})(\text{vol\%/torr})}{(\text{vol\%} - \text{vol\%}) + (\text{torr} - \text{torr})(\text{vol\%/torr})} \times 100$$

$$= \frac{(\cancel{\text{torr}})(\text{vol\%}/\cancel{\text{torr}})}{(\text{vol\%}) + (\cancel{\text{torr}})(\text{vol\%}/\cancel{\text{torr}})} \times 100$$

$$= \frac{\cancel{\text{vol\%}}}{\cancel{\text{vol\%}}} \times 100$$

$\dot{Q}_S/\dot{Q}_T$ becomes a dimensionless number (all units cancel) expressed as a percent.

An important point to keep in mind when converting units is that when one quantity equals another quantity, the two quantities can be expressed as a fraction and can be equated to unity. For example

$$1 \text{ ft} = 12 \text{ in.}$$

$$\frac{1 \text{ ft}}{12 \text{ in.}} = 1$$

or

$$1 \text{ km} = 1,000 \text{ m}$$

$$\frac{1 \text{ km}}{1,000 \text{ m}} = 1$$

Again, any two quantities that are equal when represented as a fraction are equal to one.

Any quantity can be multiplied by unity (one) without changing its value. Consider the following unit conversion.

$$4 \text{ in.} = X \text{ ft}$$

$$4 \text{ in.} \times \frac{1 \text{ ft}}{12 \text{ in.}} = \frac{4}{12} \text{ ft} = \frac{1}{3} \text{ ft} = 0.33 \text{ ft}$$

When converting from English to metric units, the procedure is essentially the same. For instance, consider converting 150 lbs to kilogram (kg).

$$16 \text{ oz} = 1 \text{ lb}$$

$$1,000 \text{ g} = 1 \text{ kg}$$

$$1 \text{ oz} = 28.35 \text{ g}$$

$$\text{kg} = 150 \text{ lbs} \times \frac{16 \text{ oz}}{1 \text{ lb}} \times \frac{1 \text{ kg}}{1,000 \text{ g}} \times \frac{28.35 \text{ g}}{1 \text{ oz}}$$

$$= \frac{68,040 \text{ kg}}{1,000}$$

$$= 68 \text{ kg}$$

PRACTICE PROBLEMS

Refer to Appendix A (pages 560-561) for the solutions and answers to the practice problems.

Apply dimensional analysis to the following formulas. Cancel the units when appropriate.

83. $R_{airway} = \dfrac{1,036 \text{ cm } H_2O - 1,046 \text{ cm } H_2O}{5 \text{ liters/sec}}$

84. specific gravity of $O_2 = \dfrac{1.43 \text{ g/liter}}{1.29 \text{ g/liter}}$

85. duration of flow (compressed O_2 gas cylinder) $= \dfrac{2,200 \text{ psig} \times 2.41 \text{ L/psig}}{10 \text{ L/min}}$

86. cardiac output $= \dfrac{250 \text{ ml O}_2/\text{min}}{\left(\dfrac{19.1 \text{ ml O}_2}{100 \text{ ml plasma}}\right) - \left(\dfrac{14.1 \text{ ml O}_2}{100 \text{ ml plasma}}\right)}$

87. time constant $= (0.2 \text{ liter/cm H}_2\text{O})(2 \text{ cm H}_2\text{O/liter/sec})$

88. $\text{pH} = 6.1 + \log\left[\dfrac{24 \text{ mEq/liter}}{(40 \text{ torr})(0.03 \text{ mEq/liter/torr})}\right]$

89. total arterial oxygen content

$= [(15 \text{ g Hb}/100 \text{ ml blood})(1.34 \text{ ml O}_2/\text{g Hb})(95.5\%)] + (100 \text{ torr})(0.003 \text{ vol}\%/\text{torr})$

90. relative rate of diffusion of CO_2 to O_2 across A-C membrane

$= \dfrac{(\sqrt{1.43 \text{ g/liter}})(0.510 \text{ ml/ml plasma}/760 \text{ torr})}{(\sqrt{1.96 \text{ g/liter}})(0.023 \text{ ml/ml plasma}/760 \text{ torr})}$

91. mean airway pressure $=$

$\left[\dfrac{(30 \text{ breaths/min})(0.45 \text{ sec/breath})}{60 \text{ sec/min}}\right] \times [(40 \text{ cm H}_2\text{O} - 10 \text{ cm H}_2\text{O}) + 10 \text{ cm H}_2\text{O}]$

92. cardiac index $= \dfrac{5 \text{ liters/min}}{2.5 \text{ m}^2}$

1-7 UNITS OF MEASUREMENT

Until recently, the metric system in this country was used exclusively among scientists and within medicine. For years now, however, it has been infiltrating all aspects of our society. All one has to do is take a walk down an aisle in the supermarket to see 1- and 2-liter bottles of soft drinks, or 750-ml, 1.5-liter, and 3.0-liter bottles of adult beverages, or to view a baseball telecast from Montreal with the distances from home plate painted on the outfield walls in meters (99 m down the left field line) to realize that the use of the metric system is gradually permeating our everyday lives. This evolution has produced obvious confusion in some instances; for example, gasoline prices indicated for liters, rather than the customary gallons, created practical problems at the pump, leading to the abandonment of this particular effort in the United States.

To avoid confusion, an international agreement was reached in 1960 concerning the use of measurements on an international scale. That agreement stipulated that certain metric system units should be used by all scientists. From this agreement the International System of Units (SI)* was established. Seven basic metric units form the foundation of the International System of Units. These seven basic units are listed in Table 1-6. (The SI system is synonymous with the *MKS* [meter-kilogram-second] system.)

*The official abbreviation (SI) for the International System of Units is from the French *Le système internationale d'unités.*

TABLE 1-6   Basic SI Units

Scientific Quantity	Unit Name	Symbol
mass	kilogram	kg
length	meter	m
time	second	sec
electric current	ampere	A
temperature	Kelvin	K
luminous intensity	candela	cd
amount of substance	mole	mol

All other SI quantities are derived from these basic SI units. For example, speed is the ratio distance per time, or m/sec; volume is expressed as m^3, i.e., m × m × m. The SI unit for pressure is kilopascal (kPa).

Like the metric system, the SI system uses a variety of prefixes to indicate decimal fractions, or multiples, or the different units. Table 1-7 illustrates a number of the SI units that are derived from the basic units.

The SI units incorporate the metric system, thereby taking advantage of the decimal system. Various prefixes are used to change SI units by powers of 10. For example, with the meter as the fundamental unit of length, one-tenth of a meter is a *deci*meter, one-hundredth of a meter is a *centi*meter, and one-thousandth of a meter is a *milli*meter. Each of these components can be located on a meterstick. The metric units for all quantities (i.e., gram, liter, etc.) use the same prefixes. For example, one-thousandth of a gram is a *milli*gram, and one-tenth of a liter is a *deci*liter.

TABLE 1-7   Derived SI Unit Prefixes

Prefix	Symbol	Exponential Form	Example
pico-	p	10^{-12}	picometer (pm) = 10^{-12} m
nano-	n	10^{-9}	nanometer (nm) = 10^{-9} m
micro-	μ	10^{-6}	micrometer (μm) = 10^{-6} m
milli-	m	10^{-3}	millimeter (mm) = 10^{-3} m
centi-	c	10^{-2}	centimeter (cm) = 10^{-2} m
deci-	d	10^{-1}	decimeter (dm) = 10^{-1} m
deka-	da	10^1 or 10	dekameter (dam) = 10^1 m
hecto-	h	10^2	hectometer (hm) = 10^2 m
kilo-	k	10^3	kilometer (km) = 10^3 m
mega-	M	10^6	megameter (Mm) = 10^6 m
giga-	G	10^9	gigameter (Gm) = 10^9 m
tera-	T	10^{12}	terameter (Tm) = 10^{12} m

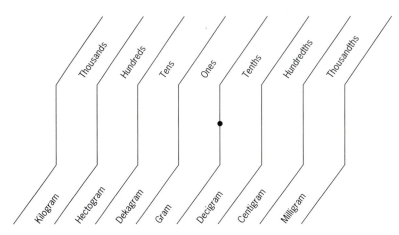

Figure 1-12 *Relationship between some metric system prefixes and their corresponding numerical values. Note the decimal point between gram and decigram.*

Figure 1-12 demonstrates the relationship between some of the prefixes in the metric system and their corresponding numerical values. The large dot between the gram and decigram columns signifies a decimal point.

The CGS (centimeter-gram-second) system uses the centimeter as the fundamental unit of length, the gram as the unit mass, and the second as the unit of time.

Table 1-8 illustrates the more common linear measurements encountered. Some of the common units of weight that are used are given in Table 1-9. A few of the more frequently encountered units of volume are found in Table 1-10.

Ordinarily, 1 ml is equal to 1 cubic centimeter (cc or cm^3). However, 1 liter is equal to 1000.027 cm^3. Therefore the cubic centimeter is somewhat smaller than the milliliter. Nonetheless, the cc, cm^3, and ml may be used interchangeably.

Figure 1-13 on page 62 illustrates the relationship between the linear dimensions length, (*l*), width (*w*), height (*h*) and volume (*V*). The product of these linear dimensions constitutes a volume; that is,

$$\text{volume} = \text{length} \times \text{width} \times \text{height}$$

$$1 \text{ cm} \times 1 \text{ cm} \times 1 \text{ cm} = 1 \text{ cubic centimeter}$$

$$= (1 \text{ cc or } 1 \text{ cm}^3)$$

$$= 1 \text{ ml}$$

$$1000 \text{ ml} = 1000 \text{ cc} = 1000 \text{ cm}^3 = 1 \text{ liter (L)}$$

$$10 \text{ cm} \times 10 \text{ cm} \times 10 \text{ cm} = 1000 \text{ cc}$$

$$= 1000 \text{ cm}^3$$

$$= 1000 \text{ ml}$$

$$= 1.0 \text{ L}$$

TABLE 1-8   Linear Measurements

Unit	Number	Exponential Form
kilometer (km)	1,000 m	10^3 m
meter (m)	1 m	10^0 m
decimeter (dm)	0.1 m	10^{-1} m
centimeter (cm)	0.01 m	10^{-2} m
millimeter (mm)	0.001 m	10^{-3} m
micrometer (μm)	0.000001 m	10^{-6} m
nanometer (nm)	0.000000001 m	10^{-9} m
Ångstrom (Å)	0.0000000001 m	10^{-10} m

TABLE 1-9   Units of Weight

Unit	Number	Exponential Form
kilogram (kg)	1,000 g	10^3 g
gram (g)	1 g	10^0 g
decigram (dg)	0.1 g	10^{-1} g
centigram (cg)	0.01 g	10^{-2} g
milligram (mg)	0.001 g	10^{-3} g
microgram (μg)	0.000001 g	10^{-6} g

TABLE 1-10   Units of Volume

Unit	Number	Exponential Form
liter (L)	1 liter	10^0 liter
deciliter (dl)	0.1 liter	10^{-1} liter
centiliter (cl)	0.01 liter	10^{-2} liter
milliliter (ml)	0.001 liter	10^{-3} liter

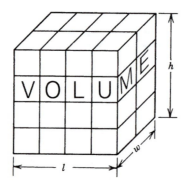

Figure 1-13   *A cube demonstrating the relationship among the linear dimensions—length (l), width (w), and height (h)—and volume (V).*

Table 1-11 shows a variety of metric equivalents and their respective units.

When converting units within the metric system, students often have difficulty remembering when to divide and when to multiply one unit by the other to make the proper conversion. The procedure described below represents a method of performing metric system conversions to alleviate confusion about when to multiply and when to divide.

Figure 1-14 illustrates the powers of 10 that are used to multiply or divide when changing metric units. An example of how to use Figure 1-14 follows.

Figure 1-14 shows five circles divided into a top half and a bottom half by the metric abbreviations. The top half of the circles (heavier lines) represents the process of converting a larger metric unit to a smaller metric unit (e.g., km to m, mm to μm, and m to nm). Also, the exponent designated at the top indicates the power of 10 by which to multiply the larger metric unit to obtain the number of decimal places in the smaller metric unit.

TABLE 1-11   Equivalents Relating Metric Units

meters $\times$ 10^2 cm/m	=	centimeters (cm)
meters $\times$ 10^3 mm/m	=	millimeters (mm)
meters $\times$ 10^6 μ/m	=	microns (μ), or micrometers (μm)
meters $\times$ 10^9 nm/m	=	nanometers (nm)
meters $\times$ 10^{10} Å/m	=	Ångstroms (Å)
centimeters $\times$ 10^8 Å/cm	=	Ångstroms (Å)
millimeters $\times$ 10^3 μ/mm	=	microns (μ)
kilograms $\times$ 10^9 μg/kg	=	micrograms (μg)
kilograms $\times$ 10^6 mg/kg	=	milligrams (mg)
grams $\times$ 10^3 mg/g	=	milligrams (mg)
liters $\times$ 10^3 ml/liter	=	milliliters (ml)
deciliters $\times$ 10^2 ml/dl	=	milliliters (ml)

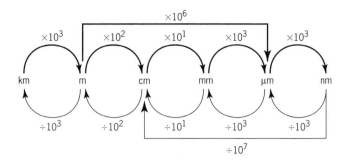

Figure 1-14 *The heavier lines on the top half of the figure signify changing from larger units to smaller units and indicate the power of 10 by which the larger unit is multiplied. The thinner lines on the bottom half of the figure represent converting smaller units to larger units and show the power of 10 by which the smaller unit is divided. The units gram and liter and their respective subdivisions (prefixes) can substitute for the unit meter in this scheme.*

So, when converting km to m, multiply the number of km by 10^3, or when converting from mm to μm, multiply the number of mm by 10^3. Also, when converting m to nm, multiply the number of m by 10^9 (i.e., $10^2 \times 10^1 \times 10^3 \times 10^3 = 10^9$).

EXAMPLE 1:

Convert 536 m to μm.

Step 1: Determine the direction of change.
The conversion here is from a larger unit to a smaller unit; therefore, the larger unit will be multiplied by some power of 10.

Step 2: Determine the power of 10 to be used in this problem.
From Figure 1-14 it can be determined that 10^6 will be needed to solve this problem.

Step 3: Multiply the value of the larger unit by 10^6.

$$(536 \; \cancel{m})(10^6 \; \mu m/\cancel{m}) = 536 \times 10^6 \; \mu m$$

$$= 5.36 \times 10^8 \; \mu m$$

Consider the curved lines with the arrow located along the bottom half of Figure 1-14. Notice that the arrows point in the opposite direction compared to those in the upper half. The bottom half of the circles represents the process of converting smaller metric units to larger metric units (e.g., nm to μm, mm to cm, and nm to m). The exponent designated along the arc of the bottom of the curved lines indicates the power of 10 by which the smaller metric unit must be divided to provide the larger metric unit.

Therefore, when converting from nm to μm, divide the number of nm by 10^3 to obtain the number of μm, or when converting mm to cm, divide the number of mm by 10^1. Also, when converting nm to m, divide the nm by 10^9. There are 9 decimal places from nm to m (i.e., $3 + 3 + 1 + 2 = 9$).

EXAMPLE 2:

Convert 7.95×10^3 nm to cm.

Step 1: Determine the direction of change.
The conversion here is from a smaller unit to a larger unit; therefore, the smaller unit will be divided by some power of 10.

Step 2: Determine the power of 10 to be used in this problem.
From Figure 1-14 it can be determined that 10^7 will be used to solve this problem.

Step 3: Divide the value of the smaller unit by 10^7.

$$\frac{(7.95 \times 10^3 \ \text{nm})}{10^7 \ \text{nm}/\text{cm}} = (7.95 \times 10^3)(10^{-7} \ \text{cm})$$

$$= 7.95 \times 10^{-4} \ \text{cm}$$

Keep in mind that units of mass (kg, g, cg, mg, μg, and ng) and volume (kl, l, cl, ml, μl, and nl) can substitute for the linear units in Figure 1-14.

Metric-English Conversion

Table 1-12 on page 65 illustrates select equivalents relating metric and English units.
    As in the previous section, the student is urged to maintain the units along with the numerical values while performing the calculations. In essence the factor-unit method previously described is encouraged.

EXAMPLE 1:

Convert 0.5 lb to grams.

Step 1: State the problem.

$$0.5 \ \text{lb} = X \ \text{g}$$

Step 2: Multiply 0.5 lb by the appropriate unity factors to cancel all the units except the one desired, i.e., grams.

$$0.5 \ \text{lb} \times \frac{1 \ \text{kg}}{2.20 \ \text{lb}} \times \frac{1000 \ \text{g}}{1 \ \text{kg}}$$

Step 3: Perform the necessary mathematical operations on the quantities in the problem.

$$\frac{0.5 \times 1000 \ \text{g}}{2.20} = 227 \ \text{g}$$

TABLE 1-12		Equivalents Relating Metric and English Units		
1 meter	×	39.37 in/m	=	39.37 inches
1 meter	×	3.28 ft/m	=	3.28 feet
1 inch	×	2.54 cm/in	=	2.54 centimeters
1 kilogram	×	2.20 lbs/kg	=	2.20 pounds
1 ounce	×	28.35 g/oz	=	28.35 grams

EXAMPLE 2:

Convert 5.43×10^{-3} ft to microns.

Step 1: State the problem.

$$5.43 \times 10^{-3} \text{ ft} = X \mu$$

Step 2: Multiply 5.43×10^{-3} ft by the appropriate unity factors to cancel all the units except the one desired, that is, microns.

$$5.43 \times 10^{-3} \text{ ft} \times \frac{12 \text{ in}}{1 \text{ ft}} \times \frac{2.54 \text{ cm}}{1 \text{ in}} \times \frac{1 \mu}{10^{-4} \text{ cm}}$$

Step 3: Perform the necessary mathematical operations on the quantities in the problem.

$$\frac{(5.43 \times 10^{-3})(12)(2.54)(1 \mu)}{10^{-4}} = 1655 \mu$$

EXAMPLE 3:

Convert 400 mg to pounds.

Step 1: State the problem.

$$400 \text{ mg} = X \text{ lbs}$$

Step 2: Multiply 400 mg by the appropriate unity factors to cancel all the units except the one desired, that is, pounds.

$$400 \text{ mg} \times \frac{1 \text{ g}}{1000 \text{ mg}} \times \frac{1 \text{ pound}}{16 \text{ oz}} \times \frac{1 \text{ oz}}{28.35 \text{ g}}$$

Step 3: Perform the necessary mathematical operations on the quantities in the problem.

$$\frac{(400)(1 \text{ pound})}{(1000)(16)(28.35)} = 0.00088 \text{ lb}$$

PRACTICE PROBLEMS

Refer to Appendix A (pages 561-562) for the solutions and answers to the practice problems.

Perform the following unit conversions:

    93. 1 Å = _____ cm
    94. 416 cm = _____ mm
    95. 4.96 g = _____ kg
    96. 2×10^{-2} nm = _____ cm
    97. 0.00937 m = _____ Å
    98. 609 mg = _____ kg
    99. 8.96×10^3 ml = _____ L
    100. 19 L = _____ ml
    101. 0.219 kg = _____ mg
    102. 0.000006 μ = _____ km
    103. 2 lbs 2 ounces = _____ kg
    104. 6.2×10^{-2} ft = _____ cm
    105. 232 lbs = _____ kg
    106. 693 m = _____ ft
    107. 4.96×10^6 g = _____ lbs
    108. 10^{39} kg = _____ ounces
    109. 150 lbs = _____ kg
    110. 1 ft = _____ cm
    111. 84 lbs = _____ g
    112. 325 ft = _____ m

1–8 LOGARITHMS

This section will introduce the reader to the fundamentals of **logarithms,** which will be useful in understanding certain acid-base concepts as well as in solving problems using the Henderson-Hasselbalch equation (Chapter 3, Section 3-4). Information about using a calculator to perform logarithmic functions will also be included.

Three elements comprise a logarithmic expression. These elements are (1) the logarithm, (2) the base, and (3) a number. For example,

$$\text{base}^{\text{logarithm}} = \text{number}$$

$$a^x = b$$

$$5^2 = 25$$

From the examples one should be able to recognize that a logarithm (abbreviated *log*) is an *exponent;* it is a *power.* A logarithmic expression represents a base raised to a power (exponent or logarithm) to obtain a number.

Since the applicability of logarithms to respiratory care is limited to the base 10, only the base 10 will be discussed. Keep in mind, however, that a base can be any number except the number one.

Logarithmic expressions can be written in two forms.

I. Exponential form ($10^2 = 100$)

II. Logarithmic form ($\log_{10} 100 = 2$)

Table 1-13 outlines how the same logarithmic expressions can be expressed in exponential and logarithmic forms.

The logarithmic form can be verbalized as, "the log of 100 to the base 10 is 2." In this form,

$$10 = \text{base}$$

$$2 = \text{logarithm (power or exponent)}$$

$$100 = \text{number}$$

Let us repeat a few times the question associated with the logarithmic form in order to determine a pattern. To what power (logarithm or exponent) must the base 10 be raised to obtain the following numbers: 10; 100; 1,000; 10,000?

A. $\log_{10} 10 = 1.000$; $1.000 = $ power, logarithm, or exponent

   Base 10 must be raised to the power of 1 to obtain the number 10; that is, $10^1 = 10$.

B. $\log_{10} 100 = 2.000$; $2.000 = $ power, logarithm, or exponent

   Base 10 must be raised to the power of 2 to obtain the number 100; that is, $10^2 = 100$.

C. $\log_{10} 1,000 = 3.000$; $3.000 = $ power, logarithm, or exponent

   Base 10 must be raised to the power of 3 to obtain the number 1,000; that is, $10^3 = 1,000$.

D. $\log_{10} 10,000 = 4.000$; $4.000 = $ power, logarithm, or exponent

   Base 10 must be raised to the power of 4 to obtain the number 10,000; that is, $10^4 = 10,000$.

TABLE 1-13   Logarithmic Expressions

Exponential Form	Logarithmic Form
$10^2 = 100$	$\log_{10} 100 = 2$
$10^0 = 1$	$\log_{10} 1 = 0$
$10^{-2} = 0.01$	$\log_{10} 0.01 = -2$

Therefore, each time the logarithm (exponent or power) increases by a factor of one, the number increases 10-fold. For example, 10^2 is 10 times greater than 10^1, and 10^3 is 10 times greater than 10^2, and so on.*

Now, how does one go about finding the logarithm (power or exponent) of the base 10 for numbers between 10 and 100, or between 100 and 1,000, and so on? For instance, how does one find the logarithm of 33? To what power must the base 10 be raised to obtain 33? That is

$$10^{\text{logarithm}} = 33$$

To find the logarithm of such a number, a log table needs to be consulted. A discussion of log tables follows shortly.

Earlier in this section it was mentioned that a logarithmic expression is comprised of three elements—logarithm, base, and number. Not to be confused with these three elements, the logarithm itself has two components. These two components are the **characteristic** and the **mantissa.**

For clarification, reconsider the expression

$$10^{\text{logarithm}} = 33$$

The logarithm of this number (33) is 1.5185. The base 10 must be raised to the power (logarithm) of 1.5185 to produce the number 33; that is, $10^{1.5185} = 33$.

The characteristic of the logarithm 1.5185 is 1, and the mantissa is .5185.

$$\text{log of 33} = \underline{1.5185}$$

mantissa

characteristic

The characteristic represents the integer portion of the logarithm; the mantissa is the decimal portion.

DETERMINING CHARACTERISTICS

There are two rules for determining the characteristic of a logarithm. One rule pertains to numbers that are equal to or greater than one, and the other rule refers to purely decimal numbers. The rule governing obtaining the characteristic of numbers equal to or greater than one will be discussed first.

Rule 1: If the number is equal to or greater than one, count the number of digits to the left of the decimal point and subtract one. The remainder is the characteristic of the logarithm. The formula used for determining a positive characteristic is $(x - 1)$, where x equals the number of integers positioned to the left of the decimal point in the number.

*The subscript 10, for example, in the expression $\log_{10} 10 = 1$ will be deleted and base 10 will be understood. Therefore, log 10 = 1 will substitute for $\log_{10} 10 = 1$.

Rule 2: If the number is less than one (i.e., a purely decimal number), count the number of places (*n*) the decimal point must be moved to the right to obtain a number between 1 and 9, inclusively, and insert that number in the general formula $(10 - n) - 10$.

Positive Characteristics:

Table 1-14 shows how to obtain the characteristic for four representative numbers greater than one.

It is important to be aware that specific groups of numbers share the same characteristic. Having the same characteristic is merely based on the amount of digits to the left of the decimal point that a number has. The log of the numbers from 1 to 9, inclusively, have a characteristic of zero because they all have one digit to the left of the decimal point. Because $1 - 1 = 0$, the characteristic for this group of numbers is zero. Note the pattern that develops for the groups of numbers in Table 1-15.

This table demonstrates the mechanics or the pattern that is followed for obtaining the characteristic of numbers greater than, or equal to, one. Because the pattern iw repetitive and rather straightforward, only a few representative groups of numbers have been included in the table.

TABLE 1–14   CHARACTERISTICS OF NUMBERS ≥1

Number	Total Digits to Left of Decimal	Formula $(x - 1)$	Chacteristic
5	1	1 − 1	0
20	2	2 − 1	1
714	3	3 − 1	2
1114	4	4 − 1	3

TABLE 1–15   CHARACTERISTICS OF GROUPS OF NUMBERS ≥1

Groups of Numbers	Total Digits to Left Left of Decimal	Formula $(x - 1)$	Characteristic
1 to 9	1	1 − 1	0
10 to 99	2	2 − 1	1
100 to 999	3	3 − 1	2
1,000 to 9,999	4	4 − 1	3
10,000 to 99,999	5	5 − 1	4

EXAMPLE:

Find the characteristic of the logarithm of 3,330.00.

Step 1: According to *Rule 1,* count the digits (integers) in the number located to the left of the decimal point.

$$3,3\,3\,0.00$$

4 digits

Step 2: Use the formula $(x - 1)$ to obtain the characteristic.

$$(x - 1) = \text{characteristic of the log of 3,330.00}$$

$$4 - 1 = 3$$

A series of examples illustrating positive characteristics follows.

$$\log 6.30 = \boxed{0}.7993$$
$$\log 63.00 = \boxed{1}.7993$$
$$\log 630.00 = \boxed{2}.7993$$
$$\log 6{,}300.00 = \boxed{3}.7993$$
$$\log 63{,}000.00 = \boxed{4}.7993$$
$$\log 630{,}000.00 = \boxed{5}.7993$$

CHARACTERISTIC

Negative Characteristics:

Table 1-16 shows how to obtain the characteristic for four representative numbers less than one.

A negative characteristic can be expressed two ways, as shown in the last column in Table 1-16.

EXAMPLE:

Obtain the characteristic of the logarithm of 0.0000595.

Step 1: According to *Rule 2,* count the places that the decimal point needs to be moved to the right to encounter a number between 1 and 9, inclusively.

$$0.0\,0\,0\,0\,5.95$$

1 2 3 4 5

TABLE 1-16   CHARACTERISTICS OF NUMBERS <1

Number	# of Decimal Places to Right	Formula $(10 - n) - 10$	Chacteristic
0.1	1	$(10 - 1) - 10$	$9 - 10$, or $\bar{1}$
0.09	2	$(10 - 2) - 10$	$8 - 10$, or $\bar{2}$
0.007	3	$(10 - 3) - 10$	$7 - 10$, or $\bar{3}$
0.0005	4	$(10 - 4) - 10$	$6 - 10$, or $\bar{4}$

Step 2: Apply the formula $(10 - n) - 10$ to determine the characteristic of the decimal number.

$$(10 - n) - 10 = \text{characteristic of the log of } 0.0000595.$$

$$(10 - 5) - 10 = 5 - 10, \text{ or -5, or } \bar{5}$$

The line (bar) overscoring the characteristic indicates that the characteristic is negative.

LOG TABLE

Now that the process of determining the characteristic of a logarithm has been presented, attention will be focused on how to find the mantissa. As we have just seen, the characteristic can be either positive or negative. However, the mantissa (the decimal component of a logarithm) will always be positive.

The table of logarithms (log table) referred to earlier can be described as a table of mantissas. It is from the log table that a mantissa of a logarithm is obtained. After the characteristic has been determined, the log table (Appendix B) completes the answer to the question, "To what power (logarithm or exponent) must the base 10 be raised to obtain a certain number?"

In order to find the log of a number, the vertical column on the extreme left of the log table provides a sequence of digits. The numbers shown horizontally at the top provide the next digit in the sequence. For example, to find the log of the number 556 find 55 on the far left vertical column, then find 6 on the uppermost, horizontal column. The mantissa is the figure located where these two points intersect, that is, 7451.

The mantissa 7451 must be preceded by the appropriate characteristic. In this example, the characteristic for 556 is 2. Therefore,

$$\log 556 = 2.7451$$

The ensuing discussion describes how to determine the log of a purely decimal number (i.e., a number less than 1). Finding the logarithm of a decimal number involves a process different from that just described. The example below outlines the steps involved in determining the log of a number less than 1.

EXAMPLE:

Determine the log of 0.000688.

Step 1: Apply the formula $(10 - n) - 10$ for providing the characteristic.

$$0 . \underbrace{0\ 0\ 0\ 6}_{1\ 2\ 3\ 4} . 8\ 8$$

$$(10 - n) - 10 = \text{characteristic of number} < 1$$

$$(10 - 4) - 10 = 6 - 10, \text{ or } \bar{4}$$

Step 2: Consult the log table to find the mantissa corresponding to the sequence of digits 688.

Common Logarithms

N.	0	1	2	3	4	5	6	7	⑧	9
55	7404	7412	7419	7427	7435	7443	7451	7459	7466	7474
56	7482	7490	7497	7505	7513	7520	7528	7536	7543	7551
57	7559	7566	7574	7582	7589	7597	7604	7612	7619	7627
58	7634	7642	7649	7657	7664	7672	7679	7686	7694	7701
59	7709	7716	7723	7731	7738	7745	7752	7760	7767	7774
60	7782	7789	7796	7803	7810	7818	7825	7832	7839	7846
61	7853	7860	7868	7875	7882	7889	7896	7903	7910	7917
62	7924	7931	7938	7945	7952	7959	7966	7973	7980	7987
63	7993	8000	8007	8014	8021	8028	8035	8041	8048	8055
64	8062	8069	8075	8082	8089	8096	8102	8109	8116	8122
65	8129	8136	8142	8149	8156	8162	8169	8176	8182	8189
66	8195	8202	8209	8215	8222	8228	8235	8241	8248	8254
67	8261	8267	8274	8280	8287	8293	8299	8306	8312	8319
⑥⑧	8325	8331	8338	8344	8351	8357	8363	8370	⑧⑧⑦⑥	8382
69	8388	8395	8401	8407	8414	8420	8426	8432	8439	8445
70	8451	8457	8463	8470	8476	8482	8488	8494	8500	8506
71	8513	8519	8525	8531	8537	8543	8549	8555	8561	8567
72	8573	8579	8585	8591	8597	8603	8609	8615	8621	8627
73	8633	8639	8645	8651	8657	8663	8669	8675	8681	8686
74	8692	8698	8704	8710	8716	8722	8727	8733	8739	8745
75	8751	8756	8762	8768	8774	8779	8785	8791	8797	8802
76	8808	8814	8820	8825	8831	8837	8842	8848	8854	8859

Refer to 68 along the extreme left vertical column, and 8 along the uppermost horizontal row. The mantissa for 688 is located where this column and row intersect.

mantissa = 8376

Step 3: Algebraically, add the mantissa to the characteristic.

$$-4.0000 \text{ (characrteristic)}$$
$$+0.8376 \text{ (mantissa)}$$
$$-3.1624 \text{ (logarithm)}$$

Alternatively, after the mantissa is obtained in *Step 2,* use the $6 - 10$ form of the characteristic, and place the mantissa after the 6. That form will then become

$$6.8376 - 10$$

In this instance, algebraically add 6.8376 to -10.0000. This calculation is as follows:

$$-10.0000$$
$$+6.8376$$
$$-3.1624$$

When expressing these logarithms in the exponential form, they become

$$10^{6.8376-10} = 0.000688$$

or

$$10^{\bar{3}.1624} = 0.000688$$

IF YOU HAVE A CALCULATOR WITH A LOG FUNCTION,

The log of 0.000688 can be quickly determined using any calculator having a log function. For example, press the following calculator keys.

PRESS: .000688 $\boxed{\log}$

Antilogarithms

The last process described in this section is that of determining **antilogarithms.** The process of determining the number when the exponent (logarithm or power) is known is called finding the antilogarithm. The process is simply the opposite of finding the logarithm.

EXAMPLE 1:

Find the antilog of $\bar{1}.2592$.

Step 1: Subtract $\bar{1}.2592$ from 10.

$$10.0000$$
$$-1.2592$$
$$8.\boxed{7408} - 10$$

desired mantissa

Step 2: From the log table, find the range of mantissas within which the desired mantissa (7408) lies and determine the high-low mantissa difference.

Common Logarithms

N.	0	1	2	3	4	5	6	7	8	9
55	7404	7412	7419	7427	7435	7443	7451	7459	7466	7474
56	7482	7490	7497	7505	7513	7520	7528	7536	7543	7551
57	7559	7566	7574	7582	7589	7597	7604	7612	7619	7627
58	7634	7642	7649	7657	7664	7672	7679	7686	7694	7701
59	7709	7716	7723	7731	7738	7745	7752	7760	7767	7774
60	7782	7789	7796	7803	7810	7818	7825	7832	7839	7846
61	7853	7860	7868	7875	7882	7889	7896	7903	7910	7917
62	7924	7931	7938	7945	7952	7959	7966	7973	7980	7987
63	7993	8000	8007	8014	8021	8028	8035	8041	8048	8055
64	8062	8069	8075	8082	8089	8096	8102	8109	8116	8122
65	8129	8136	8142	8149	8156	8162	8169	8176	8182	8189
66	8195	8202	8209	8215	8222	8228	8235	8241	8248	8254
67	8261	8267	8274	8280	8287	8293	8299	8306	8312	8319
68	8325	8331	8338	8344	8351	8357	8363	8370	8376	8382
69	8388	8395	8401	8407	8414	8420	8426	8432	8439	8445
70	8451	8457	8463	8470	8476	8482	8488	8494	8500	8506
71	8513	8519	8525	8531	8537	8543	8549	8555	8561	8567
72	8573	8579	8585	8591	8597	8603	8609	8615	8621	8627
73	8633	8639	8645	8651	8657	8663	8669	8675	8681	8686
74	8692	8698	8704	8710	8716	8722	8727	8733	8739	8745
75	8751	8756	8762	8768	8774	8779	8785	8791	8797	8802
76	8808	8814	8820	8825	8831	8837	8842	8848	8854	8859

Low mantissa 7404

High mantissa 7412

```
   7412 high mantissa
 − 7404 low mantissa
   8 high-low mantissa difference
```

Step 3: From the log table, find the range of corresponding numbers within which the desired mantissa resides and determine the high-low number difference.

Common Logarithms

N.	0	1	2	3	4	5	6	7	8	9
55	7404	7412	7419	7427	7435	7443	7451	7459	7466	7474
56	7482	7490	7497	7505	7513	7520	7528	7536	7543	7551
57	7559	7566	7574	7582	7589	7597	7604	7612	7619	7627
58	7634	7642	7649	7657	7664	7672	7679	7686	7694	7701
59	7709	7716	7723	7731	7738	7745	7752	7760	7767	7774
60	7782	7789	7796	7803	7810	7818	7825	7832	7839	7846

Low number 5500

High number 5510

61	7853	7860	7868	7875	7882	7889	7896	7903	7910	7917
62	7924	7931	7938	7945	7952	7959	7966	7973	7980	7987
63	7993	8000	8007	8014	8021	8028	8035	8041	8048	8055
64	8062	8069	8075	8082	8089	8096	8102	8109	8116	8122
65	8129	8136	8142	8149	8156	8162	8169	8176	8182	8189
66	8195	8202	8209	8215	8222	8228	8235	8241	8248	8254
67	8261	8267	8274	8280	8287	8293	8299	8306	8312	8319
68	8325	8331	8338	8344	8351	8357	8363	8370	8376	8382
69	8388	8395	8401	8407	8414	8420	8426	8432	8439	8445
70	8451	8457	8463	8470	8476	8482	8488	8494	8500	8506
71	8513	8519	8525	8531	8537	8543	8549	8555	8561	8567
72	8573	8579	8585	8591	8597	8603	8609	8615	8621	8627
73	8633	8639	8645	8651	8657	8663	8669	8675	8681	8686
74	8692	8698	8704	8710	8716	8722	8727	8733	8739	8745
75	8751	8756	8762	8768	8774	8779	8785	8791	8797	8802
76	8808	8814	8820	8825	8831	8837	8842	8848	8854	8859

$$
\begin{array}{r}
5510 \text{ high number} \\
- 5500 \text{ low number} \\
\hline
10 \text{ high-low number difference}
\end{array}
$$

Step 4: Calculate the difference between the desired mantissa (7408) and the low mantissa.

$$
\begin{array}{r}
7408 \text{ desired mantissa} \\
- 7404 \text{ low mantissa} \\
\hline
4 \text{ desired-low mantissa difference}
\end{array}
$$

Step 5: Set up the following proportion to solve for X, which represents the difference between the desired number and the low number.

$$\frac{\text{desired-low mantissa difference}}{\text{high-low mantissa difference}} = \frac{X}{\text{high-low number difference}}$$

$$\frac{4}{8} = \frac{X}{10}$$

$$X = 5$$

Step 6: Add X to the low number to obtain the desired sequence of digits.

$$
\begin{array}{r}
5500 \text{ low number} \\
+ \quad 5 \text{ desired-low number difference} \\
\hline
5505 \text{ desired sequence of digits}
\end{array}
$$

Step 7: Position the decimal point in the appropriate location according to the characteristic

$(8 - 10, \text{ or } \bar{2})$ of the logarithm.

$$0 . \underset{2 \quad 1}{\underbrace{0\ 5}}\ 5\ 0\ 5$$

Therefore, the antilog of $\bar{1}.2592$ is 0.05505.

IF YOU HAVE A CALCULATOR WITH A LOG FUNCTION,

The antilog of $\bar{1}.2592$ can be quickly determined using any calculator having a log function. For example, press the following calculator keys.

PRESS: $\boxed{-}$ 1.2592 $\boxed{-}$ $\boxed{\text{INV}}$ $\boxed{\text{log}}$

EXAMPLE 2:

Find the antilog of $\bar{2}.6176$.

Step 1: Subtract 2.6176 from 10.

$$
\begin{array}{r}
10.0000 \\
-\,2.6176 \text{ low mantissa} \\
\hline
7.\boxed{3824}\ -\ 10
\end{array}
$$

—desired mantissa

Step 2: From the log table find the range of mantissas within which the desired mantissa (3824) lies and determine the high-low mantissa difference.

$$
\begin{array}{r}
3838 \text{ high mantissa} \\
-\,3820 \text{ low mantissa} \\
\hline
18 \text{ high-low mantissa difference}
\end{array}
$$

Common Logarithms

N.	0	①	②	3	4	5	6	7	8	9
10	0000	0043	0086	0128	0170	0212	0253	0294	0334	0374
11	0414	0453	0492	0531	0569	0607	0645	0682	0719	0755
12	0792	0828	0864	0899	0934	0969	1004	1038	1072	1106
13	1139	1173	1206	1239	1271	1303	1335	1367	1399	1430
14	1461	1492	1523	1553	1584	1614	1644	1673	1703	1732
15	1761	1790	1818	1847	1875	1903	1931	1959	1987	2014
16	2041	2068	2095	2122	2148	2175	2201	2227	2253	2279
17	2304	2330	2355	2380	2405	2430	2455	2480	2504	2529
18	2553	2577	2601	2625	2648	2672	2695	2718	2742	2765
19	2788	2810	2833	2856	2878	2900	2923	2945	2967	2989
20	3010	3032	3054	3075	3096	3118	3139	3160	3181	3201
21	3222	3243	3263	3284	3304	3324	3345	3365	3385	3404
22	3424	3444	3464	3483	3502	3522	3541	3560	3579	3598
23	3617	3636	3655	3674	3692	3711	3729	3747	3766	3784
24	3802	3820	3838	3856	3874	3892	3909	3927	3945	3962
25	3979	3997	4014	4031	4048	4065	4082	4099	4116	4133
26	4150	4166	4183	4200	4216	4232	4249	4265	4281	4298
27	4314	4330	4346	4362	4378	4393	4409	4425	4440	4456
28	4472	4487	4502	4518	4533	4548	4564	4579	4594	4609
29	4624	4639	4654	4669	4683	4698	4713	4728	4742	4757

Low number 2410

High number 2420

Low mantissa

High mantissa

Step 3: From the log table find the range of corresponding numbers within which the desired mantissa resides and determine the high-low mantissa difference.

2420 high number
− 2410 low number
_____
10 high-low number difference

Common Logarithms

N.	0	1	2	3	4	5	6	7	8	9
10	0000	0043	0086	0128	0170	0212	0253	0294	0334	0374
11	0414	0453	0492	0531	0569	0607	0645	0682	0719	0755
12	0792	0828	0864	0899	0934	0969	1004	1038	1072	1106
13	1139	1173	1206	1239	1271	1303	1335	1367	1399	1430
14	1461	1492	1523	1553	1584	1614	1644	1673	1703	1732
15	1761	1790	1818	1847	1875	1903	1931	1959	1987	2014
16	2041	2068	2095	2122	2148	2175	2201	2227	2253	2279
17	2304	2330	2355	2380	2405	2430	2455	2480	2504	2529
18	2553	2577	2601	2625	2648	2672	2695	2718	2742	2765
19	2788	2810	2833	2856	2878	2900	2923	2945	2967	2989
20	3010	3032	3054	3075	3096	3118	3139	3160	3181	3201
21	3222	3243	3263	3284	3304	3324	3345	3365	3385	3404
22	3424	3444	3464	3483	3502	3522	3541	3560	3579	3598
23	3617	3636	3655	3674	3692	3711	3729	3747	3766	3784
24	3802	3820	3838	3856	3874	3892	3909	3927	3945	3962
25	3979	3997	4014	4031	4048	4065	4082	4099	4116	4133
26	4150	4166	4183	4200	4216	4232	4249	4265	4281	4298
27	4314	4330	4346	4362	4378	4393	4409	4425	4440	4456
28	4472	4487	4502	4518	4533	4548	4564	4579	4594	4609
29	4624	4639	4654	4669	4683	4698	4713	4728	4742	4757

Low number 2410

High number 2420

Step 4: Calculate the difference between the desired mantissa (3824) and the low mantissa.

3824 desired mantissa
− 3820 low mantissa
_____
4 desired-low mantissa difference

Step 5: Set up the following proportion to solve for X, which represents the difference between the desired number and the low number.

$$\frac{4}{18} = \frac{X}{10}$$

$$X = 2$$

Step 6: Add the value of X (2) to the low number to obtain the sequence of digits in the desired number.

$$
\begin{array}{r}
2410 \text{ low number} \\
+ \; 2 \text{ desired-low number difference} \\
\hline
2412 \text{ sequence of digits in desired number}
\end{array}
$$

Step 7: Position the decimal point in the appropriate location according to the characteristic $(7 - 10, \text{ or } \bar{3})$ of the logarithm.

$$
0 \; . \; 0 \; 0 \; 2 \; 4 \; 1 \; 2
$$
$$
 3 \; 2 \; 1
$$

The antilog of $\bar{2}.6176$ is 0.002412.

IF YOU HAVE A CALCULATOR WITH A LOG FUNCTION,

The antilog of $\bar{2}.6176$ can be quickly determined using any calculator having a log function. For example, press the following calculator keys.

PRESS: $\boxed{-}$ 2.6176 $\boxed{-}$ $\boxed{\text{INV}}$ $\boxed{\text{log}}$

In Chapter 3 it will be necessary to perform multiplication and division using logarithms when working problems concerning the Henderson-Hasselbalch equation. Therefore, the rules governing these two operations in relationship to logarithms will be presented here.

RULES GOVERNING USE

A. Multiplication of Logarithms

When the logs of two or more numbers are to be multiplied, add the logs. This rule can be shown as

$$
\log (A \times B \times C) = \log A + \log B + \log C
$$

EXAMPLE:

Multiply $\log (180 \times 623 \times 30)$.

$$
\begin{array}{rl}
\log (180 \times 623 \times 30) = & \log 180 + \log 623 + \log 30] \\
\log 180 = & 2.2553 \\
\log 623 = & 2.7945 \\
\log \; 30 = & +1.4771 \\
\hline
& 6.5269
\end{array}
$$

$$
6.5269 = \log \text{ of the product of } 180 \times 623 \times 30
$$

$$
3{,}364{,}200 = \text{product of } 180 \times 623 \times 30
$$

and

$$
3{,}364{,}200 = \text{antilog of } 6.5269
$$

IF YOU HAVE A CALCULATOR WITH A LOG FUNCTION,

The log (180 × 623 × 30) can be quickly determined using any calculator having a log function. For example, press the following calculator keys.

PRESS: 180 $\boxed{\times}$ 623 $\boxed{\times}$ 30 $\boxed{=}$ $\boxed{\log}$

B. Division of Logarithms

When the logs of two numbers are to be divided, subtract the logs. This rule may be shown as

$$\log\left(\frac{A}{B}\right) = \log A - \log B$$

EXAMPLE:

Divide log (400/200).

$$\log\frac{400}{200} = \log 400 - \log 200$$

$$\log 400 = \quad 2.6021$$
$$\log 200 = \frac{-2.3010}{.3011}$$

.3011 = log of the quotient of 400 ÷ 200

2 = the quotient of 400 ÷ 200

2 = antilog of .3011

IF YOU HAVE A CALCULATOR WITH A LOG FUNCTION,

The log (400/200) can be quickly determined using any calculator having a log function. For example, press the following calculator keys.

PRESS: 400 $\boxed{\div}$ 200 $\boxed{=}$ $\boxed{\log}$

PRACTICE PROBLEMS

Refer to Appendix A (pages 562-569) for the solutions and answers to the practice problems.

Label the terms in each of the following expressions:

113. $p^r = t$

p: _____

r: _____

t: _____

114. $9^2 = 81$

      9: _____

      2: _____

     81: _____

Write the following exponential forms in the logarithmic form:

115. $p^r = t$ _____

116. $6^3 = 216$ _____

117. $10^0 = 1$ _____

Find the characteristic of the log of the following numbers.

118. 0.00003 _____

119. 987654.3 _____

120. 8142 _____

121. 10^{-10} _____

122. 0.0009×10^{-5} _____

123. 385.264 _____

124. 10 _____

125. 0.090006 _____

126. 3.06×10^{-8} _____

127. 5 _____

Find the log of the following numbers. Use the log table in **Appendix B (pages 626-628).**

128. 6.870 _____

129. 0.000979 _____

130. 0.0000347×10^6 _____

131. 55.5×10^{-4} _____

132. 175.6 _____

133. 1.00 _____

134. 20 _____

135. 0.0000621 _____

136. 9.55×10^{-7} _____

137. 0.00452×10^6 _____

138. 6.00×10^{-11} _____

Find the antilog of the following logs. Use the log table in **Appendix B (pages 626-628).**

139. 1.30 _____

140. .9320 _____

141. $\bar{2}.2765$ _____

142. $\bar{4}.5670$ _____

143. 3.0043 _____

144. $\bar{8}.1904$ _____

145. 8.6693 _____

146. $\bar{3}.7305$ _____

147. $\bar{1}.6513$ _____

148. $\bar{5}.8625$ _____

149. 6.2399 _____

150. 4.4444 _____

Perform the designated mathematical operation (See **Appendix B (pages 626-628)**).

151. log (0.5241 ÷ 0.2142) _____

152. log (20 ÷ 1) _____

153 log (34 ÷ 9) _____

154. log (25 × 15) _____

155. log (1532 × 777) _____

156. log (333 × 0.456) _____

157. log (24/1.2) _____

158. log (8496/451) _____

159. log (50 × 100 × 10³) _____

160. log (10⁻² × 10⁴ × 36) _____

1-9 GRAPHS

Graphs are used in all disciplines. They are pictorial representations of quantitative relationships. They often allow a great deal of information to be visually assimilated, thus reducing verbal or written descriptions. They may also save time and labor in making calculations by allowing conclusions to be drawn by comparison.

Aside from these and perhaps other advantages, there are disadvantages associated with the use of graphs. They may be less accurate than the numbers upon which they are based and may be visually misrepresented to reflect the author's biases.

Figure 1-15 illustrates the **Cartesian coordinate system.** The horizontal line labelled by the lower case letter x is called the **abscissa,** and the vertical line designated by y is the **ordinate.** The point of intersection of the ordinate and abscissa is called the **origin.**

The intersection of the x- and y-axes produces four quadrants within the plane in which they are drawn. The four quadrants are labelled I, II, III, and IV. Values that are plotted in the different quadrants have positive or negative signs. Negative values on the x-axis are located to the left of the origin in quadrants II and III. Negative values for y reside below the origin in quadrants III and IV.

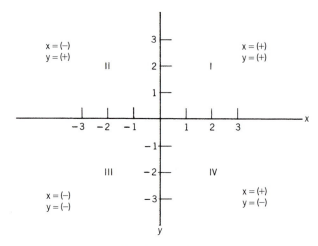

Figure 1-15 *Cartesian coordinate system showing x- and y-axes and quadrants I-IV.*

Specifically, values located in quadrant I have positive designations for x and y. Points plotted in quadrant II have a negative x value and a positive y value. Quadrant III locations possess negative designations, whereas quadrant IV points have negative y values and positive x values. Each point in a coordinate plane is assigned a unique **ordered pair** of real numbers (x and y). The two numbers, paired with a given point, are called the **coordinates** of that point. Note the examples below in Figure 1-16.

Quadrant I: $x = 4$, $y = 2$; coordinates $(4, 2)$

Quadrant II: $x = -4$, $y = 2$; coordinates $(-4, 2)$

Quadrant III: $x = -4$, $y = -2$; coordinates $(-4, -2)$

Quadrant IV: $x = 4$, $y = -2$; coordinates $(4, -2)$

Quite often the relationship between two variables is plotted along the x- and y-axes. The nature of the relationship is determined by maintaining all quantities constant except the two being investigated. One of those two quantities is then varied and the corresponding change (response) in the other is measured. The quantity that is deliberately altered is termed the **independent variable** and is plotted on the x-axis. The quantity that changes because of the variation in the independent variable is called the **dependent variable.** The dependent variable is plotted on the y-axis.

Four graphic representations will be discussed here to exemplify the different types of relationships that exist between the dependent and independent variables. These graphs are (1) a straight line, (2) a **hyperbola,** (3) a **parabola** (4) **a sigmoid curve.**

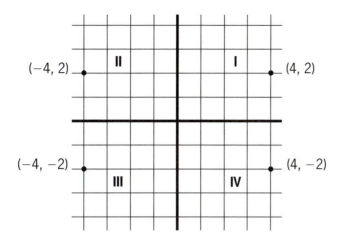

Figure 1-16 *Cartesian coordinate system illustrating data points (x and y) located in quadrants I, II, III, and IV.*

STRAIGHT LINE GRAPH

A graph consisting of a straight line intersecting the origin results when the dependent variable (*y*-axis) varies directly with the independent variable. Hooke's law describes the response of a spring to which forces of the same mass are applied, resulting in directly proportional elongation of the spring. In other words, when the spring is acted upon by a unit of force, the spring will stretch one unit of length. When acted upon by two units of force, the spring will stretch two units of length. This direct relationship will continue until the elastic limit of the spring is reached or exceeded. Figure 1-17 illustrates this direct relationship (straight line through origin), as the elongation of the spring (dependent variable) is plotted on the *y*-axis against the force (independent variable) applied to the spring shown on the *x*-axis.

The general formula for a direct relationship is shown in Figure 1-17 along the straight line connecting the data points. This formula is frequently expressed as follows:

$$y = k\,x$$

As *k* is a constant, the expression demonstrates how *y* changes with respect to changes in *x*. Therefore, for each change in *x*, the force (independent variable), there will be a directly proportional change in *y*, the elongation (dependent variable).

In the linear relationship just described, the line plotted passes through the origin. The point where the plotted line intersects the *y*-axis is called the *y-intercept*. The equation that governs a linear relationship when the straight line does not intersect the origin is

$$y = mx + b$$

where *m* and *b* are constants called the slope and *y*-intercept, respectively.

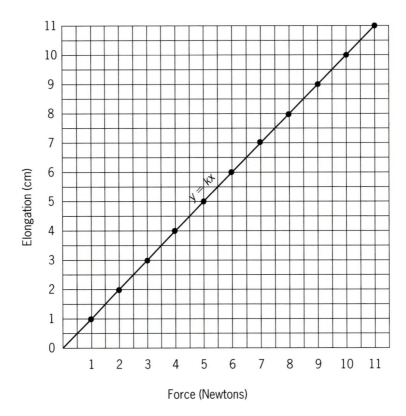

Figure 1-17 *Graphic illustration of Hooke's law demonstrating a straight line intersecting the origin when dependent variable (y-axis) varies directly with independent variable (x-axis).*

Assume that the constants m and b have the following values:

$$m = 3$$
$$b = 5$$

The equation now reads,

$$y = 3x + 5$$

The data listed in Table 1-17 represent values that can be substituted for x and y in the equation and are plotted on the graph in Figure 1-18.

The slope (m) of the line plotted in Figure 1-18 can be calculated by dividing a change (Δ) in y by a change (Δ) in x. The slope can be expressed as a ratio.

$$m = \frac{\Delta y}{\Delta x}$$

TABLE 1-17

Values for *x* and *y*
(*y* = 3*x* + 5)

x	y
0	5
1	8
2	11
3	14
4	17
5	20

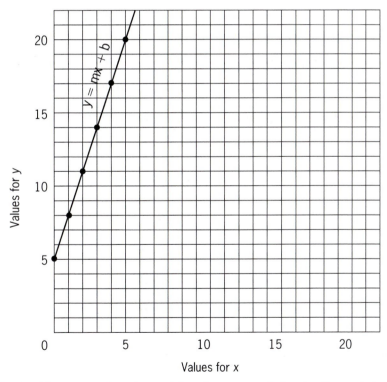

Figure 1-18 *Graphic representation of general formula y = mx + b showing linear relationship (straight line) not intersecting the origin. The plotted data are from Table 1-17.*

The horizontal change (Δx) for $x = 2$ and $x = 4$ is 2 (i.e., $4 - 2 = 2$). The corresponding vertical change (Δy) for $y = 11$ and $y = 17$ is 6 (i.e., $17 - 11 = 6$).

The slope of the line is calculated as follows:

$$m = \frac{\Delta y}{\Delta x} = \frac{(4 - 2 = 2)}{(17 - 11 = 6)} = \frac{2}{6} = \frac{1}{3} \text{ or } 0.33$$

The slope is one over three, which means that for 1 unit change along the y-axis, there will be 3 units of change along the x-axis. The y-intercept for the straight line in this situation is 5.

The formula that is used to evaluate the relationship of the carbon monoxide diffusing capacity (DLCO) and its components is shown below.

$$\frac{1}{\text{DLCO}} = \frac{1}{\theta V_C} + \frac{1}{D_M}$$

where

DLCO = carbon monoxide diffusing capacity (ml/min/mm Hg)

θ = rate of reaction between carbon monoxide and hemoglobin

V_C = pulmonary capillary blood volume

D_M = alveolar-capillary membrane resistance

This formula is analogous to the equation $y = mx + b$. Figure 1-19 on page 87 illustrates how the DLCO equation is plotted.

The reciprocal of the carbon monoxide diffusion capacity (1/DLCO) is plotted along the y-axis, and the reciprocal of the rate of the reaction between carbon monoxide and hemoglobin ($1/\theta$) is plotted on the x-axis. The three data points that comprise the straight line are the mean pulmonary capillary P_{O_2} values at 21%, 60%, and 100% oxygen.

The slope (hypotenuse of dotted right triangle) of this line is the reciprocal of the pulmonary capillary blood volume ($1/V_C$), which is a constant. The y-intercept is the reciprocal of the alveolar-capillary membrane resistance ($1/D_M$). The units for D_M itself (pressure/flow rate) indicate that this value is a resistance. Therefore, since it is the reciprocal of D_M (i.e., $1/D_M$) that it used in the equation, the factor actually represents a conductance (flow rate/pressure).

When working with graphs, a process called **extrapolation** is sometimes used. Extrapolation is the inference of an unknown value or values based on known data. Extrapolation is usually applied to estimation beyond the range of observed or known data points. Extrapolation is the opposite of **interpolation.** Interpolation is the estimation of an unknown value or values between known data points.

Extrapolation can lead to erroneous conclusions. Let's view Charles' law, an ideal gas law, as an example. Charles' law states that when the pressure and the mass of an ideal gas are constant, the gas volume is directly proportional to the gas' temperature. Figure 1-20 illustrates the behavior of a gas based on the relationship between its volume (ml) and temperature (°C), according to Charles' law.

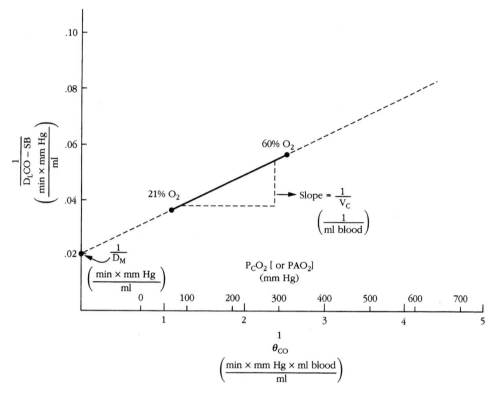

Figure 1-19 *Plotting of DLCO illustrating application of equation y = mx + b. (From Madama, Pulmonary Function Testing and Cardiopulmonary Stress Testing, 1993. Delmar Publishers.)*

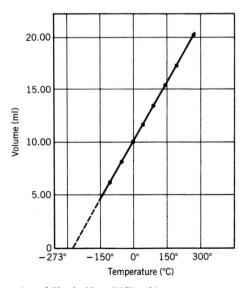

Figure 1-20 *Graphic illustration of Charles' law (V/T = k).*

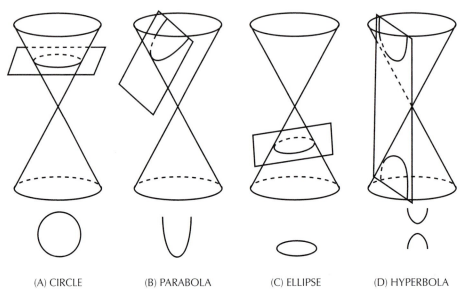

(A) CIRCLE   (B) PARABOLA   (C) ELLIPSE   (D) HYPERBOLA

Figure 1-21   *Four conic sections are depicted, depending on the inclination at which the plane intersects the cone.*

The solid portion of the line represents known data points. These known data points reflect actual gas behavior, i.e., as gas temperature decreases, gas volume also decreases. However, the dotted portion of the line represents extrapolated values. These values are based on the known values plotted on the solid portion of the line.

The inference is that as the temperature of the gas continues to fall, the gas volume decreases proportionately. Ultimately, when the gas temperature is extrapolated to −273°C, the extrapolated volume is 0 ml. Such a phenomenon does not occur, because the gas will experience a change of state and become a liquid well before this point. Furthermore, Charles' law is a gas law and does not apply to liquids. Therefore, the inference from the graph in Figure 1-20 that a −273°C gas volume becomes 0 ml is false.

HYPERBOLIC CURVE

A hyperbolic curve is described as a **conic section.** It bears this description because it is formed as a result of a plane intersecting a cone at a certain inclination. Figure 1-21 shows four conic sections. Each conic section is different, based on the inclination of the intersecting plane.

The four conic sections shown in Figure 1-21 are (a) circle, (b) parabola, (c) ellipse, and (d) hyperbola.

A hyperbola is formed when a cross section intersects both portions of the double cone (Figure 1-21D). A hyperbola contains two distinct, symmetric branches.

When the dependent variable is inversely related to the independent variable, a hyperbolic tracing develops. Figure 1-21 demonstrates the data plotted based on Boyle's law which states that when the temperature and mass of an ideal gas are constant, the pressure

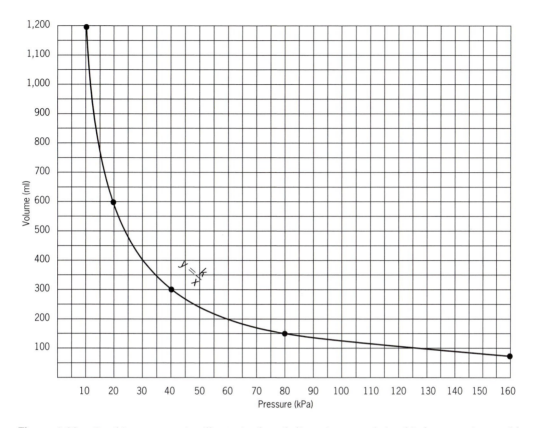

Figure 1-22   *Graphic representation illustrating hyperbolic, or inverse, relationship from equation y = k/x.*

and volume of the gas are inversely related. In Figure 1-22, the gas volume (dependent variable) is plotted on the *y*-axis and the gas pressure (independent variable) is plotted along the *x*-axis.

For hyperbolic relationships, the general equation is

$$y = \frac{k}{x}$$

which is presented in Figure 1-22 along the hyperbola. In this instance (Boyle's law), as the gas pressure in kPa doubles, the gas volume reduces by one-half.

PARABOLIC CURVE

As was previously mentioned, a parabolic curve is a conic section. The result of a cross section passing through the base of a cone and intersecting only one portion is a parabola.

Figure 1-23 on page 90 represents a parabolic graph. A parabola results when the dependent variable is directly related to the square of the independent variable. The *y*-axis in

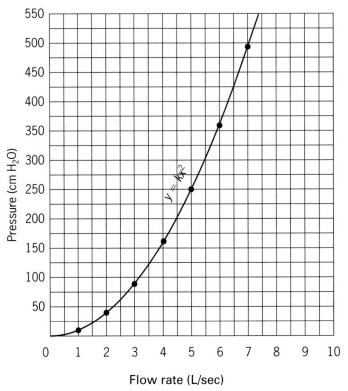

Figure 1-23 *Graphic representation demonstrating parabolic relationship resulting from equation* $y = kx^2$.

this example will be the driving pressure (ΔP), or pressure gradient, that is needed to sustain a turbulent flow pattern, as the flow rate ($\dot{V}$) of the gas increases.

The equation that characterizes this parabolic relationship is as follows:

$$y = k\,x^2$$

In this equation k is constant, and it illustrates how fast y changes with respect to x^2. The mathematical example used to demonstrate this relationship is presented below.

$$\Delta P = k\,\dot{V}^2$$

The constant k is inversely related to the square of the flow rate ($\dot{V}$). The product of this relationship provides the pressure change (driving pressure) that is needed to maintain different flow rates.

Figure 1-24 on page 91 illustrates the shape of a graph resulting from plotting two variables that are inversely proportional.

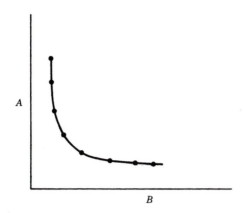

Figure 1-24 *Inverse proportion representing equation A/B = k.*

SIGMOID CURVE

A sigmoid curve is an S-shaped curve.

A number of formulas produce sigmoid curves. One such formula produces a plot of the response functions called *logistic response functions*. This formula generates a sigmoid curve.

$$E(Y) = \frac{\exp(\beta_0 + \beta_1 X)}{1 + \exp(\beta_0 + \beta_1 X)}$$

The mathematics associated with this formula and the topic of logistic response function are beyond the scope of this book. However, this information has been included here to allow the reader to appreciate the complexity of formulas associated with a sigmoid curve.

We will move along at this point to discuss a couple physiologic and clinical applications of sigmoid curves.

The oxyhemoglobin dissociation curve (Figure 1-25) is a sigmoid curve. The partial pressure of dissolved oxygen (torr or mm Hg) is plotted along the *x*-axis, and the percentage of hemoglobin saturated with oxygen, known as the oxygen saturation (S_{O_2}), is plotted on the y-axis. This curve is generated by exposing whole blood, which contains 15 grams of hemoglobin per 100 ml of blood (15 g%), to gas mixtures with progressively higher partial pressures of oxygen ($P_{O_2}s$). Certain physiologic factors, such as, the P_{CO_2}, pH, body temperature, and 2,3 DPG levels are held constant during the process.

If the whole blood sample equilibrates with a gas sample containing no oxygen (P_{O_2} 0 torr), then the hemoglobin saturation will be zero (0%). On the other hand, if the whole blood sample is exposed to gas containing a P_{O_2} of 150 torr, the percentage of hemoglobin saturated with oxygen will be approximately 100%.

The reason the oxyhemoglobin dissociation curve is sigmoid shaped is because of the phenomenon known as cooperativity (Chapter 6, Physiologic Chemistry, page 433).

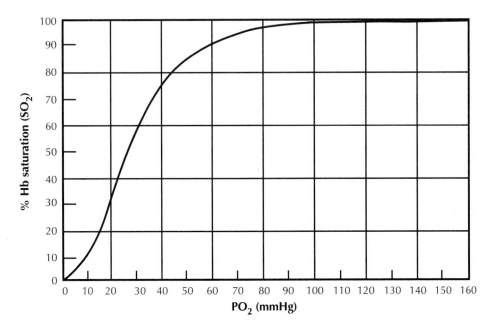

Figure 1-25 *Normal configuration (sigmoid) of the oxyhemoglobin dissociation curve.*

Cooperativity is a property displayed by the hemoglobin molecule. Each hemoglobin molecule is capable of binding with four oxygen molecules. In the lungs during oxygenation when one oxygen binding site on the hemoglobin molecule becomes occupied, hemoglobin's affinity for oxygen increases. When two binding sites are occupied by oxygen, the affinity for a third oxygen molecule becomes even greater. The same process occurs for the fourth binding site when three oxygen molecules bind to hemoglobin. In essence what happens is hemoglobin's affinity for oxygen progressively increases with the binding of oxygen molecules to hemoglobin.

At the tissue level where hemoglobin releases oxygen, the same effect takes place but in reverse. For example, when one oxygen molecule is released to the tissues, hemoglobin's affinity for oxygen decreases. This situation favors the release of oxygen to the tissues. Similarly, hemoglobin-oxygen affinity decreases with the release of each successive oxygen molecule. The hemoglobin molecule undergoes a conformational change as oxygen molecules bind or are released, creating the curvilinear shape of the oxyhemoglobin dissociation curve.

Basically, two areas of interest are located on the oxyhemoglobin dissociation curve, i.e., a flat portion and a steep portion (Figure 1-26).

Let's focus first on the flat portion of the curve. We will consider a 20 torr change in P_{O_2}, or a Δx of 20 torr. What is the consequence on the dependent variable (S_{O_2}) when the independent variable (P_{O_2}) decreases 20 torr, represented by a decreased P_{O_2} from 100 torr to 80 torr as shown in Figure 1-27? A P_{O_2} of 100 torr corresponds with an S_{O_2} of 97.5%, and a P_{O_2}

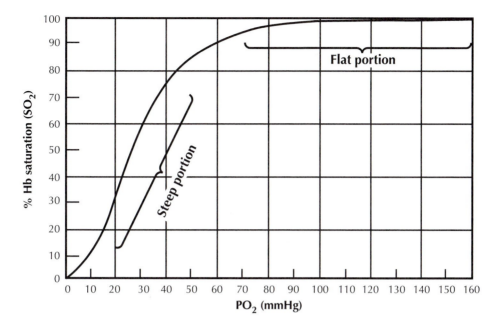

Figure 1-26 *Normal oxyhemoglobin dissociation curve highlighting the steep portion (tissue level) and the flat portion (lung level) of the curve.*

of 80 torr corresponds with an SO_2 of 95%. On the flat part of the curve, a Δx of 20 torr (independent variable), resulted in a Δy of 2.5% (dependent variable).

So, how does a Δx of 20 torr on the steep portion of the oxyhemoglobin dissociation curve affect the dependent variable (SO_2)? A PO_2 of 60 torr corresponds with an SO_2 of 90%, and a PO_2 of 40 torr corresponds with an SO_2 of 74%. The Δy along the steep segment of the curve for a 20-torr change from 60 torr to 40 torr is 16%.

To review, we saw that a Δx of 20 torr along the x-axis on the flat part of the sigmoid curve was associated with a Δy of 2.5%. On the steep portion of the curve we observed that a Δx of 20 torr produced a Δy of 16%.

Therefore, the following generalization can be made about a sigmoid curve. The same magnitude of change in the independent variable, i.e., the PO_2, along the flat and steep segments of the curve is associated with a greater change in the dependent variable (SO_2) along the steep part of the curve than along the flat portion of the curve. Both segments of the oxyhemoglobin dissociation curve have important physiologic consequences.

Another physiologic example of a sigmoid curve is the compliance curve. The compliance curve is generated by ventilating a patient at different lung volumes and recording lung pressure changes.

Varying tidal volumes will be deposited into a patient's lungs. This will be accomplished by changing the tidal volume setting on a ventilator within a range of 6 to 16 ml per kilogram of ideal body weight.

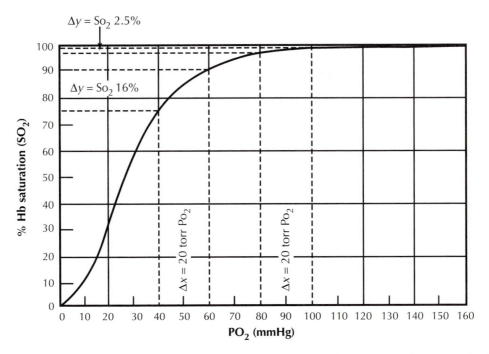

Figure 1-27 *An illustration of the oxyhemogloblin dissociation showing how a 20-torr PO_2 change affect the SO_2 along the steep and flat portions of the curve.*

The pressures involved here will be viewed from two perspectives. One is from the standpoint of the flowing gas. The other is from that of lung inflation. A pressure is developed from gas flowing through the tubing and through the patient's airways. This pressure is described as the pressure generated to overcome airway resistance (P_{Raw}). The other pressure develops from lung inflation. This pressure is similar to that produced inside a balloon filled with air and knotted at the opening. The pressure inside the balloon results from the air trapped in the balloon. Once the lung is inflated, the volume of air in the 300,000,000 alveoli exerts a pressure at end-inspiration.

Each of these two pressures has a specific name. The peak inspiratory pressure (PIP) is the sum of the pressure generated to overcome airway resistance plus the pressure produced by the volume of air in the lungs at end-inspiration. The other pressure is called the plateau or static pressure ($P_{plateau}$). The $P_{plateau}$ is the pressure exerted in the lungs by the volume of air at end-inspiration. The difference between the PIP and the $P_{plateau}$ provides the value of the P_{Raw}, the pressure generated to overcome airway resistance.

The curve that develops from plotting these data points on a pressure-volume coordinate is a sigmoid curve, called the compliance curve. The pressure is plotted on the x-axis and the volume on the y-axis.

Three clinical measurements are required for this curve to be generated. They are (1) the tidal volume (V_T), (2) the PIP which encompasses the pressure developed to overcome airway resistance and the pressure to maintain lung inflation at end-inspiration, and (3) the

$P_{plateau}$ which is the pressure developed to maintain lung inflation at end-inspiration. These measurements will be plotted on a pressure-volume axis shown in Figure 1-28.

Let's consider an example of the process. Our hypothetical patient has an ideal body weight of 60 kg. She has a static compliance of 36 ml/cm H_2O and an airway resistance of 10 cm H_2O/L/min. The ventilator is delivering the tidal volume at an inspiratory flow rate of 60 L/min.

Table 1-18 below contains data for the three measurements.

TABLE 1-18

V_T (ml)	PIP (cm H_2O)	$P_{plateau}$ (cm H_2O)
360	20	10
480	23	13
600	27	17
720	30	20
840	45	35
960	60	55

The data from Table 1-18 are plotted on the curve in Figure 1-28 on the next page.

Notice how along the steep part of the curve smaller pressure changes produce greater volume changes. However, as the flat portion of the curve is approached, greater pressure changes are required to produce the same volume changes. The volume change (Δy) has been held constant at 120 ml, but the pressure changes to produce that volume change progressively increased. (See Chapter 4 Physics, 4–7 Mechanics of Ventilation, Hooke's Law.) In other words, the $\Delta x / \Delta y$ became smaller along the flat segment of the curve compared to the steep part.

How does this information apply to the clinical setting? Put simply, over-inflating the lungs makes the alveoli less compliant. In other words, a low volume-pressure relationship can move the alveoli higher on the compliance curve (i.e., on or toward the flat portion of the sigmoid curve). Beyond a certain point, large tidal volumes associated with high pressures tend to decrease the lung's compliance (Figure 1-29 on page 97).

Another clinical application associated with the foregoing discussion of the sigmoid compliance curve is the use of positive end-expiratory pressure (PEEP) with mechanical ventilation. PEEP is the application of positive pressure to the lungs at end-exhalation. During normal, spontaneous breathing, the pressure in the lungs at end-exhalation equals atmospheric pressure. When PEEP is applied to the lungs, the pressure inside the lungs at end-exhalation is supra-atmospheric.

PEEP is used to increase a patient's functional residual capacity (FRC). As a consequence of increasing the FRC, the patient's alveoli are more inflated at end-expiration than normal (the end-expiratory lung volume is elevated). If too high PEEP levels are applied, the plateau pressure rises and the pulmonary compliance can decrease. When PEEP levels are too high, the alveoli contain a much greater volume than they do at end-exhalation

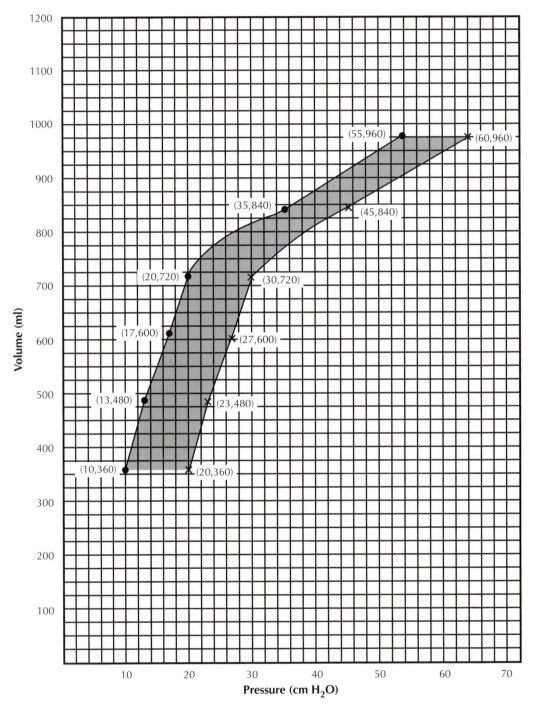

Figure 1-28 *Compliance curve resulting from the plotting of the data listed in Table 1-18.*

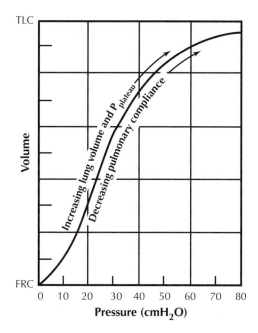

Figure 1-29 *Pulmonary compliance curve, showing the relationship between lung volume and pulmonary compliance.*

during normal breathing (FRC). Therefore, higher peak inspiratory pressures will be required to inflate the lungs further. Because the lungs become over-inflated, the patient's risk for barotrauma, and cardiovascular compromise increases. Barotrauma refers to injury, e.g., pneumothorax, done to the lung tissue caused by high intra-alveolar pressures. Cardiovascular compromise includes decreased venous return and decreased cardiac output as a result of the PEEP raising the intrathoracic pressures to high levels.

The application of PEEP often improves pulmonary compliance in these conditions. However, there is an optimum point for the application of PEEP. If that optimum point is exceeded, the pulmonary compliance actually decreases because the alveoli are so overdistended that they have a difficult time accepting more volume. Gas exchange is then impaired. In fact, when the optimum PEEP level is exceeded, numerous adverse physiologic events tend to occur. These may include a decreased PaO_2, increased $PaCO_2$, a widened $P(A-a)O_2$ gradient, a decreased C.O., and barotrauma.

PRACTICE PROBLEMS

Refer to Appendix A (pages 569-573) for the solutions and answers to the practice problems.

161. Calculate the pressure generated to overcome airway resistance if the peak inspiratory pressure is 45 cm H_2O and the plateau pressure is 20 cm H_2O.
P_{Raw} = _____

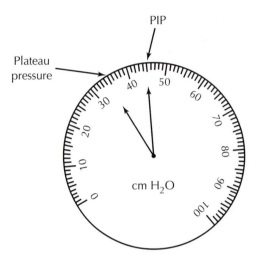

Figure 1-30 *Pressure manometer indicating a plateau pressure of 35 cm H₂O and a peak inspiratory pressure (PIP) of 45 cm H₂O.*

162. Calculate the P_{Raw} when the PIP is 35 cm H_2O and the $P_{plateau}$ is 25 cm H_2O.
P_{Raw} = _____

163. Given the ventilator pressure manometer in Figure 1-30, determine the P_{Raw}.
P_{Raw} = _____

164. Given the data in Table 1-19, plot the static compliance and dynamic compliance curves on the grid provided in Figure 1-31.

TABLE 1-19

V_T (ml)	PIP (cm H_2O)	$P_{plateau}$ (cm H_2O)
400	22	10
500	26	14
600	31	19
700	38	26
800	48	36
900	68	56

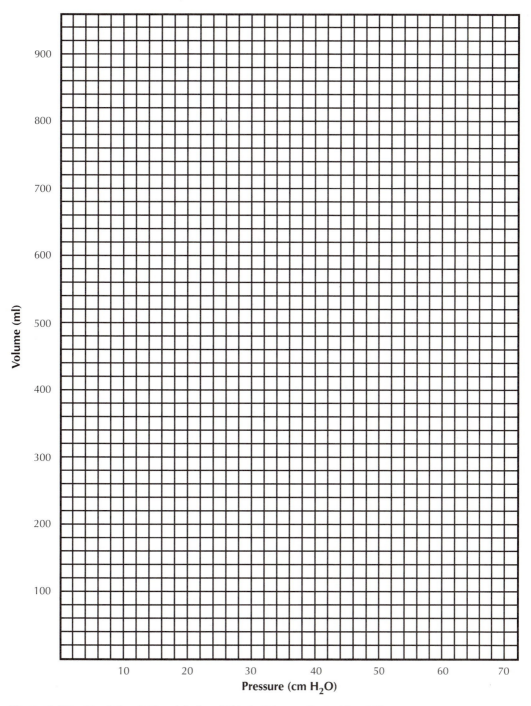

Figure 1-31 *Graph for plotting data from Table 1-19 in practice problem 164.*

165. Calculate the C_{static} values for all the points (Table 1-20) plotted on the static compliance curve in Figure 1-31.

TABLE 1-20

V_T (ml)	PIP (cm H_2O)	$P_{plateau}$ (cm H_2O)	C_{static} (ml/cm H_2O)
400	22	10	
500	26	14	
600	31	19	
700	38	26	
800	48	36	
900	68	56	

166. Calculate from Table 1-21 the $C_{dynamic}$ values for all the points plotted on the dynamic compliance curve in Figure 1-31.

TABLE 1-21

V_T (ml)	PIP (cm H_2O)	$P_{plateau}$ (cm H_2O)	$C_{dynamic}$ (ml/cm H_2O)
400	22	10	
500	26	14	
600	31	19	
700	38	26	
800	48	36	
900	68	56	

167. Calculate the P_{Raw} for each PIP-$P_{plateau}$ difference in Table 1-22.

TABLE 1-22

PIP (cm H_2O)	−	$P_{plateau}$ (cm H_2O)	=	P_{Raw} (cm H_2O)
22		10		
26		14		
31		19		
38		26		
48		36		
68		56		

168. Plot the static compliance and dynamic compliance curves on the grid provided in Figure 1-32 (page 102) using the data from Table 1-23.

TABLE 1-23

V_T (ml)	PIP (cm H_2O)	$P_{plateau}$ (cm H_2O)
400	16	10
500	20	14
600	25	19
700	32	26
800	42	36
900	62	56

169. Calculate the $C_{dynamic}$ values for all the points plotted on the dynamic compliance curve in Figure 1-32.

TABLE 1-24

V_T (ml)	PIP (cm H_2O)	$P_{plateau}$ (cm H_2O)	$C_{dynamic}$ (ml/cm H_2O)
400	16	10	
500	20	14	
600	25	19	
700	32	26	
800	42	36	
900	62	56	

170. Calculate the P_{Raw} for each PIP-$P_{plateau}$ difference in Table 1-25.

TABLE 1-25

PIP (cm H_2O)	−	$P_{plateau}$ (cm H_2O)	=	P_{Raw} (cm H_2O)
16		10		
20		14		
25		19		
32		26		
42		36		
62		56		

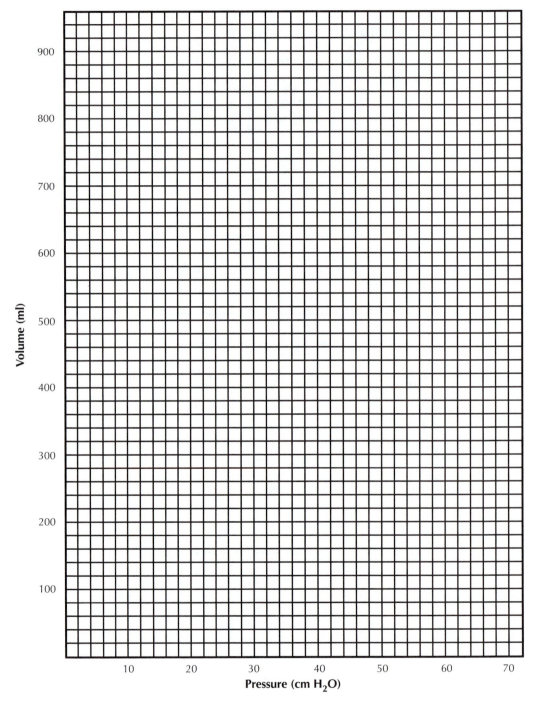

Figure 1-32 *Graph for plotting data from Table 1-23 in practice problem 168.*

CHAPTER SUMMARY

Scientific notation involves moving the decimal point to the right or left to manipulate the number and exponent to simplify the use of extremely large and small numbers in mathematical operations. When adding and subtracting numbers using scientific notation, the exponents must be equal. When multiplying and dividing, the exponents do not need to be equal.

The number of significant digits contained by a number is imposed by the precision of the measuring instrument, as well as by the least precise number involved in a calculation. Specific rules apply to the determination of significant digits contained in a number.

Ratios are a comparison of like quantities set up as a fraction having a numerator and a denominator. For a ratio to exist, the quantities must possess the same units.

A proportion is a relationship that involves two ratios. The two ratios in a proportion are equal. Therefore, knowing the values of three of the four factors, one can determine the unknown, or fourth, value.

A ratio can be converted to a percent by multiplying the ratio by 100. However, for a ratio to be converted to a percent, the ratio must contain like units. Otherwise, even multiplied by 100, it would not produce a true percent.

During any mathematical operation units are extremely important. Involving units in the actual calculation helps conceptualize the process. Retaining the units in a calculation helps with setting up the equation correctly.

A number without a unit is like a person without a name. Some numbers, of course, are derived from calculations wherein the units cancel. Such values are called dimensionless numbers. But most numbers have units to label the significance of the value. Conversion factors are valuable devices allowing one to change from unit to unit for a variety of reasons.

A logarithm is an exponent to the base 10. The pH of the blood is quantified according to a logarithmic scale. Therefore, when the pH of the blood changes by 1 pH unit, the hydrogen ion concentration actually changes 10-fold. After all, the pH is a measurement of the H^+ ion concentration.

A coordinate system, comprised of an x-axis (abscissa) and a y-axis (ordinate), consists of four quadrants into which ordered pairs can be located. The point of intersection of the abscissa and ordinate is called the origin.

A graph can take on various configurations. Different configurations include (1) a straight line, (2) a hyperbola, (3) a parabola, and (4) a sigmoid curve.

The formula $y = k x$ produces a straight line graph which intersects with the origin. The formula $y = m x + b$ results in a straight line which does not pass through the origin.

A hyperbolic curve is derived from the expression $y = k/x$, and a parabolic curve arises from the relationship $y = k x^2$.

Charles' law results in a straight line graph. Boyle's law produces a hyperbola.

A sigmoid curve is an S-shaped configuration with a steep segment and a flat portion. Two physiologic and clinical applications of a sigmoid curve are the oxyhemoglobin dissociation curve and the pulmonary compliance curve.

REVIEW QUESTIONS

1-1 SCIENTIFIC NOTATION AND EXPONENTS

Questions

1. List the expression that represents the general format for using scientific notation.
2. Explain the rule for expressing extremely large numbers in scientific notation.
3. Explain the rule governing the expression of extremely small numbers in scientific notation.
4. List each of the place values for a 10-digit number.
5. List each of the place values for a 10-digit decimal number.
6. Define *exponent.*
7. Explain how exponents are manipulated during multiplication, division, addition, and subtraction.

1-2 SIGNIFICANT DIGITS

Questions

1. Distinguish between precision and accuracy.
2. Provide an example of some diagnostic instrumentation lacking (a) precision and (b) accuracy.
3. What is the significant of the last digit of any measured value?
4. Are all zeros significance figures? Explain.
5. State the rules that govern the process of determining significant figures.
6. Explain how the number of significant figures is determined when performing mathematical operations involving measured values.
7. Differentiate between random and systematic errors.
8. Define *parallax.*
9. How can the problem of parallax be overcome?

1-3 RATIOS

Questions

1. How do the units of a ratio relate to each other.
2. What does the colon (punctuation mark) represent in a ratio?
3. Why is the physiologic measurement compliance not a true ratio?
4. Name the two components of a ratio.
5. How can unlike units be manipulated for a ratio to occur?
6. Describe how to set up a "magic box" to obtain an air/O_2 ratio for a given O_2 concentration.

7. Provide two clinical examples of measurements that are not true ratios but are expressed as if they were.
8. Provide two clinical examples of measurements that are true ratios.

1-4 PROPORTIONS

Questions

1. Define *proportion.*
2. Name the component parts of a proportion.
3. Using the letters or factors *l, f, b,* and *w,* illustrate the four forms by which a proportion can be represented.
4. Name three ideal gas laws that can be solved using the proportion method.
5. What is the meaning of the symbol $\propto$?
6. Differentiate between an inverse and a direct proportion.

1-5 PERCENTS

Questions

1. What does the % sign indicate?
2. List the three types of percent problems.
3. List the formula used for the calculation of both SO_2 and relative humidity.
4. Define the terms *content* and *capacity,* and list the units that can be used to express them.
5. Why is a ratio solution not a true percent solution?
6. What two expressions are commonly written as percents but actually are not true percentages?
7. Distinguish among the terms *dissolved oxygen, combined oxygen,* and *total oxygen content.*
8. Write the physiologic shunt equation and the clinical shunt equation.
9. Why can the $P_{A}O_2$ be substituted for by the end-pulmonary capillary oxygen tension in the physiologic shunt equation?
10. What factors are required to calculate the % shunt using the physiologic shunt equation?
11. What clinical conditions must be met before the clinical shunt equation can be used?
12. List two ways by which a patient's $PaCO_2$ can be altered while receiving controlled mechanical ventilation.
13. What is the general guideline for establishing the tidal volume of a mechanically ventilated COPD patient?
14. When considering changing the arterial Pco_2, why is the tidal volume evaluated before considering changing the ventilatory rate?

1-6 DIMENSIONAL ANALYSIS

Questions

1. What is meant by a *dimension?*
2. What is a conversion factor?
3. Why does a true ratio render a dimensionless quantity?
4. List the rules governing the use of dimensions in addition, subtraction, multiplication, and division.
5. What is the factor-units method?

1-7 UNITS OF MEASUREMENT

Questions

1. Describe the International System of Units (SI).
2. Define the MKS system.
3. Define the CGS system.
4. List the exponential form for the following SI unit prefixes: (a) nano-, (b) centi-, (c) mega-, (d) kilo-, and (e) micro-.
5. State the basic SI units.
6. What are the decimal equivalents of the following SI unit prefixes: (a) deci-, (b) micro-, and (c) milli-?

1-8 LOGARITHMS

Questions

1. List the three elements of a logarithmic expression.
2. List two synonyms of the word *logarithm.*
3. What are the two methods by which a logarithm can be expressed?
4. What are the two elemental parts of a logarithm?
5. State the differences between obtaining a positive and a negative characteristic.
6. Which part of a logarithm does a log table represent?
7. Define the term *antilog.*
8. State the rules governing the multiplication and division of logarithms.

1-9 GRAPHS

Questions

1. Draw and label a Cartesian coordinate system.
2. Define the following terms: (a) *abscissa,* (b) *ordinate,* and (c) *origin.*

3. Plot the following coordinates on the Cartesian coordinate system drawn in Question 1: (a) $(-1,0)$, (b) $(2,2)$ (c) $(2,-3)$, (d) $(-3,-3)$.
4. Define *extrapolation*.
5. Describe the graph resulting from the plotting of a direct relationship.
6. Describe the graph resulting from the plotting of an inverse relationship.
7. Define *independent variable* and *dependent variable*.
8. List the general formula that represents a direct relationship.
9. List the general formula that plots a straight line that does not pass through the origin.
10. List the ratio that describes the slope of a straight line.
11. Describe how the reciprocal of the DLCO and its components correlate with the formula $y = mx + b$.
12. List the general formula that plots a hyperbolic relationship.
13. Define a *hyperbola*.
14. Write the general equation that produces a hyperbolic curve.
15. Define a *parabola*.
16. Describe the shape of the oxyhemoglobin dissociation curve.
17. List the distinguishing features of a sigmoid curve.
18. Compare the flat portion to the steep portion of the oxyhemoglobin dissociation curve.
19. Describe the pulmonary compliance curve.
20. With the basal alveoli residing on the steep portion of the pulmonary compliance curve, and the apical alveoli approaching the rounded portion, compare the volume change in both anatomic locations when the same ΔP initiates inspiration.

Bibliography

Barnes, Thomas. *Core Textbook of Respiratory Care Practice.* 2nd ed. St. Louis: Mosby-Year Book, Inc., 1994.

Branson, R., et al. *Respiratory Care Equipment.* 2nd ed. Philadelphia: J. B. Lippincott Company, 1999.

Brooks, Stewart. *Integrated Basic Science.* 4th ed. St. Louis: The C. V. Mosby Co., 1979.

Burton, G., et al. *Respiratory Care: A Guide to Clinical Practice.* 3rd ed. Philadelphia: J. B. Lippincott Company, 1992.

Dantzker, D., et al. *Comprehensive Respiratory Care.* Philadelphia: W. B. Saunders Company, 1995.

Kacmarek, Robert, et al. *The Essentials of Respiratory Care.* 3rd ed. St. Louis: Mosby-Year Book, Inc., 1990.

Madama, Vincent. *Pulmonary Function Testing.* Albany, New York: Delmar Publishers, 1993.

Pierson, D., and Kacmarek, R. *Foundations of Respiratory Care.* New York: Churchill Livingstone, 1992.

Scanlan, Craig, et al. *Egan's Fundamentals of Respiratory Care.* 7th ed. St. Louis: Mosby-Year Book, 1998.

Shapiro, Barry, et al. *Clinical Applications of Blood Gases.* 5th ed. St. Louis: Mosby-Year Book, Inc., 1994.

CHAPTER TWO

ALGEBRA

Throughout the clinical practice of cardiorespiratory care and the study of cardio-pulmonary physiology, respiratory care students and practitioners frequently encounter quantitative problems that contain one or more unknown variables. The purpose of this chapter is to provide students and practitioners with certain algebraic principles that can be applied to help solve these problems and to better understand quantitative relationships.

CHAPTER OBJECTIVES

Upon completing this chapter, the reader will be able to apply algebraic principles to physiologic and clinical computations and will be able to

2-1 ALGEBRAIC EXPRESSIONS

- Define a *variable*.
- Define a variable expression.
- Recognize different forms of algebraic expressions.
- Convert an algebraic expression to a numerical expression.
- Solve algebraic expressions when given the values of the variables.

2-2 REAL NUMBERS

- Identify real numbers on a number line.
- State the rules for (1) addition, (2) subtraction, (3) multiplication, and (4) division of real numbers.
- Perform calculations using real numbers.

2-3 COMPARING NUMBERS

- Define the term *origin*.
- Locate positive and negative numbers located on a number line.
- Compare positive and negative numbers located on a number line.
- Find the opposite value for numbers located on a number line.
- Determine absolute values using a number line.
- Add and subtract numbers on a number line.
- Apply the concept of absolute values to the transpulmonary pressure gradient.
- Apply the concept of absolute values to physiologic examples.

2-4 SIMPLIFYING NUMERICAL EXPRESSIONS

- State the rules for order of operations.
- Simplify numerical expressions using the rules for order of operations.
- Apply the rules for order of operations to cardiopulmonary equations.

2-5 COMBINING LIKE TERMS

- Identify terms in an algebraic expression.
- Combine like terms in an algebraic expression.
- Combine like terms in cardiopulmonary equations that have more than one unknown.

2-6 EVALUATING FORMULAS

- Describe a formula.
- Transpose formulas to solve for various terms in a formula.
- Evaluate formulas.

2-7 RECIPROCALS

- Define a reciprocal relationship
- List the general format of a multiplicative inverse.
- Solve cardiopulmonary equations that contain reciprocal relationships.

FORMULAS USED IN THIS CHAPTER

$$°C = (°F - 32)\frac{5}{9}$$ (page 113)

$$C.O. = SV \times HR$$ (page 113)

$$P_{transpulmonary} = P_{alv} - P_{pl}$$ (page 126)

$P_{thorax} = P_{alv} - P_B$ (page 128)

$P_{chest\,wall} = P_{pl} - P_B$ (page 128)

$P_{transmural} = P_{airway} - P_{pl}$ (page 128)

$$P_{AO_2} = F_{IO_2}(P_B - P_{H_2O}) - P_{ACO_2}\left(F_IO_2 + \frac{1 - F_IO_2}{R}\right)$$ (page 131)

$(C_S \times \dot{V}_S) + (C_{ent} \times \dot{V}ent) = (C_{DEL} \times \dot{V}_{DEL})$ (page 134)

$\dot{V}_{DEL} = \dot{V}_S + \dot{V}_{ENT}$ (page 134)

$$P = \frac{2\,ST}{r}$$ (page 137)

$$V_D/V_T = \frac{P_{ACO_2} = P\bar{E}CO_2}{P_{ACO_2}}$$ (page 137)

$$C_{dynamic} = \frac{V_T - V_{lost}}{PIP - (PEEP_{applied} + PEEP_{auto})}$$ (page 138)

$$C = \frac{\Delta V}{\Delta P}$$ (page 141)

$$E = \frac{\Delta P}{\Delta V}$$ (page 141)

$$\frac{1}{C_T} = \frac{1}{C_L} + \frac{1}{C_{CW}}$$ (page 142)

$E_T = E_L + E_{CW}$ (page 143)

$$R_{aw} = \frac{\Delta P}{\dot{V}}$$ (page 143)

$$G_{aw} = \frac{\dot{V}}{\Delta P}$$ (page 143)

$$\frac{1}{D_L CO} = \frac{1}{D_M} + \frac{1}{\theta \times V_C}$$ (page 144)

2-1 ALGEBRAIC EXPRESSIONS

Algebra is considered a method of shortening mathematical problems. By using unknown quantities in equations, algebra offers a way to make these unknown quantities known.

Algebraic expressions contain one or more variables. A variable is defined as a symbol used to represent one or more numbers. Usually, a lower case letter (i.e., *a, m, x*, etc.) is used as a variable. The algebraic expression that contains the variable(s) is called a variable expression.

TABLE 2-1   Algebraic Expressions and Mathematical Operations

Algebraic Expressions			
Addition	**Subtraction**	**Multiplication***	**Division****
$10 + y$	$6 - x$	$\frac{3}{4} \times f$	$n \div 4$
$a + c$	$b - p$	$t \times w$	$s \div d$

*Multiplication can be represented a number of ways in algebra: A dot between the variables, such as t · w; parentheses around each variable, such as (t)(w); or simply as tw.
**Division can be signified as a fraction s/d.

Table 2-1 illustrates different mathematical operations and forms of algebraic expressions.

To find the solution to an algebraic expression, a numerical value must be given to substitute for the variable. Once a number is inserted into an algebraic expression for each variable, the expression is called a numerical expression.

For example, the algebraic expressions in Table 2-2 can be solved when the value of the variable(s) in each expression is (are) given. Solve each algebraic expression based on the values assigned to the variables below.

$y = 5$	$x = 4$	$f = 8$	$n = 16$
$a = 3$	$b = 7$	$t = \frac{1}{2}$	$s = 0.77$
$c = 2$	$p = 6$	$w = 0.6$	$d = 0.11$

TABLE 2-2   Solving Algebraic Expressions When Variables Are Known

Algebraic Expression	Numerical Expression	Solution
$10 + y$	$10 + 5$	15
$a + c$	$3 + 2$	5
$6 - x$	$6 - 4$	2
$b - p$	$7 - 6$	1
$\frac{3}{4} \times f$	$\frac{3}{4} \times 8$	6
$t \times w$	$\frac{1}{2} \times 0.6$	0.3
$n \div 4$	$16 \div 4$	4
$s \div d$	$0.77 \div 0.11$	7

The relationships among lung volumes and capacities are algebraic expressions. Figure 2-1 shows how the lung is subdivided into different volumes and capacities. Notice how each lung capacity is a combination of two or more lung volumes.

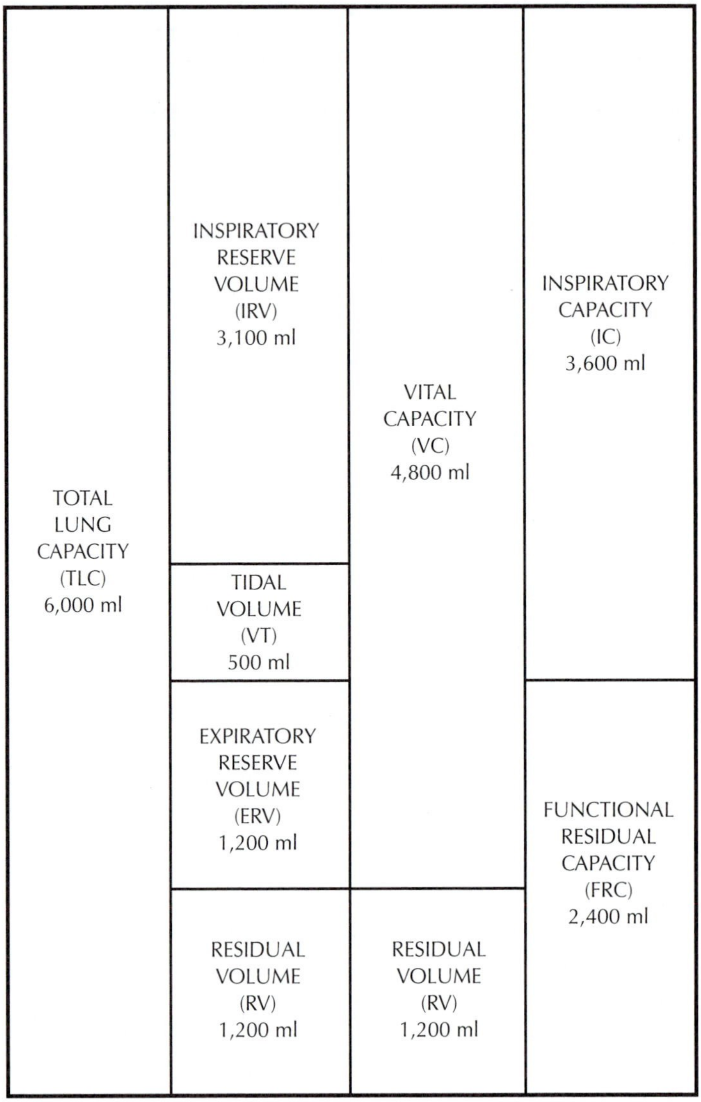

Figure 2-1 *Model showing the various lung volumes and lung capacities along with their normal values.*

A few examples of how the relationships among the lung volumes and capacities represent algebraic expressions follow.

EXAMPLE 1:

Calculate the TLC based on the following data.

$$\text{IRV} = 3,100 \text{ ml}$$

$$V_T = 500 \text{ ml}$$

$$ERV = 1,200 \text{ ml}$$

$$RV = 1,200 \text{ ml}$$

Step 1: Use the following algebraic equation.

$$TLC = IRV + V_T + ERV + RV$$

Step 2: Insert the known values and solve for TLC.

$$TLC = 3,100 \text{ ml} + 500 \text{ ml} + 1,200 \text{ ml} + 12,00 \text{ ml}$$

$$= 6,000 \text{ ml}$$

EXAMPLE 2:

Calculate the RV given the data below.

$$TLC = 6,000 \text{ ml}$$

$$IC = 3,600 \text{ ml}$$

$$ERV = 1,200 \text{ ml}$$

Step 1: Use the following algebraic expression.

$$RV = TLC - (ERV + IC)$$

Step 2: Insert the known values and solve for RV.

$$RV = 6,000 \text{ ml} - (1,200 \text{ ml} + 3,600 \text{ ml})$$

$$= 1,200 \text{ ml}$$

The formula that is used to convert degrees **Fahrenheit** to degrees **Celsius** is another example of an algebraic expression that has one variable (i.e., °F). The formula is

$$°C = (°F - 32)\frac{5}{9}$$

This equation can be solved only when the value for °F, the variable, is known. If °F = 32, the solution will be

$$°C = (32° - 32)\frac{5}{9}$$

$$= (0°)\left(\frac{5}{9}\right)$$

$$= 0°C$$

The formula used to calculate the cardiac output (C.O.), based on the variables stroke volume (SV) and heart rate (HR), exemplifies an algebraic expression that contains more than one variable. The expression is shown as

$$C.O. = SV \cdot HR$$

In this expression the stroke volume and heart rate are inversely related to one another. Therefore, this algebraic expression can be solved when the values for SV and HR are given. For instance, if SV = 70 ml/beat and HR = 72 beats/minute, then

$$C.O. = (70 \text{ ml/beat})(72 \text{ beats/min})$$

$$= 5,040 \text{ ml/min}$$

or

$$= 5.04 \text{ L/min}$$

Furthermore, the cardiac output and the heart rate are directly related to each other. Be mindful that because this formula contains three variables, the equation can be rearranged to solve for any one of them, as long as the value of the other two variables is known. Therefore, this equation can be solved for the stroke volume by dividing both sides of the equation by the heart rate (HR), and canceling like factors, that is,

$$\frac{C.O.}{HR} = \frac{SV \cdot \cancel{HR}}{\cancel{HR}}$$

$$\frac{C.O.}{HR} = SV$$

Additionally, the cardiac output and stroke volume are directly related. Consequently, the equation can be rearranged again by dividing both sides of the equation by the stroke volume (SV) and canceling like factors, that is,

$$\frac{C.O.}{SV} = \frac{\cancel{SV} \cdot HR}{\cancel{SV}}$$

$$\frac{C.O.}{SV} = HR$$

PRACTICE PROBLEMS

Refer to Appendix A (pages 573-576) for the solutions and answers to the practice problems.

Solve each algebraic expression if $x = 10$.

1. $6 + x =$ _____

2. $x + 15 =$ _____

3. $x + x =$ _____

4. $\dfrac{100}{x} =$ _____

5. $x \cdot x =$ _____

6. $\dfrac{x}{2} =$ _____

7. $\frac{1}{2}(x) =$ _____

8. $90 - x =$ _____

9. $x - 5 =$ _____

10. $0 + x =$ _____

Solve each algebraic expression if $x = 4$, $y = 6$, and $z = 9$.

11. $\frac{xz}{y} =$ _____

12. $\frac{y}{(x)(z)} =$ _____

13. $\frac{z - 3}{y - x} =$ _____

14. $\frac{xyz}{8} =$ _____

15. $\frac{1}{2}(z + 3) =$ _____

16. $(y + z)\frac{1}{3} =$ _____

17. $7x - y =$ _____

18. $\frac{x + y}{10} =$ _____

19. $2xyz =$ _____

20. $\frac{xy + 2x}{10 - z} =$ _____

Solve each algebraic expression based on the data given.

21. $V_T = V_D + V_A$

   V_D (dead space volume) = 150 cc

   V_A (alveolar volume) = 350 cc

   V_T = tidal volume (cc)

22. time constant = $(R_{aw}) (C_L)$

   R_{aw} (airway resistance) = 7 cm H_2O/L/sec

   C_L (pulmonary compliance) = 0.05 L/cm H_2O

23. $E_L = \dfrac{\text{transpulmonary pressure}}{\text{volume change}}$

    transpulmonary pressure = 4 cm H_2O
    volume change = 800 ml

24. $C_L = \dfrac{\text{volume change}}{\text{transpulmonary pressure}}$

    volume change = 800 ml
    transpulmonary pressure = 4 cm H_2O

25. $\dfrac{V_D}{V_T} = \dfrac{PaCO_2 - P\bar{E}CO_2}{PaCO_2}$

    $PaCO_2$ (arterial CO_2 tension) = 50 torr
    $P\bar{E}CO_2$ (mean exhaled CO_2 tension) = 35 torr
    V_D/V_T = dead space/tidal volume ratio

26. $P = \dfrac{2ST}{r}$

    ST (surface tension) = 40 dynes/cm
    r (radius) = 0.2 cm
    P = distending pressure

27. $T_I = \dfrac{V_T}{\dot{V}_I}$

    V_T (tidal volume) = 900 cc
    $\dot{V}_I$ (inspiratory flow rate) = 1 L/sec
    T_I = inspiratory time

28. $P_{PSV} = \left(\dfrac{PIP - P_{STATIC}}{\dot{V}_{MECH}}\right)\dot{V}_{I_{max}}$

    PIP (peak inspiratory pressure) = 40 cm H_2O
    P_{STATIC} (static pressure) = 25 cm H_2O
    $\dot{V}_{MECH}$ (mechanical inspiratory flow rate) = 1.5 liters/second
    $\dot{V}_{I_{max}}$ (patient's inspiratory flow rate) = 0.5 liter/second
    P_{PSV} = pressure support ventilation pressure

29. $MAP = \dfrac{SP + 2(DP)}{3}$

    SP (systolic pressure) = 120 mm Hg
    DP (diastolic pressure) = 75 mm Hg
    MAP = mean arterial pressure

30. $G_{aw} = \dfrac{\dot{V}}{PIP - P_{STATIC}}$

   $\dot{V}$ (inspiratory flow rate) = 0.5 liter/second

   PIP (peak inspiratory pressure) = 55 cm H_2O

   P_{STATIC} (static pressure) = 30 cm H_2O

   G_{aw} = airway conductance

Use Figure 2-2 to calculate problems 31-35.

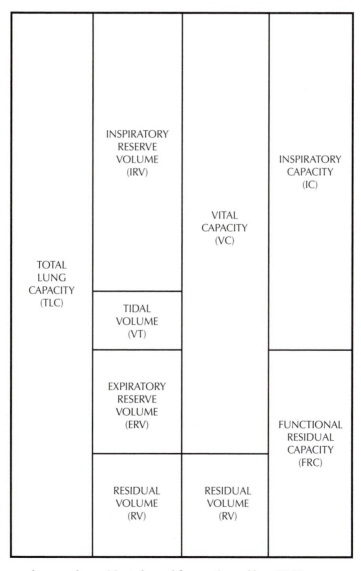

Figure 2-2 *Lung volumes and capacities to be used for practice problems 31-35.*

31. Calculate the FRC given the following data.

    TLC = 4,000 ml
    VC = 2,500 ml
    ERV = 800 ml

32. Calculate the VC based on the data shown below.

    IRV = 2,700 ml
    V_T = 350 ml
    FRC = 2,000 ml
    RV = 1,000 ml

33. Calculate the IC when the data below are known.

    VC = 2,300 ml
    FRC = 1,000 ml
    RV = 700 ml

34. Calculate the V_T from the data given below.

    VC = 4,000 ml
    ERV = 1,100 ml
    IRV = 2,700 ml

35. Calculate the RV knowing the following data.

    FRC = 2,400 ml
    VC = 4,800 ml
    IRV = 3,100 ml
    V_T = 500 ml

2-2 REAL NUMBERS

Real numbers are located all along the number line. Numbers to the left (negative) and right (positive) of the origin, including the origin (0) itself, are real numbers. Rules are applied to real numbers when they are used in mathematical operations (i.e., addition, subtraction, multiplication, and division).

Addition

Two addition rules exist. The first rule governs adding two numbers with the same sign, and the second rule refers to adding two numbers with different signs.

Addition Rule 1: (Two Real Numbers with the Same Sign)

- Add the absolute values and give the total (sum) the same sign as the numbers.

For example,

$$-5 + (-3) = -8$$

Addition Rule 2: (Two Real Numbers with Different Signs)

- Determine the absolute values.
- Subtract the smaller absolute value from the larger one.
- Give the result (sum) the same sign as the larger absolute value.

For example,

$$-30 + 25 = -5$$

Subtraction

Previously, the term *opposite* was described. When subtracting real numbers, a term synonymous with opposite is used, namely, **additive inverse**. The additive inverse of a real number is that real number's opposite absolute value. The number line that follows illustrates opposites.

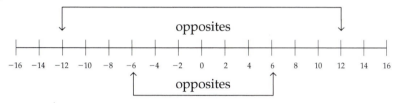

The additive inverse of −12 is +12, and the additive inverse of −6 is +6. The additive inverse of a negative number is a positive number.

Subtraction Rule:

- When subtracting a number, find its additive inverse.
- Set up the problem as an addition problem.
- Apply the addition rules.

For example, when subtracting 11 from 5, as in the problem 5 − 11, first find the additive inverse of −11. The additive inverse of −11 is +11. Now the problem can be written as an addition problem:

$$5 + (-11) = -6$$

Another form of subtraction encountered is shown in the problem below.

$$10 - (-15)$$

Again, find the additive inverse of −15. The additive inverse of −15 is +15. Now, write the problem in the form of an addition problem, as follows:

$$10 + 15 = 25$$

Multiplication

Two rules apply for multiplication. One rule describes multiplying numbers that have the same sign. The other rule refers to multiplying numbers that have different signs.

Multiplication Rule 1: (Numbers with the Same Signs)

- The product of two numbers that have the same sign is positive.

When multiplying two numbers with the same sign, two possibilities can occur: Both numbers can be positive, or both numbers can be negative. For example, when both numbers are positive, the product will be positive.

$$10 \times 3 = 30$$

When both numbers are negative, the product is also positive.

$$(-10)\,(-3) = +30$$

Multiplication Rule 2: (Numbers with Opposite Signs)

- The product of two numbers that have opposite signs will be negative.

For example,

$$(15)\,(-3) = -45$$

Division

Division is the inverse of multiplication. For example, dividing by 3 undoes multiplying by 3, i.e.,

Multiplication: $3 \times 4 = 12$

Division: $\dfrac{12}{3} = 4$

Two rules govern the division of real numbers. The first rule concerns dividing numbers that have the same sign, and the other rule deals with dividing numbers having different signs.

Division Rule 1: (Numbers with this Same Sign)

- The quotient of two real numbers (**divisor** and **dividend**) that have the same sign is positive.

For example,

$$\frac{\text{dividend}}{\text{divisor}} = \text{quotient}$$

$$\frac{+70}{+10} = +7$$

Division Rule 2: (Numbers with Different Signs)

• The quotient of two real numbers that have different signs is negative.

For example,

$$\frac{-15}{+3} = -5$$

or

$$\frac{+15}{-3} = -5$$

PRACTICE PROBLEMS

Refer to Appendix A (page 576) for the solutions and answers to the practice problems.

Perform the appropriate mathematical operation based on the sign given in the following problems:

36. $-6 + (-4) =$ _____
37. $-11 + 16 =$ _____
38. $24 + (-17) =$ _____
39. $32 - (-28) =$ _____
40. $17 - (-2) =$ _____
41. $67 + (-77) =$ _____
42. $8 \times 8 =$ _____
43. $(-13)(-10) =$ _____
44. $(-2)(14) =$ _____
45. $25 \div 5 =$ _____
46. $(-66) \div 11 =$ _____
47. $50 \div (-25) =$ _____
48. $16 \div 4 =$ _____
49. $35 \div 7 =$ _____
50. $(-18) \div 6 =$ _____

2-3 COMPARING NUMBERS

Numbers can be compared with each other if they are placed on a line in increasing order from left to right. The point where zero is located is termed the **origin**. Positive numbers reside to the right of the origin, and negative numbers are situated to the left of the origin. A line containing numbers arranged in this fashion is called a **number line**.

The number line contains real numbers. Each point on the number line corresponds to a specific real number. A number line is illustrated below.

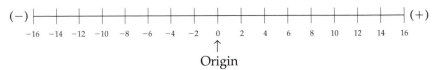

Origin

Every number on the number line has an opposite value. In other words, each value has an opposite value which is located the same distance from the origin but in the opposite direction. For example, the value 8 has an opposite value of −8. The same is true for 4 and −4, 14 and −14, etc.

Opposites

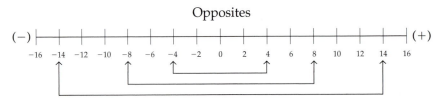

PRACTICE PROBLEMS

Refer to Appendix A (pages 576-577) for the solutions and answers to the practice problems.

Construct a number line and find the opposite of each number given below. Rank these numbers from the smallest to largest.

    51. $-6, 2, -4, 0, 5$

    52. $5, 4, -3, -1, 2.5, 0$

    53. $-3.5, -5, 1, -2, 1.5$

    54. $0.5, 0, 1, -7, 4.5$

    55. $-5.5, 3.5, -0.5, 6.5, 2$

Using the following number line, determine the opposite value of the numbers listed below.

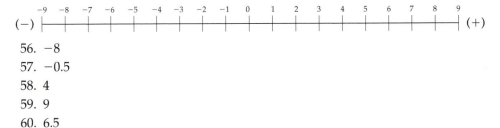

    56. -8

    57. -0.5

    58. 4

    59. 9

    60. 6.5

Absolute values can be obtained from a number line. An absolute value of a number is its distance from zero (0) on a number line. The absolute value of a number will always be positive or zero. Even though a number may reside to the left of the origin, its absolute value will be positive. It is the distance of a number from the origin that is considered, not its direction. Observe the number line below.

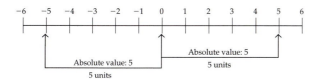

As this number line indicates, the absolute value of −5 is 5 and the absolute value of 5 is also 5. In keeping with this concept, the absolute value of −6 is 6, of 2.5 is 2.5, of 0 is 0. A number and its opposite have the same absolute value, which will either be positive or zero.

PRACTICE PROBLEMS

Refer to Appendix A (page 577) for the solutions and answers to the practice problems.

Using the following number line, find the absolute value for the numbers listed below.

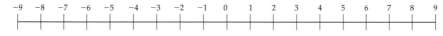

61. −8.5
62. 2
63. 9
64. −7
65. 0

Numbers on a number line can be added or subtracted. To add two numbers on a number line, begin counting from the origin (0) in the direction (left or right) indicated by the sign of the first number in the problem. Then, from that point, count in the direction of the second number. The end point on the number line is the sum of those two numbers. Note the example using the number line below.

EXAMPLE:

Add −3 and 6, or −3 + 6.

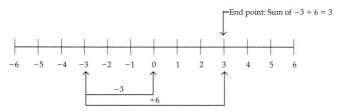

This problem is solved by moving three places to the left of zero and then moving from −3 six places in the opposite direction. The end point (six places to the right of −3) is the sum of −3 + 6. The nature of the sign associated with each number determines the direction (right or left) of movement along the number line.

PRACTICE PROBLEMS

Refer to Appendix A (pages 577-578) for the solutions and answers to the practice problems.

Use a number line to add the following numbers:

66. $3 + 5$
67. $5 + (-6)$
68. $-8 + 3$
69. $0 + (-4)$
70. $-6 + 6$

To subtract a number from another number, write the problem as an addition problem. In other words, when confronted with a problem having the general format

$$x - y$$

change it to read

$$x + (-y)$$

Therefore,

$$x - y = x + (-y)$$

Once the transition has been made from a subtraction problem to an addition problem, apply the rules for adding numbers. Follow the example below.

EXAMPLE:

Subtract -8 from 4, or $4 - 8$.
To begin, change the problem to an addition problem. Thus,

$$4 - 8 = 4 + (-8)$$

This change can be made because 4 minus 8 is the same as *positive 4 subtract positive 8*.
    The number line that follows illustrates this problem.

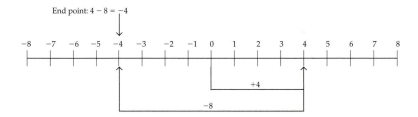

Four places from the origin were counted to the right. Then, 8 places were counted from 4 to the left because -8 was added to the $+4$.

PRACTICE PROBLEMS

Refer to Appendix A (page 578) for the solutions and answers to the practice problems.

Use a number line to subtract the following numbers:

71. $5 - 3$
72. $2 - 6$
73. $-1 - 7$
74. $-3 - 2$
75. $-4 - 7$

This concept of comparing numbers has application in the area of pulmonary mechanics relative to pressure **gradients** and in the understanding of **supra-atmospheric** and **sub-atmospheric** pressures. How absolute values, opposites, and mathematical operations relate to physiologic pressure gradients concerning pulmonary mechanics will be explored here first. Table 2-3 lists the symbols related to pulmonary mechanics.

TABLE 2-3   Symbols of Pressures Related to Pulmonary Mechanics

Symbol	Description
P_{thorax}	transthoracic pressure
P_B	barometric pressure
$P_{chest\ wall}$	pressure across the chest wall
P_{airway}	pressure inside an airway
$P_{transmural}$	pressure across the wall of an airway
P_{alv}	pressure inside alveoli
P_{pl}	pressure inside the intrapleural space
$P_{transpulmonary}$	pressure gradient across the lungs obtained by subtracting the P_{pl} from the P_{alv}

During the course of normal, spontaneous breathing, the intrapleural space maintains a subatmospheric pressure. When a tidal inspiration (from the point of end-tidal exhalation, or functional residual capacity) is taken, the **intrapleural pressure** changes from approximately -3 cm H_2O to -8 cm H_2O. The actual pressure change that occurs can be used to calculate the pulmonary compliance. In the following example, the total pressure change (ΔP) will be determined using a number line with each numerical increment representing 1 cm H_2O, as shown below.

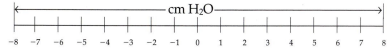

EXAMPLE:

Find ΔP.

Step 1: Express the mathematical relationship between the two pressures.

$$(-3 \text{ cm } H_2O) - (-8 \text{ cm } H_2O) = \Delta P$$

Step 2: Transform the relationship in *Step 1* to an addition problem.

$$-3 \text{ cm } H_2O + 8 \text{ cm } H_2O = \Delta P$$

Step 3: Use a number line, as demonstrated below, to determine the ΔP (i.e., the actual pressure change during inspiration).

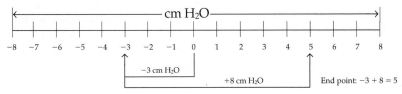

The actual pressure change that occurred within the intrapleural space in this example was 5 cm H_2O, even though both pressures (normal end-exhalation and normal end-inspiration) were given as subatmospheric.

Another physiologic application of these concepts is in determining the **transpulmonary pressure** gradient. By definition, the transpulmonary pressure ($P_{transpulmonary}$) gradient is the difference between the **intraalveolar pressure** (P_{alv}) and the intrapleural pressure (P_{pl}). Essentially, the transpulmonary pressure gradient represents an absolute pressure change based on the equation

$$P_{transpulmonary} = (P_{alv}) - (P_{pl})$$

Note Figure 2-3 which illustrates the anatomic relationship between P_{alv} and P_{pl}.

Again, P_{alv} represents the pressure in the alveoli and P_{pl} signifies the pressure in the intrapleural space. The formula for calculating $P_{transpulmonary}$ can be applied here and the variables summed algebraically using a number line.

EXAMPLE:

Determine the $P_{transpulmonary}$ when the P_{alv} is 0 cm H_2O and the P_{pl} equals -5 cm H_2O.

Step 1: Insert the known values into the formula for $P_{transpulmonary}$.

$$P_{transpulmonary} = P_{alv} - P_{pl}$$
$$= 0 \text{ cm } H_2O - (-5 \text{ cm } H_2O)$$

Step 2: Convert the subtraction problem to an addition problem.

$$P_{transpulmonary} = 0 \text{ cm } H_2O + 5 \text{ cm } H_2O$$

Step 3: Use a number line indicating units of pressure in cm H_2O to calculate the $P_{transpulmonary}$.

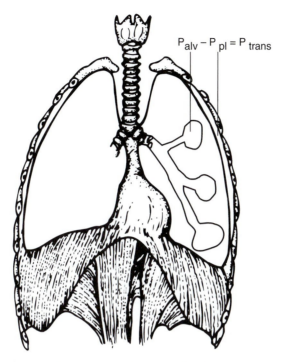

Figure 2-3. *Depiction of thorax, demonstrating the relationship between alveolar pressure (P_{alv}) and intrapleural pressure (P_{pl}) accounting for transpulmonary pressure ($P_{transpulmonary}$).*

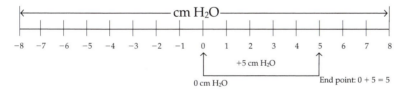

Understanding the significance of the different respiratory pressures associated with the mechanics of breathing is often difficult for students. Although the objective of this text is not to teach respiratory physiology per se, it does attempt to make clear certain physiologic concepts. Therefore, a brief discussion of various respiratory pressure gradients will be presented.

The intrapleural space is a potential space bordered by the parietal pleura adhering to the interior chest wall and by the visceral pleura, which invests the lung tissue. The opposition of elastic forces between the lungs (inward tendency) and the chest wall (outward tendency) establishes the subatmospheric pressure within the intrapleural space. The average range of normal intrapleural pressure is between -3 cm H_2O and -5 cm H_2O.

At the point of FRC, the opposition of the elastic forces between the lungs and chest wall reaches equilibrium. Also, at that point in the ventilatory cycle, no air flows through the airways. The air inside the lungs (alveoli), airways, and mouth has equilibrated with the atmosphere. The pressure in those regions is termed *atmospheric*. Atmospheric pressure can be expressed as either 1,034 cm H_2O or 0 cm H_2O. In absolute pressure terms, the value 1,034 cm H_2O can be used. In relative pressure terms, 0 cm H_2O also represents one atmosphere.

For example, an absolute pressure of 1,039 cm H_2O would be equivalent to 5 cm H_2O in relative terms, i.e.,

$$1{,}039 \text{ cm } H_2O - 1{,}034 \text{ cm } H_2O = 5 \text{ cm } H_2O$$

The value 0 cm H_2O actually results from the relationship

$$1{,}034 \text{ cm } H_2O - 1{,}034 \text{ cm } H_2O = 0 \text{ cm } H_2O$$

The pressure gradient (difference) across the lung tissue between the alveoli and the intrapleural space defines the transpulmonary pressure ($P_{transpulmonary}$). The $P_{transpulmonary}$ is quantitatively represented as

$$P_{transpulmonary} = P_{alv} - P_{pl}$$

Table 2-3 on page 125 indicates the symbols and descriptions of a few specific pressures associated with pulmonary mechanics.

These pressures are used in the determination of some of the pressure gradients related to respiratory mechanics, four of which are listed below.

- transthoracic pressure gradient

$$P_{thorax} = P_{alv} - P_B$$

- chest wall pressure gradient

$$P_{chest} = P_{pl} - P_B$$

- transmural pressure gradient

$$P_{transmural} = P_{airway} - P_{pl}$$

- transpulmonary pressure gradient

$$P_{transpulmonary} = P_{alv} - P_{pl}$$

The last concept to be used here as an example of comparing numbers is that of sub-atmospheric and supra-atmospheric pressures, and how atmospheric pressure changes are presented in actual terms.

One atmosphere of pressure at sea level, expressed in cm H_2O, is actually 1,034 cm H_2O, or zero pressure. Any pressure to the right of zero pressure is considered positive (supra-atmospheric) pressure, while a pressure reading to the left of zero is a negative (sub-atmospheric) pressure. These relationships are demonstrated on the following number line expressed in cm H_2O pressure.

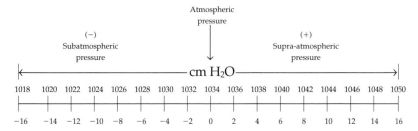

A number line can also be used to illustrate an intrapleural pressure change that occurs during a normal, spontaneous breath. If the intrapleural pressure changes from 1,030 cm H_2O at end-tidal exhalation to 1,024 cm H_2O at end-tidal inspiration, an absolute pressure change of 6 cm H_2O will have resulted, i.e., $-4 - (-10)$ or 1,030 cm H_2O − 1,024 cm H_2O.

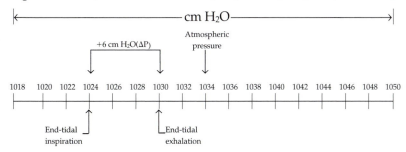

Alternatively, a number line can be constructed to calculate the 6 cm H_2O intrapleural pressure change that occurred from end-tidal exhalation to end-tidal inspiration.

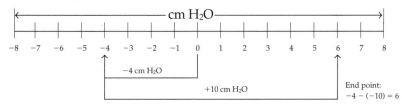

Even though the pressure changes from -4 cm H_2O to -10 cm H_2O, the magnitude of the change in pressure is 6 cm H_2O, i.e., -4 cm H_2O + 10 cm H_2O.

PRACTICE PROBLEMS

Refer to Appendix A (pages 579-580) for the solutions and answers to the practice problems.

Using a number line, determine the following pressure gradients:

76. Calculate $P_{transpulmonary}$ when P_{alv} is $+5$ cm H_2O and P_{pl} is -3 cm H_2O. _____

77. Calculate the $P_{transmural}$ when the pressure in a segmental bronchus is $+20$ cm H_2O and the P_{pl} is $+20$ cm H_2O. _____

78. Calculate the pressure change that occurs when the atmospheric pressure changes from 765 torr to −1 torr. _____

79. Calculate the transthoracic pressure gradient when P_{alv} is +5 cm H_2O and P_B is 1,034 cm H_2O. _____

80. Calculate the pressure across the chest wall when the P_{pl} is −5 cm H_2O and the atmospheric pressure is 1,034 cm H_2O. _____

2-4 SIMPLIFYING NUMERICAL EXPRESSIONS

During the clinical practice of cardiorespiratory care, the need to perform various mathematical calculations often arises. Many of these calculations require simplification to facilitate obtaining the solution. This section will present rules that can be used to simplify numerical and algebraic expressions. The rules below describe how simplification should proceed.

> *Rules for Order of Operations*
>
> - Perform operations within parentheses, i.e., ( ).
> - Perform operations within brackets, i.e., [ ].
> - Perform operations within braces, i.e., { }.
> - Multiply and divide from left to right.
> - Add and subtract from left to right.

EXAMPLE:

Simplify the following equation:

$$\{50 - [4(6 + 4)] \cdot 3\}$$

Step 1: Perform operations within parentheses (i.e., add 6 to 4).

$$\{50 - [4(10)] \cdot 3\}$$

Step 2: Perform operations within brackets (i.e., multiply 4 by 10).

$$\{50 - [40] \cdot 3\}$$

Step 3: Multiply left to right.

$$\{50 - 40 \times 3\}$$

Step 4: Perform operations within braces (i.e., subtract 120 from 50).

$$\{50 - 120\}$$

Step 5: Subtract from left to right.

$$-70$$

In the context of respiratory care, the alveolar air equation may be used to help exemplify the process of simplifying a numerical expression. The alveolar air equation is

$$P_{A}O_2 = F_{I}O_2(P_B - P_{H_2O}) - P_{A}CO_2\left[F_{I}O_2 + \left(\frac{1 - F_{I}O_2}{R}\right)\right]$$

At first sight, simplifying this formula may seem rather complicated. However, when the appropriate data are provided, and when the rules for order of operations are followed, the equation becomes manageable.

EXAMPLE:

Place the data given below in the alveolar air equation.

$F_{I}O_2 = 0.5$

$P_B = 760$ torr

$P_{H_2O} = 47$ torr

$P_{A}CO_2 = 40$ torr

$R = 0.8$

$$P_{A}O_2 = 0.5(760 \text{ torr} - 47 \text{ torr}) - 40 \text{ torr}\left[0.5 + \left(\frac{1 - 0.5}{0.8}\right)\right]$$

This expression can be simplified by following the rules for order of operations.

Step 1: Perform the operations within parentheses.

$$P_{A}O_2 = 0.5(760 \text{ torr} - 47 \text{ torr}) - 40 \text{ torr}\left[0.5 + \left(\frac{1 - 0.5}{0.8}\right)\right]$$

$$= 0.5(713 \text{ torr}) - 40 \text{ torr} [0.5 + 0.625]$$

Step 2: Perform the operations within brackets.

$$P_{A}O_2 = 0.5(713 \text{ torr}) - 40 \text{ torr}[0.5 + 0.625]$$

$$= 0.5(713 \text{ torr}) - 40 \text{ torr} [1.125]$$

Step 3: Multiply from left to right.

$$P_{A}O_2 = 0.5(713 \text{ torr}) - 40 \text{ torr}[1.125]$$

$$= 357 \text{ torr} - 45 \text{ torr}$$

Step 4: Subtract from left to right.

$$P_{AO_2} = 357 \text{ torr} - 45 \text{ torr}$$

$$= 312 \text{ torr}$$

PRACTICE PROBLEMS

Refer to Appendix A (page 580) for the solutions and answers to the practice problems.

Simplify the following numerical expressions:

81. $CaO_2 = [(Hb \times 1.34)SaO_2] + (PaO_2 \times 0.003 \text{ vol\%/torr})$
     when
     > $Hb = 15 \text{ g\%}$
     > $SaO_2 = 97.5\%$
     > $PaO_2 = 100 \text{ torr}$

82. $\dot{Q}_T = \dfrac{\dot{V}_{O_2}}{(CaO_2 - C\bar{v}O_2)}$
     when
     > $\dot{V}_{O_2} = 250 \text{ ml/min}$
     > $CaO_2 = 19.1 \text{ vol\%}$
     > $C\bar{v}O_2 = 14.1 \text{ vol\%}$

83. $\dfrac{\dot{Q}_S}{\dot{Q}_T} = \dfrac{[P_{(A-a)}O_2]0.003 \text{ vol\%/torr}}{[P_{(A-a)}O_2]0.003 \text{ vol\%/torr} + (CaO_2 - C\bar{v}O_2)}$
     when
     > $P_{AO_2} = 450 \text{ torr}$
     > $PaO_2 = 250 \text{ torr}$
     > $CaO_2 = 19.85 \text{ vol\%}$
     > $C\bar{v}O_2 = 13.95 \text{ vol\%}$

84. IBW (female) $= 105 + [5(ht - 60)]$
     when
     > height (ht) $= 65 \text{ inches}$

85. $pH = 6.10 + \log\left[\dfrac{HCO_3^-}{(PaCO_2)(0.03m \text{ Eq/L/torr})}\right]$
     when
     > $HCO_3^- = 48 \text{ mEq/L}$
     > $PaCO_2 = 80 \text{ torr}$

2-5 COMBINING LIKE TERMS

A term in an algebraic expression can take on many forms. A term can be any of the following entities:

- a number, e.g., 10
- a variable, e.g., x
- a product of numbers and variables, e.g., $2 \cdot y$
- a quotient of numbers and variables, e.g., $\dfrac{x}{4}$

The algebraic expression $4y^2 + y - 2$ contains three terms. They are $4y^2$, y, and -2. Some terms contain coefficients. The coefficient for the terms $4y^2$ and y are 4 and 1, respectively. The coefficient 1 for the term y is understood and is generally omitted. Remember, though, $y = 1y$.

Terms within an algebraic expression can often be combined, thus simplifying the equation and facilitating the computation.

EXAMPLE:

The algebraic expression

$$3[4x + 2(3y - x)] + 5y$$

can be simplified as follows by combining like terms. Remember to also use the rules for order of operations.

Step 1: Clear the parentheses by multiplying left to right.

$$3[4x + 2(3y - x)] + 5y$$
$$3[4x + 6y - 2x] + 5y$$

Step 2: Clear the brackets by multiplying left to right.

$$3[4x + 6y - 2x] + 5y$$
$$12x + 18y - 6x + 5y$$

Step 3: Add left to right.

$$12x + 18y - 6x + 5y$$
$$12x - 6x + 23y$$

Step 4: Subtract left to right.

$$12x - 6x + 23y$$
$$6x + 23y$$

Therefore,

$$3[4x + 2(3y - x)] + 5y = 6x + 23y$$

The preceding example is probably a bit more involved than one would experience clinically. However, the gas entrainment equation discussed in the following chapter (Section 4-6, "Fluid Dynamics") sometimes contains two unknowns and requires simplification by combining like terms. That equation will be simplified here.

The gas entrainment equation is:

$$(C_S \times \dot{V}_S) + (C_{ENT} \times \dot{V}_{ENT}) = (C_{DEL} \times \dot{V}_{DEL})$$

The data below represent the variables in the equation.

C_S (source gas concentration) = 100%
$\dot{V}_S$ (source gas flow rate) = 10 L/min
C_{ENT} (entrained gas concentration) = 20%
$\dot{V}_{ENT}$ (entrained gas flow rate) = unknown
C_{DEL} (delivered gas concentration) = 40%
$\dot{V}_{DEL}$ (delivered gas flow rate) = unknown

When these data are inserted in the equation, the expression becomes

$$(100\% \times 10 \text{ L/min}) + (20\% \times \dot{V}_{ENT}) = (40\% \times \dot{V}_{DEL})$$

The two unknown terms in this expression are $\dot{V}_{ENT}$ and $\dot{V}_{DEL}$. Both of these terms are a function of the source gas flow rate ($\dot{V}_S$), which is given. The relationship among these three terms ($\dot{V}_S$, $\dot{V}_{ENT}$, and $\dot{V}_{DEL}$) is

$$\dot{V}_{DEL} = \dot{V}_S + \dot{V}_{ENT}$$

Based on this relationship, each of the unknown terms in the gas entrainment equation can be represented two different ways. One way, for example, begins by rearranging the relationship above to read

$$\dot{V}_{ENT} = \dot{V}_{DEL} - \dot{V}_S$$

Since $\dot{V}_S$ is 10 L/min, then

$$\dot{V}_{ENT} = \dot{V}_{DEL} - 10 \text{ L/min}$$

In the gas entrainment equation, $\dot{V}_{DEL}$ can be represented as x; therefore, $\dot{V}_{ENT}$ becomes $x - 10$ L/min.

Substituting these unknown terms in the gas entrainment equation yields

$$(100\% \times 10 \text{ L/min}) + [20\%(x - 10 \text{ L/min})] = (40\% \times x)$$

By simplifying and combining like terms, the equation reads

$$(1{,}000 \text{ L/min}) + [20x - 200 \text{ L/min}] = 40x$$

or

$$1{,}000 \text{ L/min} - 200 \text{ liters/min} = 40x - 20x$$

$$800 \text{ L/min} = 20x$$

$$\frac{800 \text{ L/min}}{20} = x$$

$$40 \text{ liters/min} = x$$

Since x represents $\dot{V}_{DEL}$, $\dot{V}_{DEL}$ equals 40L/min. Alternatively, the problem could be set up as follows, with x representing $\dot{V}_{ENT}$:

$$(100\% \times 10 \text{ L/min}) + (20\% \times x) = [40\%(x + 10 \text{ L/min})]$$

$$(1{,}000 \text{ L/min}) + (20x) = [40x + 400 \text{ L/min}]$$

$$1{,}000 \text{ L/min} - 400 \text{ L/min} = 40x - 20x$$

$$600 \text{ L/min} = 20x$$

$$\frac{600 \text{ L/min}}{20} = x$$

$$30 \text{ L/min} = x$$

Remember that x in this situation represents $\dot{V}_{ENT}$. So, to calculate $\dot{V}_{DEL}$, add the $\dot{V}_S$ to the 30 liters/min of entrained airflow, i.e.,

$$\dot{V}_{DEL} = 30 \text{ L/min} + 10 \text{ L/min}$$

$$= 40 \text{ L/min}$$

The Fick equation for calculating the cardiac output incorporates the process of factoring. The equation reads as follows.

$$\dot{Q} = \frac{\dot{V}_{O_2}}{C(a-\bar{v})O_2}$$

where,

$\dot{Q}$ = cardiac output (ml/min)

$\dot{V}_{O2}$ = oxygen consumption (ml/min)

$C(a-\bar{v})O_2$ = arterial-mixed venous oxygen content difference (vol %)

The factor in the denominator, $C(a-\bar{v})O_2$, is a combination of two factors. They are the CaO_2 (arterial oxygen content) and the $C\bar{v}O_2$ (mixed venous oxygen content). Both C (content) and O_2 (oxygen) are in the expressions CaO_2 and $C\bar{v}O_2$. Therefore, when the expressions CaO_2 and $C\bar{v}O_2$ are combined to give the arterial-mixed venous oxygen content difference, the overall expression becomes $C(a-\bar{v})O_2$. The expression $C(a-\bar{v})O_2$ is the same as $CaO_2 - C\bar{v}O_2$. Algebraically, the expression is given as $C(a-\bar{v})O_2$. Therefore, the Fick equation may also be expressed as,

$$\dot{Q} = \frac{\dot{V}_{O_2}}{CaO_2 - C\bar{v}O_2}$$

Again, the factor $C(a-\bar{v})O_2$ is a consolidation of the two factors CaO_2 and $C\bar{v}O_2$ when the $C\bar{v}O_2$ is subtracted from the CaO_2.

PRACTICE PROBLEMS

Refer to Appendix A (pages 581-582) for the solutions and answers to the practice problems.

After combining the like terms, solve the following equations:

86. According to Boyle's law, solve for V_2 when

$V_1 = 500$ cc

$P_1 = 760$ torr

$P_2 = 1,900$ torr

$$V_1 P_1 = V_2 P_2$$

87. From the formula for calculating effective static compliance, determine the value of plateau pressure ($P_{plateau}$) when

$V_T = 900$ cc

$V_{lost} = 100$ cc

$PEEP_{applied} = 10$ cm H_2O

$PEEP_{auto} = 7$ cm H_2O

$C_{static} = 100$ ml/cm H_2O

$$C_{static} = \frac{(V_T - V_{lost})}{[P_{plateau} - (PEEP_{applied} + PEEP_{auto})]}$$

88. From the Fick equation, solve for the total venous oxygen content ($C\bar{v}O_2$) when

$\dot{Q}_T = 6$ L/min

$\dot{V}O_2 = 300$ ml/min

$CaO_2 = 18.50$ vol%

$$\dot{Q}_T = \frac{\dot{V}O_2}{(CaO_2 - C\bar{v}O_2)}$$

89. From the formula below, calculate the stroke volume (SV) when

$HR = 72$ beats/min

$CI = 3.5$ L/min/m²

$BSA = 1.65$ m²

$$\frac{HR \times SV}{BSA} = CI$$

90. Compute the inspiratory time (T_I) from the equation below when

$\bar{P}_{aw} = 15$ cm H_2O

$PIP = 30$ cm H_2O

PEEP = 10 cm H_2O

TCT = 4 sec

$$\bar{P}_{aw} = K*(PIP - PEEP)(T_I/TCT) + PEEP$$

2-6 EVALUATING FORMULAS

A formula is a mathematical statement or equation that expresses a relationship between two or more quantities. When formulas are used, adequate data must be provided to solve the equation. The amount of data required to solve an equation depends on the complexity of the formula. Less data are required to solve a problem concerning the **law of LaPlace**, for example,

$$P = \frac{2ST}{r}$$

than for solving the Bohr equation,

$$\frac{V_D}{V_T} = \frac{PaCO_2 - P\bar{E}CO_2}{PaCO_2}$$

Regarding the law of LaPlace, if any two of the three variables (P, ST, and r) in the equation are known, the third can be obtained. In other words, the law of LaPlace can be expressed three different ways:

(1) $P = \dfrac{2ST}{r}$

(2) $ST = \dfrac{(P)(r)}{2}$

(3) $r = \dfrac{2ST}{P}$

Again, formulas are mathematical expressions representing the quantitative relationships among the variables. All formulas and equations can be manipulated and transposed to solve for any variable in the formula, depending on which quantities or factors are known.

The ease with which the law of LaPlace can be manipulated has already been demonstrated. Formulas that are more complex generally require more steps to transpose.

---

*Assume that the ventilator in use delivers a square wave, or rectangular, pressure pattern; therefore, the value of K is 1.

Consider the formula for calculating the effective dynamic compliance:

$$C_{dynamic} = \frac{(V_T - V_{lost})}{PIP - (PEEP_{applied} + PEEP_{auto})}$$

In the form presented here, $C_{dynamic}$ can be determined when the following five factors, or variables, are known: (1) tidal volume (V_T), (2) volume compressed ("lost") in the ventilator tubing (V_{lost}), (3) peak inspiratory pressure (PIP), (4) therapeutically applied PEEP ($PEEP_{applied}$), and (5) inadvertant or auto PEEP ($PEEP_{auto}$).

However, the equation can be transposed to solve for any of the factors in the formula when any of the other five are known. For example, the equation may be rearranged to solve for the PIP when

$C_{dynamic} = 20$ ml/cm H_2O

$V_T = 850$ ml

$V_{lost} = 50$ ml

$PEEP_{applied} = 5$ cm H_2O

$PEEP_{auto} = 5$ cm H_2O

After substituting the variables, note where the unknown factor (PIP) is located in the equation.

$$20 \text{ ml/cm } H_2O = \frac{(850 \text{ ml} - 50 \text{ ml})}{PIP - (5 \text{ cm } H_2O + 5 \text{ cm } H_2O)}$$

The equation can be rearranged as follows to solve for the PIP:

$$(20 \text{ ml/cm } H_2O)[PIP - (5 \text{ cm } H_2O + 5 \text{ cm } H_2O)] = (850 \text{ ml} - 50 \text{ ml})$$

$$PIP - (5 \text{ cm } H_2O + 5 \text{ cm } H_2O) = \frac{(850 \text{ ml} - 50 \text{ ml})}{(20 \text{ ml/cm } H_2O)}$$

$$PIP - 10 \text{ cm } H_2O = \frac{(800 \text{ ml})}{(20 \text{ ml/cm } H_2O)}$$

$$PIP - 10 \text{ cm } H_2O = 40 \text{ cm } H_2O$$

$$PIP = 40 \text{ cm } H_2O + 10 \text{ cm } H_2O$$

$$PIP = 50 \text{ cm } H_2O$$

To verify the calculation, insert the value for PIP into the original formula and solve for $C_{dynamic}$:

$$C_{dynamic} = \frac{(850 \text{ ml} - 50 \text{ ml})}{50 \text{ cm } H_2O - (5 \text{ cm } H_2O + 5 \text{ cm } H_2O)}$$

$$= \frac{800 \text{ ml}}{40 \text{ cm } H_2O}$$

$$= 20 \text{ ml/cm } H_2O$$

Another example that will be provided here is the Bohr equation. Ordinarily, the Bohr equation solves for the $V_D : V_T$ ratio, i.e.,

$$\frac{V_D}{V_T} = \frac{PaCO_2 - P\bar{E}CO_2}{PaCO_2}$$

However, if all the variables except the $P\bar{E}CO_2$ are known, the equation can be transposed to solve for the $P\bar{E}CO_2$.

$$P\bar{E}CO_2 = PaCO_2 - \left[\left(\frac{V_D}{V_T} \right) (PaCO_2) \right]$$

Therefore, given the following values, the $P\bar{E}CO_2$ can be determined:

$PaCO_2 = 40$ torr

$V_D = 150$ cc

$V_T = 500$ cc

$$P\bar{E}CO_2 = 40 \text{ torr} - \left[\left(\frac{150 \text{ cc}}{500 \text{ cc}} \right) (40 \text{ torr}) \right]$$

$$= 40 \text{ torr} - [(0.3)(40 \text{ torr})]$$

$$= 40 \text{ torr} - 12 \text{ torr}$$

$$= 28 \text{ torr}$$

PRACTICE PROBLEMS

Refer to Appendix A (pages 582-583) for the solutions and answers to the practice problems.

Transpose the following formulas to solve for the identified unknown.

91. Calculate the central venous pressure (CVP) from the formula.

$$SVR = \frac{MAP - CVP}{C.O.}$$

when

$SVR = 20$ mm Hg/L/min

$MAP = 90$ mm Hg

$C.O. = 5$ L/min

92. From Graham's law of diffusion of a gas through a liquid medium, calculate the square root of the molecular weight of CO_2 when

O_2 solubility coefficient = 0.023 ml O_2/ml plasma/760 torr PO_2

CO_2 solubility coefficient = 0.510 ml CO_2/ml plasma/760 torr PCO_2

O_2 molecular $= 32$ a.m.u.

$R_{CO_2}{:}R_{O_2} = 19{:}1$

$$\frac{R_{CO_2}}{R_{O_2}} = \frac{(\sqrt{O_2\text{ molecular wt}})(CO_2\text{ solubility coefficient})}{(\sqrt{CO_2\text{ molecular wt}})(O_2\text{ solubility coefficient})}$$

93. From the formula below, determine the inspiratory flow rate ($\dot{V}_I$) when

   $T_I = 0.75$ sec

   $V_T = 450$ cc

$$T_I = \frac{V_T}{\dot{V}_I}$$

94. Calculate the minute ventilation ($\dot{V}_E$) when

   $f = 16$ breaths/min.

   $V_A = 400$ cc

   $V_D = 200$ cc

$$f(V_A) = f(V_T) - f(V_D)$$

95. Determine the hemoglobin concentration, [Hb], from the formula below when

   $S\bar{v}O_2 = 65\%$

   $C\bar{v}O_2 = 13.75$ vol%

   $P\bar{v}O_2 = 35$ torr

$$C\bar{v}O_2 = (1.34 \times [Hb]S\bar{v}O_2 + P\bar{v}O_2(0.003)$$

2-7 RECIPROCALS

Frequently in cardiorespiratory physiology and clinical practice, reciprocal relationships are encountered. To assist in the understanding of this concept, this section will provide the fundamental mathematical basis for reciprocal relationships and supply a number of examples of their practical application, including compliance, elastance, resistance, and conductance.

Two numbers whose product is unity, or 1, are called **reciprocals**. For example,

$$\frac{1}{3} \times \frac{3}{1} = \frac{3}{3} = \frac{1}{1} = 1$$

Because the product of 1/3 and 3 is equal to 1, 1/3 and 3 are reciprocals of each other. Another expression meaning reciprocal is **multiplicative inverse**.

The general format demonstrating a reciprocal, or multiplicative inverse, is as follows:

$$(x)\left(\frac{1}{x}\right) = 1, \text{ or } \left(\frac{1}{x}\right)(x) = 1$$

The symbol x represents any real number other than zero. The numbers x and $1/x$ are reciprocals of each other because their product equals 1. The number zero (0) does not have a reciprocal because the product of any number and 0 equals 0, not 1.

PRACTICE PROBLEMS

Refer to Appendix A (page 583) for the solutions and answers to the practice problems.

Find the reciprocal of each of the following numbers:

96. $7 = $ _____

97. $0.5 = $ _____

98. $\dfrac{1}{4} = $ _____

99. $-6 = $ _____

100. $-\dfrac{2}{3}9 = $ _____

Within the context of respiratory mechanics, the concepts of *compliance* and *elastance* represent prominent examples of reciprocal relationships. Qualitatively, compliance refers to the degree of difficulty or ease associated with the inflation of the lungs. Elastance, on the other hand, represents the recoil property of the lungs (i.e., the degree of difficulty or ease of deflation).

Simply stated, it is easier to inflate the lungs when they are more compliant. The more stiff the lungs are, the more difficult they are to inflate, the easier they are to deflate. When the lungs are easier to inflate (more compliant), they have less recoil, i.e., a lower elastance. When the lungs are more difficult to inflate (less compliant or stiff), they are more elastic—a higher elastance. So stiff lungs tend to have a greater recoil.

From these descriptions, the reciprocal nature of these two physiologic concepts emerges. Compliance (C) of the lungs relates to lung volume changes (ΔV) associated with transpulmonary pressure changes (ΔP), that is,

$$C = \frac{\Delta V}{\Delta P}$$

or

$$C = \frac{ml}{cm\ H_2O}$$

Elastance (E) associates transpulmonary pressure changes (ΔP) with lung volume changes (ΔV), that is,

$$E = \frac{\Delta P}{\Delta V}$$

or

$$E = \frac{cm\ H_2O}{ml}$$

The two components of the respiratory system (lungs and chest wall) have their own compliance and elastance values. Regarding compliance, the relationship between lung compliance (C_L) and chest wall compliance (C_{CW}) can be written as

$$\boxed{\frac{1}{C_L} + \frac{1}{C_{CW}} = \frac{1}{C_T}}$$

where

C_L = lung compliance (ml/cm H_2O)

C_{CW} = chest wall compliance (ml/cm H_2O)

C_T = total, or system, compliance (ml/cm H_2O)

Lung and chest wall compliance values are normally about 0.2 ml/cm H_2O. Therefore, to calculate C_T, add the reciprocals of lung and chest wall compliance, i.e.,

$$\frac{1}{C_T} = \frac{1}{0.2\ ml/cm\ H_2O} + \frac{1}{0.2\ ml/cm\ H_2O}$$

$$\frac{1}{C_T} = 5\ cm\ H_2O/ml + 5\ cm\ H_2O/ml$$

$$\frac{1}{C_T} = 10\ cm\ H_2O/ml$$

$$C_T = \frac{1}{10\ cm\ H_2O/ml}$$

$$C_T = 0.1\ ml/cm\ H_2O$$

Because the lung compliance and chest wall compliance are added reciprocally, the total compliance will always be less than the individual lung and chest wall compliance values. A closer look at how this equation was used to solve for the total compliance reveals the reciprocal relationship between compliance and elastance. For lung compliance note that

$$\frac{1}{C_L} = \frac{1}{0.2\ ml/cm\ H_2O} = 5\ cm\ H_2O/ml$$

The value 5 cm H_2O/ml is the lung elastance (E_L). Consequently, for lung compliance, it can be said that

$$\frac{1}{C_L} = E_L \quad \text{or} \quad \frac{1}{E_L} = C_L$$

and

$$\frac{1}{0.2 \text{ ml/cm } H_2O} = 5 \text{ cm } H_2O/\text{ml} \quad \text{or} \quad \frac{1}{5 \text{ cm } H_2O/\text{ml}} = 0.2 \text{ ml/cm } H_2O$$

Observe how the units for compliance and elastance have been rearranged in the process.

Because of the reciprocal relationship between compliance and elastance, the following equation can be developed:

$$\boxed{E_L + E_{CW} = E_T}$$

where

E_L = lung elastance (cm H_2O/ml)

E_{CW} = chest wall elastance (cm H_2O/ml)

E_T = total, or system, elastance (cm H_2O/ml)

Consider the situation when lung elastance is 4 cm H_2O/ml and chest wall elastance is 6 cm H_2O/ml. Total elastance is calculated as follows:

$$4 \text{ cm } H_2O/\text{ml} + 6 \text{ cm } H_2O/\text{ml} = 10 \text{ cm } H_2O/\text{ml}$$

Any of these values can be converted to their corresponding compliances by dividing the elastance into 1. Because lung elastance and chest wall elastance are added as whole numbers, or integers, the total elastance will always be greater than the values of lung and chest wall elastance individually. See Chapter 4 Physics, 4-7 Mechanics of Ventilation, for a more detailed discussion on compliance and elastance.

The dynamic measurements pertaining to ventilatory mechanics (i.e., airway *resistance* and airway *conductance*) are reciprocally related as well (See Chapter 4 Physics, 4-6 Fluid Dynamics, Resistance to Ventilation for more information.). Airway resistance (R_{aw}), which is present only when a fluid is flowing, is defined as a change in driving pressure (ΔP) divided by the flow rate ($\dot{V}$), or

$$R_{aw} = \frac{\Delta P}{\dot{V}} = \frac{\text{cm } H_2O}{\text{L/sec}}$$

Airway conductance (G_{aw}), therefore, is

$$G_{aw} = \frac{\dot{V}}{\Delta P} = \frac{\text{L/sec}}{\text{cm } H_2O}$$

Hence,

$$R_{aw} = \frac{1}{G_{aw}}$$

and

$$G_{aw} = \frac{1}{R_{aw}}$$

Note, again, how the units for R_{aw} and G_{aw} become rearranged.

The reciprocal relationship between resistance and conductance can also be demonstrated in the measurement of gas diffusion across the alveolar-capillary membrane. Carbon monoxide (CO) gas is used in the process to determine gas conductance along this diffusion pathway. As gas diffuses across the alveolar-capillary membrane, it encounters certain physical and chemical pathway characteristics that offer resistance to gas diffusion or conductance. These characteristics are quantitatively arranged as

$$\frac{1}{D_LCO} = \frac{1}{D_M} + \frac{1}{\theta \times V_C}$$

where

D_LCO = CO diffusing capacity (L/min/mm Hg)

D_M = membrane diffusing capacity

θ = reaction rate of CO and hemoglobin

V_C = pulmonary capillary blood volume

The factor $1/D_M$ and the reciprocal of the product of $\theta \cdot V_C$ ($1/\theta V_C$) are resistances to diffusion across the alveolar-capillary membrane; therefore, the factor $1/D_LCO$ equals a resistance. Because resistance and conductance are reciprocals of each other, i.e.,

$$\frac{1}{G} = R$$

then, D_LCO equals G, or conductance.

PRACTICE PROBLEMS

Refer to Appendix A (pages 583-584) for the solutions and answers to the practice problems.

101. If lung compliance is 0.4 ml/cm H_2O, calculate lung elastance. _____
102. Calculate the chest wall compliance when the total compliance is 0.15 ml/cm H_2O and the pulmonary compliance equals 0.30 ml/cm H_2O. _____
103. Find lung compliance when the chest wall elastance and the total elastance are 3.5 cm H_2O/ml and 5.5 cm H_2O/ml, respectively. _____

104. Plethysmographic measurement of airway resistance is 0.85 cm H_2O/L/sec. Convert this measurement to airway conductance. _____

105. Determine the resistance to diffusion for CO across the alveolar-capillary membrane if the DlCO is 23 ml/min/mm Hg. _____

CHAPTER SUMMARY

Algebraic expressions contain one or more variables, which are symbols used to signify one or more numbers. Number lines are used to assist locating real numbers. Numbers to the left of the origin are negative values and numbers to the origin's right are positive values. A line containing numbers arranged in this manner is a number line. Rules apply to the addition, subtraction, multiplication, and division of real numbers.

The rules for order of operations allow for the systematic simplification of numerical expressions. Algebraic expressions often contain multiple terms. Sometimes combining like terms is necessary when solving algebraic expressions.

Formulas are mathematical statements describing relationships among quantities. Formulas require that data be provided for the calculation to be completed.

Some physiologic measurements have a reciprocal relationship, for example, compliance (C) and elastance (E) are reciprocally related. Airway resistance (R_{aw}) and airway conductance (G_{aw}) are also reciprocally related. Two numbers whose product is one are reciprocally related to each other.

REVIEW QUESTIONS

2-1 ALGEBRAIC EXPRESSIONS

Questions

1. Define the term *variable*.
2. What is an algebraic expression that contains a variable called?
3. Explain how the solution to an algebraic expression is found.
4. What is a numerical expression?
5. Write an algebraic expression (a) with one variable, (b) with two variables, and (c) with three variables.
6. Find three formulas or equations from clinical practice or from cardiopulmonary physiology that contain (a) one variable, (b) two variables, and (c) three variables.

2-2 REAL NUMBERS

Questions

1. State the two rules that govern the addition of real numbers.
2. Describe what is meant by *additive inverse*.

3. State the rule that governs the subtraction of real numbers.
4. State the two rules that govern the multiplication of real numbers.
5. How can division be described?
6. State the two rules that govern the division of real numbers.
7. Identify the (a) dividend, (b) divisor, and (c) quotient in a division problem.

2-3 COMPARING NUMBERS

Questions

1. Describe a number line.
2. What is the significance of the origin on a number line?
3. What type of numbers are contained on a number line?
4. Define the term *opposite value*.
5. Construct a number line and label the following components: (a) origin and (b) positive and negative values.
6. Define the term *absolute value*.
7. Differentiate between *distance* and *direction* from zero on a number line.
8. Describe how numbers on a number line can be (a) added and (b) subtracted.
9. How can a subtraction problem be transformed to an addition problem?
10. Construct a number line calibrated in mm Hg and cm H_2O. Consider the best location for atmospheric pressure.
11. Construct a number line for determining the transpulmonary pressure in the apices of the lungs at FRC when the intrapleural pressure is -10 cm H_2O.

2-4 SIMPLIFYING NUMERICAL EXPRESSIONS

Questions

1. State the rules for order of operations used for simplifying numerical and algebraic expressions.
2. Simplify a numerical or algebraic expression used in cardiorespiratory care.

2-5 COMBINING LIKE TERMS

Questions

1. Define the word *term* as it applies to an algebraic expression.
2. Provide four examples of a term in an algebraic expression.
3. Write an algebraic expression that contains five terms.
4. Explain how the rules for order of operations are used to help combine like terms.

2-6 EVALUATING FORMULAS

Questions

1. Define *formula*.
2. Find a cardiopulmonary physiology or clinical formula that has at least three variables and evaluate the expression for each variable.

2-7 RECIPROCALS

Questions

1. Define a reciprocal.
2. What is a multiplicative inverse?
3. Write the general format representing a reciprocal.
4. What is the reciprocal of zero?
5. What is the reciprocal of (a) elastance and (b) conductance?
6. Is the factor $1/\text{DLCO}$ a resistance or a conductance? Why?

Bibliography

Davison, D., et al. *Pre-Algebra*. Englewood Cliffs, New Jersey: Prentice Hall, Inc., 1992.

Fair, J., and Bragg, Sadie. *Algebra 1*. Englewood Cliffs, New Jersey: Prentice Hall, Inc., 1991.

Price, J., et al. *Applications of Mathematics*. Columbus, Ohio: Merrill Publishing Co., 1988.

CHAPTER THREE

CHEMISTRY

A variety of concepts associated with clinical respiratory care and pulmonary physiology demand an understanding of certain fundamental inorganic chemistry principles. The goal of this chapter is to highlight these principles by discussing them in their basic science form and by relating them to clinical practice and pulmonary physiology.

—————— CHAPTER OBJECTIVES ——————

Upon completing this chapter, the reader will be able to relate basic concepts of chemistry to clinical respiratory care and pulmonary physiology and will be able to

3-1 ATOMIC STRUCTURE AND ELECTRON CONFIGURATION

- Name the three fundamental subatomic particles comprising an element.
- Distinguish atomic weight from atomic mass.
- Discuss electron configuration.
- Describe the significance of electron configuration.
- Explain the three types of chemical bonding.
- State the rule of eight.
- Discuss the organization of the periodic table

3-2 CHEMICAL LAWS

- State Henry's law of solubility.
- Apply Henry's law of solubility physiologically.
- Derive the conversion factor for changing P_{O_2} in the plasma from torr, or mm Hg, to volumes percent.
- Derive three conversion factors pertaining to carbon dioxide transported in the blood:
  (1) converting P_{CO_2} from torr, or mm Hg, to volumes percent.

(2) converting volumes percent of carbon dioxide to millimoles of CO_2/liter, or milliequivalents of CO_2/liter.
(3) converting P_{CO_2} from torr, or mm Hg, to millimoles of CO_2/liter, or milliequivalents of CO_2/liter.
- Perform conversion calculations among the different units used to express carbon dioxide concentration in the blood.
- Compute the total carbon dioxide level in the blood.
- State the two forms of Graham's law of diffusion.
- Apply the two forms of Graham's law of diffusion physiologically.
- Calculate the relative rate of diffusion for gases (1) diffusing within a gaseous medium and (2) diffusing across a liquid medium.

3-3 MOLARITY AND NORMALITY

- Define the following terms:
  (1) solution
  (2) solute
  (3) solvent
  (4) mole, or gram molecular weight
- Calculate the number of moles of various compounds.
- Calculate the molarity of different solutions.
- Define gram equivalent weight.
- Calculate the number of gram equivalents of various substances.
- Calculate the normality of different solutions.

3-4 LAW OF MASS ACTION AND HENDERSON-HASSELBALCH EQUATION

- Relate the law of mass action to the Henderson-Hasselbalch equation.
- Calculate hydrogen ion concentration in terms of pH, moles/liter, and nanomoles/liter.
- Apply the law of mass action and the concepts of chemical equilibrium physiologically.
- Discuss the various blood buffer systems.
- Perform acid-base calculations using the Henderson-Hasselbalch equation.

3-5 DENSITY AND SPECIFIC GRAVITY

- Compute the density and specific gravity for gases and liquids.

3-6 TEMPERATURE SCALES

- Define thermal energy.
- Define temperature.
- Differentiate among the three types of temperature scales presented.
- Solve problems involving temperature scale conversions.

3-7 ELECTROCHEMISTRY

- Define the components of an electrochemical cell.
- Distinguish between oxidation and reduction.
- Describe the flow of current through an electrochemical cell.
- Explain the purpose of applying an external polarizing voltage to a polarographic cell.
- Discuss oxidation and reduction potentials.
- State the half-reaction for the standard hydrogen electrode.
- Relate electrochemical principles to the operation of the galvanic and polarographic oxygen analyzers.

FORMULAS USED IN THIS CHAPTER

$(P_{O_2}$ torr$)(0.003$ vol %/torr$)$ (page 163)

$(P_{CO_2}$ torr$)(0.067$ vol %/torr$)$ (page 166)

$\left[HCO_3^-\right] + (P_{CO_2} \times 0.03 \text{ mEq/L/torr}) = \text{total } CO_2$ (page 166)

$r_1(\sqrt{D_1}) = r_2(\sqrt{D_2})$ (page 169)

$\dfrac{r_1}{r_2} = \dfrac{\sqrt{D_2} \times C_{S_1}}{\sqrt{D_1} \times C_{S_2}}$ (page 170)

$M = $ moles/liter   (page 173)

$N = $ gew/liter   (page 176)

$pH = \log\left(\dfrac{1}{H^+}\right)$ (page 178)

moles/L $= 9 - \log(\text{nmol/L})$ (page 182)

$(\text{nmol/L}) = \text{antilog}(9 - pH)$ (page 183)

$pH = 6.1 + \log \dfrac{HCO_3^-}{(P_{CO_2})(0.03 \text{ mEq/L/torr})}$ (page 192)

density of a solid & liquid $= $ g/ml   (page 197)

density of a gas $= $ gram mol. wt./22.4 L   (page 199)

$K = {}^{\circ}C + 273$ (page 203)

${}^{\circ}F = \dfrac{9}{5}({}^{\circ}C) + 32$ (page 203)

${}^{\circ}C = ({}^{\circ}F - 32)5/9$ (page 204)

3-1 ATOMIC STRUCTURE AND ELECTRON CONFIGURATION

This section will present information about atomic structure, electron configuration, and chemical bonding to help the reader understand relevant chemical and physical behavior of atoms and molecules.

Atoms

Developments in nuclear physics have revealed a number of subatomic particles, including the proton, neutron, electron, meson, positron, hyperon, and neutrino. The subatomic particles that will be discussed here are the proton, neutron, and electron.

All atoms contain these three particles with one exception: an atom of hydrogen contains one proton, one electron, and no neutrons. Atoms differ from one another because the number and arrangement of these subatomic particles are different. For example, the most common atom of chlorine contains 17 protons, 17 electrons, and 18 neutrons, whereas the most common atom of oxygen has 8 protons, 8 electrons, and 8 neutrons.

Where are these three subatomic particles positioned within an atom? The **proton**, which is positively charged and possesses a mass of one atomic mass unit (amu), is located within the nucleus of the atom. The number of protons contained in the nucleus of an atom (**atomic number**) determines the element. The element hydrogen has one proton, helium has two, lithium has three, etc. So, again, the number of protons in an atom constitutes its atomic number. Hydrogen has an atomic number of 1. Helium's is 2, and that for lithium is 3. Elements can be identified on the basis of their atomic number. For example, the oxygen atom has an atomic number of 8. No other element has that atomic number.

Neutrons also occupy a position within the atom's nucleus. They possess no charge (neutral) and have a mass of 1 amu. The arithmetic sum of the number of protons and the number of neutrons inside the nucleus of an atom constitutes that atom's **atomic mass.**

Compared to their basic structures most atoms of elements can accommodate additional neutrons in their nucleus. For instance, three varieties of oxygen atoms have been identified in nature (Figure 3-1).

Form A with a mass of 16 amu is the most prevalent, comprising about 99.80% of all oxygen atoms in the atmosphere. Forms B and C constitute approximately 0.04% and 0.16% of the remaining 0.20%, respectively.

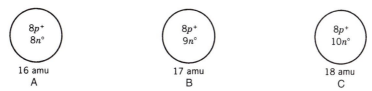

Figure 3-1. *Three types of oxygen atoms based on the atomic mass. Each form has 8 protons; however, (A) has 8 neutrons, (B) has 9 neutrons, and (C) has 10 neutrons.*

All three of these forms of oxygen have eight protons (p^+). However, forms B and C possess more neutrons (n°) than form A. In other words, all the atoms have the same atomic number but differ in their atomic mass. Types of oxygen of atomic mass 17 amu and 18 amu are said to be **isotopes** of oxygen. An isotope of any element is an atom that has the same atomic number but differs in atomic mass.

The third subatomic particle that will be described here is the **electron.** Electrons have a negative charge and contribute essentially nothing to the atomic mass of the atom. They are positioned at various levels around and away from the nucleus.

All atoms are electrostatically neutral. In the neutral atom the number of protons in the nucleus equals the number of electrons revolving about the atom's nucleus. Therefore, when the atomic number of a neutral atom is known, the number of electrons in that atom can be determined by deduction.

Electrons are so distant from the nucleus that they contribute little to the mass of the atom. In fact, the electron's mass has been determined to be about 1/1,838 of the hydrogen atom; that of the proton is 1,837/1,838 of the hydrogen atom. In other words, it would take 1,838 electrons to equal the mass of one hydrogen atom.

Electron Shells and Orbitals

As was previously mentioned, electrons are positioned at varying distances from the atom's positively charged nucleus. The electrons position themselves in an orderly fashion. For instance, radiating away from the nucleus are electron shells or principal energy levels. These energy levels are labelled numerically (1, 2, 3, etc.). Figure 3-2 shows electron shells situated about a nucleus.

The electron shell is designated by the letter n. For example, the designation $n = 4$ refers to the fourth electron shell. Each electron shell consists of at least one orbital. Orbitals are designated by the lower case letters s, p, d, and f. Within each orbital there

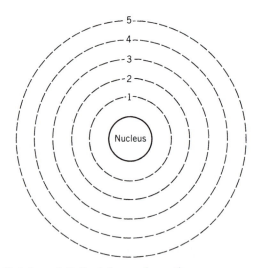

Figure 3-2. *Electron shells 1 through 5 situated around a nucleus.*

TABLE 3-1   Electron Shells and Orbitals

Electron Shell	Orbital	Subshell	Maximum No. of Electrons in Each Orbital	Maximum No. of Electrons in Each Electron Shell
1	s	1s	2	2
2	s	2s	2	8
	p	2p	6	
3	s	3s	2	18
	p	3p	6	
	d	3d	10	
4	s	4s	2	32
	p	4p	6	
	d	4d	10	
	f	4f	14	

are specific electron pathways. Only one pair of electrons (two electrons) can maximally occupy each orbital. Table 3-1 shows the relationship between the electron shells and their orbitals.

The table reveals that each successive electron shell following $n = 1$ (closest to the nucleus) becomes more complex as more orbitals become incorporated. The most complex electron shell shown on Table 3-1 is 4.

The lower case letters in the "Orbital" column designate the specific type of orbital. There are four different orbitals shown in the table—s, p, d, and f. The letters stand for sharp (or spin), principal, diffuse, and fundamental, respectively. These names were given based on the spectral lines corresponding to each orbital and were established before the advent of quantum mechanics. Each electron shell contains different numbers of orbitals. Similarly, each orbital resides in a specific subshell within an electron shell. For example, subshell $1s$ signifies that one s orbital resides in the first electron shell, and subshell $2p$ indicates that the p orbitals reside in the second electron shell.

The number of orbitals in a subshell depends on the complexity of the atom. For example, if electron shell 4 contained its full complement of subshells, it would have one s orbital, three p orbitals, five d orbitals, and seven f orbitals. Electron shells 1, 2, and 3 do not have the capability of possessing all those orbitals.

Based on probability (electron density), the shapes of the s and p orbitals have been theorized. The s orbital is considered to be spherical, and that for the p orbital is said to take on a dumbbell, or figure-8, shape. Each of the three p orbitals lie in a plane 90° from the other two. One p orbital can be considered to be positioned along an x-axis, the second one positioned along a y-axis, and the third p orbital positioned along a z-axis (oriented 90° to the x and y coordinates). The contour diagram Figure 3-3 depicts this three-dimensional electron orientation. The p orbital along the z-axis can be considered as running into and out of the page. Each p orbital is designated by the axis along which it lies, that is, p_x, p_y, and p_z.

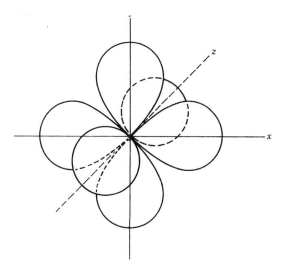

Figure 3-3. *Contour diagram illustrating relationship among p_x, p_y, and p_z.*

The three-dimensional contour diagrams representing the electron densities of the *d* and *f* orbitals are complicated and difficult to visualize. Therefore, they will not be addressed here.

The maximum number of electrons possible in any electron shell can be determined by the formula, $2(n^2)$. The lower case *n* represents the numerical value of the electron shell. For example, when $n = 1$, $2(n^2)$, or $2(1^2)$, equals 2. That means that a maximum of 2 electrons can reside in the first electron shell. Further, when $n = 2$, $2(n^2)$, or $2(2^2)$, equals 8 (i.e., a maximum of 8 electrons can position themselves in the second electron shell).

Two atoms will be used to exemplify the order of electron filling. The first is the chlorine atom (Table 3-2), which has an atomic number of 17. Therefore, it also contains 17 electrons. Notice that electron shells 1 and 2 are completely filled in this case but that the 3 level is not. The electron filling terminates when the number of electrons is depleted. The three

TABLE 3-2 Electron Filling for Chlorine Atom

Atom	No. of Electrons	Electron Shell	Orbital	No. of Electrons in Orbital	No. of Electrons in Electron Shell
Chlorine	17	1	s	2	2
		2	s	2	8
			p	6	
		3	s	2	7
			p	5	

TABLE 3-3   3 p Filling in Cl Atom

Electron Shell	Type of p Orbital	No. of Electrons in Each p Orbital
3	x	2
	y	2
	z	1

TABLE 3-4   Electron Filling for Oxygen Atom

Atom	No. of Electrons	Electron Shell	Orbital	No. of Electrons in Orbital	No. of Electrons in Electron Shell
Oxygen	8	1	s	2	2
		2	s	2	6
			p	4	

p orbitals in electron shell 3 have only five electrons. A proposed model for the electron arrangement in the three p orbitals in energy level 3 is shown in Table 3-3. The order of filling for the three p orbitals proceeds in an orderly fashion. For example, each individual p orbital (x, y, and z) must have one electron in residence before any one of the three can possess its full complement of electrons, that is, two.

The second example of electron filling is the oxygen atom. The purpose here is to show how the two unpaired electrons account for the property of **paramagnetic susceptibility** possessed by the oxygen atom. Consider Table 3-4.

Table 3-4 indicates that the number of electrons available in the oxygen atom complete electron shell 1 and partially fill the 2 shell. A closer look at the filling of the electron 2 shell, specifically in terms of its orbitals, is in order. The s orbital fills to its maximum. However, the three p orbitals do not fill to capacity. A proposed order of filling of the p orbitals is presented as follows:

$$p_x\ 1e^-,\ 1e^-$$

$$p_y\ 1e^-$$

$$p_x\ 1e^-$$

In this proposed electron arrangement, both the p_y and p_z orbitals remain incompletely filled because of the unavailability of more electrons. Consequently, the oxygen atom has two unpaired electrons in its outermost shell. This electron configuration accounts for the paramagnetic property of oxygen because the lone electrons in the p_y and p_z orbitals rotate about their respective axes in the same direction as they move through their respective paths. When an orbital is filled to capacity (two electrons), one electron rotates about its axis clockwise, and the other rotates counterclockwise. Consequently, no net magnetic effect results. But, in the case of oxygen, the two unpaired, outermost electrons rotating in the same direction result in the atom's paramagnetism (see the discussion in Chapter 4, "Paramagnetic Susceptibility").

The order of electron filling in the orbital presented here for the oxygen atom is only a proposed sequence. Any of the individual *p* orbitals can be the first to accommodate an electron. However, none of the *p* orbitals can have its full complement until all three *p* orbitals have one electron.

Table 3-5 indicates a representative number of examples of electron filling. From the examples one can see that some of the electron shells overlap, as is the case with potassium. Electrons enter electron shell 4 before the 3 shell is completely filled. Specifically, the *s* orbital in the 4th electron shell fills before the *d* orbitals in the 3rd shell are completely filled. A similar situation exists concerning the electron shells 4 and 5 in the element molybdenum.

The overlapping of electron shells does not occur until the transition from shell 3 to shell 4 is encountered. No overlapping is experienced among the first three shells.

The schematic Figure 3-4 represents a more detailed depiction of electron filling than that indicated in Table 3-5.

It can be seen that the *s* orbital of the ensuing electron shell fills before the *d* orbitals and immediately after the filling of the *p* orbitals in the previous shell. Overlapping of electron shells occurs after the 2 shell completely fills.

A recapitulation of some of the more salient points regarding electron configuration will now be presented.

- Electrons are positioned in different electron shells at varying distances from the atom's nucleus.

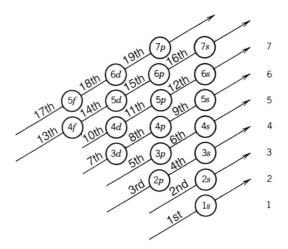

Figure 3-4. *Order of electron filling for electron shells 1 through 7. Notice that some lower shells remain below capacity as some higher shells begin filling, e.g., electron shell 4 (4s) begins filling before shell 3 (3d) completely fills.*

TABLE 3-5 Electron Configuration of Representative Atoms

Electron Configuration — Orbitals: (Number of Electrons)

Element (Symbol)	Atomic No.	No. of Electrons	1 s	2 s	2 p_x	2 p_y	2 p_z	3 s	3 p_x	3 p_y	3 p_z	3 d[b]	4 s	4 p_x	4 p_y	4 p_z	4 d	4 f[c]	5 s	5 p_x	5 p_y	5 p_z	5 d	5 f
Hydrogen (H)	1	1	1																					
Helium (He)	2	2	2																					
Carbon (C)	6	6	2	2	1	1																		
Nitrogen (N)	7	7	2	2	1	1	1																	
Oxygen (O)	8	8	2	2	2	1	1																	
Sodium (Na)	11	11	2	2	2	2	2	1																
Chlorine (Cl)	17	17	2	2	2	2	2	2	2	2	1													
Potassium (K)	19	19	2	2	2	2	2	2	2	2	2		1											
Calcium (Ca)	20	20	2	2	2	2	2	2	2	2	2		2											
Iron (Fe)	26	26	2	2	2	2	2	2	2	2	2	6	2											
Molybdenum (Mo)	42	42	2	2	2	2	2	2	2	2	2	10	2	2	2	2	4		2					

[a]Note that some of the electron shells overlap. For example, for potassium the 4s orbital houses an electron before the 3d orbital. Likewise, for molybdenum the 5s orbital fills before the 4f orbital. The 4f orbital accepts electrons.

[b]The d orbital is comprised of five individual pathways capable of accommodating 10 electrons. This arrangement is similar to the p orbital, which has three pathways with accommodations for six electrons (p_x, p_y, p_z).

[c]The f orbital is comprised of seven individual pathways capable of accommodating 14 electrons.

- The electrons revolve around the atom's nucleus and rotate about their own axes.
- The positioning of electrons around the nucleus is orderly.
- All atoms have electron shells within which the electrons reside.
- The maximum number of electrons that can occupy any given electron shell is shown by the formula $2(n^2)$.
- Electrons occupy orbitals within each electron shell.
- The electron shells are designated numerically as 1, 2, 3, etc.
- The orbitals are designated by the lower case letters s, p, d, and f, of which there are one s orbital, three p orbitals, five d orbitals, and seven f orbitals when present.
- No more than two electrons can occupy any orbital.
- Electron filling begins at electron shell 1 ($n = 1$) and proceeds outward.

Chemical Bonding

Equipped with an understanding of electron configuration, the reader is now prepared to understand the nature of bonding between and among atoms to form compounds. There are three types of chemical bonds that can form. These bonds include (1) electrovalent (ionic) bonds, (2) covalent bonds, and (3) ionic-covalent bonds.

An electrovalent or ionic bond results when the atoms of two or more elements combine with each other by transferring electrons. What actually happens is one electron leaves the outermost electron shell of one of the atoms and enters the outermost electron shell of the atom with which it is reacting. Consider the reaction between a sodium (Na) atom and a chlorine (Cl) atom.

The chlorine atom (atomic number 17) was previously seen to have seven electrons in its outermost shell. One of the p orbitals was one electron short of being completely filled.

Let's view the sodium atom (atomic number 11) and its electron configuration. Two electrons enter electron shell 1 (s orbital); eight electrons enter shell 2 (s and p orbitals). The remaining electron occupies the s orbital in the 3rd shell by itself.

There is a tendency in nature for all atoms to seek eight electrons in their outermost electron shell when they participate in a chemical reaction. This tendency is called the **rule of eight.** This, of course, is a general rule giving way to certain exceptions when the number of electrons involved is small; for example, reactions involving hydrogen, which has only one electron. However, with such exceptions aside, the rule of eight prevails.

By observing the electron configurations of Na and Cl, we see that Cl has seven electrons in its outermost shell and Na has only 1. When these two species react, Na transfers its lone electron from shell 3 to Cl. The transferred electron enters the partially filled p orbital in shell 4 of the Cl atom.

Recall that previous to this electron transfer we dealt with electrostatically neutral entities. Subsequently, Cl has accepted 1 electron; therefore, it now has an excess of electrons. It has become negatively charged. Sodium, on the other hand, has donated one electron; therefore, it now has an excess of protons. It has become positively charged.

Such charged bodies, those having unequal numbers of protons and electrons, are called **ions.** Ions having an excess number of protons (positively charged) are termed **cations.** Those with an excess of electrons (negatively charged) are **anions.**

By virtue of this electron transfer, we now have an Na$^+$ ion (cation) and a Cl$^-$ ion (anion). The bond that holds the NaCl molecules together is called an **electrovalent** or **ionic bond.** The electrostatic attraction between these opposite charges maintains molecular integrity. Sodium chloride (NaCl) is called an **electrovalent** or **ionic compound.**

Also, note that, by accepting the electron from Na, Cl achieved eight electrons in its outermost electron shell ($n = 3$). At the same time, Na is left with eight electrons within its outermost shell ($n = 2$); hence, the rule of eight applies.

The second type of bond to be discussed is the **covalent bond,** which results from the sharing of one or more pairs of electrons. Covalent bonding results in the formation of covalent molecules.

Let us look at the diatomic molecule of oxygen (O_2). Earlier we saw that the oxygen atom (atomic number 8) has two unpaired electrons in its outermost shell ($n = 2$). Specifically, two of the p orbitals in electron shell 2 have one electron each. Therefore, when two oxygen atoms unite to form molecular O_2, electron sharing occurs between the two atoms. As a result of this sharing, each oxygen atom actually receives its octet, albeit the shared electrons spend equal time between the two oxygen atoms. Traditionally, covalent bonding between oxygen atoms has been shown as follows (Figure 3-5):

$$A \quad O=O \qquad B \quad \overset{\cdot\cdot}{O}::\overset{\cdot\cdot}{O}$$

Figure 3-5. *Two representations of covalent bonding in an oxygen molecule. Two pairs of shared electrons are indicated by (A) two dashes and (B) four dots between the two oxygen atoms.*

However, such depictions do not account for oxygen's magnetic properties because they imply that the two pairs of shared electrons spend an equal amount of time revolving about each atom. Such an implication is not consistent with oxygen's paramagnetic qualities. No representation of molecular oxygen seems to display this property.

Aside from compounds that are either bound by electrovalent or covalent bonds, some compounds are held together by a combination of both. For example, the compound NH_4Cl (ammonium chloride) contains the two bond types. The covalent bonds are located within the ammonium ion (NH_4^+), and the electrovalent bond is between the NH_4^+ and Cl$^-$.

As elements react to form compounds, electrons are either transferred or shared, or both. The electrons involved in these processes are, as we said, the outermost electrons. These are called the **valence electrons.** The **valence** of an atom is the number of electrons transferred (donated or received) in forming ions or the number shared in forming molecules. For example, Na has a valence of 1 because it donates on electron and forms the Na$^+$ cation. The Cl$^-$ anion also has a valence of 1; it receives one electron and becomes Cl$^-$. Oxygen has a valence of 2 because two electrons are involved in the covalent bond formation. Some atoms can share or transfer electrons in more than one way when they react. Iron (Fe), for instance, can have valences of either 2 or 3. The physiologic significance of the oxidation number* change in iron from Fe^{2+} to Fe^{3+} will be discussed in Chapter 6 "Physiologic Chemistry" (Section 6-7, Hemoglobin Biochemistry).

*The oxidation number of an anion or cation is identical to the electrovalence or charge of the ion. However, a sign (+ or −) is shown for the oxidation number, whereas no sign is associated with the valence.

PERIOD TABLE OF ELEMENTS

The periodic table of elements contains over 100 elements. Development of the periodic table began in the late 1700s. The most detailed classification of elements came in 1869 when Mendeleev published his work on the subject. He arranged the elements in periods based on increasing atomic masses. Today's periodic table lists the elements in horizontal rows based on increasing atomic numbers, and provides a large amount of information. Along with each element's symbol, the periodic table lists its atomic number, atomic mass, electron configuration, and oxidation state(s).

The periodic table is comprised of seven horizontal rows called **periods.** The first element in each row or period is an active metal, and the last element in each, save the seventh row, is a noble (inert) gas.

The periodic table can also be viewed as having 18 vertical columns called **groups** or **families.** The elements in each group or family possess similar chemical and physical properties. Because each element is a member of a horizontal row and a vertical column, each element belongs to a period and a group (family).

The electron configuration for the members of each group or family are related. In fact, every group or family member has the same electron configuration in the valence (outer) shell. Helium is an exception to this rule because helium contains only two electrons. The student is directed to the periodic table located on the back cover of this book to view this pattern.

Another noteworthy pattern has to do with the period of elements. The number of the period wherein an element is situated corresponds with the energy level of the element's valence electrons. For example, potassium (K) is situated in period IV and has four principal energy levels (valence electrons in energy level four).

Many other trends, such as electronegativity, atomic radius, and ionic radius, are obtained by the periodic table of elements. However, these and other trends are beyond the scope of this text.

3-2 CHEMICAL LAWS

Within this section the physiologic application of Henry's law of solubility and Graham's law of diffusion will be developed. Henry's law will be applied to oxygen and carbon dioxide gas transport in the plasma. Additionally, conversion factors for changing the partial pressure expressed in torr and mm Hg to volumes percent will be derived for both of these gases. The computation of total carbon dioxide in the blood will also be demonstrated.

Two physiologic applications of Graham's law of diffusion will be presented: (1) for gases within gases and (2) for gases across the alveolar-capillary membrane. Calculations pertaining to the diffusion of gases through these two media (gases and liquids) will be shown.

Henry's Law of Solubility

Henry's law states that the amount of gas that dissolves in a liquid at a given temperature is directly proportional to the partial pressure of the gas above the surface of the liquid. This law applies only to gases that do not chemically react with the solvent.

Figure 3-6 illustrates the effect of an increased pressure on the solubility of a gas. Figure 3-6A represents a dynamic equilibrium state between the gas and the liquid. The double arrows inside the container indicate that the rate at which gas molecules are dissolving in the liquid equals that of the gas molecules escaping the solution.

As the pressure above the liquid's surface increases, as depicted by the large arrow atop the piston in Figure 3-6B, the solubility of the gas increases, and more gas molecules physically dissolve in the liquid.

The amount of oxygen physically dissolved in plasma serves as a physiologic example of Henry's law. Oxygen transported in this form does not chemically combine with plasma. It merely dissolves in the liquid component (plasma) of the blood and exerts a partial pressure in that solution (PaO_2 and $P\bar{v}O_2$).

During the breathing of atmospheric air, an oxygen tension gradient is established between the alveoli and the pulmonary capillary blood. Because a higher oxygen tension is present in the alveoli, oxygen molecules diffuse across the alveolar-capillary membrane

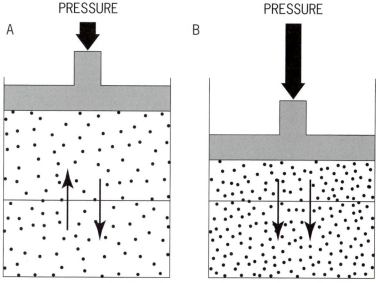

Figure 3-6. *Henry's law of solubility: (A) represents a state of equilibrium between gas dissolving in the liquid and gas escaping from solution (arrows); (B) depicts increased pressure of gas above the liquid (piston forced downward) and more gas molecules dissolving in solution. If the increased pressure is held constant, a new equilibrium state would be established.*

into the pulmonary capillary blood. The pressure gradient for oxygen across the alveolar-capillary membrane is 60 torr. This gradient is comprised of an oxygen partial pressure of 100 torr in the alveoli and approximately 40 torr in the mixed venous blood entering the pulmonary capillaries (i.e., 100 torr − 40 torr = 60 torr).

Henry's law is therapeutically manifested when a patient's FIO_2 is increased in order to increase the PaO_2. What occurs is that more oxygen molecules enter the alveoli (increased PAO_2) because of the increased FIO_2. The increased FIO_2 causes the amount of gas (oxygen) above the surface of the liquid (blood) to increase. Consequently, more oxygen molecules diffuse across the alveolar-capillary membrane and physically dissolve in the plasma, producing a higher PaO_2.

All gases that physically dissolve in plasma obey Henry's law, for example, carbon dioxide and nitrogen.

Each gas has its own **solubility coefficient.** The solubility coefficient is a measurement that depends on the following factors: (1) the solvent (dissolving medium), (2) the temperature, and (3) the pressure. Essentially, the solubility coefficient is the amount of gas that, at a given temperature, can be dissolved by 1 ml of a given liquid at standard pressure.

Physiologically, the solubility coefficient of oxygen is determined in terms of (1) plasma as the solvent, (2) 760 torr Po_2 (standard pressure), and (3) body temperature (37°C). Under these conditions oxygen's solubility coefficient has a value of 0.023. The meaning of this value is that 0.023 ml of oxygen can be dissolved by 1 ml of plasma when oxygen gas exerts a pressure of 760 torr on the plasma at normal body temperature. This description can be shown as

$$0.023 \text{ ml } O_2/\text{ml plasma}/760 \text{ torr } Po_2$$

The solubility coefficient of oxygen has practical applications. An important one is its use in the derivation of the factor for converting dissolved oxygen expressed in terms of *mm Hg* or *torr* to *volumes percent*. Being able to convert the partial pressure of oxygen expressed in mm Hg or torr to volumes percent is useful when one calculates other physiologic measurements such as (1) total arterial oxygen content (CaO_2), (2) total mixed venous oxygen content ($C\bar{v}O_2$), (3) arterial-mixed venous oxygen content difference [$C(a-\bar{v})O_2$], etc. The derivation of this factor follows.

Because 0.023 ml of oxygen dissolves in 1 ml of plasma under a pressure of 760 torr of oxygen, the amount of oxygen able to be dissolved in 1 ml of plasma for each torr of oxygen can be determined by dividing 0.023 ml O_2/ml plasma by 760 torr Po_2. This relationship is shown below.

$$\frac{0.023 \text{ ml } O_2/\text{ml plasma}}{760 \text{ torr}} = 0.00003 \text{ ml } O_2/\text{ml plasma}/\text{torr } Po_2$$

The string of units *ml O_2/ml plasma/torr Po_2* is unwieldy and can be reduced to a more manageable one. However, the cumbersome measurement above can be somewhat simplified by multiplying it by 100 to expand the volume of plasma incorporated in the measurement from 1 to 100 ml. Therefore,

$$0.00003 \text{ ml } O_2/\text{ml plasma}/\text{torr } Po_2 \times 100 \text{ ml plasma} = 0.003 \text{ ml } O_2/100 \text{ ml plasma}/\text{torr } Po_2$$

Physiologic gas volumes are often expressed in terms of volumes percent (vol%). The unit volumes percent means "X" amount of gas (in ml) dissolved in 100 ml of plasma. Therefore, the units ml O_2/100 ml plasma can be expressed as vol%. Hence,

$$0.003 \text{ ml } O_2/100 \text{ ml plasma/torr } P_{O_2}$$

becomes

$$0.003 \text{ vol\%/torr } P_{O_2}$$

Now any P_{O_2} (P_{aO_2} or $P\bar{v}O_2$) value obtained from a sample of blood can be converted to its equivalent in volumes percent. For example, a P_{aO_2} of 100 torr would be changed to volumes percent as follows:

$$(0.003 \text{ vol\%/torr})(100 \text{ torr}) = 0.3 \text{ vol\%}$$

Let's stop for a moment here to consider exactly what 0.3 volumes percent means. Volumes percent refers to some volume of gas dissolved in 100 ml of plasma. So, 0.3 volumes percent means that three-tenths (3/10) of a ml of oxygen is dissolved in 100 ml of plasma. Three-tenths of a ml of oxygen per 100 ml of plasma is very little oxygen.

Consider the left ventricular stroke volume which is the volume of blood pumped out of the left ventricle during each beat of the heart. The left ventricular stroke volume (60 to 80 ml/beat) contains less than 0.3 ml oxygen in the dissolved state.

Generally, we evaluate a patient's oxygenation status by measuring the dissolved oxygen in mm Hg or torr, not in volumes percent. The normal partial pressure of dissolved arterial oxygen is 80 to 100 mm Hg. That value may seem like a large amount of oxygen, but in actuality it is not. A P_{aO_2} of 100 mm Hg represents only 0.3 ml of dissolved oxygen per 100 ml of blood. Thankfully, we have hemoglobin.

The following box highlights the conversion factor that is used to convert any P_{O_2} expressed in torr, or mm Hg, to volumes %.

Formula for Converting P_{O_2} (torr or mm Hg) to vol%
(P_{O_2} torr)(0.003 vol%/torr) = vol%

Another gas of physiologic importance that will be dealt with here is carbon dioxide. The solubility coefficient for carbon dioxide in plasma at 37°C and at 760 torr P_{CO_2} is 0.510, that is,

$$0.510 \text{ ml } CO_2/\text{ml plasma}/760 \text{ torr } P_{CO_2}$$

Reducing this expression to reflect the amount of CO_2 dissolved per ml of plasma per 1 torr P_{CO_2}, it becomes

$$\frac{0.510 \text{ ml } CO_2/\text{ml plasma}}{760 \text{ torr } P_{CO_2}} = 0.00067 \text{ ml } CO_2/\text{ml plasma/torr } P_{CO_2}$$

Incorporating the unit volumes percent, the expression is shown as

$$0.00067 \text{ ml } CO_2/\text{ml plasma/torr } P_{CO_2} \times 100 \text{ ml plasma} = 0.067 \text{ vol\%/torr } P_{CO_2}$$

The factor 0.067 vol%/torr P_{CO_2} can be multiplied by any P_{CO_2} ($PaCO_2$ or $P\bar{v}CO_2$) to provide the volumes percent equivalent for that measurement. For example, a $P\bar{v}CO_2$ of 40 torr would be changed to vol% as follows:

$$(0.067 \text{ vol%/torr})(40 \text{ torr}) = 2.68 \text{ vol%}$$

However, dissolved carbon dioxide quite often needs to be converted to millimoles per liter (mmol/liter), or milliequivalents/liter (mEq/L), rather than being expressed as volumes percent for the purpose of calculating the total CO_2 in the blood. Total blood CO_2 is obtained by adding the amount of physically dissolved CO_2 and the quantity of CO_2 carried in the form of the bicarbonate ion (HCO_3^-). Total CO_2 is expressed in terms of mmol CO_2/liter of blood.

$$
\begin{array}{rcl}
\text{combined } CO_2 = & & HCO_3^- \\
+\text{dissolved } CO_2 = & & +P_{CO_2} \\
\hline
\text{total } CO_2 & & \text{total } CO_2 \text{ (mmol/liter)}
\end{array}
$$

Therefore, the combined CO_2, that is, amount carried as HCO_3^-, is obtained in terms of volumes percent and is converted to mmol CO_2/liter. The dissolved CO_2, obtained as torr or mm Hg, is converted to mmol CO_2/liter.

Volumes percent can be converted to mmol/liter, or mEq/L, as follows:

Step 1: Determine the conversion factor needed to convert volumes percent to millimoles of CO_2 per liter.

$$1 \text{ mmol } CO_2/\text{liter} = X \text{ volumes percent}$$

Step 2: Under standard conditions 1 g molecular weight, or **mole,** of CO_2 occupies a volume of 22.3 liters.*

$$1 \text{ mole } CO_2 \text{ @ STP} = 22.3 \text{ liters, or } 22,300 \text{ ml}$$

Step 3: If a mole of CO_2 occupies 22,300 ml STP, then a millimole (one one-thousandth of a mole) of CO_2 at STP will occupy 22.3 ml.

$$\text{mmol } CO_2 = \frac{22,300 \text{ ml}}{1,000} = 22.3 \text{ ml}$$

Step 4: Now that a millimole of CO_2 has been defined, it is necessary to apply this unit physiologically (i.e., in terms of one liter of plasma). Therefore,

$$1 \text{ mmol } CO_2/\text{liter plasma} = \frac{22.3 \text{ ml } CO_2}{1,000 \text{ ml plasma}}$$

Recall from Step 3 that the volume 22.3 ml represents that volume occupied by a millimole of CO_2 at STP.

---

*Carbon dioxide is not an ideal gas. Therefore, it deviates slightly from the volume (22.4 liters) occupied by an ideal gas at standard temperature (0°C) and standard pressure (760 torr). It occupies 22.3 liters of volume at STP. STP represents standard temperature and standard pressure.

Step 5: Ordinarily, gas volumes in plasma are expressed as volumes percent (ml/100 ml plasma) and not as ml/1,000 ml plasma. Therefore,

$$22.3 \text{ ml } CO_2/1{,}000 \text{ ml plasma} = 2.23 \text{ ml } CO_2/100 \text{ ml plasma}$$

Note the difference in the placement of the decimal point.

Step 6: Recall that the expression *volumes percent*, which represents some volume of gas dissolved in 100 ml of plasma, is abbreviated as *vol%*. Hence,

$$2.23 \text{ ml } CO_2/100 \text{ ml plasma} = 2.23 \text{ vol\%}$$

Step 7: Therefore, 1 mmol CO_2 per liter of plasma equals 2.23 vol% of CO_2. Consequently,

$$\text{mmol } CO_2/\text{liter} = \frac{\text{vol\%}}{2.23 \text{ vol\%/mmol } CO_2/\text{liter}}$$

Therefore, there are 2.23 vol% of CO_2 per mmol CO_2/liter. When dividing this factor into the amount of combined CO_2 (i.e., HCO_3^-), the units vol% cancel and the answer is expressed as mmol CO_2/liter.

EXAMPLE 1:

Convert 53.5 vol% of CO_2 to mmol/liter.

Step 1: Recall the relationship between volumes percent (vol%) and millimoles/liter (mmol/liter) for carbon dioxide.

$$\text{mmol } CO_2/\text{liter} = \frac{\text{vol\%}}{2.23 \text{ vol\%/mmol } CO_2/\text{liter}}$$

Step 2: Divide 53.5 vol% by 2.23 vol%/mmol CO_2/liter and cancel units accordingly.

$$\text{mmol } CO_2/\text{liter} = \frac{53.5 \text{ vol\%}}{2.23 \text{ vol\%/mmol } CO_2/\text{liter}}$$

$$= 24 \text{ mmol } CO_2/\text{liter}$$

EXAMPLE 2:

Convert 1.2 mmol CO_2/liter to vol%.

Step 1: Rearrange the original relationship between vol% and mmol/liter to solve for vol%.

$$\text{vol\%} = (\text{mmol } CO_2/\text{liter})(2.23 \text{ vol\%/mmol } CO_2/\text{liter})$$

Step 2: Multiply (1.2 mmol CO_2/liter) by (2.23 vol%/mmol CO_2/liter) and cancel units accordingly.

$$\text{vol\%} = (1.2 \text{ mmol } CO_2/\text{liter})(2.23 \text{ vol\%/mmol } CO_2/\text{liter})$$

$$= 2.68 \text{ vol\%}$$

The factor used for changing mm Hg or torr to mmol CO_2/liter is derived from the carbon dioxide solubility coefficient mentioned previously, that is, 0.510 ml CO_2/ml plasma/760 torr P_{CO_2}. The CO_2 solubility coefficient was reduced to 0.067 vol%/torr P_{CO_2}. Therefore,

$$\frac{0.067 \text{ vol\%/torr } P_{CO_2}}{2.23 \text{ vol\%/mmol } CO_2/\text{liter}} = 0.03 \text{ mmol } CO_2/\text{liter/torr } P_{CO_2}$$

Any P_{CO_2} can now be converted to mmol CO_2/liter by

$$(P_{CO_2})(0.03 \text{ mmol } CO_2/\text{liter/torr})$$

Note the following equation illustrating a P_{CO_2} of 40 torr being converted to mmol CO_2/liter.

$$(40 \text{ torr})(0.03 \text{ mmol } CO_2/\text{liter/torr}) = 1.2 \text{ mmol } CO_2/\text{liter}$$

EXAMPLE:

Calculate the total CO_2 when the $PaCO_2$ is 30 torr and the combined CO_2 is 60 vol%.

Step 1: Convert the $PaCO_2$ of 30 torr to mmol CO_2/liter.

$$(30 \text{ torr})(0.03 \text{ mmol } CO_2/\text{liter/torr}) = 0.9 \text{ mmol } CO_2/\text{liter}$$

Step 2: Convert 60 vol% to mmol CO_2/liter.

$$\frac{60 \text{ vol\%}}{2.23 \text{ vol\%/mmol } CO_2/\text{liter}} = 26.9 \text{ mmol } CO_2/\text{liter}$$

Step 3: Add the combined CO_2 to the dissolved CO_2 to determine the total CO_2.

$$\begin{array}{l} 26.9 \text{ mmol } CO_2/\text{liter (combined } CO_2) \\ + \ 0.9 \text{ mmol } CO_2/\text{liter (dissolved } CO_2) \\ \hline 27.8 \text{ mmol } CO_2/\text{liter (total } CO_2) \end{array}$$

The following box highlights the conversion factors used in conjunction with carbon dioxide transport calculations.

Conversion Factors Associated with CO_2 Transport Calculations	
• to convert P_{CO_2} (torr or mm Hg) to vol%	$(P_{CO_2} \text{ torr})(0.067 \text{ vol\%/torr}) = \text{vol\%}$
• to convert CO_2 in vol% to mmol/L, or mEq/L	$\dfrac{CO_2 \text{ vol\%}}{2.23 \text{ vol\%/mmol/L}} = \text{mmol/L}$
• to convert P_{CO_2} (torr or mm Hg) to mmol/L, or mEq/L	$(P_{CO_2} \text{ torr})(0.03 \text{ mmol/L/torr}) = \text{mmol/L}$

PRACTICE PROBLEMS

Refer to Appendix A (pages 584-586) for the solutions and answers to the practice problems.

Convert the following partial pressures of oxygen to vol%:

1. 60 mm Hg _____
2. 100 torr _____
3. 40 torr _____
4. 1,900 mm Hg _____
5. 760 mm Hg _____

Convert the following partial pressures of carbon dioxide to vol%:

6. 40 torr _____
7. 75 mm Hg _____
8. 25 torr _____
9. 63 mm Hg _____
10. 760 torr _____

Convert the following carbon dioxide levels expressed as vol% to mmol/L (mEq/L):

11. 2.68 vol% _____
12. 56.20 vol% _____
13. 53.52 vol% _____
14. 18.37 vol% _____
15. 37.81 vol% _____

Convert the following partial pressures of carbon dioxide to mmol/L (mEq/L):

16. 40 mm Hg _____
17. 25 mm Hg _____
18. 65 torr _____
19. 90 torr _____
20. 760 torr _____

Calculate either the dissolved, combined, or total CO_2 in the following problems:

21. Calculate the combined CO_2 in mmol/liter, when the $PaCO_2$ is 40 mm Hg and the total CO_2 is 53.50 vol%. _____
22. Calculate the $PaCO_2$ in torr when the total CO_2 is 35 mmol/liter and the combined CO_2 is 75.05 vol%. _____
23. Calculate the combined CO_2 in mmol/L when the dissolved CO_2 is 4.0 vol% and the total CO_2 is 44.0 vol%. _____

24. Calculate the dissolved CO_2 in torr when the combined CO_2 is 27.1 mEq/L and the total CO_2 is 63.6 vol%. _____

25. Calculate the total CO_2 in mEq/L when the dissolved CO_2 is 1.7 mEq/L and the combined CO_2 is 42.37 vol%. _____

Graham's Law of Diffusion

The movement of gas molecules from one area of a system to another resulting from random molecular motion is called **diffusion.** Gas molecules move independently of one another continually bombarding the walls of the containing vessel and colliding with each other. After impacting with each other and/or with the container walls, the gas molecules rebound elastically, that is, with no net loss of kinetic energy. Their chaotic, random motion carries them to regions of higher or lower concentration. There is no way of predicting the location or direction of a specific gas molecule. Over time, however, a mixture of gases will equilibrate because gases diffuse from an area of high partial pressure (concentration) to a region of low partial pressure (concentration). Gas diffusion depends on concentration gradients and not on volume differences.

Despite the extremely rapid velocity possessed by gas molecules (average velocity of N_2 gas at room temperature is 1,150 miles/hour), gaseous diffusion proceeds at a much slower rate than anticipated. Molecular collisions slow the diffusion process. Because of frequent molecular collisions, gas molecules are constantly changing their direction of travel. The motion of gas molecules is characterized as zig-zag, random, and chaotic, thereby impeding the diffusion process.

Figure 3-7 illustrates the hypothetical pathway of one gas molecule within a container. The black dot represents the point of origin in tracing this gas molecule's hypothetical pathway. Note the jagged (zig-zag) nature of this molecular path. Each jagged point represents a collision with another gas molecule and a change of direction. The ultimate path taken by a gas molecule is comprised by innumerable short, straight-line segments. The dashed line with the arrow indicates the net displacement, or distance traveled, by the gas molecule.

Two aspects of Graham's law will be considered. The first concerns the diffusion of a gas within a gas and the second the diffusion of a gas through a liquid.

The law governing the diffusion of a gas within a gas states that lighter molecules will diffuse and equilibrate faster than heavier molecules when both intermingle with one another within a container. Quantitatively speaking, the relative rates of diffusion (r) are inversely proportional to the square root of the densities (D). For example,

$$\frac{r_1}{r_2} = \frac{\sqrt{D_2}}{\sqrt{D_1}}$$

or

$$r_1 \sqrt{D_1} = r_2 \sqrt{D_2}$$

Because the mass of the gas molecule is reciprocally related to the square of the gas molecule's velocity, the square root of the densities can be replaced by the square root of the molecular weights.

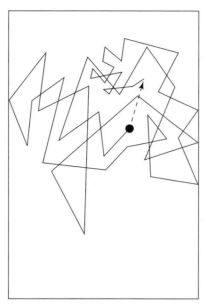

Figure 3-7. *Motion of a hypothetical gas molecule in a container. The black dot signifies the starting point. Each jagged point in the path represents a molecular collision. Each straight line indicates unimpeded motion. The dashed line with the arrow signifies the net distance traveled by the gas molecule. Molecular collisions slow the diffusion process.*

The relative rates of diffusion of O_2 and CO_2 will be used to demonstrate this substitution. The density of molecular oxygen is 1.43 g/liter and that of CO_2 is 1.96 g/liter. Oxygen's rate of diffusion will be represented by ro_2 and rco_2 will represent the carbon dioxide diffusion rate.

$$\frac{ro_2}{rco_2} = \frac{\sqrt{1.96 \text{ g/liter}}}{\sqrt{1.43 \text{ g/liter}}}$$

$$= \frac{1.400}{1.195}$$

$$ro_2 = 1.17 \, rco_2$$

Substituting the square root of the molecular weights for the square roots of the densities yields the expression

$$\frac{ro_2}{rco_2} = \frac{\sqrt{44}}{\sqrt{32}}$$

$$= \frac{6.633}{5.657}$$

$$ro_2 = 1.17 \, rco_2$$

Both expressions show that oxygen diffuses 1.17 times faster than the carbon dioxide. Therefore, when considering the activity of these two gases within an alveolus, Graham's law relating to the diffusion of a gas within a gas shows that oxygen diffuses faster than carbon dioxide.

On the basis of the kinetic theory of matter, increasing gas temperature increases gas velocity and accelerates the rate of diffusion. Physiologically, gas temperature would not be much of a consideration because, under ordinary circumstances, body temperature does not fluctuate to a great extent. Therefore, the average kinetic energy, $1/2\ mv^2$, for gas molecules in the alveoli can be considered constant throughout the lungs.

The diffusion rate of gases through a liquid can be determined by examining factors peculiar to the situation under consideration. Graham's law of diffusion relating to the diffusion of gases into a liquid incorporates the *solubility coefficient* of each gas, which, in turn, takes into consideration (1) the nature of the solvent, (2) the temperature, and (3) the pressure.

Mathematically, Graham's law describing gaseous diffusion through a liquid medium is

$$\frac{r_1}{r_2} = \frac{\sqrt{D_2}(Cs_1)}{\sqrt{D_1}(Cs_2)}$$

where

r = rate of gas diffusion

D = gas density (molecular weights can also be substituted)

Cs = solubility coefficient of the gas

The equation shows that the relative rates of diffusion of two gases are inversely proportional to the square roots of their densities (molecular weights) and directly proportional to their solubility coefficients. Comparing the relative rates of diffusion of carbon dioxide and oxygen across the alveolar-capillary membrane, a fluid barrier, the equation is shown as

$$\frac{r_{CO_2}}{r_{O_2}} = \frac{(\sqrt{D_{O_2}})(Cs_{CO_2})}{(\sqrt{D_{CO_2}})(Cs_{O_2})}$$

$$= \frac{(\sqrt{1.43\ g/L})(0.510)}{(\sqrt{1.96\ g/L})(0.023)}$$

$$= \frac{(1.195)(0.510)}{(1.400)(0.023)}$$

$$= \frac{0.609}{0.032}$$

$$r_{CO_2} = 19\ r_{O_2}$$

The equation shows that carbon dioxide is 19 times more diffusible across the alveolar-capillary membrane than is oxygen.

It is important to make a distinction here between the relative rates of diffusion of carbon dioxide and oxygen, as gases diffusing within a gas mixture and as gases diffusing

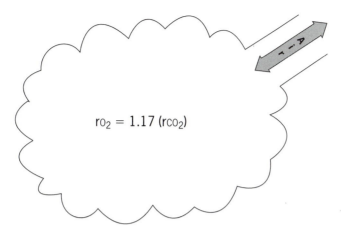

$$r_{O_2} = 1.17\ (r_{CO_2})$$

Figure 3-8. *An alveolus within which O_2 molecules diffuse 1.17 times faster than CO_2 molecules, (i.e., $r_{O_2} = 1.17 \times r_{CO_2}$), based on Graham's law governing the diffusion of gases within a gaseous medium.*

through a liquid. Oxygen diffuses 1.17 times faster than carbon dioxide within a gas mixture, for example, *within* an alveolus. Carbon dioxide diffuses 19 times faster than oxygen *across* the alveolar-capillary membrane.

Figure 3-8 represents an alveolus within which oxygen and carbon dioxide gas move (diffuse) via the kinetic energy imparted on the gas molecules by the body's temperature. Bear in mind that within an acinus (respiratory bronchioles, alveolar ducts, and alveolar sacs) air movement is accomplished by way of molecular diffusion, not by convection or bulk flow. Oxygen molecules move faster within these structures then do carbon dioxide molecules.

Figure 3-9 depicts an alveolar-capillary membrane across which oxygen and carbon dioxide molecules diffuse as a result of concentration gradients for these two gases between the alveolus and the blood in the pulmonary capillary. Because of its greater lipid solubility, carbon dioxide diffuses faster than oxygen across the alveolar-capillary membrane.

Another application of Graham's law regarding gases diffusing through a liquid medium is in determining the factor used for converting the carbon monoxide (CO) diffusing capacity across the alveolar-capillary membrane in terms of oxygen. By multiplying the carbon monoxide diffusing capacity by 1.23, one can convert the carbon monoxide diffusing capacity to that of oxygen. This factor (1.23) is obtained by using Graham's law as follows:

$$\frac{r_{O_2}}{r_{CO}} = \frac{(\sqrt{\text{molecular wt. CO}})(C_sO_2)}{(\sqrt{\text{molecular wt. O}_2})(C_sCO)}$$

$$= \frac{(\sqrt{28})(0.023)}{(\sqrt{32})(0.0175)}$$

$$= \frac{(5.292)(0.023)}{(5.650)(0.0175)}$$

$$r_{O_2} = 1.23\ r_{CO}$$

The utility of this factor is to convert the measured carbon monoxide lung diffusing capacity (D_LCO) to that for oxygen. By multiplying the D_LCO by 1.23, the D_LO_2 can be

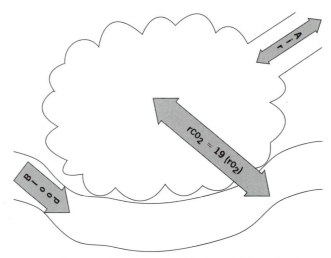

Figure 3-9. *An alveolar-capillary membrane across which O_2 and CO_2 molecules traverse. CO_2 molecules passively diffuse 19 times faster than O_2 molecules, based on Graham's law governing the diffusion of gases through a liquid medium.*

estimated. For example, the average D_LCO for a normal, resting subject is about 30 ml/min/mm Hg (STPD). The approximate D_LO_2 can be obtained as follows:

$$D_LCO \times 1.23 = D_LO_2$$

$$(30 \text{ ml/min/mm Hg})(1.23) = 37 \text{ ml/min/mm Hg}$$

PRACTICE PROBLEMS

Refer to Appendix A (pages 586-587) for the solutions and answers to the practice problems.

Calculate the following problems according to Graham's law of diffusion for either a gas within a gas or a gas through a liquid:

26. How much more diffusible is gaseous hydrogen (2 amu) than gaseous oxygen (32 amu)? _____

27. Calculate the relative rate of diffusion for methane gas (CH_4 = 16 amu) and phosgene gas ($COCl_2$ = 99 amu).

28. The solubility coefficients for CO_2 and O_2 in water at 38°C are 55.0 and 2.4, respectively. How much more diffusible is CO_2 than O_2 in this medium? _____

29. Determine the relative rate of diffusion for nitrous oxide (N_2O: solubility coefficient 0.41, molecular weight 44 amu) and cyclopropane (C_3H_6: solubility coefficient 0.011, molecular weight 42 amu) in water at 38°C. _____

30. Compare the rate of diffusion of O_2 (molecular weight 32 amu; solubility coefficient 0.023) to CO (molecular weight 28 amu; solubility coefficient 0.0175) across the alveolar-capillary membrane. _____

3-3 MOLARITY AND NORMALITY

Two forms of expressing the concentration of solutions (i.e., molarity and normality) will be discussed. The topics are offered here to aid the reader in understanding the concepts of drug concentrations and physiologic solutions.

Before molarity and normality are discussed a number of definitions need to be presented. A **solution** is a homogeneous substance formed by the mixture of one or more solutes and a solvent. The **solute** is the substance being dissolved, and the **solvent** is the medium in which the solute is dissolved. A **dilute** solution is one in which a relatively small amount of solute is present in proportion to solvent.

Molar Solutions

A molar solution is defined as the number of gram molecular weights, gram-moles, or moles of solute per liter of solution. A mole is the quantity of a substance whose weight in grams is numerically equal to the substance's molecular weight in atomic mass units (amu). For example, 32 g of oxygen, 44 g of carbon dioxide, or 98 g of sulfuric acid (H_2SO_4) all represent 1 mole. The following formula shows how the number of moles can be calculated when the weight (grams) and the gram molecular weight of a compound are given.

$$\text{No. of moles} = \frac{\text{No. of grams}}{\text{gram molecular weight}}$$

EXAMPLE 1:

Determine the number of moles of chlorine present in 106.5 g (gram molecular weight of $Cl_2 = 71$ g).

$$(106.5 \cancel{g})\left(\frac{1 \text{ mole}}{71 \cancel{g}}\right) = 1.5 \text{ moles}$$

The formula for calculating molarity is

$$\text{molarity (M)} = \frac{\text{moles (m)}}{\text{liter (L)}}$$

EXAMPLE 2:

Calculate the molarity of a 200 ml solution containing 16 g of CH_3OH. (See Periodic Table on inside back cover for atomic weights.)

Step 1:   Convert 16 g of CH_3OH to moles (molecular weight of $CH_3OH = 32$ amu).

$$\frac{16 \text{ g}}{32 \text{ amu}} = 0.5 \text{ mole } CH_3OH$$

Step 2: Convert 200 ml to liters.

$$1 \text{ ml} = 10^{-3} \text{ liter}$$

$$200 \text{ ml} \times 10^{-3} \text{ liter/ml} = 0.2 \text{ liter}$$

Step 3: Apply the molarity formula.

$$M = \text{mole/liter}$$

$$= \frac{0.5 \text{ mole CH}_3\text{OH}}{0.2 \text{ liter}}$$

$$= 2.5 \text{ M}$$

PRACTICE PROBLEMS

Refer to the Periodic Table on the inside back cover for atomic weight values and to Appendix A (pages 587-588) for the solutions and answers to the practice problems.

Calculate the number of moles contained in the following substances:

31. 98 g H_3PO_4 _____

32. 513 g $C_{12}H_{22}O_{11}$ _____

33. 138,000 mg C_2H_6O _____

34. 68 g $C_3H_8O_3$ _____

35. 133,400 g Hb _____

Calculate the following molarity problems. **(Refer to the Periodic Table on the inside back cover for atomic weights.)**

36. Calculate the molarity of a solution containing 60 g of acetic acid (CH_3COOH) in 1,000 ml.

_____

37. Determine the weight (g) of $C_{12}H_{22}O_{11}$ in 60 ml of a 3 M solution.

_____

38. How many milliliters of a 0.1 M NaOH solution contain 8 grams?

_____

39. What is the molarity if a KOH solution in which 10 grams of KOH are added to 1 liter of water?

_____

40. How many grams of H_3PO_4 are present in a 0.110 M solution?

_____

Normal Solutions

A normal solution is defined as the number of gram equivalent weights of solute per liter of solution. The term **gram equivalent weight** can be defined numerous ways, for instance, as the weight in grams of an acid that contains 1 mole of replaceable hydrogen ions or as the weight in grams of a base that contains 1 mole of replaceable hydroxyl ions (OH^-). Usually, the simplest method for obtaining the gram equivalent weight (Eq) of any substance (acid, base, salt, radical, or element) is to divide the gram molecular weight of the substance by the valence of that substance. If the valence is negative, disregard the negative sign and divide the gram molecular weight by the numerical value. Note the following examples.

EXAMPLE 1:

Find the weight Eq of one gram equivalent weight of H_2SO_4.

$$H_2SO_4 \rightarrow 2H^+ + SO_4^{-2}$$

Since H_2SO_4 ionizes into two H^+ ions (two positive charges) and one sulfate radical (two negative charges), divide the gram molecular weight by 2.

$$(98 \text{ g/mole})\left(\frac{1 \text{ mole}}{2 \text{ Eq}}\right) = 49 \text{ g/Eq}$$

Forty-nine grams of H_2SO_4 represent one gram equivalent weight (Eq) of H_2SO_4. Ninety-eight grams of H_2SO_4 would be two Eq, and 24.5 g would be 0.5 Eq for this substance.

EXAMPLE 2:

Find the weight Eq of one gram equivalent weight of NaOH.

$$NaOH \rightarrow Na^+ + OH^-$$

Since NaOH ionizes into one Na^+ ion (one positive charge) and one OH^- ion (one negative charge), divide the gram molecular weight by one. Because NaOH is a monovalent compound, its gram molecular weight (40 g) is identical to its gram equivalent weight.

$$(40 \text{ g/mole})\left(\frac{1 \text{ mole}}{1 \text{ Eq}}\right) = 40 \text{ g/Eq}$$

This situation is true for all monovalent compounds, that is, their molecular weights and gram equivalent weights are equal. Therefore, 40 g of NaOH is 1 Eq and 1 mole; 80 g would be 2 gram equivalent weights and 2 moles; 20 g would be 0.5 Eq of each.

EXAMPLE 3:

Find the weight Eq of one gram equivalent weight of $Al_2(SO_4)_3$.

$$Al_2(SO_4)_3 \rightarrow Al^{+3} + 3 SO_4^{-2}$$

Since $Al_2(SO_4)_3$ ionizes into two cations (six positive charges) and three anions (six negative charges), divide the gram molecular weight by 6. The gram molecular weight of $Al_2(SO_4)_3$ is 342 g. Thus,

$$(342 \text{ g/mole})\left(\frac{1 \text{ mole}}{6 \text{ Eq}}\right) = 57 \text{ g/Eq}$$

Hence, 57 g of $Al_2(SO_4)_3$ represent 1 Eq of $Al_2(SO_4)_3$, 114 g would be 2, and 28.5 g would be 0.5 Eq of this compound.

The formula for determining normality is

$$\text{normality (N)} = \frac{\text{gram equivalent weight (Eq)}}{\text{liter (L)}}$$

EXAMPLE 4:

Calculate the normality of a liter solution containing 100 g of $Al_2(SO_4)_3$.

Step 1:   Calculate the gram molecular weight of $Al_2(SO_4)_3$.

$$Al = 27 \text{ g}$$
$$S = 32 \text{ g}$$
$$O = 16 \text{ g}$$

Gram atomic weights of constituent atoms of $Al_2(SO_4)_3$.

$$(2 \times 27 \text{ g}) + (3 \times 32 \text{ g}) + (12 \times 16 \text{ g}) = 342 \text{ g}$$

↑	↑	↑
2 Al	3 S	12 O
atoms	atoms	atoms

Step 2:   Calculate the weight of 1 Eq of $Al_2(SO_4)_3$.

$$(342 \text{ g/mole})\left(\frac{1 \text{ mole}}{1 \text{ Eq}}\right) = 57 \text{ g/Eq} = 1 \text{ Eq}$$

Because this compound would ionize as $Al_2(SO_4)_3 \rightarrow 2Al^{+3} + 3SO_4^{-2}$, the gram molecular weight is divided by 6.

Step 3:   Determine the number of Eq of $Al_2(SO_4)_3$ that are present in 100 grams of $Al_2(SO_4)_3$.

$$\frac{100 \text{ g}}{57 \text{ g/Eq}} = 1.75 \text{ Eq}$$

Step 4:   Calculate the normality.

$$N = \frac{Eq}{L}$$

$$= \frac{1.75 \text{ Eq}}{1 \text{ L}}$$

$$= 1.75 \text{ N}$$

PRACTICE PROBLEMS

Refer to the Periodic Table on the inside back cover for atomic weight values and to Appendix A (pages 588-590) for the solutions and answers to the practice problems.

Determine the number of equivalents in the weights of the following substances. (Assume complete dissociation or ionization.)

41. 24 g H_2SO_4 _____

42. 28 g $AlCl_3$ _____

43. 200 g H_3PO_4 _____

44. 100 g $Zn(OH)_2$ _____

45. 62 g H_2CO_3 _____

Calculate the following problems concerning normality. (Assume complete dissociation or ionization.)

46. What is the normality of a solution containing 2.45 g of H_2SO_4 in 800 ml of solution?

_____

47. Calculate the normality of a 1 M solution of H_2SO_4.

_____

48. How many grams of NaOH need to be added to 2 liters of solution to prepare a 0.25 N NaOH solution?

_____

49. Find the number of grams of KOH that are needed to prepare 1 liter of 0.3 N KOH solution.

_____

50. What weight (mg) of solute is contained in 50 ml of a 0.01 N $Ca(OH)_2$ solution?

_____

3-4 LAW OF MASS ACTION AND HENDERSON-HASSELBALCH EQUATION

The physiologic importance of limiting the change in the hydrogen ion concentration within body fluid compartments is well recognized. Wide pH shifts can interfere with various metabolic processes. This section discusses the chemical and mathematical basis for acid-base relationships. The reader should consult any respiratory physiology text for presentations of acid-base physiology.

pH Concepts

An acid can be defined as a substance that releases hydrogen ions (H^+), or donates protons. In other words, an acid is a substance that increases the hydrogen ion concentration of a solution. A base is described as a compound that provides hydroxyl ions (OH⁻). Solutions that have greater amounts of H⁺ ions, as compared to the number of OH⁻ ions present, are said to be **acidic.** Conversely, solutions having a greater concentration of OH⁻ ions relative to their H⁺ ion concentration are termed **basic** or **alkaline.**

The acidity and alkalinity of a solution can be quantitatively expressed as either **pH** or **pOH,** respectively. Specifically, what these measurements represent is the molar concentration (moles/liter) of hydrogen ions (H⁺) and hydroxyl ions (OH⁻) in solution.

For example, the concentration of both H⁺ and OH⁻ ions in a pure water solution is the same; that is, in a liter of such a solution the weight of the H⁺ ions is 0.0000001 g, (10^{-7} moles/liter), and the weight of the OH⁻ ions is 0.0000017 g (10^{-7} moles/liter). Thus, water solutions are neutral; they contain equal amounts of acid and base components.

If the pH of a solution increases, the pOH decreases. Conversely, if the pH decreases, the pOH increases. For example, a pH of 3 is the same as a pOH of 11.

A pH scale is shown in Figure 3-10. The range of the pH scale is 0–14. As mentioned, a pH of 7 is neutral, for instance, the pH of water. As the numerical value for pH diminishes, the solution becomes more acidic and less alkaline. The converse is also true.

The mathematical expressions indicating pH are

$$pH = \log\left(\frac{1}{[H^+]}\right)$$

that is, the logarithm of the reciprocal of the hydrogen ion concentration, or

$$pH = -\log\ [H^+]$$

that is, the negative logarithm of the hydrogen ion concentration. The symbol [ ] indicates concentration expressed in moles/liter.

Recall (Chapter 1, Section 1-8, "Logarithms") that the logarithm of a quantity (number) is the power to which the base 10 must be raised to equal that number. For example, the log of 0.001, or 10^{-3}, is −3.

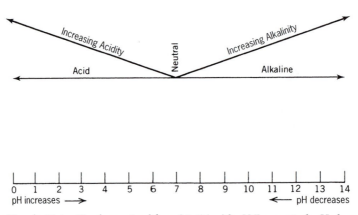

Figure 3-10. *pH scale. Note pH values extend from 0 to 14 with pH 7 as neutral. pH above 7 is alkaline and pH below 7 is acid.*

Problems involving pH can be solved by using either equation. For example, determine the pH of a solution having a hydrogen ion concentration of 0.000001 M (10^{-6} moles/liter).

$$pH = \log\left(\frac{1}{[H^+]}\right)$$

$$= \log\left(\frac{1}{10^{-6}}\right) \qquad \text{Note:} \quad \frac{1}{10^{-6}} = 10^6$$

$$= \log 1 + \log 10^6$$

$$= \log 10^6$$

$$= 6$$

Alternatively,

$$pH = -\log [H^+]$$

$$= -\log (10^{-6})$$

$$= \log 10^6$$

$$= 6$$

IF YOU HAVE A CALCULATOR WITH A LOG FUNCTION,

The log $\dfrac{1}{10^{-6}}$ can be quickly determined using any calculator having a log function. For example press the following calculator keys.

PRESS: 10 $\boxed{y^x}$ 6 $\boxed{+/-}$ $\boxed{=}$ $\boxed{\log}$ $\boxed{+/-}$

However, knowing that

$$\frac{1}{10^{-6}} = 10^6$$

you may **PRESS:** 10 $\boxed{y^x}$ 6 $\boxed{=}$ $\boxed{\log}$

Remember that the expression $\log 10^6 = 6$ asks the question, "To what power (logarithm or exponent) must the base 10 be raised to obtain one million (10^6)?" The value 6 to the right of the equal sign represents the power to which the base 10 must be raised to produce the number 1,000,000, that is, 10^6.

The hydrogen ion concentration is not always present in integer powers of 10. Consequently, their logarithms must be obtained by referring to a log table or by using a calculation. Consider the following example. Find the pH of a solution having a hydrogen ion concentration of 0.000053 M.

Step 1: Use either mathematical expression to solve for pH.

$$pH = -\log [H^+]$$

Step 2: Insert the value given for [H⁺].

$$pH = -\log (0.000053)$$
$$= -\log (5.30 \times 10^{-5})$$
$$= -\log 5.30 + (-\log 10^{-5})$$
$$= -.7243 - (-5)$$
$$= -.7243 + 5$$
$$= 4.28$$

Alternatively,

$$pH = \log\left(\frac{1}{[H^+]}\right)$$
$$= \log\left(\frac{1}{0.000053}\right)$$
$$= \log 18867.9$$
$$= 4.28$$

IF YOU HAVE A CALCULATOR WITH A LOG FUNCTION,

The -log (0.000053) can be quickly determined using any calculator having a log function. For example, press the following calculator keys.

PRESS: .000053 ⌊log⌋ ⌊+/−⌋

Keep in mind that a pH change of one represents a 10-fold change in hydrogen ion concentration. For example,

A.
$$[H^+] = 10^{-7} \text{ mole/liter}$$
$$pH = -\log 10^{-7}$$
$$= \log 10^7$$
$$= 7$$

B.
$$[H^+] = 10^{-6} \text{ mole/liter}$$
$$pH = -\log 10^{-6}$$
$$= \log 10^6$$
$$= 6$$

Example A shows a pH of 7 and example B shows a pH of 6. A pH drop from pH 7 to pH 6 is equivalent to a 10-fold increase in the hydrogen ion concentration. Furthermore, a decrease of 0.3 pH reflects a doubling of the hydrogen ion concentration. These relationships are a result of the logarithmic nature of the pH scale.

TABLE 3-6 Hydrogen Ion Concentration: nmol/L vs. pH

pH	nanomoles/liter	pH	nanomoles/liter
8.00	10	7.37	43
7.52	30	7.36	44
7.50	32	7.35	45
7.45	35	7.34	46
7.44	36	7.33	47
7.43	37	7.32	48
7.42	38	7.31	49
7.41	39	7.30	50
7.40	40	7.26	55
7.39	41	7.25	56
7.38	42	7.00	100

To avoid using logarithms when expressing the hydrogen ion concentration of a solution, the unit **nanomoles** (nmol) is sometimes used. The Greek prefix "nano-" represents one one-billionth, or 10^{-9}. The unit nanomole, therefore, indicates one one-billionth of a mole, or 10^{-9} mole.

Table 3-6 compares the hydrogen ion concentration expressed in pH units (logarithmic units) and in nanomoles per liter.

Normal arterial blood pH 7.40 corresponds to 40 nanomoles/liter, or 40×10^{-9} mole/liter. The normal arterial blood pH range of 7.35 to 7.45 is equivalent to a nanomole/liter range of 45 to 35. As pH increases, the number of nanomoles/liter decreases. Likewise, as pH decreases the hydrogen ion concentration in nanomoles/liter increases.

Table 3-6 also indicates that a 0.01 pH unit change within the range of 7.35 to 7.45 (normal range for arterial blood) is associated with a hydrogen ion concentration change of approximately 1 nanomole/liter. This relationship between pH units and nanomoles/liter is useful in its clinical application. However, it is an approximation only.

Figure 3-11 shows the relationship between the Pco_2 in arterial blood and arterial blood hydrogen ion concentration in nanomoles/liter. This relationship is represented at three different blood bicarbonate concentrations, namely 12 mmol/liter, 24 mmol/liter, and 48 mmol/liter.

When the Pco_2 is 40 mm Hg and the HCO_3^- is 24 mmol/liter, the $[H^+]$ is 40×10^{-9} moles/liter or 40 nanomoles/liter. Since a Pco_2 of 40 mm Hg and a $[HCO_3^-]$ of 24 mmol/liter result in a combined CO_2/dissolved CO_2 ratio of 20:1,* the pH will be 7.40. Therefore, a hydrogen ion concentration of 40 nanomoles/liter is equivalent to a pH of 7.40.

---

*The following ratios refer to the base-to-acid ratio in the blood:

$$\frac{\text{kidney function}}{\text{lung function}} = \frac{\text{combined } CO_2}{\text{dissolved } CO_2} = \frac{24 \text{ mmol/liter}}{40 \text{ mm Hg} \times 0.03} = \frac{24 \text{ mmol/liter}}{1.2 \text{ mmol/liter}} = \frac{20}{1}$$

In this physiologic example, millimoles CO_2/liter = milliequivalents CO_2/liter.

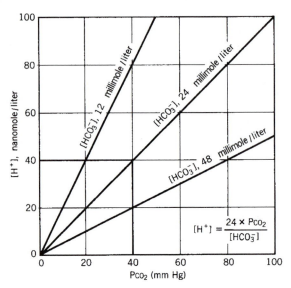

Figure 3-11. *Graphic representation of the relationship between* P_{CO_2} *(mm Hg) and the* [H^+] *in nanomoles/ liter at* [HCO_3^-] *of 12, 24, and 48 mmol/liter. From Adams, A. P., Hahn, C. E. W.: Principles and Practice of Blood Gas Analysis, Franklin Scientific Projects, Ltd., 1979, London, England. Used with permission.*

Hydrogen ion concentrations given in nanomoles/liter can be easily converted to pH units as follows:

$$pH = 9 - \text{log of the } H^+ \text{ ion concentration in nanomoles/liter}$$

For example, convert 40 nanomoles/liter to its corresponding pH unit.

$$pH = 9 - \log 40$$
$$= 9 - 1.60$$
$$= 7.40$$

IF YOU HAVE A CALCULATOR WITH A LOG FUNCTION,

The expression $9 - \log 40$ can be quickly determined using any calculator having a log function. For example, press the following calculator keys.

PRESS: 9 $\boxed{-}$ $\boxed{(}$ 40 $\boxed{\log}$ $\boxed{)}$ $\boxed{=}$

Similarly, hydrogen ion concentration expressed as pH can be changed to moles/liter by the equation

$$\text{moles/liter} = \text{antilog} (-pH)$$

For instance, given pH 7.40, find the number of moles of hydrogen ions per liter.

$$\text{moles/liter} = \text{antilog} (-7.40)$$

$$= \left(\frac{1}{\text{antilog pH}} \right)$$

$$= \left(\frac{1}{\text{antilog } 7.40} \right)$$

$$= \frac{1}{.250 \times 10^8}$$

$$= 4.0 \times 10^{-8}$$

$$= 40 \times 10^{-9}$$

IF YOU HAVE A CALCULATOR WITH A LOG FUNCTION,

The antilog (-7.40) can be quickly determined using any calculator having a log function. For example, press the following calculator keys.

PRESS: 7.4 $\boxed{\text{INV}}$ $\boxed{\text{log}}$ $\boxed{1/x}$

Alternatively, hydrogen ion concentration expressed in pH units can be converted to nanomoles/liter as follows:

$$\text{nanomoles/liter} = \text{antilog } (9 - \text{pH})$$

For example, convert pH 7.40 to nanomoles of H^+ ions per liter.

$$\text{nanomoles/liter} = \text{antilog } (9 - 7.40)$$

$$= \text{antilog } 1.60$$

$$= 40$$

IF YOU HAVE A CALCULATOR WITH A LOG FUNCTION,

The antilog (9 − 7.40) can be quickly determined using any calculator having a log function. For example, press the following calculator keys.

PRESS: 9 $\boxed{-}$ 7.4 $\boxed{=}$ $\boxed{\text{INV}}$ $\boxed{\text{log}}$

pK CONCEPTS

The pK is defined as the negative logarithm of the dissociation constant of an acid. That is,

$$pK = -\log K_D$$

Acids are categorized as either weak or strong. Weak acids tend not to dissociate readily, therefore, they liberate few free H+ ions. Carbonic acid (H_2CO_3) is a good example of a weak acid. It does not dissociate readily. The dissociation of H_2CO_3 is shown below.

$$H_2CO_3 \rightleftharpoons H^+ + HCO_3^-$$

Strong acids, on the other hand, readily dissociate, and liberate many free H^+ ions. Sulfuric acid (H_2SO_4) is a strong acid because it readily dissociates into its component ions. The dissociation of H_2SO_4 is as follows.

$$H_2SO_4 \rightleftharpoons 2H^+ + SO_4{}^{2-}$$

The equilibrium reaction for a generic acid (HA) shown where will further illustrate the difference between weak and strong acids.

$$HA \rightleftharpoons H^+ + A^-$$

where,

   HA = undissociated acid

   H^+ = hydrogen ion (acid component)

   A^- = negative ion (base component)

For weak acids, fewer H^+ ions and A^- ions will form, therefore, more HA molecules will be present. For strong acids, more H^+ ions and A^- ions will form, consequently, fewer HA molecules will exist.

The pK value of an acid represents the pH at which the acid is 50% dissociated and 50% undissociated. In other words, the pK is the pH corresponding to half neutralization. That is, equal concentrations of acid (H^+) and base (A^-) will be present. Different acids have different pK values, depending on the acid's tendency to dissociate. In practical terms, the lower the pK, the stronger the acid, and the higher the pK, the weaker the acid.

Another practical pH-pK relationship is as follows. When the pH is less than the pK, the acid is less than 50% dissociated. Conversely, when the pH is greater than the pK, the acid is more than 50% dissociated.

Law of Mass Action and Chemical Equilibrium

When two or more chemical substances react, one or more substances different from the reacting species will form. As an example, consider the reaction

$$A + B \rightarrow C + D$$

where substances A and B chemically react to form the products C and D. It has been experimentally found that a definite relationship exists between the speed, or rate, of the reaction and the concentration of the reacting species. The law of mass action describes this relationship. The rate of a chemical reaction is proportional to the concentration of the reactants.

In the hypothetical reaction shown above, the reaction rate is proportional to the number of moles per liter of the reactants A and B. If the number of moles/liter of A increases by a factor of three (triples) and that of B doubles, the rate of reaction increases six-fold.

Because the reaction rate varies according to a number of other factors besides the concentration of reactants—for example, the chemical nature of the reactants, catalysis, and the system temperature—the rate of the reaction can be equated to some quantity k multiplied by the molar concentrations of the reactants. This expression can be shown as

$$R = k[A][B]$$

The quantity k is constant for a given reaction at a specified temperature and is called the **rate constant** for the reaction.

Up to this point the reaction

$$A + B \rightarrow C + D$$

has been considered only as favored to the right. However, many chemical reactions are reversible. Therefore, we need to consider the reverse reaction

$$C + D \rightarrow A + B$$

This reaction also has a rate based on the factors previously indicated and can be shown as

$$R' = k'[C][D]$$

The quantity k' is a term incorporating the chemical nature of C and D and the system temperature. Therefore, because the chemical nature of A and B differs from that of C and D, k' does not equal k.

Let us return to the original reaction

$$A + B \rightarrow C + D$$

Now that we have established this reaction as reversible, yield symbols representing the forward and reverse nature of this reaction need to be included. The reaction can now be represented as

$$A + B \rightleftharpoons C + D$$

Experimentation has revealed that, as a reaction proceeds, the concentration of the reactants decreases. The reactants usually are present at definite concentrations. As time passes, their concentrations stabilize and become constant. This state in which concentrations no longer change is called the state of **chemical equilibrium.**

For the model reaction used here, the state of chemical equilibrium can be shown as

$$k[A][B] = k'[C][D]$$

or

$$k[\text{reactants}] = k'[\text{products}]$$

Rearranging this expression produces

$$\frac{k}{k'} = \frac{[\text{products}]}{[\text{reactants}]}$$

or

$$\frac{k}{k'} = \frac{[C][D]}{[A][B]}$$

The ratio k/k' can be replaced by the term K since a constant divided by a constant produces yet another constant.

Substituting K for k/k' changes the expression to

$$K = \frac{[C][D]}{[A][B]}$$

where the term K is the **equilibrium constant.**

Therefore, when the reaction is in a state of equilibrium, the equilibrium constant is numerically equal to the product of the molar concentrations of the products divided by the product of the molar concentrations of the reactants. At the same time, the rate of the forward reaction $(A + B \rightarrow C + D)$ is equal to the rate of the reverse reaction $(A + B \leftarrow C + D)$. This relationship represents the law of mass action.

To illustrate the validity of this relationship, that is,

$$K = \frac{[products]}{[reactants]}$$

study Table 3-7.

TABLE 3-7

Trial*	moles/liter				K
	A	B	C	D	
1	4.00	2.00	2.00	2.00	0.5
2	4.50	2.50	2.375	2.375	0.5
3	8.26	0.50	1.44	1.44	0.5
4	5.00	16.00	6.33	6.33	0.5

Constant system temperature maintained.

The equilibrium constant for the hypothetical reaction $A + B \rightleftharpoons C + D$ is 0.5. Each of the four trials for this reaction illustrates differing equilibrium concentrations for the products and reactants. Despite the varying equilibrium concentrations, K remains 0.5. In a closed system, the equilibrium constant will remain the same as long as the temperature does not change.

The preceding discussion has described the rate of reaction and the concept of chemical equilibrium in a static or closed system. If the system were an open one, the following factors would affect the equilibrium state:

- addition ($\uparrow$) of reactants would favor the forward reaction ($\uparrow A + \uparrow B \rightleftharpoons C + D$)
- removal ($\downarrow$) of products would favor the forward reaction ($A + B \rightleftharpoons \downarrow C + \downarrow D$)

- removal ($\downarrow$) of reactants would favor the reverse reaction ($\downarrow$A + $\downarrow$B $\rightleftharpoons$ C + D)
- addition ($\uparrow$) of products would favor the reverse reaction (A + B $\rightleftharpoons$ $\uparrow$C + $\uparrow$D)

Physiologic reactions occur essentially in an open system. When physiologic reactions are in a balanced state, the condition is referred to as a **dynamic equilibrium.** In physiologic systems or reactions, the same principles of chemical equilibrium that apply to a static environment apply to one that is dynamic.

Let us consider one physiologic condition to illustrate how (1) the concentration of the reactants and products, (2) catalysis, (3) temperature, and (4) the chemical nature of the reactants and products influence the rate of reaction. The physiologic example to be discussed is that associated with the **chloride shift.**

At the tissue level, arterial blood deposits oxygen and picks up the metabolic waste product carbon dioxide. Carbon dioxide is transported a number of ways in the plasma and the erythrocyte. Here we will be concerned only with the hydration of CO_2 in the red blood cell (RBC). The reaction in the RBC at the tissue level is

$$CO_2 + H_2O \overset{CA}{\rightarrow} H_2CO_3 \rightarrow H^+ + HCO_3^-$$

Notice that the two yield signs (arrows) are directed rightward, implying that this reaction is nonreversible. When one considers blood gas transport *in toto*, including transport from the lungs to the tissues, this reaction is indeed reversible. However, the discussion here is limited to the events occurring at the tissue level. Consequently, the reaction is favored to the right at that point. Keep in mind that these reactions will be favored to the left in the lungs.

The catalyst, carbonic anhydrase (CA), in the erythrocyte causes the hydration of CO_2 to proceed at a rate 13,000 times more rapidly as compared to the hydration of carbon dioxide in the plasma, where CA is absent. Therefore, catalysis contributes to the rightward movement of this reaction.

At this point in its transit through the systemic circulation, the arterial blood yields approximately 25% of its O_2 supply to the tissues and now increases its capacity for CO_2. Therefore, the greater concentration of CO_2 influences the movement of this reaction to the right. At the same time, the HCO_3^- that forms from the dissociation of the H_2CO_3 (carbonic acid) is removed from the red blood cells as part of the chloride shift. For each HCO_3^- ion that leaves the RBC, one chloride (Cl^-) ion enters. Additionally, deoxygenated hemoglobin buffers the H^+ ions produced as H_2CO_3 dissociates. These events further cause the hydration of CO_2 reaction in the RBC at the tissue level to be favored to the right. Note Figure 3-12.

In summary, the following factors favor the hydration of CO_2 to the right at the tissue level.

- The continuous production of CO_2 as a metabolic waste product (addition of reactant)
- The continuous removal of the products of CO_2 hydration
    a. H^+ ions buffered by hemoglobin
    b. HCO_3^- ions removed from the RBC via the chloride shift
- The catalytic activity of carbonic anhydrase

The temperature and the chemical nature of the reactants and products remain constant throughout this reaction.

Buffered by
hemoglobin in
RBC

$$CO_2 + H_2O \xrightarrow{CA} H_2CO_3 \rightarrow H^+ + HCO_3^-$$

Aerobic
metabolism
waste product
enters RBC for
transport

Leaves RBC
during chloride
shift

Figure 3-12. *Hydration of CO₂ in red blood cells at the tissue level. The aerobically produced CO₂ passively diffuses from the cells into the erythrocyte where it chemically combines with H₂O in the presence of carbonic anhydrase (CA). The resultant H⁺ ions are buffered by hemoglobin, as the HCO₃⁻ ions (combined CO₂) passively diffuse into the plasma in exchange for Cl⁻ ions.*

Buffer Solutions

The pH of human blood is normally maintained within the narrow pH range of 7.35 to 7.45. Significant deviations outside this range can result in serious cellular dysfunction or even death. It is obvious then that human physiology must provide mechanisms protecting against large pH changes, since acid and alkaline substances continually pass into circulation.

Such systems—those resistant to pH shifts—are called **buffer solutions** or **buffers.** These solutions are mixtures of a weak acid and the salt (the anion of an acid plus the cation of a base) of that weak acid. Human blood possesses a number of buffer systems. These buffers are shown in Table 3-8.

TABLE 3-8 Physiologic Buffer Systems

Weak Acid	Salt of Weak Acid
1. HHb (acid hemoglobin)	KHB (potassium hemoglobin)
2. KH_2PO_4 (potassium acid phosphate)	K_2HPO_4 (potassium alkaline phosphate)
3. H_2CO_3 (carbonic acid)	$NaHCO_3$ (sodium bicarbonate)
4. H protein (acid proteinate)	Na protein (sodium proteinate)
5. NaH_2PO_4 (sodium acid phosphate)	Na_2HPO_4 (sodium alkaline phosphate)

The carbonic acid/sodium bicarbonate (H_2CO_3/$NaHCO_3$) buffer system will be used to illustrate this protective mechanism.

If more acid, HCl for example, was added to a solution containing H_2CO_3 and $NaHCO_3$, the HCO_3^- ions would react with the H⁺ ions to form the weak acid H_2CO_3* and sodium (Na⁺) and chloride (Cl⁻) ions.

---

*The K of H_2CO_3 is approximately 5.0×10^{-7} at 37°C. Therefore, less than 0.2% of H_2CO_3 dissociates to form H⁺ and HCO_3^-.

These reactions are demonstrated below.

$$\text{NaCl (neutral salt)}$$

$$
\begin{array}{lll}
\text{NaHCO}_3 & \rightarrow & \boxed{\text{Na}^+} \; + \; \boxed{\text{HCO}_3^-} \\
\text{HCl} & \rightarrow & \boxed{\text{Cl}^-} \; + \; \boxed{\text{H}^+}
\end{array}
$$

$$\text{H}_2\text{CO}_3 \text{ (weak acid)}$$

Therefore, when a strong acid is added to a buffer system, the products will be a weak acid and a neutral salt. Any pH change will be small and gradual.

On the other hand, consider the addition of a strong base (NaOH) to the H_2CO_3/NaHCO$_3$ buffer system. The products would be NaHCO$_3$, which is a weak alkaline salt, and H_2O. Again, the pH change will be slight and unabrupt.

Note the example of these reactions that follows.

$$\text{H}_2\text{O (water)}$$

$$
\begin{array}{lll}
\text{H}_2\text{CO}_3 & \rightarrow & \boxed{\text{H}^+} \; + \; \boxed{\text{HCO}_3^-} \\
\text{NaOH} & \rightarrow & \boxed{\text{OH}^-} \; + \; \boxed{\text{Na}^+}
\end{array}
$$

$$\text{NaHCO}_3 \text{ (weak alkaline salt)}$$

When examining buffer systems further, we find that the weak acid (H_2CO_3) is slightly ionized and that the salt of that weak acid is almost completely ionized. This relationship can be shown quantitatively as

$$K = \frac{[\text{H}^+][\text{HCO}_3^-]}{[\text{H}_2\text{CO}_3]}$$

indicating that the product of the molar concentrations of the H^+ and HCO_3^- ions (products) divided by the molar concentration of H_2CO_3 (reactant) equals an **ionization** (equilibrium) **constant.** Be reminded that this expression represents the law of mass action.

Buffer systems are maximally effective at the pH corresponding to their pK. Furthermore, their effectiveness usually covers a range of 1.0 pH unit above and below their pK, or pK $\pm$ 1 pH unit.

In reference to the NaHCO$_3$/H$_2$CO$_3$ (or the more physiologically appropriate HCO$_3^-$/CO$_2$) buffer system, a pK of 6.1 (7.85×10^{-7} mole/liter or 785 nanomoles/liter) means that maximum buffering by this system will occur at pH 6.1. Therefore, since a pH of 6.1 is incompatible with human existence and since the normal range for blood pH is 7.35 to 7.45, the HCO$_3^-$/CO$_2$ buffer system does not seem as though it would be physiologically effective. Likewise, consider this buffer system's effective range, which is 5.10 to 7.10 (i.e., pK 6.1 $\pm$ 1 pH unit).

So, what is the physiologic utility of the HCO_3^-/CO_2 buffer system? Two extremely important functions will be mentioned. First, is the high concentration of HCO_3^- in the plasma, i.e., 22 to 26 mEq/L, and the low dissolved carbon dioxide levels in the plasma, i.e., 1.05 to 1.35 mEq/L, or 35 torr × 0.03 mEq/L/torr and 40 torr × 0.03 mEq/L/torr, respectively. The bicarbonate ion effectively buffers H+ ions produced by nonvolatile acids in the body, for example

$$HCl + NaHCO_3 \rightleftharpoons NaCl + H_2CO_3$$

The nonvolatile acid HCl is a very strong acid; it readily dissociates into H^+ and Cl^-. In the reaction shown above, H_2CO_3 forms. H_2CO_3 is also an acid, but it is an extremely weak acid in comparison to HCl. Therefore, the H^+ ion concentration increases (pH decreases) slightly because fewer H^+ ions are dissociated.

Second, the HCO_3^-/CO_2 buffer system provides an effective mechanism for CO_2 excretion via the lungs. The HCO_3^-/CO_2 buffer system is an open buffer system, as opposed to a closed system.

Table 3-9 lists four physiologic buffers, their corresponding pKs and their effective pH range.

TABLE 3-9   Physiologic Buffers (37°C)

Buffer System	pK	Effective pH Range
HCO_3^-/CO_2	6.1	5.10–7.10
$HbO_2^-/HHbO_2$	6.7	5.70–7.70
$HPO_4^{-2}/H_2PO_4^-$	6.8	5.80–7.80
Hb^-/HHb	7.9	6.90–8.90

Henderson-Hasselbalch Equation

Essentially, the Henderson-Hasselbalch equation is based on the law of mass action. Here it will be applied to the carbonic acid/sodium bicarbonate buffer system. The equilibrium constant for the carbonic acid/sodium bicarbonate buffer system can be calculated as follows:

$$K = \frac{[H^+][HCO_3^-]}{[H_2CO_3]}$$

Solving for $[H^+]$, the equation will read

$$[H^+] = K\frac{[H_2CO_3]}{[HCO_3^-]}$$

The purpose of rearranging the equation to solve for the hydrogen ion concentration is to ultimately arrive at a value for the pH of the system.

The next step is to take the logarithm of each side of the equation.

$$\log[H^+] = \log K + \log\frac{[H_2CO_3]}{[HCO_3^-]}$$

Each side of the equation is then multiplied by -1 to give

$$-\log [H^+] = -\log K + \left(-\log \frac{[H_2CO_3]}{[HCO_3^-]}\right)$$

which is the same as

$$-\log [H^+] = -\log K + \log \frac{[HCO_3^-]}{[H_2CO_3]}$$

Recall that $-\log [H^+]$ defines pH. Therefore, the term *pH* can substitute for $-\log [H+]$. Also, by definition $-\log K$ defines pK. Consequently, after making these substitutions, this equation now becomes

$$pH = pK + \log \frac{[HCO_3^-]}{[H_2CO_3]}$$

Under normal physiologic conditions, the equilibrium constant K for the entire carbonic acid/bicarbonate buffer system is 7.85×10^{-7}. Since $pK = -\log K$, then $pK = -\log 7.85 \times 10^{-7}$ which becomes

$$pK = -\log 7.85 + \log 10^{-7}$$

$$= -.8949 + 7$$

$$= 6.10$$

Therefore, pK for this system is 6.10. The equation now reads

$$pH = 6.10 + \log \frac{[HCO_3^-]}{[H_2CO_3]}$$

The pK of 6.1 actually represents the sum of the two pKs in the overall CO_2 hydration reaction. The first pK, which is 3.4, results from the reaction between CO_2 and H_2O to form carbonic acid, that is,

$$CO_2 + H_2O \xrightarrow[3.4]{pK_1} H_2CO_3$$

The second pK (2.7) comes from the ionization of carbonic acid into its component species hydrogen and bicarbonate ions.

$$H_2CO_3 \xrightarrow[2.7]{pK_2} H^+ + HCO_3^-$$

The pK for the overall reaction equals pK_1 plus pK_2, or

$$pK = pK_1 + pK_2$$

$$= 3.4 + 2.7$$

$$= 6.10$$

To expedite calculations, thus facilitating the clinical utility of this equation, the dissolved arterial carbon dioxide (PaCO$_2$) replaces H$_2$CO$_3$ in the expression. This substitution is possible because the concentration of H$_2$O in the two-part reaction shown below is considered constant. Therefore, the CO$_2$ level, measured as the PaCO$_2$, directly affects the H$_2$CO$_3$ concentration and, ultimately, the H$^+$ concentration (pH). H$_2$CO$_3$ is a transitory intermediate in the CO$_2$ hydration reaction. Because H$_2$CO$_3$ is a transitory intermediate in the overall reaction,

$$CO_2 + H_2O \rightleftharpoons H_2CO_3 \rightleftharpoons H^+ + HCO_3^-$$

then

$$K = \frac{[H^+][HCO_3^-]}{[CO_2][H_2O]}$$

When the concentration of H$_2$O is assumed to be constant, the factor [H$_2$O] is removed from the equation, which becomes

$$pH = pK + \log \frac{[HCO_3^-]}{[CO_2]}$$

Furthermore, the use of Pco$_2$ is convenient because it is easily measured via blood gas analysis and can be rapidly converted to a mmol/liter by being multiplied by the factor 0.03 mmol/liter/torr.* The relationship is now shown as

$$pH = 6.10 + \log \frac{[HCO_3^-]}{(Pco_2)(0.03)}$$

Table 3-10 illustrates the eight steps used here to derive the Henderson-Hasselbalch equation as it applies to the carbonic acid/sodium bicarbonate buffer system.

From the discussion of Henry's law (Section 3-2), the reader will recall that HCO$_3^-$ is reported clinically in terms of millimoles/liter and that this measurement represents the amount of carbon dioxide in the combined state. The ratio of combined to dissolved CO$_2$ in the arterial blood is ordinarily 20:1, that is, HCO$_3^-$ 24 mmol/liter and Pco$_2$ 40 torr $\times$ 0.03 = 1.2 mmol/liter. Therefore,

$$\frac{[HCO_3^-]}{[(Pco_2)(0.03)]} = \frac{combined\ CO_2}{dissolved\ CO_2} = \frac{24\ mmol/liter}{1.2\ mmol/liter} = \frac{20}{1}$$

Substituting 20 for the [HCO$_3^-$]/(Pco$_2$)(0.03) ratio in the Henderson-Hasselbalch equation yields

$$pH = 6.10 + \log 20$$
$$= 6.10 + 1.30$$
$$= 7.40$$

---

*The reader may wish to review Section 3-2, "Chemical Laws"—Henry's Law of Solubility for the derivation of the factor (0.03 mmol/liter/torr) used for changing the partial pressure of carbon dioxide expressed as either mm Hg or torr to mmol/liter.

TABLE 3-10 Summary of Henderson-Hasselbalch
Equation Derivation

Step 1:
$$K = \frac{[H^+][HCO_3^-]}{[H_2CO_3]}$$

Step 2:
$$[H^+] = \frac{K[H_2CO_3]}{[HCO_3^-]}$$

Step 3:
$$\log[H^+] = \log K + \log \frac{[H_2CO_3]}{[HCO_3^-]}$$

Step 4:
$$-\log[H^+] = -\log K + \left(-\log \frac{[H_2CO_3]}{[HCO_3^-]}\right)$$

Step 5:
$$-\log[H^+] = -\log K + \log \frac{[HCO_3^-]}{[H_2CO_3]}$$

Step 6:
$$pH = pK + \log \frac{[HCO_3^-]}{[H_2CO_3]}$$

Step 7:
$$pH = 6.10 + \log \frac{[HCO_3^-]}{[H_2CO_3]}$$

Step 8:
$$pH = 6.10 + \log \frac{[HCO_3^-]}{(P_{CO_2})(0.03)}$$

The Henderson-Hasselbalch equation allows for the calculation of either the pH, HCO_3^- (combined CO_2), or P_{CO_2} (dissolved CO_2) provided that any two of the three factors are known. From this relationship, it can now be understood how the HCO_3^-/P_{CO_2} ratio influences the pH of the blood.

EXAMPLE 1:

Calculate the pH when the combined CO_2 is 21 mmol/liter and the dissolved CO_2 is 25 mm Hg.

Step 1: Set up the Henderson-Hasselbalch equation.

$$pH = 6.10 + \log \frac{[HCO_3^-]}{(0.03)(P_{CO_2})}$$

Step 2: Insert known values and calculate for pH.

$$pH = 6.10 + \log \left[\frac{21 \text{ mmol/liter}}{(0.03 \text{ mmol/liter/torr})(25 \text{ torr})}\right]$$

$$= 6.10 + \log \left[\frac{21 \text{ mmol/liter}}{0.75 \text{ mmol/liter}} \right]$$

$$= 6.10 + \log 28$$

$$= 6.10 + 1.45$$

$$= 7.55$$

IF YOU HAVE A CALCULATOR WITH A LOG FUNCTION,

The equation $6.10 + \log \left[\frac{21 \text{ mEq/L}}{(0.03 \text{ mEq/L/torr})(25 \text{ torr})} \right]$ can be quickly determined using any calculator having a log function. For example, press the following calculator keys.

PRESS: .03 $\boxed{\times}$ 25 $\boxed{=}$ $\boxed{\text{STO}}$ 21 $\boxed{\div}$ $\boxed{\text{RCL}}$ $\boxed{=}$ $\boxed{\log}$ $\boxed{+}$ 6.1

EXAMPLE 2:

Determine the $PaCO_2$ when the pH is 7.24 and the HCO_3^- is 26 mmol/liter.

Step 1: Set up the Henderson-Hasselbalch equation.

$$pH = 6.10 + \log \frac{[HCO_3^-]}{(0.03)(Pco_2)}$$

Step 2: Insert known values.

$$7.24 = 6.10 + \log \left[\frac{26 \text{ mmol/liter}}{(0.03 \text{ mmol/liter/torr})(Pco_2)} \right]$$

Step 3: Simplify the equation.

$$7.24 - 6.10 = \log \left[\frac{26 \text{ mmol/liter}}{(0.03 \text{ mmol/liter/torr})(Pco_2)} \right]$$

$$1.14 = \log 26 - \log[(0.03)(Pco_2)]$$

$$1.14 = 1.42 - \log[(0.03)(Pco_2)]$$

$$\log[(0.03)(Pco_2)] = 1.42 - 1.14$$

$$\log[(0.03)(Pco_2)] = 0.28$$

Step 4: Find the antilogarithm of 0.28 and calculate the Pco_2.

$$(0.03)(Pco_2) = \text{antilog } 0.28$$

$$(0.03)(Pco_2) = 1.90$$

$$Pco_2 = \frac{1.90}{0.03}$$

$$Pco_2 = 63 \text{ torr}$$

The Henderson-Hasselbalch equation can be rearranged in the following manner to solve for the $PaCO_2$ (i.e., when the pH and the $[HCO_3^-]$ are given).

$$PaCO_2 = \frac{[HCO_3^-]}{[0.03 \text{ mEq/L/torr} \times \text{antilog (pH} - 6.1)]}$$

IF YOU HAVE A CALCULATOR WITH A LOG FUNCTION,

The expression $\dfrac{[26 \text{ mEq/L}]}{[0.03 \text{ mEq/L/torr} \times \text{antilog } (7.24 - 6.1)]}$ can be quickly determined using any calculator having a log function. For example, press the following calculator keys.

PRESS: 7.24 $\boxed{-}$ 6.1 $\boxed{=}$ $\boxed{\text{INV}}$ $\boxed{\text{log}}$ $\boxed{\times}$ .03 $\boxed{\text{STO}}$ 26 $\boxed{\div}$ $\boxed{\text{RCL}}$

The Henderson-Hasselbalch equation can be rearranged a third way to solve for the $[HCO_3^-]$ when the pH and the $PaCO2$ are known. Hence,

$$[HCO_3^-] = (0.03 \text{ mEq/L/torr} \times PaCO_2)[\text{antilog (pH} - 6.1)]$$

The following box illustrates the various forms by which the pH can be calculated.

Forms Used to Calculate pH
• $pH = \log\left(\dfrac{1}{[H^+]}\right)$
• $pH = -\log [H^+]$
• $pH = 9 - \log H^+ \text{ nmol/L}$
• $pH = pK + \log \dfrac{[HCO_3^-]}{(Pco_2)(0.03)}$

The expressions listed in the box below represent the three variations of the Henderson-Hasselbalch equation based on which two of the three variables are known.

Variations of Henderson-Hasselbalch Equation
• $pH = pK + \log \dfrac{[HCO_3^-]}{(Pco_2)(0.03)}$
• $Pco_2 = \dfrac{[HCO_3^-]}{[0.03 \times \text{antilog (pH} - 6.1)]}$
• $[HCO_3^-] = (0.03 \times Pco_2)[\text{antilog (pH} - 6.1)]$

PRACTICE PROBLEMS

Refer to Appendix A (pages 591-594) for the solutions and answers to the practice problems.

Determine the pH of the following hydrogen ion concentrations [H^+]:

51. [H^+] = 10^{-11} _____
52. [H^+] = 2.30×10^{-4} _____
53. [H^+] = 4.80×10^{-10} _____
54. [H^+] = 6.30×10^{-1} _____
55. [H^+] = 4.60×10^{-4} _____

Convert the following hydrogen ion concentrations in nanomoles/liter to pH:

56. 33 nanomoles/liter _____
57. 34 nanomoles/liter _____
58. 57 nanomoles/liter _____
59. 58 nanomoles/liter _____
60. 100 nanomoles/liter _____

Convert the following hydrogen ion concentrations given in pH units to nanomoles/liter:

61. pH 7.49 _____
62. pH 7.48 _____
63. pH 7.29 _____
64. pH 7.35 _____
65. pH 7.10 _____
66. pH 8.00 _____
67. pH 8.53 _____
68. pH 6.21 _____
69. pH 14 _____
70. pH 1 _____

Use the Henderson-Hasselbalch equation to solve the following problems:

71. Calculate the pH when the combined and dissolved CO_2 are 15 mEq/liter and 25 torr, respectively.

_____

72. Determine the $PaCO_2$ when the combined CO_2 is 20 mmol/liter and the pH is 7.48.

_____

73. Find the dissolved carbon dioxide value when the bicarbonate value is 26 mmol/liter and the pH is 7.42.

_____

74. Calculate the $[HCO_3^-]$ at pH 7.46 and $PaCO_2$ 26 mm Hg.

_____

75. Determine the total CO_2 when the pH is 7.24 and the dissolved CO_2 is 28 mm Hg.

_____

76. Obtain the pH of an arterial blood sample that has a $PaCO_2$ of 75 torr and a HCO_3^- ion concentration of 36 mEq/L. _____

77. Calculate the HCO_3^- ion concentration of a sample of blood that has a dissolved CO_2 tension of 30 torr and a pH of 7.48. _____

78. Determine the $[HCO_3^-]$ of a patient whose pH is 7.33 and has a partial pressure of dissolved CO_2 of 35 mm Hg. _____

79. What is the pH of a patient whose bicarbonate ion concentration is 18 mEq/L and whose $PaCO_2$ is 55 mm Hg? _____

80. What is the $[HCO_3^-]$ of a blood sample with a pH of 7.22 and $PaCO_2$ of 20 torr?

_____

3-5 DENSITY AND SPECIFIC GRAVITY

The respiratory care practitioner often employs the concepts of **density** and **specific gravity** in his work without, perhaps, actually realizing the scientific basis of the therapeutic application. For instance, substituting a helium-oxygen (He-O_2) gas mixture for an air-oxygen mixture when working with patients who have an airway obstruction is theoretically founded on the concept that a helium-oxygen mixture is less dense than a mixture of air-oxygen. The less dense gas mixture supposedly allows for more gas molecules to move beyond areas that are partially obstructed in the tracheobronchial tree.

Additionally, the influence density has upon the comparative rates of diffusion of O_2 and CO_2 across the alveolar-capillary membrane was observed in Section 3-2 in the discussion of Graham's law of diffusion.

Liquids and Solids

Density is defined as mass per unit volume, that is, the amount of mass of a substance per amount of volume occupied by that substance. Quantitatively, this relationship reads

$$\text{density (D)} = \frac{\text{mass (g)}}{\text{volume (ml)}} \text{ or } \frac{\text{mass (g)}}{\text{volume (cc)}}$$

The density of solids and liquids is determined in the same manner and is expressed in the same units. It is important to interject here the distinction between the terms *mass* and *weight*. Mass can be described as the amount of matter a substance contains; weight is the gravitational attraction between the earth and matter. Therefore, the mass of an object is constant, and its weight varies with its distance from the earth. For example, a 70-kg astronaut leaving the earth and traveling to the moon will weigh just under 12 kg upon reaching his destination because the moon's gravity is about one-sixth that of earth's. However, the amount of matter comprising the astronaut remains constant.

A simple problem may be useful in illustrating the relationship between mass and volume. Determine the density of 0.00654 liter of a substance weighing 89 grams.

Step 1: Convert 0.00654 liter to milliliters.

$$(0.00654 \text{ liter}) \left(\frac{1000 \text{ ml}}{1 \text{ liter}} \right) = 6.54 \text{ ml}$$

Step 2: Use the formula for calculating density.

$$D = \frac{\text{mass}}{\text{volume}}$$

$$= \frac{89 \text{ g}}{6.54 \text{ ml}}$$

$$= 13.6 \text{ g/ml}$$

This particular substance happens to be mercury (Hg).

One milliliter of water has been found to weigh 1 gram at STP. Hence, the density of water is 1 g/ml.

Recall that 1,034 cm H_2O and 760 mm Hg equal one atmosphere of pressure. Quite often the need arises to convert pressure expressed as mm Hg to cm H_2O and vice versa. The relationship between these two units of pressure is based on the comparison of the density of H_2O to that of Hg. For example,

$$\frac{1,034 \text{ cm } H_2O}{760 \text{ mm Hg}} = 1.36 \text{ cm } H_2O/\text{mm Hg}$$

The factor 1.36 cm H_2O/mm Hg represents one-tenth the density of Hg because the denominator was expressed in millimeters (mm) of Hg instead of centimeters (cm) of Hg. More plainly,

$$\frac{1,034 \text{ cm } H_2O}{76 \text{ cm Hg}} = 13.6 \text{ cm } H_2O/\text{cm Hg}$$

Comparing cm H_2O to cm Hg clearly shows that Hg is 13.6 times more dense than H_2O.

The densities of solids and liquids are compared to the density of water to determine the value for the specific gravity of a substance. The specific gravity of a substance is essentially a ratio of densities. Therefore, as is the case for all ratios, only like entities can be compared. A dimensionless value results. For example, the specific gravity of mercury can be determined thus:

$$\frac{13.6 \text{ g/ml}}{1 \text{ g/ml}} = 13.6$$

It can readily be seen that the specific gravity for any solid or liquid will be the same quantity as its density but without units.

Gases

The density of gases is computed differently from that of the other two states of matter primarily because gas volumes are greatly influenced by changes in temperature and pressure. Consequently, gas densities are determined under standard temperature and pressure (STP) conditions. Gas density is calculated by dividing the volume occupied by 1 mole of gas at STP, that is, 22.4 liters, into the gram molecular weight of that gas. The expression is shown as

$$\text{density (D)} = \frac{\text{gram molecular weight}}{22.4 \text{ liters}}$$

The units for gas density are grams per liter.

As an example, the density of oxygen can be obtained by dividing its gram molecular weight (32 g) by its volume at STP (22.4 liters). The expression is

$$\text{density of O}_2 = \frac{32 \text{ g}}{22.4 \text{ liters}}$$

$$= 1.43 \text{ g/liters}$$

The specific gravity of a gas is determined by comparing the density of the gas to the density of the standard. The standard used for gases is the density of air, which is 1.29 g/liter. Therefore, the specific gravity of oxygen is obtained as follows:

$$\frac{1.43 \text{ g/liter}}{1.29 \text{ g/liter}} = 1.11$$

Once again, the value for specific gravity is dimensionless because the quantity is obtained from a ratio.

It is noteworthy that the specific gravity of air is 1.00 (1.29 g/liter ÷ 1.29 g/liter). Oxygen has a higher specific gravity than air. Therefore, oxygen molecules added to an air environment will tend to accumulate at the lowest point of the environment. For example, when a mist tent is in operation, the oxygen molecules added to the enclosure gravitate toward the mattress because of the relationship between the specific gravities of air and oxygen.

The density of a gas mixture can also be obtained. This process will be discussed here. In addition to requiring the value of the gram molecular weight (GMW) of each gas in the mixture, the percentage of each gas in the mixture is also necessary. The general formula for calculating the density of a gas mixture is shown below.

$$D = \frac{(C_{gas} \times GMW)_1 + (C_{gas} \times GMW)_2 + \ldots (C_{gas} \times GMW)_n}{22.4 \text{ liters}}$$

where,

D = gas density
C = gas concentration (%)
GMW = gram molecular weight of gas

Let's apply this formula to two gas mixtures that have clinical and physiologic applications. The two gas mixtures are air (N_2 and O_2) and heliox (He and O_2).

For the purpose of the discussion here, only the major components of atmospheric air will be considered in the air mixture, i.e., N_2 and O_2. Air contains essentially 79% N_2 and 21% O_2. Nitrogen has a gram molecular weight of 28 a.m.u. and oxygen's GMW is 32 a.m.u. These values will be inserted in the density formula for gas mixtures as shown below.

DENSITY OF NITROGEN-OXYGEN (AIR) GAS MIXTURE

$$D = \frac{\left(\frac{79}{100} \times 28 \text{ g}\right) + \left(\frac{21}{100} \times 32 \text{ g}\right)}{22.4 \text{ liters}}$$

$$= \frac{22.12 \text{ g} + 6.72 \text{ g}}{22.4 \text{ liters}}$$

$$= 1.29 \text{ g/liter}$$

Now, let's consider an 80-20 helium-oxygen gas mixture. Helium has a GMW of 4 a.m.u. and oxygen has a GMW of 32 a.m.u. In this particular gas mixture helium comprises 80% of the mixture and air comprises 20%.

DENSITY OF 80-20 HELIUM-OXYGEN GAS MIXTURE

$$D = \frac{\left(\frac{80}{100} \times 4 \text{ g}\right) + \left(\frac{20}{100} \times 32 \text{ g}\right)}{22.4 \text{ liters}}$$

$$= \frac{3.2 \text{ g} + 6.4 \text{ g}}{22.4 \text{ liters}}$$

$$= 0.43 \text{ g/liter}$$

Comparing the two gas mixture densities, we see that the He-O_2 mixture is 3 times less dense than air, that is

$$\frac{\text{air D}}{\text{He} - O_2 \text{ D}} = \frac{1.29 \text{ g/liter}}{0.43 \text{ g/liter}} = 3$$

Heliox (80-20) is sometimes used to help ventilate patients who have upper or large airway obstruction. The theory of the clinical application of helium-oxygen therapy is discussed in Chapter 4 Physics on page 243.

PRACTICE PROBLEMS

Refer to Appendix A (page 594-595) for the solutions and answers to the practice problems.

81. Calculate the density of carbon dioxide gas.

82. Compute the specific gravity of gaseous carbon dioxide.

   _____

83. Calculate the density of nitrous oxide (N_2O).

   _____

84. Determine the density of a metal cube weighing 90 g and measuring 3.0 cm along each side.

   _____

85. Compute the specific gravity of carbon monoxide gas.

   _____

3-6 TEMPERATURE SCALES

This section will present three commonly used temperature scales, as well as describe differences between thermal energy and temperature. Formulas will be given to allow for the conversion from one temperature scale to another.

Thermal Energy and Temperature

All matter is comprised of molecules that are in constant motion. The degree of this motion differs among the three states of matter (solid, liquid, and gas). The movement of molecules within a solid is restricted by the intermolecular forces holding the solid together. A liquid possesses more molecular activity than a solid. However, a gas has the greatest molecular motion of the three states of matter because the forces holding the gas molecules together have been entirely overcome, allowing the gas molecules complete freedom of movement, except for the limitation imposed by the walls of its container. The movement of these molecules is referred to as **kinetic energy.** These molecules also possess **potential energy** which depends on the vibratory movement of the molecules.

According to the kinetic theory of matter, a hot object contains more thermal energy than a cold object of the same size. What this statement means is the molecules comprising the hot object possess a greater amount of energy (kinetic energy and potential energy) than the molecules of the cold object.

The **thermal energy** of any object is the sum of the kinetic energy (KE) and potential energy (PE) of the object's molecules. That is,

$$\text{molecular KE} + \text{molecular PE} = \text{thermal energy}$$

The molecules comprising the hot object do not all have an equal amount of energy. Some molecules have a greater amount of kinetic energy and some have a lesser amount. Furthermore, some molecules within the hot object have a greater potential energy than others. The same situation applies to the cold object as well.

The molecules of any object possess an average energy. In the example discussed here, the molecules of the hot object contain an average energy greater than the average energy of the molecules comprising the cold object.

Temperature is a measure of the average kinetic energy of the molecules of an object. Temperature is independent of the number of molecules in an object, whereas thermal

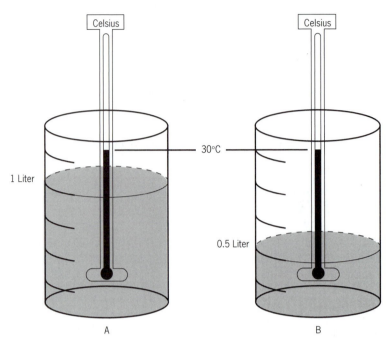

Figure 3-13. *Two equal-sized containers partially filled with different volumes of water at the same temperature (30°C). Both containers have the same* average *kinetic energy. Because container A holds twice the volume of B, A has twice the* total *kinetic energy as container B.*

energy (KE + PE) depends on the number of molecules constituting an object. Consider two equal-sized containers, each partially filled with water (Figure 3-13).

Container A is filled with 1.0 liter of water and container B is filled with 0.5 liter of water. Both of these volumes of water have the same temperature (30°C), which means that the *average* kinetic energy of the molecules of these two volumes of water is equal. However, the water in container A has more thermal energy (KE + PE) than the water in container B because the number of water molecules in container A is greater than the number of molecules of water in container B.

Here is another point to contemplate concerning Figure 3-13: Because the volume of water in container A is twice the volume in container B (temperature A = temperature B), the water in container A has twice the *total* kinetic energy compared with the water in container B. Remember that temperature is a measure of the *average* kinetic energy of a body, not the *total*.

Different temperature scales are used to measure the average kinetic energy of matter. Three temperature scales will be described in this section: (1) the Fahrenheit scale, (2) the Celsius scale, and (3) the Kelvin, or Absolute scale. In the United States, the Fahrenheit scale is in widespread use. It is predominantly used in nonscientific, everyday temperature situations. However, the Celsius scale is used primarily in science and medicine. The Kelvin, or Absolute, scale is also used in science. Based on the SI convention, a degree sign is omitted when the Kelvin scale is used. Therefore, when reference is made to the equivalent of 0°C on the Kelvin scale, 273K is written, not 273°K. The Kelvin is the SI unit of temperature.

TABLE 3-11 Comparison of Temperature Scales

°C	K	°F	Temperature scales
100°	373	212°	Boiling point of water
0°	273	32°	Freezing point of water
−273°	0	−459°	Absolute zero

The following discussion will demonstrate how these three temperature scales interrelate. Table 3-11 compares the three temperature scales just mentioned.

The table shows that for the Celsius and Kelvin scales there are 100 calibrations between the boiling point and freezing point of water. Furthermore, because the Kelvin scale begins at 0° (absolute zero), and because the Celsius scale starts at −273°, any Celsius reading will always be 273° lower than an equivalent temperature on the Kelvin scale. Therefore, the conversion from Celsius to Kelvin is

$$K = °C + 273$$

and conversely

$$°C = K - 273$$

When comparing the Celsius and Fahrenheit scales, one finds that the Fahrenheit degree is only five-ninths ($\frac{5}{9}$) as large as the Celsius degree. This fractional relationship results from the fact that on the Fahrenheit scale there are 180 calibrations between 32°F (freezing point of water) and 212°F (boiling point of water), whereas between the same two points (0°C and 100°C) on the Celsius scale the number of calibrations amounts to 100. Therefore,

$$\frac{100°C}{180°F} = \frac{5}{9} °C/°F$$

or

$$\frac{180°F}{100°C} = \frac{9}{5} = 1.8°F/°C$$

The quantitative relationships among the three temperature scales discussed here are illustrated in Figure 3-14.

The interconversion of Fahrenheit and Celsius temperatures is based on this fractional relationship. Again, an interval of 1°F = $\frac{5}{9}$°C, and an interval of 1°C = $\frac{9}{5}$°F, or 1.8°F.

The formula to convert from Celsius to Fahrenheit temperatures is

$$°F = \frac{9}{5}(°C) + 32$$

or

$$°F = 1.8(°C) + 32$$

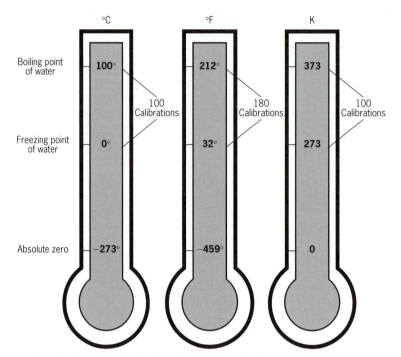

Figure 3-14. *Celsius (°C), Fahrenheit (°F), and Kelvin or Absolute (K) temperature scales. Note that between the boiling and freezing points of water both the Celsius and Kelvin scales have 100 calibrations and that the Fahrenheit scale has 180 calibrations between those two points. These scalar relationships serve as the basis for the formulas used to convert from one temperature scale to another.*

The equation used to convert from Fahrenheit to Celsius temperatures is

$$°C = (°F - 32)\frac{5}{9}$$

Temperatures on the Fahrenheit scale can be converted to degrees Kelvin thus:

$$K = (°F - 32)\frac{5}{9} + 273$$

The expression **absolute zero** represents the lowest temperature measurement possible. According to Charles' law (an **ideal gas** law), all gases have zero volume at absolute zero (−273°C or 0 K). Refer to Chapter 4, Figure 4-16, which illustrates the relationship between volume and temperature for an ideal gas.

PRACTICE PROBLEMS

Refer to Appendix A (pages 595-598) for the solutions and answers to the practice problems.

Convert the following Celsius temperatures to degrees Fahrenheit:

86. 1°C _____
87. 89°C _____

88. −89°C _____
89. −40°C _____
90. 40°C _____

Convert the following Fahrenheit temperatures to degrees Celsius:

91. 98.6°F _____
92. −65°F _____
93. −459°F _____
94. −32°F _____
95. 43°F _____

Convert the following Fahrenheit and Celsius temperatures to the Kelvin scale:

96. 98.6°F _____
97. −40°F _____
98. −273°C _____
99. −118°C _____
100. 273°C _____
101. 32°F _____
102. −459°F _____
103. −40°F _____
104. 72°F _____
105. 22°C _____

3-7 ELECTROCHEMISTRY

Respiratory care practitioners routinely determine the oxygen concentration delivered by a variety of oxygen appliances and also obtain the partial pressure of oxygen from arterial and venous blood samples. This section is written to provide the clinical practitioner with the fundamental principles and concepts of electrochemistry, which serve as the functional basis for most of the equipment used for such analysis.

Terminology

Electrochemistry concerns itself with (1) chemical reactions that produce an electric current and (2) chemical reactions produced by an electric current. Chemical reactions that produce an electric current represent the process occurring in a cell ("battery"); chemical reactions resulting from exposure to an electric current represent the process of electrolysis.

Before launching into a discussion of these two mechanisms, certain terms and expressions require definitions for the sake of clarity.

Commonly, respiratory care practitioners use expressions such as *polarographic electrode,* or *Po₂ electrode,* when referring to the actual electrochemical sensors used to measure the partial pressure of oxygen (Po_2) in blood samples. However, those expressions are misnomers and do not precisely describe the measuring instrument. The term **electrode** specifically refers to the cathode and the anode, which are the terminals of an electrochemical cell where oxidation-reduction reactions occur.

The entire electrochemical sensor—the cathode, the anode, and the electrolyte solution—should be termed an **electrochemical cell**.

The disparity in terminology will be overlooked here to conform to the common practice in the use of these terms and to avoid confusion. However, precise electrochemical terminology will be used when discussing the components of the electrochemical cell.

Electrochemical Cells

The electrochemical cells discussed here will have the following constituents: (1) a cathode, (2) an anode, (3) an electrolyte solution, and (4) a current meter (ammeter). Figure 3-15 illustrates these components in relation to each other.

The cathode is the electrode at which reduction occurs. **Reduction** is the process whereby a molecule, or an atom, gains one or more electrons. Therefore, the cations in the electrolyte solution migrate to the cathode to become reduced (gain electrons).

Meanwhile, at the anode the anions from the electrolyte solution undergo oxidation. **Oxidation** is the process whereby a molecule or an atom loses one or more electrons. The electrons at the anode travel through that terminal, through the wire to the ammeter, and, finally, to the cathode where they are used in the reduction reaction.

A complete circuit is present. The oxidation reaction at the anode provides the electrons. The current meter (ammeter) senses the electron flow through the wires. The cathode uses the electrons to "fuel" the reduction reaction, which takes place at that terminal. The

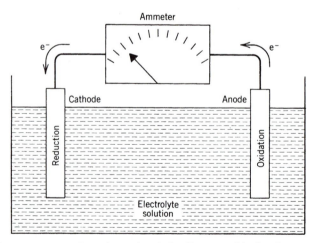

Figure 3-15. *Basic components of an electrochemical cell responsible for the generation of an electron flow (current).*

current (flow of electrons) results from the oxidation-reduction reactions. The cell will continue to provide a current until one of the cations becomes depleted.

Keep in mind that the electron flow (current) travels through the wire from the anode to the cathode, whereas in the electrolyte solution the cations move to the cathode and the anions migrate to the anode.

A more practical example follows. Figure 3-16 illustrates an electrochemical cell with a zinc (Zn) anode and a copper (Cu) cathode dipped into an electrolyte solution of copper sulfate ($CuSO_4$).

Reduction occurs at the copper cathode. Electrons travel through the wire from the zinc anode to the copper cathode where they react with the copper ions (Cu^{+2}) in solution according to the following half-reaction:

$$Cu^{+2} + 2e^- \rightarrow Cu$$

In electrochemistry a half-reaction represents what takes place at either the anode or cathode. A half-reaction demonstrates the gain of electrons (reduction) or the loss of electrons (oxidation). Eventually, the copper ions in solution will become depleted as copper is deposited on the cathode.

Zinc ions (Zn^{+2}) and two electrons ($2e^-$) are formed during the oxidation of zinc at the anode as shown by the half-reaction

$$Zn \rightarrow Zn^{+2} + 2e^-$$

The zinc ions (Zn^{+2}) then migrate through the electrolyte solution in the direction of the copper cathode, and the electrons move through the wire to the cathode. During the course of this reaction, the zinc electrode breaks down and eventually disappears.

This electrochemical cell, also called a galvanic cell, will produce an electric current until either the zinc anode or copper ions in the original solution is depleted. The overall reaction for this galvanic cell is

$$Zn + CuSO_4 \rightarrow ZnSO_4 + Cu$$

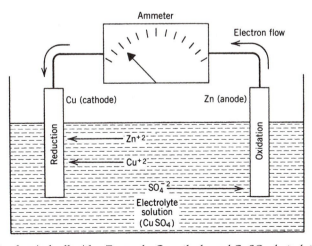

Figure 3-16. *Electrochemical cell with a Zn anode, Cu cathode, and $CuSO_4$ electrolyte solution.*

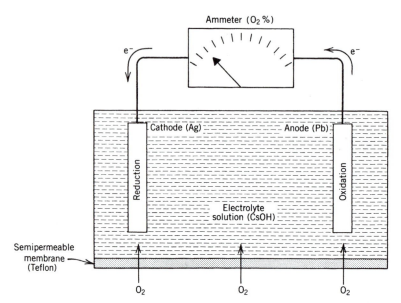

Figure 3-17. *Galvanic fuel cell. O_2 molecules diffusing across the Teflon membrane participate in a reduction reaction at the cathode; OH^- ions migrate to the anode where they react with Pb to produce electrons, which are measured as current by the ammeter.*

Galvanic Cell Analyzer

The electrochemical cells illustrated and discussed in the previous section represent the operational principles of the galvanic cell oxygen analyzer, commonly called the **galvanic fuel cell** (another misnomer).

The galvanic fuel cell differs somewhat from the basic electrochemical cell shown in Figure 3-15.

Galvanic fuel cell components include:

1. Silver (Ag) or gold (Au) cathode
2. Lead (Pb) anode
3. Cesium hydroxide (CsOH) or potassium hydroxide (KOH) electrolyte solution
4. Ammeter calibrated in terms of oxygen percentage
5. A membrane permeable to oxygen molecules (Teflon or polypropylene)

Figure 3-17 illustrates a galvanic fuel cell.

Oxygen molecules are brought into contact with the Teflon membrane (permeable essentially only to oxygen molecules) as the gas is being sampled. The oxygen molecules diffuse across the membrane into the electrolyte solution because of the partial pressure gradient existing between the P_{O_2} of the sample gas and the P_{O_2} of the electrolyte solution. Once inside the electrochemical cell, the oxygen molecules react with water according to the following reduction reaction at the cathode:*

---

*Because water molecules are involved in this double decomposition reaction at the cathode, it could be said that oxygen molecules undergo *hydrolysis.*

$$O_2 + 2H_2O + 4e^- \rightarrow 4OH^-$$

The hydroxyl ions (OH^-) produced migrate to the anode where they participate in the oxidation of lead, as shown by the reaction

$$Pb + 4OH^- \rightarrow 2H_2O + 4e^-$$

It can be seen from these two half-reactions (reduction at the cathode and oxidation at the anode) that four hydroxyl (OH^-) ions are formed for each oxygen molecule that is reduced and that four electrons ($4e^-$) are provided by the oxidation of lead (Pb) at the anode.

Keep in mind that this oxidation-reduction reaction involves the transfer of electrons from the cathode to the anode via the electrolyte solution, thereby completing the electrical circuit. The ammeter will register this electron flow only when the circuit is complete.

Therefore, an electric current (electron flow from the lead anode to the silver cathode) is proportional to the rate of diffusion of oxygen molecules across the semipermeable Teflon membrane. The electric current is directly proportional to the number of oxygen molecules moving into the electrolyte solution. The number of oxygen molecules is directly proportional to the partial pressure of oxygen (Po_2) in the sample gas. Consequently, the greater the Po_2 of the sample gas, the greater the number of oxygen molecules there are diffusing across the semipermeable membrane, which, in turn, results in an increased electron flow, or electric current, as measured by the ammeter calibrated in percentage of oxygen.

Polarographic Analyzer

The **polarographic cell** is composed of the same basic components that constitute the galvanic cell. The polarographic cell, however, contains an external circuit providing a polarizing voltage. The external polarizing voltage (-0.6 volt) is supplied by a battery to the cathode to accelerate the reduction of oxygen. Figure 3-18 shows a polarographic cell.

In a process similar to the process in the galvanic cell analyzer, oxygen molecules from the sample gas or liquid diffuse across the semipermeable membrane and migrate toward the platinum electrode (cathode), where they react with water and electrons (reduction reaction).

The voltage delivered to the cathode by the external circuit facilitates this reduction reaction. The reduction reaction (hydrolysis of oxygen) is shown as

$$O_2 + 2H_2O + 4e^- \rightarrow 4OH^-$$

The hydroxyl (OH^-) ions produced by the reduction reaction at the cathode travel to the silver anode. The silver is oxidized at the silver anode providing more electrons ($4e^-$) for the reduction reaction taking place at the cathode. The reaction at the anode is

$$4OH^- + 2Ag \rightarrow 2H_2O + 2AgO + 4e^-$$

Once again, the amount of current flowing through the ammeter is directly proportional to the Po_2 of the sample gas or liquid. The greater the Po_2 of the sample fluid, the greater the number of O_2 molecules diffusing across the semi-permeable membrane and migrating to the cathode. The readout on the ammeter can be calibrated according to either O_2 percentage or partial pressure of oxygen.

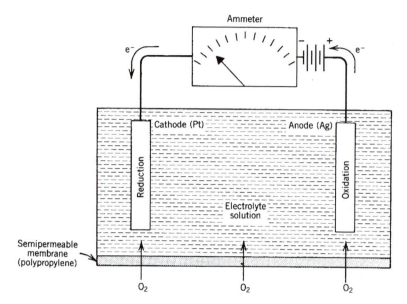

Figure 3-18. *Polarographic cell. The reduction rate of O_2 at the cathode is increased by an external polarizing voltage.*

The utility of the external circuit incorporated in the polarographic analyzer is that it accelerates the rate of oxygen consumption. A polarographic analyzer will consume oxygen without an external electric source, but the rate of such a reaction will be quite slow.

The electrochemical cell just discussed is the one used in blood gas analyzers and in some oxygen analyzers. This cell is commonly known by a variety of names, which include *Po_2 electrode,* **Clark electrode** (named after the person who originally designed this electrode in the early 1950s), and *polarographic electrode.*

Oxidation Potentials

Oxidation potentials indicate the tendency of a substance to undergo either reduction or oxidation reactions. Oxidation potentials are obtained by comparing an electrode made of a given substance—for example, silver, lead, gold, or platinum—to a hydrogen electrode that serves as the standard electrode. The standard hydrogen electrode, where the reference half-reaction is the reduction of H^+ to H_2, is assigned a standard reduction potential of 0.0 volt. That is,

$$2H^+ + 2e^- \rightarrow H_2$$

The voltage of the battery (cell) is indicated by a voltmeter. The voltage and the direction of the current represent the substance's tendency to undergo either reduction or oxidation.

Oxidation potentials are actually obtained by setting up a galvanic cell with hydrogen (the standard) as one electrode and some other substance as the other electrode. For example, when comparing copper to hydrogen, the hydrogen electrode acts as the anode and the copper electrode functions as the cathode. Therefore, the current flows through the wires from the hydrogen electrode to the copper electrode; that is, oxidation occurs at the hydrogen electrode, and reduction takes place at the copper electrode.

During the course of this reaction the voltmeter indicates 0.34 volt. What the voltmeter represents is that the oxidation reaction

$$H_2 \rightarrow 2H^+ + 2e^-$$

has a greater tendency to occur than the oxidation reaction

$$Cu \rightarrow Cu^{+2} + 2e^-$$

by 0.34 volt.

The actual cell reactions are as follows:

$$Anode: H_2 \rightarrow 2H^+ + 2e^- \text{ (oxidation)}$$

$$Cathode: Cu^{+2} + 2e^- \rightarrow Cu \text{ (reduction)}$$

$$Cell \ reaction: H_2 + Cu^{+2} \rightarrow 2H^+ + Cu$$

When zinc is compared to hydrogen, the hydrogen electrode acts as the cathode, the zinc electrode functions as the anode, and the voltmeter reads 0.76 volt. In this instance, zinc has a greater tendency to lose electrons than does hydrogen. Therefore, the oxidation reaction

$$Zn \rightarrow Zn^{+2} + 2e^-$$

has a greater tendency to occur than does the oxidation reaction

$$H_2 \rightarrow 2H^+ + 2e^-$$

by 0.76 volt.

The actual cell reactions for this electrochemical cell are as follows:

$$Anode: Zn \rightarrow Zn^{+2} + 2e^- \text{ (oxidation)}$$

$$Cathode: 2H^+ + 2e^- \rightarrow H_2 \text{ (reduction)}$$

$$Cell \ reaction: Zn + 2H^+ \rightarrow H_2 + Zn^{+2}$$

Table 3-12 lists the oxidation potentials of various substances, including some that are used in galvanic and polarographic analyzers.

The voltage of an electrochemical cell can be determined by obtaining the algebraic sum of the oxidation potential and the reduction potential, that is,

$$E^\circ = E^\circ_{oxidation} + E^\circ_{reduction}$$

where

E° = total voltage of electrochemical cell (volts)

$E^\circ_{oxidation}$ = total voltage at the anode (volts)

$E^\circ_{reduction}$ = reduction potential at the cathode (volts)

TABLE 3-12   Oxidation Potentials

Anode	Anode Reaction	Oxidation Potential (Standard Hydrogen Electrode = 0.00 volt)
Zn;Zn^{+2}	Zn $\rightarrow$ Zn^{+2} + 2e$^-$	+0.76 volt
Pb;Pb^{+2}	Pb $\rightarrow$ Pb^{+2} + 2e$^-$	+0.13 volt
H$_2$;H$^+$	**H$_2$ $\rightarrow$ 2H$^+$ + 2e$^-$**	**0.00 volt**
Cu;Cu^{+2}	Cu $\rightarrow$ Cu^{+2} + 2e$^-$	−0.34 volt
Hg;Hg^{+2}	Hg $\rightarrow$ Hg^{+2} + 2e$^-$	−0.79 volt
Ag;Ag^{+1}	Ag $\rightarrow$ Ag^{+1} + 1e$^-$	−0.80 volt
Pt;Pt^{+2}	Pt $\rightarrow$ Pt^{+2} + 2e$^-$	−1.20 volts
Au;Au^{+3}	Au $\rightarrow$ Au^{+3} + 3e$^-$	−1.50 volts

For example, the voltage of the electrochemical cell having a zinc anode and a copper cathode shown in Figure 3-16 can be calculated in the following manner:

$$E^\circ = E^\circ_{oxidation} + E^\circ_{reduction}$$

$$E^\circ = E^\circ_{Zn;Zn^{+2}} + E^\circ_{Cu^{+2};Cu}$$

where

E° = total voltage of electrochemical cell (volts)

$E^\circ_{Zn;Zn^{+2}}$ = oxidation potential of the zinc anode, which is 0.76 volt (Table 3-12)

$E^\circ_{Cu^{+2};Cu}$ = reduction potential of the copper cathode, which is 0.34 volt (Table 3-12)

Therefore, the voltage for the electrochemical cell illustrated in Figure 3-16 is

$$E^\circ = E^\circ_{Zn;Zn^{+2}} + E^\circ_{Cu^{+2};Cu}$$

$$= 0.76 \text{ volt} + 0.34 \text{ volt}$$

$$= 1.10 \text{ volts}$$

The voltage for the galvanic cell analyzer previously discussed can be obtained as follows:

$$E^\circ = E^\circ_{oxidation} + E^\circ_{reduction}$$

$$= E^\circ_{Pb;Pb^{+2}} + E^\circ_{Ag^+;Ag}$$

$$= 0.13 \text{ volt} + 0.80 \text{ volt}$$

$$= 0.93 \text{ volt}$$

If the voltage of an electrochemical cell, as determined in the examples above, is positive, the cell will spontaneously produce a flow of electrons (current). Hence the $E^\circ_{Pb;Pb^{+2}}$ + $E^\circ_{Ag^+;Ag}$ gives a positive 0.93 volt, and the reaction

$$Pb + 2Ag^+ \rightarrow Pb^{+2} + 2Ag$$

is spontaneous and current-producing. If a negative value is obtained for the voltage, the forward reaction will not occur spontaneously. However, the reverse reaction will take place and cause current to flow in the opposite direction. In order for the appropriate reactions to take place an external current must be applied. The process of applying an electric current to cause an oxidation-reduction reaction (one that will not occur spontaneously) to occur is called electrolysis.

The reduction potential is numerically equal to the oxidation potential for the same reaction but is opposite in sign. Therefore, for the same reaction,

$$E^o_{oxidation} = -E^o_{reduction}$$

For example, consider the following half-cell reactions:

A. For the oxidation of Zn to Zn^{+2},

$$Zn \rightarrow Zn^{+2} + 2e^-$$

the voltage is 0.76 volt.

B. For the reduction of Zn^{+2} to Zn,

$$Zn^{+2} + 2e^- \rightarrow Zn$$

the voltage is -0.76 volt.

Galvanic vs. Polarographic

Both the galvanic fuel cell and the polarographic cell are electrochemical cells. Both of these electrochemical cells undergo spontaneous oxidation-reduction reactions and produce an electric current.

As described in the discussion on the polarographic analyzer, the external polarizing circuit accelerates the reduction of oxygen. Therefore, because the reaction proceeds spontaneously in the polarographic cell, one should not construe the process occurring within that cell as electrolysis despite the presence of an external current.

The voltage for the polarographic cell shown in Figure 3-18 can be calculated as follows:

$$E^o = E^o_{Ag;Ag^+} + E^o_{Pt^{+2};Pt}$$

$$= -0.80 \text{ volt} + 1.20 \text{ volts}$$

$$= 0.40 \text{ volt}$$

The voltage for the polarographic cell having a silver (Ag) anode and a platinum (Pt) cathode is 0.40 volt. Because the voltage is positive, the reaction takes place spontaneously and produces an electric current. However, the voltage is low, indicating a slow reaction. Applying an external electric source causes this reaction to proceed more rapidly.

Once again, the purpose of the external polarizing circuit is to facilitate the cathode (reduction) reaction.

CHAPTER SUMMARY

With the exception of hydrogen (one proton and one electron), atoms contain protons, neutrons, and electrons. These subatomic particles are arranged in an orderly fashion. The nucleus houses the protons and neutrons, and the electrons are positioned in various energy levels around the nucleus. The valence electrons are located in an atom's outer energy level. They influence much of the behavior and properties exhibited by an atom. The periodic table of elements is a listing of the known elements. The atoms are categorized in periods and families or groups based on numerous chemical characteristics.

Henry's law of solubility describes the ability of a gas to dissolve in a liquid. This law applies to the dissolved oxygen and carbon dioxide (other gases as well) in the plasma portion of whole blood. Under normal physiologic conditions, if the amount of O_2 breathed by a person increases, the amount of O_2 dissolving in the plasma also increases.

Graham's law of diffusion has two physiologic applications. One refers to gas behavior inside a container, e.g., the alveoli in the lungs. The other refers to the diffusion of gases across fluid barriers (membranes). The alveolar-capillary membrane allows O_2 and CO_2 to diffuse. These gases diffuse through (across) this membrane at different rates because of their solubility differences.

The relationship between a solute and a solvent can be expressed many ways. Molarity and normality provide two methods for doing so. Molarity involves using the number of gram molecular weights per liter of solution, while normality incorporates the number of gram equivalent weights per liter of solution.

The logarithmic pH scale ranges from 0 to 14. A pH of 7 is neutral; human blood has a pH of 7.40. The pH is quantified as the log of the reciprocal of the H^+ ion concentration. The H^+ ion concentration can be measured as (1) pH, (2) moles/liter, and (3) nanomoles/liter. These forms are interconvertible.

The law of mass action describes the relationship between the rate (speed) of a chemical reaction and the concentration of the reacting species. All chemical reactions at a specific temperature have a rate constant. During the course of a chemical reaction, the reactant concentrations decrease, stabilize, and become constant. The point at which a chemical reaction's reactants stabilize is called a chemical equilibrium.

Buffer solutions are solutions that resist pH changes despite the addition of either acids or bases to the solution. The pH of a buffer solution does change, but the change is minimal. Buffers are comprised of a weak acid and the salt of that weak acid. Human blood contains H_3CO_2/HCO_3^-, HHb/Hb, NaH_2PO_4/HPO_4^{2-}, and protein buffers to help stabilize the body's pH.

The Henderson-Hasselbalch equation can be used to calculate the pH of the blood when the $PaCO_2$ and the $[HCO_3^-]$ are known. Actually, any of these three (pH, $PaCO_2$, and $[HCO_3^-]$) can be calculated from the Henderson-Hasselbalch equation, as long as any two of the three variables are known.

The density of the three states of matter can be calculated knowing the mass per unit volume of any substance. For liquids and solids, the mass divided by the volume the substance occupies provides the density. Gas density is obtained by dividing the gas's gram molecular weight by its gram molecular volume, i.e., 22.4 liters at STP. Specific gravity is a ratio of densities. For liquid and solids, the specific gravity is the ratio of the density of some liquid or solid divided by the standard density, i.e., H_2O, or 1 g/cc. The specific gravity of a gas is obtained by dividing the density of a gas by the standard density for gases (air density = 1.29 g/L).

Three temperature scales are often used in science. They are the Fahrenheit, Celsius, and Kelvin (Absolute) temperature scales. Each scale uses different boiling and melting points for water. Additionally, the Fahrenheit scale has different divisions or calibrations compared to the other two scales. These temperature scales can be converted from one to another.

Electrochemical cells (galvanic cell and polarographic analyzers) are used to analyze oxygen in gas samples. These cells contain an anode and a cathode in contact with an electrolyte solution. Through oxidation (anode) and reduction (cathode) reactions electrons are formed and flow through a "circuit", and measured by an ammeter calibrated to read O_2%.

REVIEW QUESTIONS

3-1 ATOMIC STRUCTURE AND ELECTRON CONFIGURATION

Questions

1. List the subatomic particles located inside an atom's nucleus.
2. Define the terms (a) *atomic mass* and (b) *atomic number*.
3. List the atomic number and the atomic mass for the three forms of oxygen atoms found in nature.
4. Describe an isotope.
5. Differentiate an atom from an ion.
6. What is the spatial relationship among electron shells, subshells, and orbitals?
7. What is the general formula used to determine the maximum number of electrons that can occupy an electron shell?
8. List the maximum number of electrons that can occupy electron shells (a) 1, (b) 2, (c) 3, and (d) 4.
9. How many electrons can maximally reside in subshells (a) $4s$, (b) $4p$, (c) $4d$, and (d) $4f$?
10. Describe the spatial orientation that each of the three p orbitals has with one another.
11. Plot the electron configuration for each of the following atoms: carbon (atomic number 6), neon (atomic number 10), and iron (atomic number 26).
12. What is the maximum number of electrons that can reside in each orbital?
13. What accounts for an oxygen atom's paramagnetic property?
14. Differentiate between electrovalent (ionic) and covalent bonding.
15. Describe the rule of eight.
16. Distinguish between cations and anions.
17. What are valence electrons?
18. What is the name given to the horizontal rows on the periodic table?

19. What name is given to the vertical columns on the periodic table?
20. Describe the electron configuration pattern moving down from the top of a vertical column.

3-2 CHEMICAL LAWS

Questions

1. State Henry's law of solubility.
2. Provide a physiologic example of Henry's law.
3. How does increasing a patient's F_IO_2 represent a manifestation of Henry's law?
4. The determination of a solubility coefficient is based on what three factors?
5. What is meant by the unit *volumes percent*?
6. What is the factor that is used to convert the partial pressure of dissolved oxygen from *torr* or *mm Hg* to vol%.
7. Show the derivation of that factor.
8. Show the derivation of the factor used to convert any P_{CO_2} in torr or mm Hg to volumes %.
9. Indicate the manner in which total CO_2 is expressed.
10. Total CO_2 is the mathematical sum of what two components?
11. Show the relationship between the units *volumes percent* and *millimoles of CO_2/liter*.
12. Derive the factor used to convert the amount of dissolved CO_2 expressed in *torr* or *mm Hg* to millimoles of CO_2/liter.
13. Explain what is meant by *diffusion*.
14. Distinguish between Graham's law of diffusion as it applies to a gas diffusing within another gas and as it applies to a gas diffusing within a liquid.
15. Write the formula that applies to the relative rate of diffusion for O_2 and CO_2 within an alveolus.
16. Write the formula that describes the relative rate of diffusion for O_2 and CO_2 across the alveolar-capillary membrane.
17. What term can substitute for the gas densities in both forms of Graham's laws?
18. Explain why the diffusion of a gas proceeds slower than anticipated.
19. Which form of Graham's law of diffusion applies to the D_LCO measurement? Why?
20. Write the formula that provides the factor used to convert the D_LCO to the D_LO_2?

3-3 MOLARITY AND NORMALITY

Questions

1. The following terms: (a) *solute*, (b) *solvent*, and (c) *solution*.
2. Define a mole.
3. Define a gram molecular weight.

4. Write the formula that provides the calculation of the number of moles of a substance.
5. List the formula for molarity.
6. Define a gram equivalent weight.
7. Write the formula for normality.
8. What is the relationship between the gram molecular weight and the gram equivalent for a monovalent compound?
9. How do the molarity and normality of a monovalent compound compare?
10. When is a 1 M solution equivalent to a 1 N solution?

3-4 LAW OF MASS ACTION AND HENDERSON-HASSELBALCH EQUATION

Questions

1. What do the expressions *pH* and *pOH* represent?
2. What are the molar concentrations of H^+ and OH^- ions in a pure water solution?
3. How do pH and pOH relate to each other?
4. Present two mathematical expressions that would allow for the calculation of pH.
5. A pH change from 9 to 7 would represent what degree of change in the $[H^+]$ in that solution? Would the solution be alkaline or acidic?
6. An increase of 0.3 pH unit represents what degree of $[H^+]$ change?
7. Define the Greek prefix "*nano-.*"
8. What is a nanomole?
9. Given a $PaCO_2$ of 40 mm Hg and $[HCO_3^-]$ of 12 mmol/liter, determine the $[H^+]$ in nanomoles/liter.
10. How many nanomoles of H^+ ions/liter produce a pH of 7.40?
11. Given a dissolved carbon dioxide tension of 30 mm Hg and a combined carbon dioxide value of 24 millimoles/liter, find the hydrogen ion concentration in nanomoles per liter.
12. What pH value corresponds to the $[H^+]$ in nanomoles/liter in question 11?
13. Ah $[H^+]$ of 60 nanomoles per liter corresponds to a $[H^+]$ of how many moles per liter?
14. As the pH increases, the hydrogen ion concentration in nanomoles/liter
   _____ .
15. If the pH of human blood changed from 7.35 to 7.37, what would be the corresponding $[H^+]$ change expressed in nanomoles/liter?
16. Write the equation used to convert pH expressed in logarithmic units to the equivalent of $[H^+]$ in nanomoles/liter.
17. Show how $[H^+]$ expressed as pH can be changed to moles/liter.
18. What is the law of mass action?
19. What factors influence the rate of a chemical reaction?

20. Describe what is meant by a state of chemical equilibrium.
21. Distinguish between the terms *products* and *reactants.*
22. Define *equilibrium constant.*
23. Explain how the law of mass action applies to the chloride shift at the tissue level.
24. List the two products that result when a strong acid (e.g., HCl) is added to a buffer solution comprised of a weak acid and the salt of that weak acid.
25. List the two products that result when a strong base (e.g., NaOH) is added to a buffer solution as described in question 24.
26. How can human blood be considered a buffer solution?
27. What law is the basis for the Henderson-Hasselbalch equation?
28. Show the derivation of the Henderson-Hasselbalch equation.
29. Define the term *pK.*
30. Write the overall CO_2 hydration reaction.
31. What two pK values comprise the pK for the overall CO_2 hydration reaction?

3-5 DENSITY AND SPECIFIC GRAVITY

Questions

1. Differentiate between mass and weight.
2. How is density quantitatively defined?
3. Compare the method for determining the density of solids and liquids to that used for gases.
4. Compare the units used to express the density of solids and liquids to those used for gases.
5. Why is the value for specific gravity a dimensionless entity?
6. What is the standard used for finding (a) the specific gravity of solids and liquids and (b) the specific gravity of gases?
7. What are the values for these two standards?
8. How does the density of O_2 relate to the density of air?
9. How does the specific gravity of O_2 relate to the specific gravity of air?
10. What is the specific gravity of (a) the substance used as the standard for determining the specific gravity of solids and liquids and (b) the substance used as the standard for obtaining the specific gravity of gases?

3-6 TEMPERATURE SCALES

Questions

1. Define thermal energy.
2. Differentiate *average* kinetic energy from *total* kinetic energy.

3. Define temperature.

4. Compound A weighs 2 grams; compound B weighs 1 gram. Both compounds have a temperature of 50°C. Which compound has more thermal energy? Why?

5. Which compound in question 4, A or B, has the higher *total* kinetic energy? Why?

6. Using the freezing and boiling points of water as references, compare the Fahrenheit, Celsius, and Kelvin temperature scales.

7. Show the formula for converting from the Celsius scale to the Kelvin scale.

8. List the quantitative expressions used for changing degrees Fahrenheit to degrees Celsius and vice versa.

9. List the formulas used for converting degrees Fahrenheit to degrees Kelvin and vice versa.

10. Define *absolute zero*.

3-7 ELECTROCHEMISTRY

Questions

1. Define the terms *electrode* and *electrochemical cell*.

2. List the basic components of an electrochemical cell.

3. At which electrode does reduction occur? Oxidation?

4. Describe the processes of oxidation and reduction.

5. Describe the flow of electrons (current) in relation to the anode and cathode compared to the movement of the anions and cations in the electrolyte solution.

6. Write the half-reaction occurring at the cathode in an electrochemical cell having a Zn anode and a Cu cathode, both immersed in a $CuSO_4$ solution.

7. Write the half-reaction occurring at the anode in the same electrochemical cell.

8. What are some of the differences between the galvanic fuel cell and a basic electrochemical cell?

9. How many electrons are made available by the oxidation process at the Pb anode in the galvanic fuel cell?

10. Write the half-reaction that occurs at the anode and the cathode in the galvanic fuel cell.

11. How does the electron flow (current) in a galvanic fuel cell relate to the number of O_2 molecules diffusing into the electrolyte solution?

12. How does a polarographic cell differ from a galvanic fuel cell?

13. What is the function of the external polarizing voltage associated with a polarographic cell?

14. Write the half-reaction that takes place at the anode and cathode in the polarographic analyzer.

15. What is the relationship between the current flowing through the ammeter and the amount of O_2 molecules in the gas or liquid sample?

16. What is another name for the *polarographic electrode*?

17. What is an oxidation potential and how is it obtained?

18. How can the voltage of an electrochemical cell be determined?

19. What event will result if the voltage of an electrochemical cell has a negative value?

20. Define the symbol E^o.

21. What electrode is used as the standard to which other half-reactions are compared?

22. What is the (a) reduction potential and (b) oxidation potential of the standard electrode?

23. What is the relationship between the oxidation potential and the reduction potential?

24. Define *electrolysis*.

25. Compare the galvanic fuel cell and the polarographic electrode.

Bibliography

Adams, A., and Hahn, C. *Principles and Practices of Blood-Gas Analysis.* London: Franklin Scientific Projects, Ltd., 1979.

Adriani, J. *The Chemistry and Physics of Anesthesia*, 2nd ed. Springfield, IL: Charles C. Thomas, Publishers, 1962.

Filley, G. *Acid-Base and Blood Gas Regulations.* Philadelphia: Lea and Febiger, 1971.

Guenter, C., and Welch, M. *Pulmonary Medicine.* Philadelphia: J. B. Lippincott Company, 1977.

Kacmarek, R., et al. *The Essentials of Respiratory Therapy*, 4th ed. St. Louis: Mosby-Year Book, Inc., 1995.

Levitzky, M. *Pulmonary Physiology*, 3rd ed. New York: McGraw-Hill, Inc., 1991.

Murray, J. *The Normal Lung.* Philadelphia: W. B. Saunders, 1976.

Rattenborg, C. *Clinical Use of Mechanical Ventilation.* St. Louis: Mosby-Year Book, Inc., 1981.

Scanlan, C. *Egan's Fundamentals of Respiratory Care*, 7th ed., St. Louis: Mosby-Year Book, Inc., 1998.

Shapiro, B., et al. *Clinical Application of Blood Gases*, 5th ed. St. Louis: Mosby-Year Book, Inc., 1994.

Strauch, M. *Pharmacology of Respiratory Therapy Medications.* Mosby-Year Book, Inc. 1979.

Wojciechowski, W. *Advanced Practitioner Exam Review: Guidelines for Success.* 2nd ed., Albany: Delmar Publishers, Inc., 2000.

Wojciechowski, W. *Entry-Level Exam Review: Guidelines for Success.* 2nd ed., Albany: Delmar Publishers, Inc., 2000.

CHAPTER FOUR

PHYSICS

The field of respiratory care is permeated with technology. As a consequence, the respiratory care practitioner is in a unique position because he not only has to develop interpersonal skills to psychosocially interact with his patients, but he also must possess a working knowledge of mechanical skills to apply the technology toward the physical treatment and support of his patients.

The purpose of this chapter is to present a variety of physical principles that apply to respiratory care equipment and cardiopulmonary physiology. Some of the principles will initially be discussed out of their respiratory care context. However, these principles will later be related to physical theories and laws to ultimately bring forth their clinical and/or physiologic relevance.

CHAPTER OBJECTIVES

Upon completing this chapter, the reader will understand various physical laws, principles, and theories associated with respiratory care and will be able to

4-1 WORK

- Define *work.*
- Calculate work.
- Describe the relationship between the applied force and the direction of motion.
- Define *power.*

4-2 ENERGY

- Define *energy.*
- State the two forms of energy.
- Describe the relationship between work and kinetic energy.

- Explain the relationship between work and potential energy.
- Discuss how potential energy and kinetic energy convert from one form of energy to another.
- List the formulas for kinetic energy and potential energy.

4-3 KINETIC THEORY OF MATTER

- Discuss the kinetic theory of matter.

4-4 PRESSURE

- Define *pressure.*
- State the formula for pressure.
- Describe how a column of liquid relates to atmospheric pressure.
- Describe the relationship between the density of a liquid and the height of the liquid in an evacuated tube.
- State the various pressure equivalents of one atmosphere.
- Perform mathematical conversions using the various ways of expressing pressure.

4-5 GAS LAWS

- Clinically and physiologically apply Boyle's law.
- Apply Charles' law to clinical respiratory care.
- Relate Gay-Lussac's law to compressed gas cylinders.
- Use the combined gas law to correct for gas volumes collected under varying conditions.
- Discuss the graphic representation of Boyle's and Charles' laws.
- Perform calculations using Boyle's law, Charles' law, and Gay-Lussac's law.
- Apply Dalton's law of partial pressures to the gas mixtures in the atmosphere, trachea, and alveoli.
- Calculate partial pressures of gases after correcting for the presence of P_{H_2O}.
- Distinguish F_{gas} from P_{gas}.
- State the significance of Avogadro's law as it relates to gas volumes exposed to specific conditions.

4-6 FLUID DYNAMICS

- Apply principles and laws of fluid dynamics to various fluid conducting systems.
- Relate the law of continuity to ventilatory and circulatory physiology.
- Apply the Bernoulli principle to air entrainment devices and to partially obstructed airways receiving ventilation.
- Discuss the rationale for helium-oxygen therapy.

- Relate the Venturi principle to gas delivery systems.
- Perform air entrainment calculations.
- Discuss the different types of flow patterns found in the tracheobronchial tree.
- Describe the physical characteristics of the different flow patterns.
- Identify the various components that account for resistance to ventilation.
- Differentiate between series and parallel resistances.
- Solve mathematical problems relating to resistance.
- Discuss fluid viscosity.
- Apply Poiseuille's law of laminar flow to varying clinical situations.
- Relate Poiseuille's law to the concept of airway resistance.
- Discuss in the context of Poiseuille's law the influence of airway caliber on airway resistance.
- Explain how airway length affects other factors in Poiseuille's law.
- Relate the concept of Reynold's number to fluid flow pattern.

4-7 MECHANICS OF VENTILATION

- Apply physical principles and laws to the mechanics of ventilation.
- Relate Hooke's law to the concept of compliance.
- Calculate mathematical problems concerning compliance.
- Describe the role that pulmonary surfactant and surface tension have during breathing (Law of LaPlace).
- Discuss the concept of ventilation time constants.
- Calculate mathematical problems dealing with time constants.
- Describe the clinical relevance of ventilation time constants.

4-8 STARLING'S LAW OF THE CAPILLARIES

- Explain the interaction among the osmotic and hydrostatic pressures at the capillary level using Starling's law of the capillaries.
- Define *hydrostatic pressure.*
- Describe osmosis.
- Discuss normal capillary dynamics.
- Explain the fluid dynamics associated with peripheral and pulmonary edema.

4-9 PHYSICAL AND ELECTRICAL OXYGEN ANALYZERS

- Discuss the theory of operation of physical and electrical oxygen analyzers.
- Explain the application of paramagnetic susceptibility to oxygen analysis.
- Describe the principle of thermal conductivity and its utility in an electric oxygen analyzer.
- Discuss the function of the Wheatstone bridge in an electric oxygen analyzer.

FORMULAS USED IN THIS CHAPTER:

$W = F \times d$ (page 227)

$P = w/t$ (page 231)

$KE = 1/2mv^2$ (page 232)

$PE = mgh$ (page 236)

$P = \dfrac{F}{A}$ (page 241)

$P_1V_1 = P_2V_2$ (page 246)

$V/T = k$ (page 251)

$P/T = k$ (page 254)

$P_T = P_1 + P_2 + P_3 + \ldots Pn$ (page 258)

$P_B - P_{H_2O} = P_{B_{corrected}}$ (page 260)

$\dfrac{C_{gas}}{100} = F_{gas}$ (page 261)

$P_AO_2 = F_IO_2(P_B - P_{H_2O}) - P_ACO_2\left(F_IO_2 + \dfrac{1 - F_IO_2}{R}\right)$ (page 265)

$PV = nRT$ (page 267)

$A_1v_1 = A_2v_2$ (page 270)

$D(v_2^2 - v_1^2) = P_1 - P_2$ (page 279)

$(C_S \times \dot{V}_S) + (C_{ENT} \times \dot{V}_{ENT}) = (C_{DEL} \times \dot{V}_{DEL})$ (page 281)

$\dot{V}_{DEL} = \dot{V}_S + \dot{V}_{ENT}$ (page 281)

$R = \Delta P/\dot{V}$ (page 294)

$R_T = R_1 + R_2 + R_3 + \ldots R_n$ (page 297)

$\dfrac{1}{R_T} = \dfrac{1}{R_1} + \dfrac{1}{R_2} + \dfrac{1}{R_3} + \ldots \dfrac{1}{R_n}$ (page 297)

$\eta = \dfrac{P\pi r^4}{8LV}$ (page 306)

$Rn = \dfrac{v \times D \times d}{\eta}$ (page 310)

$\dfrac{1}{C_T} = \dfrac{1}{C_L} + \dfrac{1}{C_{CW}}$ (page 315)

$TC = R_{aw} \times C_L$ (page 320)

$P = \dfrac{2ST}{r}$ (page 325)

$\dot{Q}_f = K_f(P_c - P_i) - \sigma\,(\pi_c - \pi_i)$ (page 342)

4-1 WORK

The scientific definition of **work** differs significantly from the various meanings the word has in colloquial usage. For example, as you are sitting in your chair reading this book, are you doing work? Are you performing work if you go to the gym to play basketball or go to the park to play tennis? Is Atlas doing work as he supports the earth on his shoulders? (Just hope that he doesn't shrug.) Are you doing work as you sit at your computer for hours manipulating your mouse? It becomes quite clear that in everyday usage the word has a variety of meanings.

Scientifically, work has only one definition. Work is the product of a **force** exerted on an object and the **distance** the object moves in the direction of the force. The magnitude of the work performed can be calculated using the formula shown below:

$$W = F \times d$$

where

W = work

F = force (acting in the direction of motion)

d = distance

Again, F is the force applied to a body, and d is the distance the body moves parallel to the force (i.e., in the direction of the force).

From the relationship presented here, one should note that if either the force (F) or the distance (d) is equal to 0, no work (W) will be performed. The amount of work will be 0 if the direction of the force acting on the object is perpendicular to the motion. (Don't tell Atlas that he isn't working. He may be come agitated!)

If you hold a stack of respiratory therapy textbooks at waist level as you walk across the classroom (Figure 4-1), you have not done any work on those books. Despite any muscle fatigue that you may experience, you did no work on those books.

The reason no work was done on the books is that the force and the distance, or displacement (motion), were perpendicular to each other (Figure 4-2).

If, on the other hand, you carried the stack of respiratory therapy texts (at the same height, i.e., waist level) upstairs to the library, the situation changes. Figure 4-3 illustrates this activity. In walking from downstairs to upstairs, you exerted an upward force of Wt (weight of books) as you raised the books through distance h.

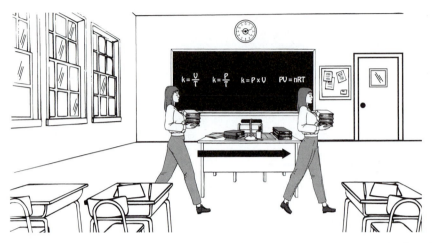

Figure 4-1 *Despite holding the books waist high, the student performs no work because the direction of the force is perpendicular to the motion.*

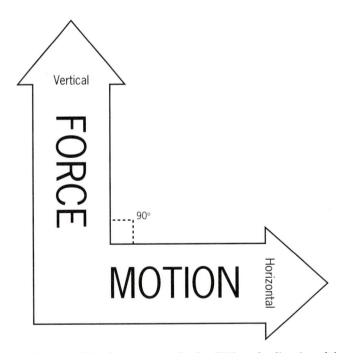

Figure 4-2 *When the direction of the force is perpendicular (90°) to the direction of the motion, no work is done.*

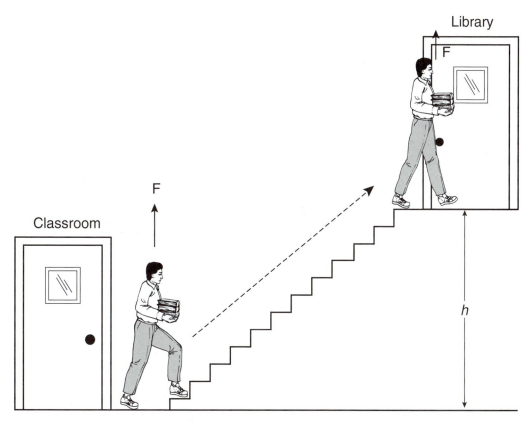

Figure 4-3 *Work is done by the student's vertical force component along the distance* h. *He is lifting the books (waist level) through the distance* h; *hence work is done.*

Remember, only a force applied in the direction of motion does work. You may wonder what results when a force is exerted at some angle to the motion. Figure 4-4 depicts this situation. As you push a box filled with respiratory therapy books along the floor, the force (F) has two components—a horizontal component (F_H) and a vertical component (F_V). Because F_V is perpendicular to the direction of the motion, F_V performs no work. However, F_H is applied parallel to the direction of the motion, therefore, F_H does work.

Consider yet another aspect of work, that is, work done against the force of gravity. This concept was alluded to somewhat in Figure 4-3. We saw that when you carried the stack of books upstairs, work was done based on the formula.

$$W = Wt \times h$$

where

W = work

Wt = weight of object

h = height

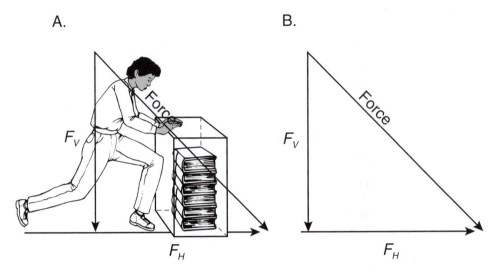

Figure 4-4 *A force applied to an object at an angle to the direction of the motion. Two force components* F_H *(horizontal) and* F_V *(vertical) result when a force is applied at an angle to the motion. In A, the* F_H *is parallel to the motion; hence* F_H *does work. This relationship is again represented in B, where* F_V *does no work as* F_H *does*

Work was done because the force was applied in the same direction as the motion, or displacement, i.e., vertically.

Think about what happens when you finally leave the library, upstairs, and return downstairs with your books to the classroom. Figure 4-5 illustrates the entire sequence of events discussed here. The same formulas apply. However, the work done on the books during the descent (B to C) is computed with the distance having a negative sign because the motion is in the opposite direction of that done on the books during the ascent (A to B). The work done on the books from A to B has the same magnitude as the work done on them from B to C. However, because the work done in these two instances is opposite in direction (i.e., positive work is done from A to B and negative work is done from B to C), the net work done on the books from A to C is zero. Quantitatively, the net work done on the books of the same weight carried upstairs, then downstairs (same distance; opposite direction), is shown as

$$\text{work A to C} = \text{work A to B} + \text{work B to C}$$
$$= (Wt \times d) + [Wt \times (-d)]$$
$$= (+Wt\, d) + (-Wt\, d)$$
$$= 0$$

Table 4-1 outlines the different units used to measure work.
Listed below are examples of calculations involving work.

EXAMPLE 1:

Calculate the net work done by a 150-lb man who climbs up and then down a 20-ft ladder.

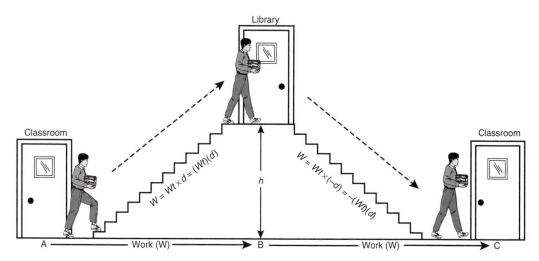

Figure 4-5 *Total work done is zero. Work against gravity is done by the person ascending the stairs; therefore work done from A to B has a positive value. Work with gravity is done by the person descending the stairs; therefore work from B to C has a negative value. As a result, the total work from A to C is 0.*

TABLE 4-1 Units Used to Measure Work ($F \times d$)

Measurement System	Work (W)	Force (F)	Distance (d)
English	foot-pound (ft-lb)	pounds (lbs)	feet (ft)
MKS	joule (J)	newton (N)	meter (m)
CGS	erg	dyne	centimeter (cm)

Step 1: Determine the force and distance for the *ascent* of the ladder.

$$F = 150 \text{ lbs}$$

$$d = 20 \text{ ft}$$

Step 2: Substitute the variables into the work formula.

$$W = F \times d$$

$$= (150 \text{ lbs})(20 \text{ ft})$$

$$= 300 \text{ ft-lbs}$$

Step 3: Determine the force and distance for the *descent* of the ladder.

$$F = 150 \text{ lbs}$$

$$d = -20 \text{ ft}$$

Step 4: Substitute the variables into the work formula.

$$W = F \times d$$
$$= (150 \text{ lbs})(-20 \text{ ft})$$
$$= -300 \text{ ft-lbs}$$

Step 5: Combine the results of *Step 2* and *Step 4* to determine the net work.

$$\text{net } W = (300 \text{ ft-lbs}) + (-300 \text{ ft-lbs})$$
$$= 0$$

EXAMPLE 2:

A person lifts a stack of bricks weighing 170 N to a height of 2.5 meters. How much work is done?

Step 1: Determine the force and distance.

$$F = 170 \text{ N}$$
$$d = 2.5 \text{ m}$$

Step 2: Solve for work.

$$W = F \times d$$
$$= 170 \text{ N} \times 2.5 \text{ m}$$
$$= 425 \text{ N-m}$$
$$= 425 \text{ J}$$

EXAMPLE 3:

A respiratory care practitioner applies a horizontal force of 1.4×10^6 dynes to move a mechanical ventilator 12 meters across the floor. How much work did she do?

Step 1: Determine the force and distance.

$$F = 1.4 \times 10^6 \text{ dynes}$$
$$d = 12 \text{ m or } 1{,}200 \text{ cm}$$

Step 2: Solve for work.

$$W = F \times d$$
$$= (1.4 \times 10^6 \text{ dynes})(1{,}200 \text{ cm})$$
$$= 1.68 \times 10^9 \text{ dyne-cm}$$
$$= 1.68 \times 10^9 \text{ ergs}$$

Power

When you carried your stack of respiratory therapy books upstairs, no consideration was given to how long it took you to travel from the classroom to the library. In other words, no mention was made of the time required to do the work. **Power** is defined as the rate of doing work and can be quantitatively expressed as

$$P = \frac{W}{t}$$

where

P = power (watts)

W = work (joules)

t = time (seconds)

A **watt** is defined as one **joule** per second. Therefore, a machine that works at a rate of one joule/second has a power of one watt. Power is often expressed in kilowatts (i.e., 1,000 watts) because a watt is a rather small unit. Power can also be expressed as horsepower, which is 550 foot-pounds of work/second.

The ability to do work is independent of time; power is work done per unit of time. Therefore, the amount of work that you did carrying the stack of books upstairs to the library will be the same whether you ascend the stairs in 5 seconds or 5 minutes. Similarly, the total work done will be the same if you carry each book upstairs separately or the whole stack at once.

PRACTICE PROBLEMS

Refer to Appendix A (page 598) for the solutions and answers to the practice problems.

Perform the calculations requested in the following problems:

1. A respiratory care practitioner is pushing a 200-lb mechanical ventilator up a 15-ft ramp. He is applying a force of 20 lbs parallel to the incline. How much work will he do?

   Answer: _____

2. A respiratory therapy student places a case of normal saline on a shelf that is 2.4 meters above the floor. The work that she did was 240 J. What force did she apply to the box?

   Answer: _____

3. A respiratory care student is supporting a full E cylinder of oxygen across his right shoulder (not the recommended technique) after lifting it 185 cm off the storage room floor. The amount of work done to lift the cylinder was 1.4×10^9 ergs. What vertical force was applied to the E cylinder?

   Answer: _____

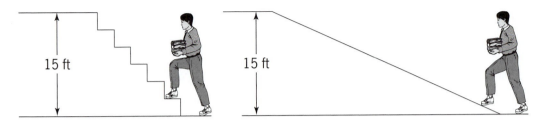

Figure 4-6

4. The student in question 3 begins walking from the storage room to the laboratory, a distance of 460 cm, with the E cylinder of oxygen still supported on his right shoulder. Calculate the amount of work that he will do.

   Answer: _____

5. Calculate the work done by the man climbing the stairs and the one ascending the ramp in Figure 4-6. Both men weigh 180 lbs, and the distance between the floors is 15 feet.

   Answer: _____ and _____

4-2 ENERGY

Work and energy are integrally related. Without this relationship a discussion of work is meaningless. **Energy** is an object's ability to do work. Work is essentially the transfer of energy by mechanical means. The more energy an object has, the greater ability the object has to do work. Therefore, energy is defined in the context of work. These two physical concepts are inseparable.

Kinetic Energy

In mechanical terms energy can be described as either **kinetic energy** or **potential energy.** This section will be devoted to (1) a further elaboration on the relationship between kinetic energy and work and (2) the derivation of the formula that quantitatively defines kinetic energy.

Kinetic energy is the energy of an object of mass (m) moving at a **velocity** (v). Basically, kinetic energy is defined as the energy resulting from the motion of an object. A moving object, that is, one possessing kinetic energy, has the ability to do work because of its motion. The formula describing kinetic energy is shown as

$$KE = \frac{1}{2}mv^2$$

The units for kinetic energy are the same as those for work, i.e., joules, ergs, or foot-pounds.

By virtue of mass being in the kinetic energy equation, the more massive an object, the greater kinetic energy it potentially can have. For example, an 18-wheeler traveling at

60 miles/hour has more kinetic energy than a Volkswagen Beetle moving down the highway at the same rate of speed. Similarly, the faster an object is moving, the more kinetic energy it has. Therefore, the ability to do work increases as the mass and/or velocity of the object increases. An overview of the derivation of the kinetic energy formula will be presented to provide a more complete understanding of this form of energy.

Work was previously defined as

$$W = F \times d \tag{1}$$

The two components of work (W) (i.e., force and distance) will be separately analyzed and derived. Then, the two analyses and derivations will be combined to form the mathematical expression for kinetic energy.

In accordance with Newton's second law of motion,*

$$F = m \times a \tag{2}$$

where

F = force (in the direction of the acceleration)

m = mass

a = acceleration (the rate of change of velocity)

The formula illustrates that the force (F) is the product of the mass (m) of an object and the object's **acceleration** (a).

An object's mass refers to the quantity of matter contained by that object; acceleration is related to the change in the speed of an object. In terms of physics, acceleration is the rate of change of an object's velocity.

Recall that velocity represents a measure of some linear distance per time, such as miles per hour (mi/hr), meters per minute (m/min), or centimeters per second (cm/sec). Since acceleration is defined as the rate of change of an object's velocity, time is introduced into the unit of acceleration twice. Consequently, acceleration becomes some linear distance per time per time (e.g., [(m/sec)/sec or m/sec^2]).

Quantitatively, for a body starting from rest, acceleration can be represented as

$$a = \frac{v}{t} \tag{3}$$

where

a = acceleration

v = velocity

t = time

This relationship shows that velocity divided by time equals acceleration, that is, the rate of change of velocity, or a linear measurement per time per time.

---

*The acceleration (rate of change of velocity) of an object is directly proportional to the force exerted on the object and inversely proportional to the object's mass.

The equivalent of acceleration a in equation 3, which is v/t, can now substitute for a in equation 2. The following relationship will result:

$$F = m\left(\frac{v}{t}\right)$$

or

$$F = \frac{m\,v}{t} \tag{4}$$

Distance d in equation 1 can be expressed as

$$d = \frac{(v_i + v_f)}{2} \cdot t \tag{5}$$

where

v_i = the initial velocity of an object

v_f = the final velocity of the same object (i.e., its velocity after a given period of time has elapsed)*

t = time

2 = allowance for the average velocity to be computed

Therefore,

$$d = (\text{average velocity})(\text{time})$$

Equation 5 shows how the distance can be determined, if within a given time interval an object's average velocity can be measured. Dimensional analysis of equation 5 reveals how the time units cancel and how the distance unit remains. The linear unit meter (m) will be used for distance, and the unit second (sec) will indicate time.

$$d = \frac{\left[\left(\dfrac{m}{sec}\right)_i + \left(\dfrac{m}{sec}\right)_f\right]\,sec}{2}$$

$$= \frac{\left(2\,\dfrac{m}{sec}\right)sec}{2}$$

$$= \text{meter}$$

Equation 5 can also be written for a body starting from rest as

$$d = \frac{vt}{2} \tag{6}$$

In such a situation $v_i = 0$ and v_f will be the object's velocity at the termination of the time interval during which the velocity was measured.

---

*The expression *final velocity* does not mean that the object comes to rest (zero velocity). It refers to the termination of the time interval. In fact, the object can continue in motion indefinitely.

What follows will be the synthesis of the individual analysis of both F and d from equation 1. Equation 4 indicates that the force F equals the product of the mass m times the velocity v divided by the time t. Therefore, mv/t from equation 4 can be substituted for F in equation 1 resulting in

$$W = \left(\frac{mv}{t}\right) d \tag{7}$$

Now, distance d from equation 7 can be replaced by $vt/2$ from equation 6, rendering

$$W = \left(\frac{mv}{t}\right)\left(\frac{vt}{2}\right) \tag{8}$$

Simplifying equation 8, we get

$$W = \left(\frac{mv}{\cancel{t}}\right)\left(\frac{v\cancel{t}}{2}\right) \tag{9}$$

$$= \frac{mv^2}{2}$$

$$= \frac{1}{2}mv^2$$

The formula for kinetic energy, $\frac{1}{2}mv^2$, has thus been derived.

Table 4-2 summarizes the steps used in the derivation of the kinetic energy formula.

TABLE 4-2 Derivation of Formula for Kinetic Energy

Step 1:	$W = F \times d$
Step 2:	$F = m \times a$
Step 3:	$W = (m \times a)d$
Step 4:	$a = \dfrac{v}{t}$
Step 5:	$W = m\left(\dfrac{v}{t}\right)d$
Step 6:	$d = \dfrac{vt}{2}$
Step 7:	$KE = \left(\dfrac{mv}{t}\right)\left(\dfrac{vt}{2}\right)$
Step 8:	$KE = \dfrac{1}{2}mv^2$

Potential Energy

The other form of mechanical energy is potential energy. It is the energy of an object resulting from its position or configuration. The potential energy acquired by an object equals the work performed on that object against gravity or against elastic forces. The classical example of a book resting on a table will serve to illustrate the concept of potential energy. Work was performed against gravity to lift the book to the level of the table. Therefore, the resting book has the potential to do work.

Similarly, winding the mainspring of a spring-operated watch compresses the atoms of the spring. Work was done to bring the atoms of the mainspring closer to each other; hence, the coiled spring now possesses potential energy.

Quantitatively, potential energy of position, or gravitational potential energy, is expressed as

$$PE = m \times g \times h \tag{1}$$

where

m = the mass of the object

g = the acceleration due to gravity for freely falling objects

h = the vertical distance (height) through which a force ($m \times g$) is applied

Recall that work was earlier defined as the product of a force times the distance through which the force acts. Also, the force (F) was defined as mass times acceleration, which is given by

$$F = m \times a$$

However, in this instance, the acceleration factor, a, that was previously used can be replaced by g, which is the gravitational acceleration constant, or the acceleration caused by gravity. Therefore, the force applied by a freely falling object can now be defined as

$$F = m \times g \tag{2}$$

Because F is merely the freely falling object's weight (w), F can be replaced by w. The expression now reads

$$w = m \times g \tag{3}$$

As an object of mass, m, freely falls and accelerates because of gravity, g, through a vertical distance, h, work is performed. Once again, the relationship between work and energy should be apparent.

Equation 1 represents the metric expression for potential energy. According to the English system, the relationship is

$$PE = w \times h \tag{4}$$

where

w = the weight that represents the force required to lift an object

h = the vertical distance (height) through which the weight (w) is exerted

TABLE 4-3	Derivation of Formula for Potential Energy
Step 1:	$W = F \times d$
Step 2:	$F = m \times g$
Step 3:	$W = (m \times g)d$
Step 4:	$PE = m \times g \times h$ (metric system expression)
Step 5:	$w = m \times g$
Step 6:	$PE = w \times h$ (English system expression)

Table 4-3 illustrates the steps involved in the derivation of the formula for potential energy.

The following example discusses the interaction between kinetic energy and potential energy, which were independently presented. The example here is intended to illustrate how these two forms of energy can transform into each other.

Notice the girl in Figure 4-7 throwing a baseball vertically into the air. (Note: The friction between the ball and the air molecules is ignored in this example.)

The girl does work to launch the ball. As the ball leaves the girl's hand, it has kinetic energy. As the ball rises, its speed gradually diminishes because of the influence of the downward force of gravity. As the speed of the ball decreases with increasing height, the kinetic energy of the ball decreases.

When the flight of the ball reaches its apex, the velocity of the ball becomes zero. At that point, the ball has no kinetic energy. The loss of kinetic energy can be quantitatively verified using the kinetic energy formula, $KE = \frac{1}{2}mv^2$. Inserting zero velocity into the equation, the kinetic energy is calculated as follows:

$$KE = \frac{1}{2} m(0)^2 = 0 \text{ J}$$

Of course, anything multiplied by zero (0) equals zero. The kinetic energy of the ball at the top of its flight (apex) is zero. At that point, the kinetic energy has completely transformed to potential energy. When the ball descends, its velocity increases under the influence of the downward force of gravity. Once the ball begins to gain velocity, potential energy begins to convert to kinetic energy—energy is transformed again. When the ball enters the girl's glove, the ball has regained its original velocity. Hence, the kinetic energy is the same as when the ball was thrown into the air. Remember that the friction between the ball and the air molecules is considered negligible in this example.

In summary, the total energy in this example is constant, that is,

$$E_T = KE + PE$$

The energy is totally kinetic at the beginning and end of the ball's flight. At the flight's apex, the energy is totally potential. Between the girl and the flight's apex (ascent and descent), the total energy is a combination of the two energy forms.

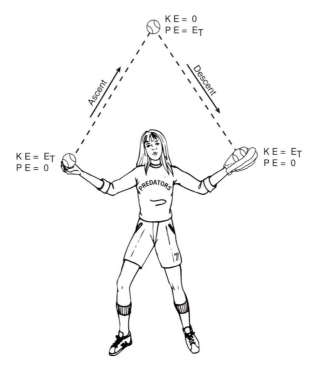

Figure 4-7   KE = *kinetic energy;* PE = *potential energy; and* E_T = *total energy. The instant the ball leaves the girl's hand,* E_T = KE *and* PE = *0. As the ball ascends,* KE *gradually decreases (velocity slows) and* PE *steadily increases. Energy continuously changes form (KE to PE) and* E_T = KE + PE. *At the flight's apex, the ball's velocity is 0; therefore,* KE = *0 and* E_T = PE. *All energy has transformed to* PE *at this point. As the ball starts falling,* PE *begins changing to* KE. *Throughout its descent, the ball gradually picks up speed and* PE *steadily changes to* KE *(*E_T = KE + PE*). When the ball enters the glove,* E_T = KE *and* PE = *0. All the energy has reconverted from* PE *to* KE.

Both kinetic energy and potential energy will be reintroduced during the discussion of Bernoulli's principle in Section 4-6, "Fluid Dynamics." However, at that point both kinetic and potential energy will be discussed in the context of fluids, incorporating the term *volume,* and not in reference to a given object's mass, *m.*

When considering the kinetic energy per volume (*V*), the previous equation 9 becomes

$$\frac{\frac{1}{2}mv^2}{V} = \frac{1}{2}Dv^2 \qquad (5)$$

since *m/V* (mass per unit volume) equals density (*D*). The factors in this expression are as follows:

m = the mass of the fluid

v = the velocity of the fluid

V = the volume of the fluid

D = the density (mass/volume) of the fluid

Therefore, in the formula for kinetic energy, density (D) can substitute for mass (m). Similarly, the formula for potential energy per volume (V), derived from equation 1, is

$$\frac{m \times g \times h}{V} = Dgh \tag{6}$$

since m/V (mass per unit volume) equals density (D). The factors in this expression are as follows:

m = the mass of the fluid

g = the acceleration due to the gravity for freely falling objects

h = the vertical distance through which a force is applied

V = the volume of the fluid

D = the density of the fluid

4-3 KINETIC THEORY OF MATTER

The kinetic theory of matter states that any given sample of matter is composed of many small particles (molecules, atoms, or ions) that are in constant motion. This theory applies to all three states of matter—solids, liquids, and gases.

Intermolecular forces (**van der Waals forces**), the forces between adjacent molecules, limit the mobility of molecules in a solid. The molecules of a solid are restricted or confined. They are chemically bound and cannot freely move about the boundaries of the solid. Rather, they oscillate about a fixed point. When the temperature of a solid is raised high enough, the bonds between the molecules or atoms comprising the solid can be disrupted, thereby allowing the molecules or atoms to move about more freely. When this situation occurs, the solid has achieved a change of state and has become a liquid.

In liquids the intermolecular forces are less than those in solids. Therefore, liquid molecules are free to move about within the confines of a container. The movement of molecules within the liquid state can be described as random, haphazard, or irregular. Such motion is synonymous with that described in 1827 by Robert Brown, a Scottish botanist; this movement is referred to as **Brownian motion.** The intermolecular forces in the liquid state are insufficient to maintain shape, but are sufficient to maintain volume.

When the temperature of a liquid is elevated to the point where most of the intermolecular forces are overcome, allowing the molecules to travel at a rapid velocity and to escape the confines of the liquid, the liquid becomes a gas. Gases have the weakest intermolecular forces, allowing them to expand indefinitely. Gas molecules move at extremely high speeds and are widely separated. The movement of gas molecules is also described as Brownian motion. Gases can be confined only when limits are placed on their expansion, that is, when they are placed in a closed container.

Confined gas molecules continue to move at a high rate of speed within their container. Under such conditions these molecules collide with one another and with the walls of the containing vessel. Consequently, a pressure is exerted by the gas. If the gas volume is decreased, molecular bombardments increase, giving rise to an increased pressure. Conversely, gas pressure decreases as the enclosed gas is allowed to expand, hence fewer molecular collisions. All gases, regardless of their chemical composition, respond in a similar fashion to temperature and pressure changes.

The kinetic theory of matter explains how gas molecules exert pressure against the walls of a closed container. The randomly moving gas molecules inside the container bombard the interior walls of the container. Each gas molecule inside the container possesses a velocity with which it strikes the container's wall. The collisions between the walls and the gas molecules are virtually elastic. (In an elastic collision the total kinetic energy of the objects is the same before and after the collision and **momentum** is conserved, e.g., two billiard balls or two marbles colliding.)

As the container wall is struck by a gas molecule, the gas molecule exerts an outward impulse against the container's wall. At the instant the molecule is in contact with the wall, the molecule exerts a force. Collisions occur between the confined gas molecules and the walls of the container every instant. The collisions are so numerous that the total force exerted by the gas is constant within any reasonable time interval.

However, if the surface area of the wall of the container was increased, more numerous molecular collisions with the wall would occur. The more frequent wall-molecule collisions would produce a greater total force exerted by the confined gas molecules. The amount of collisions per unit area is not dependent on the wall's size. Therefore, the pressure (force per unit area) is a constant that is independent of the size of the wall. The pressure exerted by the gas molecules is equal on all sides because the molecules are moving randomly in all directions.

The kinetic molecular theory of gas molecules is summarized in the following statements:

- Gases consist of large numbers of molecules in continuous, random motion.
- The volume of all the molecules of the gas is negligible compared with the total volume in which the gas is contained.
- Energy is transferred from molecule to molecule during molecular collisions (perfectly elastic). However, the average kinetic energy of the gas molecules remains constant only as long as the gas temperature does not change.
- The average kinetic energy and the absolute temperature of the gas molecules are directly proportional (i.e., at any temperature the gas molecules have the same average kinetic energy).

The ideal gas equation, discussed in Chapter 3, fails to describe the real relationship among gas molecules. For example, at high pressure real gases do not behave ideally. However, at lower pressures gas behavior deviates less from the ideal gas equation. Furthermore, gases behave more ideally at extremely high temperatures compared with their behavior at very low temperatures.

The reasons for these deviations from ideal behavior are (1) real gas molecules have a finite volume and (2) gas molecules exert attractive forces (van der Waals forces) upon one another.

4-4 PRESSURE

Pressure is quantitatively defined as a force (F) acting perpendicularly to a surface area (A), that is,

$$P = \frac{F}{A}$$

Within the atmosphere we breathe, the force results from the constant motion, that is, the kinetic energy ($\frac{1}{2}mv^2$ or $\frac{1}{2}Dv^2$), of the molecules of the constituent gases. This force is applied against the surface of the earth. The result of dividing this applied force by the surface area upon which it acts is ordinarily described as **atmospheric pressure.**

In the context of cardiopulmonary physiology and the clinical treatment of cardiopulmonary diseases, measuring various forms of pressure is of extreme importance. This section has a threefold purpose: (1) to explain the basis for atmospheric pressure, (2) to introduce various units used for measuring and expressing pressure, and (3) to demonstrate how to convert from one unit of pressure to another.

Atmospheric pressure can be measured by inverting the open end of an evacuated glass tube (which is closed at the other end) into a mercury reservoir. The pressure of the atmosphere acts on the reservoir surface causing mercury to rise into the glass tube. The glass tube is calibrated in either inches, centimeters, or millimeters to allow the height of the mercury column to be measured, as is shown in Figure 4-8.

Understanding the rationale for using an evacuated tube with one end closed is paramount. Consider Figure 4-9, which illustrates an open-ended (both ends) tube immersed in a mercury reservoir. Notice that the mercury does not rise inside the open-ended tube as it did in the evacuated tube shown in Figure 4-8.

The atmospheric pressure (P) is equal both inside and outside of the tube; therefore, the mercury level is the same throughout the system. The reason why the mercury does not rise in the open-ended tube is that when such a tube is immersed into the mercury, the atmospheric pressure acts on the surface of the liquid equally inside and outside the open-ended tube. The atmospheric pressure is equal throughout the entire reservoir, causing the liquid level to remain even.

By multiplying the density (D) of the liquid in the reservoir by the height (h) of the liquid column in the evacuated tube, the pressure acting on the reservoir's surface can be calculated. Note the apparatus shown in Figure 4-10.

For example, if the liquid is mercury, the calculation using the *weight density* (English system) is

$$\text{atmospheric pressure} = \text{height of liquid} \times \text{density of liquid}$$

$$= \text{in.} \times \text{lbs/in.}^3$$

$$= \text{lbs/in.}^2 \text{ or } \textbf{psi} \text{ (pounds per square inch)}$$

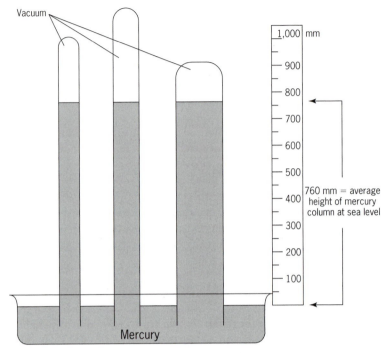

Figure 4-8 *Three evacuated glass tubes with their open ends immersed in a mercury reservoir. Mercury rises up the glass tubes because the atmospheric pressure acting on the surface of the mercury forces the mercury up the evacuated glass columns. Note that the height of the mercury column is independent of the diameter of the glass tube.*

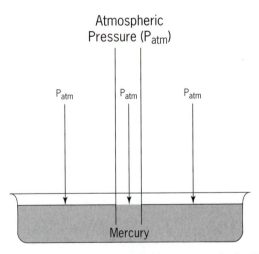

Figure 4-9 *Open-ended (both ends) glass tube immersed in a mercury basin. Note that because of the equal influence of atmospheric pressure (P_{atm}) on the mercury surface inside and outside the glass tube, the level of mercury does not rise above the level of the mercury in the basin.*

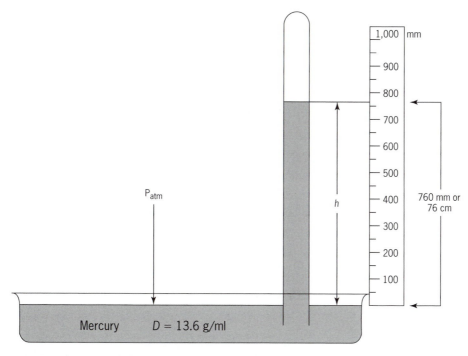

Figure 4-10 *The open end of an evacuated glass tube is immersed in a mercury reservoir exposed to P_{atm}. The P_{atm} is calculated by multiplying the density (D) of the liquid (mercury) in the reservoir by the height (h) of the mercury column in the evacuated glass tube.*

In metric-units the corresponding calculation is

$$\text{pressure} = \text{cm} \times \text{g/cm}^3$$
$$= \text{g/cm}^2$$

The unit **atmosphere** is commonly used as a unit of pressure. It represents the average pressure exerted on the earth at sea level. In fact, this measurement is used as the **standard atmospheric pressure, or barometric pressure.** The following list includes various equivalents of one atmosphere (atm).

760 mm Hg
760 torr
1034 cm H_2O
33 ft H_2O
14.7 psi
29.9 in. Hg
101.33 kPa
1.014×10^6 dynes/cm^2

EXAMPLE 1:

Convert 1 ft H_2O to cm H_2O.

Step 1: Find the corresponding equivalent units.

$$1 \text{ ft} = 12 \text{ in.}$$

$$1 \text{ in.} = 2.54 \text{ cm}$$

Step 2: Solve for cm.

$$12 \text{ in.} \times 2.54 \text{ cm/in.} = 30.48 \text{ cm}$$

Answer: 30.48 cm H_2O

EXAMPLE 2:

Convert 191.36 in. Hg to atm.

Step 1: Find the corresponding atmospheric equivalent in in. Hg.

$$29.9 \text{ in. Hg} = 1 \text{ atm}$$

Step 2: Solve for atm.

$$191.36 \text{ in. Hg} \times \frac{1 \text{ atm}}{29.9 \text{ in. Hg}} = 6.40 \text{ atm}$$

Answer: 6.40 atm

EXAMPLE 3:

Convert 100 mm Hg to kPa.

Step 1: State the problem.

$$100 \text{ mm Hg} = \underline{\quad} \text{ kPa}$$

Step 2: Set up a proportion using the pressure given (100 mm Hg) and the atmospheric equivalent of kPa and mm Hg.

$$1 \text{ atm} = 101.33 \text{ kPa}$$

$$1 \text{ atm} = 760 \text{ mm Hg}$$

$$\frac{100 \text{ mm Hg}}{760 \text{ mm Hg}} = \frac{X}{101.33 \text{ kPa}}$$

$$X = \frac{(100 \text{ mm Hg})(101.33 \text{ kPa})}{760 \text{ mm Hg}}$$

$$X = \frac{10,133 \text{ kPa}}{760} = 13.33 \text{ kPa}$$

Answer: 13.33 kPa

PRACTICE PROBLEMS

Refer to Appendix A (pages 598-599) for the solutions and answers to the practice problems.

Perform the following pressure conversions:

6. 9.21×10^6 mm Hg = _____ cm H_2O
7. 429 ft H_2O = _____ atm
8. 380 torr = _____ ft H_2O
9. 80 in. Hg = _____ cm Hg
10. 4.92×10^{-8} psi = _____ atm
11. 9.03×10^9 mm Hg = _____ in. Hg
12. 4.29×10^3 atm = _____ torr
13. 563 kPa = _____ atm
14. 9.49×10^2 kPa = _____ torr
15. 2.78×10^4 cm H_2O = _____ kPa

4-5 GAS LAWS

The physical behavior of matter in the gaseous state can be explained on the basis of the variables (1) temperature, (2) pressure, (3) volume, and (4) mass (amount of gas). The expressions *ideal gas* and *perfect gas* imply that certain physical phenomena, intermolecular forces, for example, are disregarded for the purpose of understanding or predicting gas behavior. Therefore, a number of laws that follow will be presented in the context of an ideal gas. In an ideal gas context, the relationship among the variables can be observed under conditions wherein certain factors are held constant. These variables do not change independently of one another.

Keep in mind that no real gas behaves like an ideal gas under all conditions of temperature and pressure. The ideal gas is an imaginary standard to which the behavior of a known gas is compared. Under ordinary conditions of temperature and pressure most gases conform to the gas laws, and their behavior resembles that of an ideal gas. However, under conditions of high pressures and low temperatures, significant deviations from ideal gas behavior occur.

Some gases conform better to the ideal gas laws than others. For example, oxygen and hydrogen conform fairly well. However, carbon dioxide and ammonia do not. Carbon dioxide is often referred to as a non-ideal gas.

Two of the laws, Boyle's and Charles', have been alluded to earlier in Chapter 1, Section 1-2, "Ratios." They, along with a number of other gas laws, will be discussed here in more detail. Whenever possible, clinical and/or physiologic references will be made.

Boyle's Law

Boyle's law states that for a given mass of gas the volume (V) and pressure (P) are inversely proportional when the temperature (T) is constant. This relationship is shown mathematically as

$$P \times V = k$$

where

P = pressure

V = volume

k = temperature and mass of gas (constant)

Figure 4-11 demonstrates the relationship among these variables as conditions change. The arrows represent the force applied to the piston.

Figure 4-11A shows that the gas molecules inside the cylinder occupy a certain volume and exert a certain pressure when the weightless piston is influenced by a certain weight (W). Figure 4-11B demonstrates that the pressure doubles when twice the weight is exerted on the piston. The gas volume in this case is halved. The gas molecules in the cylinder exert a greater pressure because molecule-molecule and molecule-wall collisions are more frequent. The volume is compressed and the molecules are more crowded. In Figure 4-11B the number of collisions is twice the original situation. Quantitatively, this relationship is shown as

$$(2P)\left(\frac{V}{2}\right) = k$$

where

$2P$ = twice the original pressure (P)

$\dfrac{V}{2}$ = half the original volume (V)

Conversely, Figure 4-11C shows that the original pressure is halved and the volume is doubled when half the weight (½ W) is imposed on the piston. The gas molecules in this cylinder experience less interaction among themselves and fewer collisions with the walls of the cylinder because they have more room in which to travel. The volume has been decompressed. Note the relationship

$$\left(\frac{P}{2}\right)(2V) = k$$

where

$\dfrac{P}{2}$ = half the original pressure (P)

$2V$ = twice the original volume (V)

Therefore, when an ideal gas changes from its original pressure (P_1) and volume (V_1) to a new pressure (P_2) and volume (V_2), the expression becomes

$$P_1V_1 = P_2V_2$$

or

$$\frac{P_1}{P_2} = \frac{V_2}{V_1}$$

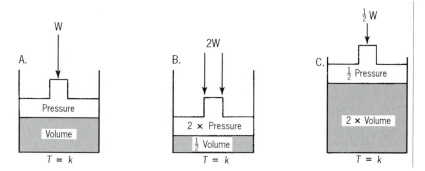

Figure 4-11 *Boyle's law. Cylinder A shows a volume-pressure relationship. Arrow atop piston denotes pressure caused by weight (W). Cylinder B indicates a twofold pressure increase (double arrows) causing a twofold volume reduction. Cylinder C depicts one half the original pressure (small arrow) resulting in twofold volume increase. Temperature and mass of the gas are constant.*

The following data (Table 4-4) are plotted on the graph in Figure 4-12 to illustrate the relationship between pressure and volume, as expressed in Boyle's law.

The original pressure and volume are 100 torr and 1,000 ml, respectively. The set of conditions immediately following represents a doubling of the original pressure and halving of the original volume. The ensuing sets of data demonstrate a threefold, fivefold and tenfold increase over the original pressure with the corresponding volumes being reduced by the same factor. Notice that when these data points are connected by a line the resulting curve is a hyperbola. A hyperbolic curve indicates that the variables plotted on the graph are inversely related.

EXAMPLE:

A constant mass of gas is confined to a cylinder by a piston (Figure 4-13) at a temperature of 25°C and is exposed to two different sets of pressure and volume conditions. The volume of gas in the cylinder was 350 ml when a pressure of 700 torr was exerted by the piston. Calculate the new volume in the cylinder as the piston pressure increases to 950 torr.

TABLE 4-4   Boyle's Law Data Plotted in Figure 4-12

Pressure (torr)	Volume (ml)
100	1,000.00
200	500.00
300	333.33
500	200.00
1,000	100.00

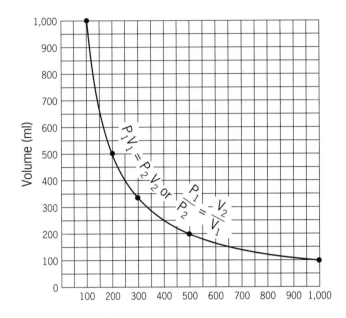

Figure 4-12 *Graphic representation of Boyle's law using data from Table 4-4. A line connecting the data produces a hyperbola.*

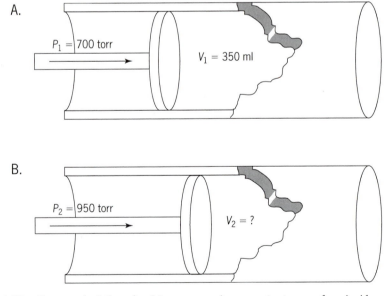

Figure 4-13 *Cutaway depiction of a piston compressing a constant mass of gas inside a cylinder at 25°C at two different pressure (P) and volume (V) conditions: A piston pressure (P_1) is 700 torr and the compressed volume (V_1) is 350 ml. B piston pressure (P_2) increased to 950 torr; the compressed volume (V_2) is unknown.*

	Constants	Pressure	Volume
TABLE 4-5 Boyle's Law Data in Figure 4-13			
Original Conditions ($P_1 V_1$)	m and T	700 torr	350ml
Changed Conditions ($P_2 V_2$)	m and T	950 torr	V_2

Step 1: Arrange the data in a table (Table 4-5) to identify the original and changed pressure-volume conditions.

Step 2: Insert the known values into the formula.

$$\frac{P_1}{P_2} = \frac{V_2}{V_1}$$

$$\frac{700 \text{ torr}}{950 \text{ torr}} = \frac{V_2}{350 \text{ ml}}$$

$$V_2 = \frac{(700 \text{ torr})(350 \text{ ml})}{950 \text{ torr}}$$

$$= 258 \text{ ml}$$

Boyle's law manifests itself within the thorax when breathing efforts are made against a closed glottis. Keep in mind that body temperature and mass of the gas are constant. Body temperature is 37°C, and the mass is constant because gas molecules cannot move past the closed glottis.

Clinically, the **body plethysmograph** (body box) is based on Boyle's law (Figure 4-14). One of the physiologic measurements provided by this device is **thoracic gas volume.** The subject sits inside the airtight body plethysmograph and breathes the air around him through a mouthpiece while the air temperature inside the body box equilibrates with the patient's body temperature. At a certain point during the subject's ventilatory cycle, usually end-exhalation, the mouthpiece is temporarily occluded by means of an electronic shutter.

Assuming that the point of normal end-exhalation is the reference point, it is known that intraalveolar pressure is equal to atmospheric pressure because no air is flowing (no pressure gradient exists). This pressure reading is the original pressure, or P_1. The original volume, or V_1, the thoracic gas volume, is unknown.

When the subject's airway becomes momentarily occluded, the thorax enlarges and intrathoracic gas decompresses during subsequent inspiratory efforts. The intrathoracic gas decompression produces a new thoracic gas volume, that is, the original volume (V_1) plus ΔV (the increase in volume due to decompression) and a new pressure (P_2).

Mathematically, the resulting relationship becomes

$$P_1 V_1 = P_2 (V_1 + \Delta V)$$

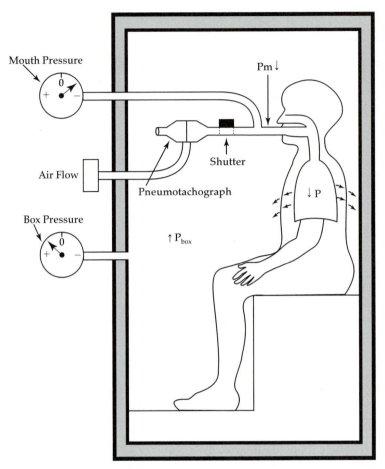

Figure 4-14 *Thoracic gas volume determination via body plethysmograph based on Boyle's law. Body box volume known, alveolar pressure measured, body box pressure measured, and thoracic gas volume unknown.*

where

P_1 = original alveolar pressure

V_1 = thoracic gas volume (TGV)

P_2 = new pressure created when airway was temporarily occluded and when the thorax was expanded

$V_1 + \Delta V$ = original TGV plus additional intrathoracic volume resulting from decompression when airway was occluded

Keep in mind that Boyle's law does not apply to the mechanics of normal, spontaneous breathing. Pressure and volume changes occur during normal inspiration and exhalation. However, the mass of the gas in the lungs changes throughout the ventilatory cycle, thereby negating one of Boyle's law requirements (i.e., a constant mass of gas).

Note the events associated with spontaneous breathing that follow. When the diaphragm contracts (descends), intrapleural pressure drops further below atmospheric pressure (becomes more negative). This subatmospheric pressure is rapidly transmitted across the relatively thin lung parenchyma, thus creating a subatmospheric pressure within the alveoli. Consequently, a pressure gradient exists (mouth pressure greater than intraalveolar pressure), causing air to move from the atmosphere into the lungs. As air enters the lungs, lung volume increases. So, during inspiration intrapleural pressure decreases and lung volume increases.

When the pressure gradient ceases and airflow terminates as a consequence of lung filling, the diaphragm passively relaxes (ascends) causing intraalveolar pressure to rise above ambient pressure. The pressure gradient then reverses direction, permitting air to leave the lungs. Therefore, during exhalation intraalveolar pressure rises and lung volume decreases.

Charles' Law

Charles' law states that for a given mass of gas the volume varies directly with the absolute temperature when the pressure is constant. Mathematically, this relationship can be shown as

$$\frac{V}{T} = k$$

where

V = volume

T = temperature (K)

k = pressure and mass of gas (constants)

Figure 4-15 illustrates Charles' law as the variables are subjected to different conditions. Figure 4-15A illustrates the volume-temperature relationship when pressure is held constant. At 0°C (273 K) the cylinder volume is 273 cc. Figure 4-15B shows the effect on the volume produced by a 1°C rise in temperature. In fact, cylinder B's volume increases 1/273 of the original volume at 0°C as the temperature of the cylinder increases 1°C.

This volume change can be shown quantitatively.*

$$\frac{V_1}{V_2} = \frac{T_1}{T_2}$$

$$\frac{273 \text{ cc}}{V_2} = \frac{273 \text{ K}}{274 \text{ K}}$$

$$V_2 = \frac{(273 \text{ cc})(274 \text{ K})}{273 \text{ K}}$$

$$= 274 \text{ cc}$$

*All calculations involving the gas laws must be performed in K. Therefore, all temperature values must be converted to K. Remember the 0°C = 273 K and that the formula for converting Celsius temperature to Kelvin scale is K = °C + 273.

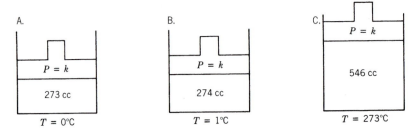

Figure 4-15 *Charles' law. Cylinder A represents a volume-temperature relationship at 0°C. Cylinder B shows the same relationship at 1°C. Note that the volume expanded by 1 cc (1/273 × 273 cc). Cylinder C demonstrates the volume doubling (546 cc) when the temperature increases from 0°C to 273°C. Pressure and mass of the gas are constant.*

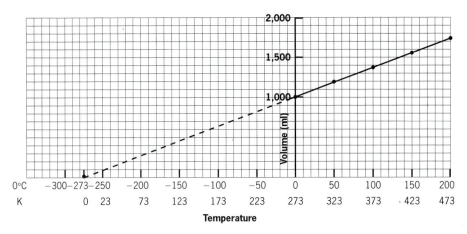

Figure 4-16 *Graphic representation of Charles' law using data from Table 4-6. A line extended through the five plotted points produces a straight line indicating a direct relationship between the variables. If the line is extended to the left (dashed line) of the plotted data, it intersects the x-axis at −273°C (0 K). Volume is said to be zero at that temperature.*

As the temperature further increases, as is shown in Figure 4-15C, the gas volume continues to expand. Cylinder C's temperature has risen to 273°C. Consequently, cylinder C's volume doubles from 273 cc to 546 cc. This volume change can be verified by using the previous relationship.

By the same token, as the temperature decreases, the gas volume decreases by 1/273 of the original volume at 0°C. The lowest temperature that Charles was able to experimentally achieve in his day was about −20°C. Therefore, he was not able to actually observe gas behavior at lower temperatures. He simply extrapolated (extending the plotted line beyond measured data points) below that temperature to −273°C (absolute zero).

Refer again to the cylinders in Figure 4-15. If the temperature dropped to −273°C (absolute zero) the original 273 cc volume would "shrink" to zero!

Figure 4-16 illustrates the plotting of the following data (Table 4-6) on a temperature-volume graph. The original volume at 0°C is 1,000 ml. The second set of data represents

TABLE 4-6 Charles' Law Data Plotted in Figure 4-16

Volume	Temperature
1,000 ml	0°C
1,183 ml	50°C
1,366 ml	100°C
1,549 ml	150°C
1,733 ml	200°C

a 50°C increase in the temperature, which resulted in a 183-ml volume increase from the original volume (i.e., 50°C × 1/273 ml/°C × 1,000 ml). In each instance, the volume will expand 1/273 of the original volume for each °C change from 0°C.

Extending a line through all the plotted temperature-volume data points produces a straight line. Recall from Chapter 1, Section 1-9, "Graphs," that plotting the general formula $y/x = k$ results in a straight line. The formula for Charles' law conforms to that format, that is, $V/T = k$.

Notice in Figure 4-16 that, when the line through the plotted data is extended to the left beyond the data points $y = 1,000$ ml and $x = 0$°C, it intersects the x-axis at a temperature of -273°C, or 0 K. That is the theoretical temperature (absolute zero) where the volume becomes zero. This hypothetical phenomenon is demonstrated as follows:

$$\frac{V_1}{V_2} = \frac{T_1}{T_2}$$

where

$T_1 = 0$°C, or 273 K

$V_1 = 273$ cc

$T_2 = -273$°C, or 0 K

$V_2 = X$

Therefore,

$$\frac{273 \text{ cc}}{X} = \frac{273 \text{ K}}{0 \text{ K}}$$

$$X = \frac{(273 \text{ cc})(0 \text{ K})}{273 \text{ K}}$$

$$X = 0 \text{ cc}$$

The following example demonstrates how to determine the new, or changed, volume when given temperature-volume data pertaining to Charles' law.

EXAMPLE:

A volume of 1.5 liters of CO_2 gas at 30°C is heated to 180°C. Assume that this heating occurs under constant pressure conditions. Calculate the new volume.

Step 1: Convert the temperatures from °C to K (K = °C + 273).

$$T_1 = 30°C + 273 = 303 \text{ K}$$

$$T_2 = 180°C + 273 = 453 \text{ K}$$

Step 2: Insert the known values into the equation for Charles' law.

$$\frac{V_1}{T_1} = \frac{V_2}{T_2}$$

$$\frac{1.5 \text{ L}}{303 \text{ K}} = \frac{V_2}{453 \text{ K}}$$

$$V_2 = \frac{(1.5 \text{ L})(453 \text{ K})}{303 \text{ K}}$$

$$= 2.24 \text{ L}$$

Gay-Lussac's Law

Gay-Lussac's law states that for a given mass of gas the pressure varies directly with the absolute temperature when the gas volume remains constant. This relationship is

$$\frac{P}{T} = k$$

Gay-Lussac experimentally discovered that when a quantity of gas at standard temperature (0°C) is heated to 1°C, the pressure increases 1/273 of the original pressure at 0°C when the volume is held constant.

Figure 4-17 demonstrates the proportional pressure changes accompanying temperature changes as the gas volume and mass remain constant.

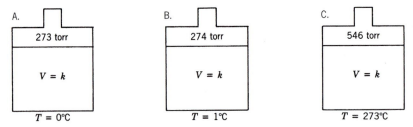

Figure 4-17 *Gay-Lussac's law. Cylinder A indicates a pressure-temperature relationship at 0°C. Cylinder B depicts the same relationship at 1°C. Note that the pressure increased by 1 torr (1/273 × 273 torr). Cylinder C shows the pressure doubling (546 torr) when the temperature increases from 0°C to 273°C. Volume and mass of the gas are constant.*

In Figure 4-17A, the cylinder contains a constant volume at 0°C (standard temperature) and at a pressure of 273 torr. Figure 4-17B demonstrates the influence that a 1°C temperature increase has on the pressure exerted on the constant volume. That pressure increased by 1 torr when the temperature changes from 0 to 1°C. Quantitatively, this can be seen as*

$$\frac{P_1}{P_2} = \frac{T_1}{T_2}$$

$$\frac{273 \text{ torr}}{P_2} = \frac{273 \text{ K}}{274 \text{ K}}$$

$$P_2 = \frac{(273 \text{ torr})(274 \text{ K})}{273 \text{ K}}$$

$$= 274 \text{ torr}$$

In other words, the pressure increased by an increment of 1/273 of the original pressure at 0°C.

Figure 4-17C exemplifies what happens to the original pressure (273 torr) as the temperature increases from 0 to 273°C. The original pressure doubles to 546 torr.

Conversely, Gay-Lussac's law also states that as a constant volume of gas experiences a 1°C drop in temperature the pressure decreases by 1/273 of the original pressure. Consequently, if a fixed quantity of gas were progressively cooled to absolute zero (−273°C), the pressure would cease to exist. This theoretical implication can be shown mathematically using cylinder A in Figure 4-17 as the starting point.

$P_1 = 273$ torr

$P_2 = X$

$T_1 = 273$ K

$T_2 = 0$ K

$$\frac{P_1}{P_2} = \frac{T_1}{T_2}$$

$$\frac{273 \text{ torr}}{X} = \frac{273 \text{ K}}{0 \text{ K}}$$

$$X = \frac{(273 \text{ torr})(0 \text{ K})}{273 \text{ K}}$$

$$X = 0 \text{ torr}$$

A clinical example of Gay-Lussac's law is a compressed gas cylinder whose contents are not being tapped. It can then be assumed that the volume and mass of the gas will remain virtually constant because the gas is confined to a steel alloy cylinder. Therefore, pressure and temperature are the two directly related variables.

*K = °C + 273.

EXAMPLE:

Suppose that a three-fourths-full G cylinder of oxygen is stored in a room at 25°C. Suddenly, the room temperature rises to 70°C. What would be the pressure in the cylinder when the temperature of the cylinder equilibrates with the room?

Step 1: Convert the temperature from °C to K (K = °C + 273).

$$T_1 = 25°C + 273 = 298 \text{ K}$$

$$T_2 = 70°C + 273 = 343 \text{ K}$$

Step 2: Insert the known values into the Gay-Lussac equation.

$P_1 = (3/4)(2,200 \text{ psig}) = 1,650 \text{ psig}$

$P_2 = \text{unknown}$

$$\frac{P_1}{P_2} = \frac{T_1}{T_2}$$

$$\frac{1,650 \text{ psig}}{P_2} = \frac{298 \text{ K}}{343 \text{ K}}$$

$$P_2 = \frac{(1,650 \text{ psig})(343 \text{ K})}{298 \text{ K}}$$

$$P_2 = 1,899 \text{ psig}$$

The combined gas law relates the pressure, volume, and temperature of a fixed mass of gas. The expression for the combined gas law is

$$\frac{PV}{T} = k$$

or

$$\frac{P_1 V_1}{T_1} = \frac{P_2 V_2}{T_2}$$

The combined gas law is essentially a combination of Boyle's law and Charles' law. It allows for the calculation of the new gas volume when both the gas temperature and pressure change, thereby eliminating the need for two calculations.

The combined gas law provides the quantitative relationship and is the basis for the calculation of gas volume conversions associated with pulmonary function testing specifically: (1) atmosphere temperature, pressure, saturated (**ATPS**) to standard temperature pressure, dry (**STPD**); (2) ATPS to body temperature, pressure, saturated (**BTPS**); and (3) STPD to BTPS. When using the combined gas law, corrections must be made for the presence of **water vapor.** For example, if a gas is saturated with water vapor, the partial pressure of the water vapor (P_{H_2O}) must be subtracted from the total pressure before the calculations are performed. Table 4-7 lists correction factors to convert gas volumes collected at ATPS to BTPS.

The following problem exemplifies how to determine the volume conversion factor needed to correct gas volumes from STPD to BTPS.

TABLE 4-7 Factors to Convert Gas Volumes from Room Temperature, Saturated, to 37°C, Saturated

Factor to Convert Vol. to 37°C Sat.	When Gas Temperature (°C) is	With Water Vapor Pressure (mm Hg)[a] of
1.102	20	17.5
1.096	21	18.7
1.091	22	19.8
1.085	23	21.1
1.080	24	22.4
1.075	25	23.8
1.068	26	25.2
1.063	27	26.7
1.057	28	28.3
1.051	29	30.0
1.045	30	31.8
1.039	31	33.7
1.032	32	35.7
1.026	33	37.7
1.020	34	39.9
1.014	35	42.2
1.007	36	44.6
1.000	37	47.0

SOURCE: Reproduced with permission from Comroe, J. H., Jr. et al. The Lung: Clinical Physiology and Pulmonary Function Tests, 2nd ed., Chicago: Yearbook Medical Publishers, Inc., ©1962 and Handbook of Chemistry and Physics, Boca Raton, FL: CRC Press, Inc.
[a]H_2O vapor pressures from Handbook of Chemistry and Physics (34th ed., Cleveland: Chemical Rubber Publishing Co., 1952), p. 1981.
NOTE: These factors have been calculated for barometric pressure of 760 mm Hg. Since factors at 22°C, for example, are 1.0904, 1.0910, and 1.0915, respectively, at barometric pressures 770, 760, and 750 mm Hg, it is unnecessary to correct for small deviations from standard barometric pressure.

EXAMPLE:

The original pressure is 760 mm Hg and the original temperature is 0°C, or 273 K; the final pressure is 755 mm Hg and the final temperature is 37°C, or 310 K. The water vapor pressure at 37°C is 47 mm Hg.

$$P_1 = 760 \text{ mm Hg} \qquad P_2 = 755 \text{ mm Hg}$$
$$T_1 = 273 \text{ K} \qquad T_2 = 310 \text{ K}$$
$$P_{H_2O} = 0 \text{ mm Hg} \qquad P_{H_2O} = 47 \text{ mm Hg}$$
$$V_1 \qquad V_2$$

Step 1: Correct the final pressure (P_2) for the presence of water vapor pressure.

$$P_2 - P_{H_2O} = \text{corrected } P_B$$

$$755 \text{ mm Hg} - 47 \text{ mm Hg} = 708 \text{ mm Hg}$$

Step 2: Apply the combined gas law and solve for V_2.

$$\frac{P_1 V_1}{T_1} = \frac{P_2 V_2}{T_2}$$

$$\frac{(760 \text{ mm Hg})(V_1)}{273 \text{ K}} = \frac{(708 \text{ mm Hg})(V_2)}{310 \text{ K}}$$

$$V_2 = \frac{(760 \text{ mm Hg})(V_1)(310 \text{ K})}{(708 \text{ mm Hg})(273 \text{ K})}$$

$$V_2 = 1.219 \, (V_1)$$

The factor needed to convert gas volume from STPD to BTPS is 1.219. Therefore, the volume (V_2) at BTPS will be 1.219 times greater than the volume (V_1) at STPD.

Therefore, if the original volume (V_1) was 4.50 liters the final volume (V_2) would be calculated as follows:

$$V_2 = 1.219 \, (V_1)$$

$$V_2 = 1.219 \, (4.50 \text{ liters})$$

$$V_2 = 5.49 \text{ liters}$$

Figure 4-18 is a visual summary relating the variables pressure, volume, and temperature and the gas laws that govern them. For Charles' law, the constant is pressure (P). The constant P is located at the apex of the triangle and is opposite the straight line (base of the triangle), indicating a direct relationship between volume (V) and temperature (T) in Charles' law.

Regarding Boyles' law, T is the constant and P and V are inversely related. Last, for Gay-Lussac's law, V is constant, and a direct relationship exists between P and T.

Dalton's Law of Partial Pressures

Dalton's law states that the total pressure exerted by a mixture of gases is equal to the sum of the partial pressures of the constituent gases. The formula for Dalton's law is

$$P_{total} = P_1 + P_2 + P_3 + \ldots P_n$$

with the subscript n implying that any number of partial pressures can be added, assuming that they are all part of the same mixture.

Applying Dalton's law to the mixture of gases, i.e., the physiologically relevant atmospheric air constituents, in the lungs could be shown as

$$P_B = P_{O_2} + P_{CO_2} + P_{N_2} + P_{H_2O}$$

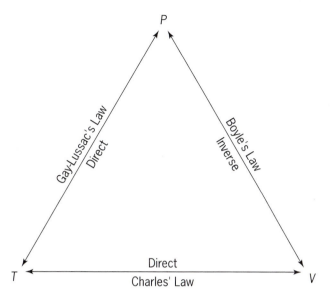

Figure 4-18 *Visual summary of Gay-Lussac's, Charles' and Boyle's laws. The factor (P, V, or T) that is opposite each straight line is the constant for the gas law on that line. The factors at the end of the double arrow line are the variables in the gas law on that line. The nature of the relationship (direct or inverse) is also indicated. For example, for Boyle's law, T is k, and the variable P and V are inversely related to each other.*

Each of these constituent gases behaves independently within the alveoli. However, the individual partial pressures of all the constituents combined comprise the atmospheric pressure within the alveoli. Numerically, at standard pressure (760 torr), the values would approximately be

$$P_B \text{ (barometric pressure)} = 760 \text{ torr*}$$
$$P_{O_2} = 100 \text{ torr}$$
$$P_{CO_2} = 40 \text{ torr}$$
$$P_{N_2} = 573 \text{ torr}$$
$$P_{H_2O} = 47 \text{ torr}$$
$$760 \text{ torr} = 100 \text{ torr} + 40 \text{ torr} + 573 \text{ torr} + 47 \text{ torr}$$

The partial pressure of water vapor (P_{H_2O}) contributes to the total pressure in the example above. Therefore, it obeys Dalton's law. Nonetheless, when calculating the fractional concentration of one of the constituents in a gas mixture containing water vapor, the

---

*Recall that 760 torr is the approximate atmospheric pressure at sea level. The barometric pressure for Denver, Colorado, though, is approximately 640 torr.

partial pressure of the water vapor must first be subtracted from the total pressure. In the case of the lungs, if one needs to determine the fractional concentration of carbon dioxide (F_{CO_2}) in the mixture, the procedure would be

Step 1:

$$P_B - P_{H_2O} = \text{corrected } P_B$$

$$760 \text{ torr} - 47 \text{ torr} = 713 \text{ torr}$$

Step 2:

$$F_{CO_2} = \frac{P_{CO_2}}{\text{corrected } P_B}$$

$$= \frac{40 \text{ torr}}{713 \text{ torr}}$$

$$= 0.056$$

$$= 0.056 \times 100, \text{ or } 5.6\%$$

The P_{H_2O} is subtracted from the total pressure because water vapor does not behave as an ideal gas. The pressure exerted by water vapor is dependent on the temperature and the relative humidity. Therefore, the P_{H_2O} will be a constant value for any given temperature and relative humidity. Table 4-8 lists various temperatures and their corresponding maximum P_{H_2O} values.

In the table it can be seen that the pressure exerted by the water vapor increases as the temperature increases. The converse is also true.

TABLE 4-8 Maximum Water Vapor Pressures (P_{H_2O}) at Different Temperatures

Temperatures (°C)	P_{H_2O} (torr)	Temperatures (°C)	P_{H_2O} (torr)
14	12.0	26	25.2
15	12.8	27	26.7
16	13.6	28	28.3
17	14.5	29	30.0
18	15.5	30	31.8
19	16.5	31	33.7
20	17.5	32	35.7
21	18.7	33	37.7
22	19.8	34	39.9
23	21.1	35	42.2
24	22.4	36	44.6
25	23.8	37	47.0

PRACTICE PROBLEMS

Refer to Appendix A (page 599) for the solutions and answers to the practice problems. Use the water vapor pressure table (Table 4-7) for these problems.

16. A saturated gas mixture with a total pressure of 730 torr is maintained at a temperature of 34°C. What is the corrected total pressure for this gas mixture?

    $PT_{corrected}$ = _____

17. Determine the corrected total pressure for a saturated gas mixture exerting a total pressure of 680 mm Hg at 22°C.

    $PT_{corrected}$ = _____

18. Find the corrected total pressure of a saturated gas mixture exerting a total pressure of 880 torr at 15°C.

    $PT_{corrected}$ = _____

19. What is the $PT_{corrected}$ for a saturated gas mixture exerting a total pressure of 1,000 torr at a temperature of 33°C?

    $PT_{corrected}$ = _____

20. A saturated gas mixture is applying a total pressure of 740 mm Hg at 26°C. What is the corrected total pressure for this gas mixture?

    $PT_{corrected}$ = _____

DRY ATMOSPHERIC AIR & AIR CONTAINING WATER VAPOR PRESSURE

Assuming that dry atmospheric air is inhaled by a normal healthy person, the respiratory mucosa provides moisture to the inspired gas. The inspired air equilibrates to body temperature (37°C) and achieves the maximum water vapor pressure (47 torr) by the time the gas molecules reach the carina.

The percentages of the constituent gases inhaled by this person are nitrogen 79.01%, oxygen 20.95%, and carbon dioxide 0.04%. Actually, atmospheric air is composed of other gases as well (ozone, helium, hydrogen, neon, argon, and so on), but they are present in extremely small amounts and will be ignored here.

The two-step process for converting the gas percentage to its partial pressure is given below.

CONVERTING GAS PERCENTAGE TO PARTIAL PRESSURE

Step 1: Convert the gas percentage to its fractional concentration.

$$\frac{\text{gas percentage}}{100} = \text{fractional concentration}$$

Step 2: Convert the fractional concentration to the partial pressure of the gas.

$$(\text{barometric pressure})(\text{fractional concentration}) = \text{partial pressure}$$

Therefore, concerning the gas mixture just given, the partial pressure of the constituent gases can be obtained as follows:

Nitrogen 79.01%:

Step 1: Convert the gas percentage to its fractional concentration.

$$\frac{79.01\%}{100} = 0.7901$$

Step 2: Convert the fractional concentration to the partial pressure of the gas.

$$(760 \text{ torr})(0.7901) = 600.48 \text{ torr}$$

$$P_{N_2} = 600.48 \text{ torr}$$

Oxygen 20.95%:

Step 1: Convert the gas percentage to its fractional concentration.

$$\frac{20.95\%}{100} = 0.2095$$

Step 2: Convert the fractional concentration to the partial pressure of the gas.

$$(760 \text{ torr})(0.2095) = 159.22 \text{ torr}$$

$$P_{O_2} = 159.22 \text{ torr}$$

Carbon dioxide 0.04%:

Step 1: Convert the gas percentage to its fractional concentration.

$$\frac{0.04\%}{100} = 0.0004$$

Step 2: Convert the fractional concentration to the partial pressure of the gas.

$$(760 \text{ torr})(0.0004) = 0.30 \text{ torr}$$

$$P_{CO_2} = 0.30 \text{ torr}$$

As this inhaled gas mixture enters the trachea, water vapor becomes one of its constituent gases, and, as a result, the partial pressures of the original constituents change. The amount of water vapor pressure that is exerted in the trachea is 47 torr. Again, recall that the sum of the individual partial pressures must equal, in this case, the barometric pressure (760 torr). Therefore, with the addition of the water vapor pressure, the remaining gases (N_2, O_2, and CO_2) in the mixture contribute less partial pressures than in the dry state.

Note how the barometric pressure is corrected for water vapor pressure in the following example.

CORRECTION FOR WATER VAPOR PRESSURE (P$_{H_2O}$)

barometric pressure − water vapor pressure = corrected barometric pressure

$$P_B - P_{H_2O} = \text{corrected } P_B$$

$$760 \text{ torr} - 47 \text{ torr} = 713 \text{ torr}$$

The individual partial pressures of moist tracheal air now become the product of the fractional concentration of each constituent and the corrected barometric pressure. The partial pressures of the constituent gases based on the corrected barometric pressure are calculated below.

Nitrogen 79.01%:

Step 1: Convert the gas percentage to its fractional concentration.

$$\frac{79.01\%}{100} = 0.7901$$

Step 2: Convert the fractional concentration to the partial pressure of the gas.

$$0.7901 \times 713 \text{ torr} = 563.34 \text{ torr}$$

$$P_{N_2} = 563.34 \text{ torr}$$

Oxygen 20.95%:

Step 1: Convert the gas percentage to its fractional concentration.

$$\frac{20.95\%}{100} = 0.2095$$

Step 2: Convert the fractional concentration to the partial pressure of the gas.

$$0.2095 \times 713 \text{ torr} = 149.37 \text{ torr}$$

$$P_{O_2} = 149.37 \text{ torr}$$

Carbon dioxide 0.04%:

Step 1: Convert the gas percentage to its fractional concentration.

$$\frac{0.04\%}{100} = 0.0004$$

Step 2: Convert the fractional concentration to the partial pressure of the gas.

$$0.0004 \times 713 \text{ torr} = 0.29 \text{ torr}$$

$$P_{CO_2} = 0.29 \text{ torr}$$

PRACTICE PROBLEMS

Refer to Appendix A (pages 599-600) for the solutions and answers to the practice problems.

21. A dry gas mixture exerts a total pressure of 670 mm Hg at 35°C. The mixture contains 20.93% oxygen. Convert the oxygen concentration to its fractional concentration.

    F_{O_2} = _____

22. A saturated gas mixture, containing 5% CO_2, exerts a total pressure of 755 mm Hg at 36°C. What is the fractional concentration of CO_2 in this mixture?

    F_{CO_2} = _____

23. A saturated gas mixture exerting a total pressure of 550 torr at 26°C contains 80% helium. What is the partial pressure of helium in this gas mixture?

    P_{He} = _____

24. A dry gas mixture contains 26% N_2 at a temperature of 18°C. Determine the P_{N_2} if this gas mixture has a P_T of 600 mm Hg.

    P_{N_2} = _____

25. A saturated gas mixture exerts a total pressure of 980 mm Hg at a temperature of 14°C. Calculate the partial pressure exerted carbon monoxide which occupies 33% of the total gas mixture.

    P_{CO} = _____

In the trachea the total pressure available for nitrogen, oxygen, and carbon dioxide is 713 torr, not 760 torr, because of the correction for water vapor pressure. Therefore, the P_{O_2} decreases from approximately 159 torr in the inspired air to about 149 torr in the trachea. Meanwhile, the P_{N_2} drops from about 600 torr to 563 torr. The partial pressure of CO_2 reduces slightly also. Table 4-9 compares the relative partial pressures of the gas mixture in the atmosphere and the trachea. The sum of the differences between the P_{O_2}, P_{N_2}, and P_{CO_2} of dry atmospheric air and moist tracheal air equals 47 torr, accounting for the addition of the water vapor pressure supplied to the inspired gas by the respiratory mucosa.

TABLE 4-9 Comparison of Dry Atmospheric Air to Tracheal Air

	Dry Atmospheric Air (torr)	Tracheal Air (torr)
P_{O_2}	159.22	149.37
P_{N_2}	600.48	563.34
P_{CO_2}	0.30	0.29
P_{H_2O}	0.00	47.00
P_B	760.00	760.00

Let us proceed with this physiologic example of Dalton's law one step further. As the gas moves from the trachea to the alveoli, it experiences further alterations. The changes that occur result from the oxygen uptake and the carbon dioxide removal at the blood-gas interface, that is, the alveolar-capillary membrane. Oxygen is continuously removed from, and carbon dioxide is continuously added to, the alveoli by pulmonary capillary blood because of the respective pressure gradients for these two gases. No additional water vapor is added because the inspired air is considered fully saturated (47 torr at 37°C) by the time the air enters the alveoli. In fact, the inspired air is essentially 100% saturated at body temperature by the time it passes the carina. Therefore, the P_{H_2O} plays no role in partial pressure changes taking place after the air leaves the trachea on its journey to the alveoli.

The alveolar air equation can be used here to determine the P_AO_2. The equation is

$$P_AO_2 = F_IO_2(P_B - P_{H_2O}) - P_ACO_2\left(F_IO_2 + \frac{1 - F_IO_2}{R}\right)$$

where

P_AO_2 = partial pressure of alveolar oxygen (torr)

F_IO_2 = fractional concentration of inspired oxygen

P_B = barometric pressure (torr)

P_{H_2O} = water vapor pressure (torr)

P_ACO_2 = partial pressure of alveolar carbon dioxide (torr)

R = respiratory quotient (carbon dioxide production/oxygen consumption); normal value is 0.8

The arterial carbon dioxide tension ($PaCO_2$) can substitute for the alveolar carbon dioxide tension (P_ACO_2) in this equation because complete equilibration across the alveolar-capillary membrane is assumed for carbon dioxide. The two values are not exactly equal; however, the $PaCO_2$ provides a close enough estimate for clinical use and for illustration in this example. Therefore, a normal $PaCO_2$ 40 torr will represent the P_ACO_2. We can now insert values into the equation.

$$P_AO_2 = 0.2095 \, (760 \text{ torr} - 47 \text{ torr}) - 40 \text{ torr}\left(0.2095 + \frac{1 - 0.2095}{0.8}\right)$$

$$= 0.2095 \, (713 \text{ torr}) - 40 \text{ torr } (1.1976)$$

$$= 149.37 \text{ torr} - 47.90 \text{ torr}$$

$$= 101.47 \text{ torr}$$

Note that the alveolar oxygen tension dropped to approximately 101 torr from about 149 torr in the trachea, and that the P_ACO_2 rose from 0.29 torr in the trachea to 40 torr in the alveoli. The alveolar oxygen percentage is around 14%, that is, (101 torr ÷ 713 torr)100; and the alveolar CO_2 percentage is 5.61%, that is, (40 torr ÷ 713 torr)100. Table 4-10 summarizes the partial pressure changes taking place as inspired air travels from the trachea to the alveoli.

TABLE 4-10 Comparison of Tracheal Air to Alveolar Air

	Tracheal Air (torr)	Alveolar Air (torr)
P_{O_2}	149.37	101.47
P_{N_2}	563.34	571.55
P_{CO_2}	0.29	40.00
P_{H_2O}	47.00	47.00
P_B	760.00	760.00

Avogadro's Law

Avogadro's law states that at equal temperatures and pressures equal volumes of different gases, regardless of their mass, contain equal numbers of molecules. For example, if the two gases oxygen (32 amu) and helium (2 amu) are confined to separate enclosures subject to the same conditions of volume, temperature, and pressure, the two enclosures will contain the same number of molecules. Note Figure 4-19.

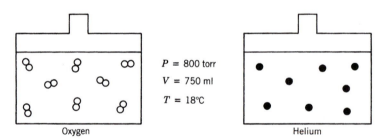

$P = 800$ torr
$V = 750$ ml
$T = 18°C$

Oxygen   Helium

Figure 4-19 *Two different gases (oxygen and helium) are illustrated in separate containers exposed to the same P, V, and T conditions. Avogadro's law states that gases under these same conditions contain the same number of molecules.*

It is now established that, if the weight of a gas in grams equal to the molecular weight of the gas (gram molecular weight, gram-mole, or mole) is subjected to conditions of standard pressure (760 torr) and temperature (0°C), the gas will occupy a volume of 22.4 liters.* Further, 6.02×10^{23} (Avogadro's number) molecules comprise that volume under standard conditions.

Quantitatively, Avogadro's law is written as

$$n = kV$$

---

*This volume applies only to ideal gases. If carbon gas is exposed to these conditions, it occupies a volume of approximately 22.3 liters. Carbon dioxide is not an ideal gas.

where

n = number of moles

k = constant

V = volume (liters)

Ideal Gas Law

The ideal gas law is written as

$$PV = nRT$$

where

P = pressure

V = volume

T = temperature (K)

n = number of moles of gas

R = universal gas (Boltzman's) constant (82.1 atm • ml/mol • K, or
8.31 Pa • m^3/mol • K)

The ideal gas law is actually based on Boyle's law, Charles' law, and Avogadro's law. It allows for the calculation of moles or grams of a gas.

EXAMPLE:

A 5.0-L sample of carbon dioxide gas at 373 K is at one atmosphere of pressure. Determine the number of moles of carbon dioxide in this sample.

Step 1:   Rearrange the ideal gas equation to solve for n.

$$n = \frac{PV}{RT}$$

Step 2:   Insert the known values into the equation.

$$n = \frac{(1 \text{ atm})(5{,}000 \text{ ml})}{(82.1 \text{ atm} • \text{ml/mol} • \text{K})(373 \text{ K})}$$

$$n = \frac{5{,}000 \text{ atm} • \text{ml}}{30{,}623.3 \text{ (atm} • \text{ml/mol} • \text{K)K}}$$

$$= 0.16 \text{ mole of } CO_2$$

PRACTICE PROBLEMS

Refer to Appendix A (pages 600-605) for the solutions and answers to the practice problems. Use the water vapor pressure table (Table 4-7) when necessary.

Perform the following calculations and identify the gas law.

26. A compressed cylinder at a pressure of 750 torr at 25°C experiences a temperature increase to 45°C. Determine the pressure in the tank under constant volume conditions.

    Answer: _____ *Gas law:* _____

27. A gas volume of 500 cc is exposed to a pressure of 900 torr. The pressure is decreased to 750 torr. Calculate the new volume when the temperature remains constant.

    Answer: _____ *Gas law:* _____

28. A gas occupying a volume of 100 ml has a temperature of 30°C. What volume will the gas occupy at 10°C if the pressure remains constant?

    Answer: _____ *Gas law:* _____

29. A gas held under constant pressure has a volume of 200 ml at 30°C. What volume will this gas occupy at −10°C?

    Answer: _____ *Gas law:* _____

30. A volume of 500 ml of gas is enclosed in a cylinder experiencing a pressure of 780 mm Hg. Determine the volume at a pressure of 2,280 mm Hg under constant temperature conditions.

    Answer: _____ *Gas law:* _____

31. A balloon filled with helium has a volume of 3.0 liters at sea level. The balloon rises to a height in the atmosphere where its volume is 9.0 liters. Calculate the pressure in kPa at this altitude as the temperature remains constant.

    Answer: _____ *Gas law:* _____

32. Determine the gas correction factor for a volume of saturated gas collected at 755 torr at a temperature of 26°C (ATPS) to a gas saturated at 760 torr and normal body temperature (BTPS).

    Answer: _____ *Gas law:* _____

33. A saturated mixture of oxygen (40 torr), nitrogen (200 torr), and carbon dioxide at 20°C exerts a total pressure of 317 torr. Determine the partial pressure of carbon dioxide in this mixture and the percentage of all three constituent gases.

    Answer: P_{CO_2} _____ ; $\%O_2$ _____ ; $\%N_2$ _____ ; $\%CO_2$ _____

    Gas law: _____

34. Determine the number of moles in a 40.0-L helium gas volume at a temperature of 50°C at a pressure of 202.66 kPa.

    Answer: _____ *Gas law:* _____

35. Find the gas correction factor for a volume of gas collected at STPD to a gas saturated at 750 torr at 37°C (BTPS).

    Answer: _____   *Gas law:* _____

36. A full E cylinder of oxygen is located in a storage room where the temperature was 22°C. The room temperature suddenly increased to 33°C. Determine the pressure inside the cylinder after the contents equilibrate with the new room temperature.

    Answer: _____   *Gas law:* _____

37. Calculate the factor for correcting V_1 collected at 100.26 kPa at 27°C (ATPS) to V_2 at 101.33 kPa (BTPS).

    Answer: _____   *Gas law:* _____

38. A sample of air at 22°C is trapped over water in the closed end of an inverted evacuated tube. The air occupies a volume of 100 ml and is at a pressure of 1,006 cm H_2O. Determine the volume that this sample of air would occupy if it were dry at the same temperature and pressure.

    Answer: _____   *Gas law:* _____

39. Correct 4.76 L collected at 758 torr and 37°C (BTPS) to 753 mm Hg and 24°C (ATPS).

    Answer: _____   *Gas law:* _____

40. Find V_2 for 3.87 L of a gas collected at 760 torr and 28°C (ATPS) to STPD.

    Answer: _____   *Gas law:* _____

41. Correct to BTPS (757 torr) 5.55 L of gas collected at STPD.

    Answer: _____   *Gas law:* _____

4-6 FLUID DYNAMICS

Respiratory care practitioners are frequently involved with gases moving through conduction systems. These systems include the movement of gases into and out of the lungs during ventilation, the transit of gases through mechanical devices, and the flow of blood through both the pulmonary and systemic vasculatures.

   This section will provide a variety of principles and concepts concerning fluid dynamics. These will include (1) the law of continuity, (2) the Bernoulli principle, (3) the Venturi principle, (4) flow patterns, (5) resistance to flow, (6) viscosity, (7) Poiseuille's law, and (8) Reynold's number. These physical aspects will be discussed to enhance the understanding of air flowing through the tracheobronchial tree and blood coursing through the vasculature.

Law of Continuity

The law of continuity, based on the **law of conservation of matter,** explains the relationship between the cross-sectional area of a tube through which a fluid is flowing and the velocity of the flowing fluid when the flow rate is constant. In quantitative terms, the product of the cross-sectional area and the velocity for a given **flow rate** is constant. Therefore, the two factors, cross-sectional area and velocity, are inversely related; that is, as the cross-sectional area decreases for a given flow rate the velocity of the flowing gas increases and vice versa.

As a practical illustration, consider the following analogy. If you threw a stick into a swiftly moving river, which ultimately joined a large lake, you may be required to run along the river bank to keep pace with the stick's movement (velocity). However, upon reaching the lake, you can catch your breath and repay your oxygen debt because the stick has slowed down (decreased velocity) upon entering the lake (because the lake has a cross-sectional area larger than that of the river).

The continuity equation can be shown as

$$A \times v = k$$

where

A = the cross-sectional area of the tube

v = the average velocity of the flowing fluid

k = a constant

or as

$$A_1 \times v_1 = A_2 \times v_2$$

which indicates that the product of the cross-sectional area and the velocity at any two points in the conducting system are the same for a constant flow rate.

Incidentally, the cross-sectional area of a tube (circle) is given by the formula

$$A = \pi r^2 \tag{1}$$

or

$$A = \frac{\pi \times d^2}{4} \tag{2}$$

where

A = the cross-sectional area

π = the constant value 3.14 (symbolized by the Greek letter pi)

r = the radius of the tube

d = the diameter of the tube

Figure 4-20 illustrates a fluid at a constant flow rate* ($\dot{V}_1 = \dot{V}_2$) moving through a conducting system in which the cross-sectional area changes from A_1 to A_2 and the velocity of the flowing fluid changes from v_1 to v_2. As the tube narrows from point 1 to point 2, the cross-sectional area decreases ($A_1 > A_2$), and the velocity (distance/time) of the flowing fluid increases ($v_1 < v_2$). Again, the flow rate through the system remains constant ($\dot{V}_1 = \dot{V}_2$).

Flow rate is defined as volume/time. It is symbolized by $\dot{V}$; the dot above the upper case V indicates time. The symbol V by itself without a dot over it signifies volume.

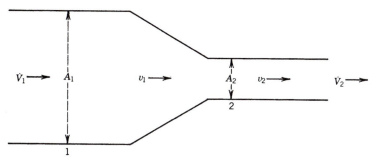

Figure 4-20 *Law of continuity. Under constant flow rate conditions ($\dot{V}_1 = \dot{V}_2$). The cross-sectional area decreases as the fluid (gas or liquid) flows from segment 1 to segment 2 of the conducting system. At the same time, the velocity of flow increases from segment 1 to segment 2 as the fluid encounters the convergence.*

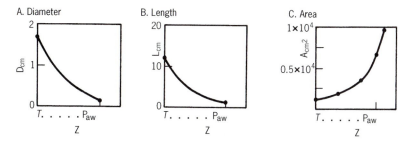

Figure 4-21 *Graphic representation of the geometric configuration of the tracheobronchial tree. Graph A shows that airway diameter progressively decreases along the airway generations (Z) from the trachea (T) to the peripheral airways (P_{aw}); graph B demonstrates how airway length diminishes from T through P_{aw}; graph C illustrates the continuous increase in cross-sectional area as the airway branches at each generation from T through P_{aw}. From Tisi, Gennaro M.: Pulmonary Physiology in Clinical Medicine, © 1980, Williams & Williams Co., Baltimore. Used with permission.*

Dimensional analysis of the continuity equation demonstrates that the product of the cross-sectional area and the velocity equals the flow rate, that is,

$$\text{cross-sectional area} \times \text{velocity} = \text{flow rate}$$

$$cm^2 \times cm/sec = cm^3/sec$$

Physiologically, the continuity equation applies to the movement of air through the tracheobronchial tree. The geometric configurations of the airways from the trachea to the alveoli differ in (1) diameter, (2) length, and (3) cross-sectional area (Figure 4-21).

Figure 4-21 shows measurements for each of these three dimensions ranging from the trachea to the peripheral airways. Figure 4-21A plots airway diameter in centimeters (D_{cm}) on the *y*-axis and airway branching from the trachea (T) to the peripheral airways (P_{aw}) on the *x*-axis. The graph clearly shows that each subsequent airway branching (generation) experiences a decrease in diameter. Figure 4-21B plots airway length in centimeters (L_{cm}) versus airway branchings and illustrates that each ensuing **airway generation** is shorter than its parent. Figure 4-21C depicts the relationship between total cross-sectional area (A_{cm^2}) and airway divisions and demonstrates that the cross-sectional area progressively increases at each airway generation (Z).

These architectural variations result in an asymmetrical pattern of branching described as **irregular dichotomous branching** (Figure 4-22).

Dichotomous branching implies that each branch gives rise to two daughter branches, each of which becomes a parent and in turn gives rise to two more daughter branches. Figure 4-23 illustrates regular dichotomous branching.

Throughout the tracheobronchial tree, which is characterized by irregular dichotomous branching, the cross-sectional area increases at each airway generation despite the formation of daughter branches with a smaller diameter and a shorter length. For example, the diameter of the trachea exceeds that of either the right or left mainstem bronchus individually. However, the sum of the diameters of both the right and left mainstem bronchi is greater than that of the trachea itself. Therefore, since the radius is a function of the diameter (radius = diameter/2), the cross-sectional area increases. This condition occurs at each successive branching until the cross-sectional area of the alveoli becomes approximately 70 m², or 700,000 cm². This area is approximately the area occupied by a tennis court! The cross-sectional area from the trachea (5 cm²) to the alveoli increases approximately 140,000-fold.

What consequence does this tremendous increase in cross-sectional area have on the velocity of the gas flowing through the tracheobronchial tree? Because the relationship between the cross-sectional area and velocity is inverse, the velocity of the inspired gas decreases at each airway generation until the gas reaches the alveoli. At this point the gas is

IRREGULAR DICHOTOMY

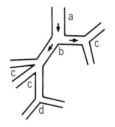

Figure 4-22 *Irregular dichotomous branching demonstrating asymmetrical branching pattern.*

REGULAR DICHOTOMY

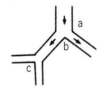

Figure 4-23 *Regular dichotomous branching demonstrating the division of each airway into two branches. Each ensuing generation with this variety of branching forms two symmetrical daughters.*

no longer under the influence of the **transairway pressure gradient** ($P_{mouth} - P_{alveoli}$) which initiated the inspiration. Alveolar gas moves via **molecular diffusion;** that is, it travels by means of the kinetic energy ($\frac{1}{2}mv^2$) imparted to it by the temperature (37°C) of the internal environment. The continuity equation for the entire tracheobronchial tree should read

$$(A_{trachea})(v_{trachea}) = (A_{alveoli})(v_{alveoli})$$

The continuity equation can also be applied to the pulmonary vasculature. Pulmonary blood flow (cardiac output = heart rate × stroke volume) can be considered constant over time. Therefore, the velocity of blood flow is greater through the pulmonary arteries and arterioles than it is in the pulmonary capillary network where the cross-sectional area is larger. The physiologic advantage of the reduced velocity of blood flow through the pulmonary capillaries is that it lengthens the time allowed for gas exchange across the alveolar-capillary membrane.

Also, the area of contact per volume of blood becomes greater, as is shown by the relationship between the formula for the area of a cylinder and that for the volume of a cylinder. The area of a cylinder is given by

$$A = \pi 2rl$$

where

A = the area of the vessel

$2r$ = the diameter of the vessel

π = 3.14 (designated by the Greek letter pi)

l = the length of the vessel

The volume of a cylinder is given by

$$V = \pi r^2 l$$

where

V = the volume of the vessel

π = 3.14

r = the radius of the vessel

l = the length of the vessel

Comparing these two formulas, we obtain

$$\frac{A}{V} = \frac{\pi 2rl}{\pi r^2 l}$$

$$\frac{A}{V} = \frac{2}{r}$$

This relationship demonstrates that, as the radius gets smaller, the ratio, A/V, becomes larger. Specifically, as the vessel volume (V) decreases, the surface area (A) increases; that is, for a given volume more surface area is available if the volume is comprised of more cylinders of smaller radii.

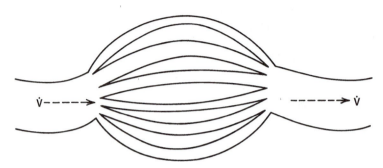

Figure 4-24 *A parallel conducting network through which a constant flow traverses. The conduits of smaller radii within the parallel circuit provide an increased surface area. From Wojciechowski, William V.:* Comprehensive Review of Respiratory Therapy, © 1981. *Reprinted by permission of John Wiley & Sons,*

Figure 4-24 shows a conducting system comprised of a cylindrical conduit of a certain radius giving way to a network of smaller conduits of smaller radii. As the smaller cylindrical conduits with their smaller radii emerge, the surface area they provide also increases.

Physiologically, Figure 4-24 refers to any capillary network. It can represent a pulmonary arteriole branching into numerous parallel pulmonary capillaries, which converge downstream to form a pulmonary venule. The essential point to obtain from this scheme is that the velocity of the flow of fluid decreases through the parallel branches as the cross-sectional area increases. If this model is applied to the pulmonary capillaries, gas exchange across the alveolar-capillary membrane is enhanced because of the decreased velocity and the increased surface area available per unit volume. In terms of a systemic capillary, the diffusion of nutrients and cellular waste products is facilitated.

Figures 4-25 and 4-26 show the relationship between the cross-sectional area and velocity, respectively, throughout the entire circulatory system.

Figure 4-25 illustrates the relationship between cross-sectional area (cm^2), indicated on the vertical axis, and specific locations in both the systemic and pulmonary vasculatures, on the horizontal axis. For example, the cross-sectional area of the aorta is less than the total cross-sectional area of the systemic capillaries.

Figure 4-26 shows how blood velocity (y-axis) changes as it travels through various parts of the circulatory system (x-axis). The y-axis (velocity) is calibrated in cm/sec; the x-axis again indicates specific locations throughout circulation. It can be seen here that the velocity of the blood flowing through the aorta is greater than that traveling through the systemic capillaries.

Considering the two figures together, they reveal that, as the sum of the cross-sectional area of the blood vessels increases from the aorta to the systemic capillaries, the velocity of the blood flow decreases.

Bernoulli Principle

The Bernoulli principle describes the relationship between **lateral wall pressure** and velocity for an incompressible fluid flowing through a tube in laminar (streamline) fashion.

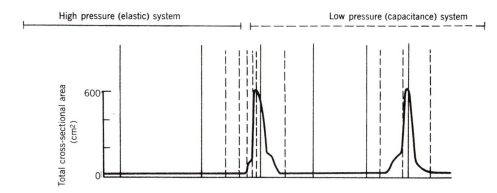

Figure 4-25 *A comparison of Figure 4-26 depicting the total cross-sectional area of the circulatory system on the y-axis and specific locations of the circulation along the x-axis starting with the aorta at the origin. The first peak (increased cross-sectional area) represents the systemic capillaries, and the second one refers to the pulmonary capillaries. Reproduced with permission from Henry, J. P., and Meehan, J. P.:* The Circulation: An Integrative Physiologic Study, *copyright © 1971 by Yearbook Medical Publishers, Inc., Chicago.*

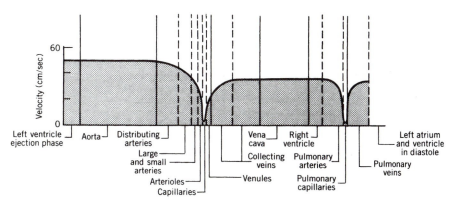

Figure 4-26 *A comparison of Figure 4-25 showing how the velocity of the blood flow throughout the entire circulatory system changes inversely with the system's cross-sectional area. Note how the two figures (4-25 and 4-26) could almost fit together like puzzle pieces and almost form a rectangle. The implication is that the product of A and v is k. Reproduced with permission from Henry, J. P., and Meehan, J. P.:* The Circulation: An Integrative Physiologic Study, *copyright © 1971 by Yearbook Medical Publishers, Inc., Chicago.*

As a fluid flows through a tube, it exerts a pressure in all directions. Hence, a lateral wall pressure results in forces acting radially on the walls of the tube, as is illustrated in Figure 4-27. Each arrow in the diagram represents the **radial force** (i.e., the lateral wall pressure) operating on the wall of a cylindrical tube.

The Bernoulli equation is based on the **law of conservation of energy.** It states that in a constant fluid flow system the sum of the pressure energy (lateral wall pressure), the potential energy per unit volume of fluid, and the kinetic energy per unit volume of fluid at one point in the system equals the sum of these energy forms at any other point downstream.

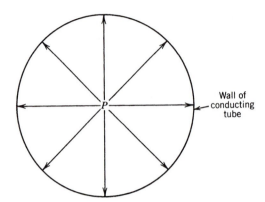

Figure 4-27 *Cross-sectional view of a conducting tube illustrating the concept of lateral wall pressure. The lines emanating from the center of the tube (P) to the conduit's wall represent the lateral wall pressure exerted by the fluid flowing through the system. This pressure radiates 360° from the center of the horizontally flowing fluid.*

Quantitatively, the equation reads

$$\left(\tfrac{1}{2}Dv^2\right)_1 + (Dgh)_1 + P_1 = \left(\tfrac{1}{2}Dv^2\right)_2 + (Dgh)_2 + P_2^* \tag{1}$$

where

$\tfrac{1}{2}Dv^2$ = formula for kinetic energy/volume

Dgh = formula for potential energy/volume

P = lateral wall pressure; sometimes described as pressure energy

In order to isolate the two factors of primary interest, namely, lateral wall pressure (P) and velocity (v), a number of assumptions can be made that simplify the overall equation. Because gas flow through the tracheobronchial tree originates from the pressure gradient between the mouth (atmosphere) and the alveoli, and because the value of h does not change appreciably, gravity will be assumed to have no influence on the flow of air through the tracheobronchial tree. Therefore, the potential energy formula can be eliminated from the equation. Thus,

$$\left(\tfrac{1}{2}Dv^2\right)_1 + P_1 = \left(\tfrac{1}{2}Dv^2\right)_2 + P_2 \tag{2}$$

or

$$\tfrac{1}{2}D(v_2^2 - v_1^2) = P_1 - P_2 \tag{3}$$

*Because density (D) is given by the formula mass/volume, $\tfrac{1}{2}Dv^2$ is the kinetic energy per unit volume of fluid, and Dgh is the potential energy per unit volume of fluid. The acceleration of gravity is designated by g, and h is the height above some reference level. Refer to Section 4-2, "Energy" in this chapter for the derivation of these formulas.

Further simplification results from the fact that gas density D will remain constant as the gas flows through the system and can be factored out of the equation. Hence,

$$\frac{1}{2}(v_2^2 - v_1^2) = P_1 - P_2 \tag{4}$$

Finally, the value ½, used to determine the average velocity in the kinetic energy formula $(Dv^2/2)$, can be factored out of the proportional expression in equation 4. Consequently, the factors lateral wall pressure and velocity remain. Therefore,

$$v_2^2 - v_1^2 \propto P_1 - P_2 \tag{5}$$

This expression indicates that the lateral wall pressure gradient (pre-obstruction lateral wall pressure minus post-obstruction lateral wall pressure) is proportional to the velocity (squared) gradient, that is, the square of the post-obstruction velocity minus the square of the pre-obstruction velocity. This relationship will now be discussed in the context of Figure 4-28.

Because the gas moves through the tube at a constant flow rate ($\dot{V}_1 = \dot{V}_3$) and with a constant driving pressure, the gas velocity must increase as the gas moves through the tube's convergence (segment 2) and must decrease as its traverses the divergence (segment 3). In segment 2 (convergence) some of the pressure energy or lateral wall pressure is converted to kinetic energy, as manifested by the velocity increase ($v_2 > v_1$). Because v_2 is greater than v_1, the kinetic energy ($\frac{1}{2}Dv^2$) is greater in segment 2. In other words, $\frac{1}{2}Dv^2$ in segment 1 is less than $\frac{1}{2}Dv^2$ in segment 2.

The reverse of this situation occurs as the conducting system in segment 3 diverges. A portion of the kinetic energy is reconverted to pressure energy as the lateral wall pressure there increases ($P_3 > P_2$) and gas velocity decreases ($v_3 < v_2$), that is, $\frac{1}{2}Dv^2$ in segment 2 is greater than $\frac{1}{2}Dv^2$ in segment 3.

Reconsider at this time the relationship between the conducting tube's cross-sectional area and the velocity of the flowing fluid discussed in the previous section. Recall also that these two factors are inversely related. As the cross-sectional area decreases, the velocity of the flowing fluid increases, and vice versa. Notice that the cross-sectional area in segment 1 in Figure 4-28 is greater than that in segment 2 (convergence). As the fluid

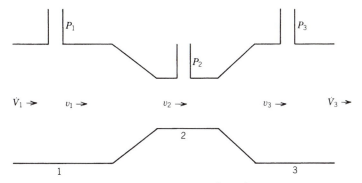

Figure 4-28 *Bernoulli principle. A constant flowing fluid ($\dot{V}_1 = \dot{V}_3$) exerts a lateral wall pressure (P_1) and has a velocity (v_1) along segment 1. At the convergence (segment 2), where the cross-sectional area decreases, P_2 decreases as v_2 increases. At the divergence (segment 3), P_3 increases as v_3 decreases (cross-sectional area increases). The relationship implied is $(P)(v) = k$.*

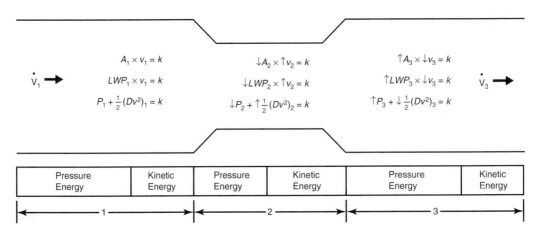

Figure 4-29 *Summary of the law of continuity, the Bernoulli principle, and the law of conservation of energy. Note that as the flow rate of the fluid remains constant ($\dot{V}_1 = \dot{V}_3$), each mathematical relationship in each segment (1, 2, and 3) throughout the system equals k and that the component energies (pressure energy and kinetic energy) change at each segment.*

flows from segment 1 to segment 2, its velocity increases ($v_2 > v_1$). Conversely, as the fluid flows from segment 2 to segment 3, the cross-sectional area increases. The velocity of the flow consequently decreases ($v_3 < v_2$).

Conceptually, what one can do here is substitute the lateral wall pressure for the cross-sectional area to try to comprehend the Bernoulli principle. Because the Bernoulli principle applies to conducting tubes experiencing either a constriction or a dilatation, the suggested substitution (lateral wall pressure for cross-sectional area) may enhance its understanding. These events and concepts are summarized in Figure 4-29.

The relationships outlined in the Bernoulli principle have therapeutic ramifications. These ramifications become manifest in the context of obstructive lung disease patients receiving medical gas therapy.

If flow rates at a constant driving pressure are applied to partially obstructed airways, the gas velocity will increase through these narrowed airways, and the lateral wall pressure will decrease. Increasing the flow rate further will magnify the problem by widening the pre- and post-obstruction velocity gradient and will decrease the lateral wall pressure further.

As lateral wall pressure decreases across a partial obstruction, less pressure becomes available for alveolar inflation distal to the stenosis (narrowing).

Keep in mind that two gradients exist at the narrowing, the velocity gradient, which is squared, and the lateral wall pressure gradient. If the flow rate through a narrowed airway, or tube, is increased, both the velocity and lateral wall pressure gradients will increase. The post-obstruction lateral wall pressure actually decreases, but its gradient increases (widens) as the difference between the pre- and post-obstruction lateral wall pressure values increases (widens).

In terms of the velocity, the actual value of the velocity increases as gas flows across the partial obstruction. Likewise, the velocity gradient increases (widens), that is, pre-obstruction velocity is less than post-obstruction velocity.

The clinical application of He-O_2 therapy is based on the Bernoulli equation. You will recall that earlier in this section the density factor D was eliminated from equation 3 because it was considered constant. However, let us reintroduce it to the proportional expression in equation 5, previously discussed. Therefore,

$$D(v_2^2 - v_1^2) \propto P_1 - P_2 \qquad (6)$$

As the equation is now written, one can appreciate how the density of a gas can influence the velocity and lateral wall pressure gradients across a stenosed, or narrowed, airway. Any gas, regardless of its density, flowing across a stricture will develop an increased velocity gradient and an increased lateral wall pressure gradient. However, the intent of administering a He-O_2 mixture in place of an air-O_2 mixture is to lessen the degree of both the velocity and lateral wall pressure gradient changes. Whether the flowing gas is a helium-oxygen mixture or an air-oxygen mixture, lateral wall pressure drops as the gas flows through a stricture. Therefore, the lateral wall pressure gradient increases (widens) at that point. However, with a helium-oxygen mixture the lateral wall pressure drops to a lesser degree (less pressure energy changes to kinetic energy) because a helium-oxygen mixture is less dense than an air-oxygen mixture. Because lateral wall pressure drops to a lesser extent when a less dense gas is flowing, more pressure is available for airway inflation beyond the narrowing.

Venturi Principle

The Venturi principle incorporates Bernoulli's principle in that the decrease in lateral wall pressure across a convergence is taken advantage of to entrain another fluid into the source flow. Observe Figure 4-30.

In the diagram,

A_1 = cross-sectional area proximal to narrowing

P_1 = lateral wall pressure exerted by source gas

v_1 = velocity (distance/time) of source gas

$\dot{V}_1$ = flow rate (volume/time) of source gas

A_2 = cross-sectional area at narrowing

P_2 = lateral wall pressure of source gas

v_2 = velocity of source gas

$\dot{V}_2$ = flow rate of entrained gas

A_3 = cross-sectional area distal to narrowing

P_3 = lateral wall pressure exerted by the source gas
    plus the entrained gas

v_3 = velocity of the source gas plus the entrained gas

$\dot{V}_3$ = flow rate of the source gas plus the entrained gas

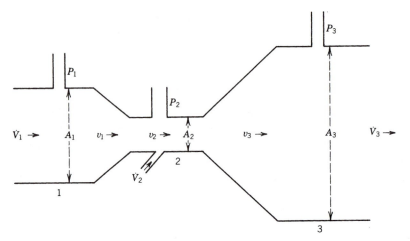

Figure 4-30 *Air entrainment system. The decreased lateral wall pressure in segment 2 (P_2) allows for the entrainment of room air ($\dot{V}_2$); therefore,$\dot{V}_1 + \dot{V}_2 = \dot{V}_3$. An air entrainment system is not a constant flow sys-*

As the gas flows ($\dot{V}_1$) from its source through cross-sectional area A_1, it exerts a lateral wall pressure P_1 and has a velocity v_1. When the fluid enters the narrowing, indicated by cross-sectional area A_2, the lateral wall pressure drops as shown by P_2 ($P_1 > P_2$), and the velocity v_2 increases. This drop in lateral wall pressure (below atmospheric pressure) is utilized to entrain another fluid into the system. Therefore,$\dot{V}_2$ joins the flow of the source gas $\dot{V}_1$. As the entrained flow and the source gas flow traverse the tube together through the divergence, represented by the cross-sectional area A_3, the lateral wall pressure P_3 increases, and the velocity v_3 decreases. The resulting delivered flow$\dot{V}_3$ is the sum of $\dot{V}_1$ plus $\dot{V}_2$. It is, therefore, greater than each of those flow rates individually.

The phenomena described above occur when a fluid flows through a **Venturi tube**. However, from an architectural standpoint a Venturi tube must be constructed according to certain specifications.

The following geometric arrangements must be applied (Figure 4-31): (1) the angle of convergence from segment 1 to segment 2 of the conducting system must be gradual,

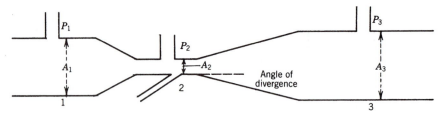

Figure 4-31 *Venturi principle. The architechtural configuration of the conducting system conforms to the requirements of the Venturi principle: (segment 1) gradual convergence, (segment 2) angle of divergence <15°, and (segment 3) adequate widening beyond divergence to accommodate entrained flow.*

(2) the angle of divergence from segment 2 to segment 3 must *not* exceed 15°, and (3) the widening (segment 3) beyond the narrowing must be large enough to accommodate the increased volume resulting from the entrained flow at segment 2.

These structural designs are needed in order for the distal lateral wall pressure to *approximate* the proximal lateral wall pressure. In Figure 4-31, P_3 approximates P_1.

It is interesting to note that respiratory care equipment does not incorporate true Venturi systems. Although gas entrainment devices are routinely employed, none of them attempts to restore prerestriction lateral wall pressure (P_1) distal to the narrowing. The third segment of Figure 4-31 is excluded from respiratory care equipment because there is no therapeutic advantage in or need for restoring the postrestriction lateral wall pressure (P_3) to its prerestriction (P_1) level. Keep in mind, however, that, even though a true Venturi is not incorporated in respiratory care equipment, gas entrainment at specific ratios is achieved by therapeutically employed oxygen delivery devices. The primary concern is the adequacy of gas entrainment.

A formula is available to calculate some of the physical events pertaining to air entrainment devices. It is based on the following algebraic relationship:

$$(C_S \times \dot{V}_S) + (C_{ENT} \times \dot{V}_{ENT}) = (C_{DEL} \times \dot{V}_{DEL})$$

where

C_S = concentration of the source gas

$\dot{V}_S$ = flow rate of the source gas

C_{ENT} = concentration of the entrained gas

$\dot{V}_{ENT}$ = flow rate of the entrained gas

C_{DEL} = concentration of the delivered gas

$\dot{V}_{ENT}$ = flow rate of the delivered gas

The equation states that the product of the concentration and flow rate of the source gas plus the product of the concentration and flow rate of the entrained gas equals the product of the delivered gas concentration and its flow rate.

The reader should note that for continuously flowing fluids the fundamental relationship among (1) the source gas flow rate, (2) the entrained gas flow rate, and (3) the delivered gas flow rate is

$$\dot{V}_S + \dot{V}_{ENT} = \dot{V}_{DEL}$$

which indicates that the sum of the source and entrained gas flow rates equals the flow rate of the delivered gas.

When the appropriate information is given, any variable in the problem can be computed. Since this equation is ordinarily applied to oxygen delivery devices, the factors C_S and C_{ENT} are considered constant. The concentration of the source gas is assumed to be 100% (FiO_2 1.0) since the oxygen delivery devices are driven by 100% oxygen. The concentration of the entrained gas (C_{ENT}) is assumed to be 21% (FiO_2 0.21) because room air is the entrained gas.

EXAMPLE 1:

Calculate the FIO_2 delivered by a jet nebulizer operating at 10 lpm and providing a total flow of 20 lpm.

Step 1: Determine the entrained flow rate $(\dot{V}_{ENT})$ from the following relationship:

$$\dot{V}_S + \dot{V}_{ENT} = \dot{V}_{DEL}$$

Transposing to solve for $\dot{V}_{ENT}$ yields

$$\dot{V}_{ENT} = \dot{V}_{DEL} - \dot{V}_S$$
$$= 20\ lpm - 10\ lpm$$
$$= 10\ lpm$$

Step 2: Calculate the FIO_2 from the following equation.

$$(C_S \times \dot{V}_S) + (C_{ENT} \times \dot{V}_{ENT}) = (C_{DEL} \times \dot{V}_{DEL})$$
$$(100\% \times 10\ lpm) + (21\% \times 10\ lpm) = (X \times 20\ lpm)$$
$$10\ lpm + 2.1\ lpm = X(20\ lpm)$$
$$\frac{12.1\ \cancel{lpm}}{20\ \cancel{lpm}} = X$$
$$0.60 = X$$
$$FIO_2 = 0.60$$

EXAMPLE 2:

Calculate both the entrained flow and the delivered flow for an oxygen delivery device operating at a flow rate of 15 liters per minute and delivering 40% oxygen.

Step 1: Use $\dot{V}_S + \dot{V}_{ENT} = \dot{V}_{DEL}$ to determine the designations for $\dot{V}_{ENT}$ and $\dot{V}_{DEL}$.

$$\dot{V}_S = 15\ lpm$$
$$\dot{V}_{ENT} = X\ lpm$$
$$\dot{V}_{DEL} = (X\ lpm + 15\ lpm)$$

Therefore, inserting the designations for $\dot{V}_{ENT}$ and $\dot{V}_{DEL}$, the equation becomes:

$$\dot{V}_S + \dot{V}_{ENT} = \dot{V}_{DEL}$$
$$15\ lpm + X\ lpm = (X\ lpm + 15\ lpm)$$

Step 2: Calculate the entrained flow rate and the delivered flow rate using the formula

$$(C_S \times \dot{V}_S) + (C_{ENT} \times \dot{V}_{ENT}) = (C_{DEL} \times \dot{V}_{DEL})$$

where

$C_S = 100\%$
$\dot{V}_S = 15\,lpm$
$C_{ENT} = 21\%$
$C_{DEL} = 40\%$
$\dot{V}_{ENT} = X\,lpm$
$\dot{V}_{DEL} = X\,lpm + 15\,lpm$

$$(100\% \times 15\,lpm) + (21\% \times X\,lpm) = 40\%\,(X\,lpm + 15\,lpm)$$

$$(15\,lpm) + (0.21 \times X\,lpm) = (0.40 \times X\,lpm) + (6\,lpm)$$

$$15\,lpm - 6\,lpm = (0.40 \times X\,lpm) - (0.21 \times X\,lpm)$$

$$9\,lpm = 0.19\,(X\,lpm)$$

$$\frac{9\,lpm}{0.19} = X\,lpm$$

$$47.4\,lpm = X\,lpm$$

Because X lpm equals $\dot{V}_{ENT}$, then $\dot{V}_{ENT}$ equals 47.4 lpm.

Step 3: Calculate the delivered flow rate using the equation from *Step 1.*

$$\dot{V}_S + \dot{V}_{ENT} = \dot{V}_{DEL}$$

$$15\,lpm + 47.4\,lpm = \dot{V}_{DEL}$$

$$62.4\,lpm = \dot{V}_{DEL}$$

The air: O_2 ratio for each FiO_2 can also be determined from two components of the equation, namely, $\dot{V}_{ENT}$ and $\dot{V}_S$. The air: O_2 ratio is obtained as follows:

$$\frac{\dot{V}_{ENT}}{\dot{V}_S} = \frac{air\ flow\ rate}{O_2\ flow\ rate}$$

For example, the air-O_2 ratio in Example 1 is calculated by dividing the entrained airflow by the oxygen (source) flow, thus,

$$\frac{air}{O_2} = \frac{\dot{V}_{ENT}}{\dot{V}_S} = \frac{10\,lpm}{10\,lpm} = \frac{1}{1} = 1{:}1$$

The FiO_2 resulting from an air:O_2 ratio of 1:1 is 0.60. Table 4-11 lists approximate air:O_2 ratios for commonly encountered FiO_2s.

The "magic box" described in Chapter 1, Section 1-3, "Ratios," is a shortcut method for obtaining air:O_2 ratios when the FiO_2 is known.

TABLE 4-11 Air:O_2 Ratios for Commonly Encountered FIO_2S and O_2%

FIO_2	O_2%	AIR:O_2
1.00	100	0:1
0.80	80	0.3:1
0.70	70	0.6:1
0.60	60	1:1
0.50	50	1.7:1
0.45	45	2:1
0.40	40	3:1
0.35	35	5:1
0.30	30	18:1
0.28	28	10:1
0.24	24	25:1

PRACTICE PROBLEMS

Refer to Appendix A (pages 605-607) for the solutions and answers to the practice problems.

Use the air entrainment formula to perform the following calculations:

42. Calculate the total flow delivered to a patient via a Puritan-Bennett all-purpose nebulizer operating at an FIO_2 of 0.70 with a liter flow of 15 liters per minute.

   _____

43. Determine the entrained air flow rate for a Venturi mask operating at a flow of 4 liters per minute and delivering 28% oxygen. _____

44. Compute the air:oxygen ratio for the Venturi mask discussed in problem 43.

   _____

45. What flow rate of oxygen would be required to produce a 0.60 FIO_2 if the entrained airflow is 10 liters per minute? _____

46. Determine the air:oxygen ratio for the oxygen delivery device presented in problem 45.

   _____

47. What is the FIO_2 of an oxygen delivery system operating at 15 liters per minute, entraining 60 liters per minute of room air? _____

48. Calculate both the source flow and the total flow of an O_2 device delivering 24% oxygen and entraining 60 liters per minute. _____

49. What is the total flow delivered by an oxygen mask providing an FIO$_2$ of 0.54 and operating at an oxygen flow of 10 liters per minute? _____

50. Compute the FIO$_2$ delivered to a patient receiving humidified oxygen from a device operating at 10 liters per minute and entraining 30 liters per minute of room air.

51. Determine the air:O$_2$ ratio for the oxygen device described in problem 50.

Laminar and Turbulent Flow

When a fluid travels through a tube system, it takes on the characteristics of one of two types of flow patterns. The two types of flow patterns are **laminar** and **turbulent flow.** Physiologically, a third type of flow pattern is thought to exist. It is called **tracheobronchial flow** and is considered to be a combination of laminar and turbulent flow. Exactly where it exists in the tracheobronchial tree is a matter of speculation. However, it is usually thought of as being in the vicinity of airway bifurcations where the velocity profile of the flowing gas differs from that of either laminar or turbulent flow. The discussion that follows will primarily concern itself with laminar and turbulent flow.

Laminar, or streamline, flow is characterized as a concentric series of thin cylindrical layers, as is shown in Figure 4-32.

Each of these cylindrical layers or laminae represents a stream of horizontally moving fluid molecules. In a continuous, one-way flow through a system of rigid, cylindrical, internally smooth, and unobstructed tubes, the layer or lamina next to the wall of the tube is essentially motionless. This layer is designated the *boundary layer* where fluid velocity is zero (*A* and *B*, Figure 4-33).

The fluid layers at *A* and *B* in Figure 4-33 represent the boundary layer. The velocity of each respective layer or lamina increases from the boundary layer toward the center of the tube. Therefore, during laminar flow the velocity of the horizontal layers of fluid is nonuniform. The velocity along the central axis (axial velocity) of the tube is greatest.

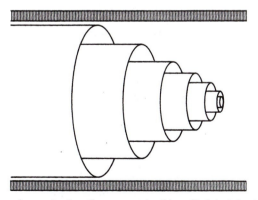

Figure 4-32 *Laminar flow; demonstrating the concentric, thin cylindrical, horizontal layers, or laminae, of flowing fluid. From Richardson, Daniel R.;* Basic Circulatory Physiology, *modification of Figure 5–4, 1976, Little, Brown & Co., Boston.*

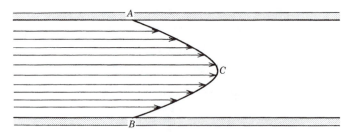

Figure 4-33 *Characteristics of laminar flow include parabolic velocity profile (A–C–B), boundary layers (A and B), axial velocity (C), and parallel, horizontally flowing gas layers (arrows).*

Consequently, the velocity among the fluid layers from A to C increases, and that from C to B decreases. This particular velocity variation results in a parabolic velocity profile for laminar flow. This characteristic velocity profile is shown by the curved line A–C–B.

During laminar flow friction develops between adjacent layers. Fluid molecules making the transition (diffusing) from fast to slow layers reduce the entire velocity of flow. This fluid property is called **viscosity** and will be discussed in more detail later in this chapter.

The development of laminar flow depends on both the architecture of the conducting system and certain properties of the flowing fluid. Tube systems that are rigid, straight, internally smooth, and unobstructed are more conducive to laminar flow than those that are flaccid, circuitous, and internally corrugated. When the velocity of flow exceeds a certain value (i.e., **critical velocity**), which is a function of the viscosity and density of the fluid, laminar flow will convert to turbulent flow. Therefore, turbulent flow can develop even in a tube whose geometry favors laminar flow (Figure 4-34).

The pressure gradient needed to produce and maintain laminar flow is proportional to the flow rate times a constant related to the viscosity of the gas. Consequently,

$$\Delta P = k_1 \times \dot{V} \tag{1}$$

where

ΔP = the **driving pressure** (pressure gradient)

k_1 = a constant related to gas viscosity and independent of gas density

$\dot{V}$ = the gas flow rate (volume/time)

As the character of flow changes from laminar to turbulent, the concentric, parallel layers no longer slide smoothly over each other. The orderly flow pattern of laminar flow degenerates into numerous vortices or **eddy currents.** There is an increased transfer or exchange of fluid mass among the degenerating concentric layers. The fluid flows through the tube essentially at uniform velocity. Figure 4-35 depicts a fluid flowing in turbulent fashion.

The velocity profile of turbulent flow is somewhat flattened compared to the parabolic shape it assumes with laminar flow. Movement of the fluid molecules is random, chaotic, and rapid.

The driving pressure required to produce turbulent flow is proportional to the square of the flow rate times a constant related to the density of the gas. Therefore

$$\Delta P = k_2 \times \dot{V}^2 \tag{2}$$

where

ΔP = the driving pressure (pressure gradient) or change in pressure

k_2 = a constant related to gas density and independent of gas viscosity

$\dot{V}^2$ = the gas flow rate (volume/time) raised to the second power

With the understanding that **airway resistance** (R) is expressed as

$$R = \frac{\Delta P}{\dot{V}} = \frac{\text{pressure gradient}}{\text{gas flow rate}} \quad\quad (3)$$

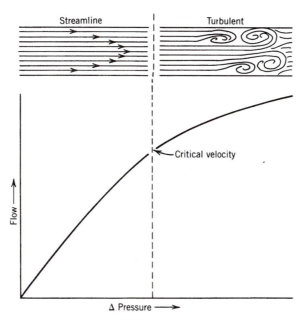

Figure 4-34 *The concentric, horizontal, parallel layers of laminar flow can decay, or degenerate, to turbulent flow if the fluid velocity exceeds a certain point. That velocity is called the critical velocity. From Smith, J., and Kampine, J.:* Circulatory Physiology: The Essentials, *© 1984, Williams & Wilkins Co., Baltimore.*

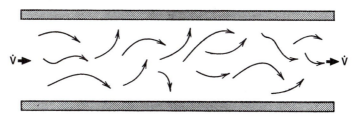

Figure 4-35 *Characteristics of turbulent flow include random, chaotic movement of gas molecules (curved arrows), blunted velocity profile, higher driving pressure required to generate flow, and increased airway resistance.*

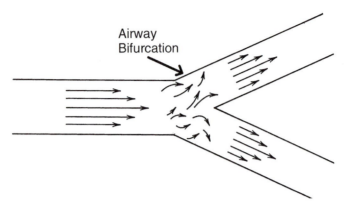

Figure 4-36 *A hypothetical airway branching showing laminar flow breaking down to tracheobronchial flow at the bifurcation and redeveloping distal to the bifurcation.*

it should be clear that the airway resistance associated with laminar flow (equation 1) will be substantially less than that resulting from turbulent flow (equation 2). At the same time, a laminar flow pattern requires a smaller pressure gradient to produce and maintain a flow rate than does a turbulent flow pattern. Recall that a pressure gradient (ΔP or driving pressure) is the necessary prerequisite for the existence of a flow ($\dot{V}$).

Since tracheobronchial flow (Figure 4-36) is a combination of both laminar and turbulent flow, the driving pressure (transairway pressure gradient) needed to produce this flow pattern can be shown as

$$\Delta P = (k_1 \times \dot{V}) + (k_2 \times \dot{V}^2) \tag{4}$$

The three forms of flow patterns described here—laminar, turbulent, and tracheobronchial—are said to develop in the large, the central, and some of the small airways throughout the tracheobronchial tree when a tidal volume enters the lungs during conventional ventilation.* Gas movement in the form of laminar, turbulent, and tracheobronchial flow through these lung regions is considered to take place by means of bulk flow or **convection.**

Airflow During High Frequency Ventilation

During both spontaneous and conventional mechanical ventilation, gas movement is accomplished primarily by two modes of transport. The first is bulk convective movement of gas molecules from an area of high pressure to one of relatively low pressure. Convection is the mechanism by which gas flows through the conductive airways. The conductive airways include the trachea through the bronchioles, inclusively, or generations 0 through 15 (Figure 4-37).

From the level of the terminal bronchioles to the acini, generations 16 through 23, gas movement no longer depends on a pressure gradient but is instead influenced by molecular diffusion. Molecular diffusion arises from the kinetic energy imparted on the gas molecules

*Conventional ventilation includes (1) low-frequency, high tidal volume, positive or negative pressure mechanical ventilation and (2) spontaneous ventilation.

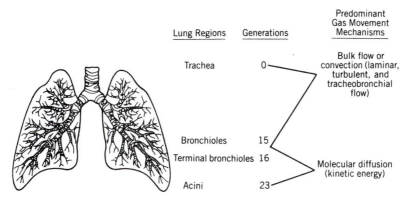

Figure 4-37 *Illustration of tracheobronchial tree showing convective gas movement through generations 0 through 15, inclusively, and molecular diffusion as the gas transport mechanism in generations 16–23.*

from the heat (body temperature) in the airways. Within the lungs, the heat produces random, thermal, molecular oscillations. This mechanism accounts for the movement of oxygen and carbon dioxide at and near the alveolar-capillary membrane.

The mechanism of gas flow during conventional ventilation is conceptualized as follows:

$$V_A = V_T - V_D$$

where

V_A = alveolar volume

V_T = tidal volume

V_D = anatomic dead space volume

This traditional model of respiratory physiology holds that as the tidal volume decreases, increasing the ventilatory rate will maintain ventilation as long as the tidal volume exceeds the anatomic dead space volume. If the tidal volume is less than the anatomic dead space volume, there is no remaining alveolar volume. Increasing the ventilatory rate at this point ($V_T < V_D$) would theoretically be of no use in increasing minute ventilation because only the anatomic dead space volume would be increased. No gas would reach the alveoli for gas exchange to occur.

Early observations of ventilation at supraphysiologic frequencies (>60 breaths/min) demonstrated that this tenet is not absolute. In fact, at very high respiratory rates, gas exchange can be accomplished at tidal volumes that are so small as to approximate the anatomic dead space volume. This apparent contradiction of the traditional model of pulmonary ventilation suggests that some other factor, or factors, must influence gas movement when high frequency ventilation (HFV) is employed. It is not accepted that specific geometric and mechanical properties of the lung may influence convection and diffusion to interact, producing other modes of gas transport.

Several different physiologic phenomena shed light on what is believed to occur. Apneic diffusion oxygenation was studied in animals and humans in the early 1950s. Subjects were paralyzed in an environment of high-flow oxygen. After periods of apnea, the $PaCO_2$ was observed to rise, as expected. However, the PaO_2 did not decrease, as one might surmise. Oxygenation was maintained by diffusion alone, in the absence of convective flow.

Another phenomenon, cardiogenic oscillation, occurs when the motion of the beating heart is transmitted to surrounding lung tissue, resulting in a five-fold increase in gas diffusion within the pulmonary regions adjacent to the cardiac structures.

The impedance of the respiratory system also influences delivered gas volumes at high frequencies. Impedance is an index of the impediment a body presents to gas flow. The point of minimal impedance corresponds to the resonant, or natural, frequency of the lung. At the resonant frequency, air movement is opposed only by airway resistance. Impedance is derived from the compliance, resistance, and inertia of the lung. Impedance is thought to have a significant impact on the mechanical efficiency of HFV.

Although gas exchange during HFV is not yet completely understood, H. K. Chang (see Bibliography at the end of this chapter) has identified five different modes of gas transport that are believed to play a role. The first is direct alveolar ventilation by bulk convection. This mode is a specific application of bulk gas flow, whereby in ventilation with a small tidal volume, some gas molecules may reach some alveoli situated near the airway opening (mouth).

The second mode of transport, as with conventional ventilation, is by molecular diffusion at the alveolar-capillary membrane.

The third mechanism is a result of asymmetric axial velocity profiles produced during laminar flow within the conducting airways. Laminar flow through a tube produces the so-called asymmetric velocity profile. The lamina, or layer, of molecules next to the wall of the tube (boundary layer) is essentially motionless because of friction. The velocity of the gas molecules of each layer progressively increases toward the center of the tube, so that the molecules in the center are moving most rapidly. In other words, the velocity of each of the horizontally moving layers of molecules is different, i.e., nonuniform velocity.

Experiments with asymmetric velocity profiles have shown that a full cycle of oscillatory flow will produce convective forward movement of the molecules in the center of the tube. The gas molecules closest to the wall are displaced backward. In relation to a reference point, a new forward movement of the gas bolus is accomplished.

Figure 4-38 shows the position and shape of a cluster of aerosol particles (dots) in reference to a point of origin at three different time segments as the aerosol and the carrier gas (arrows) flow through a tube. The three time segments are labeled (1) initial (the point of the aerosol's introduction into the flowing gas), (2) end right flow (analogous to end-inspiration), and (3) final (analogous to end-exhalation).

Initially (top portion of the diagram), the right border of the aerosol is designated the *reference origin*, as signified by the broken vertical line extending across all three time segments. As time elapses, the flat velocity profile of the aerosol assumes the shape of a parabola, as the aerosol is deformed by the nonuniform velocities of the concentrically layered molecules of the flowing (rightward) fluid. During its rightward flow, some of the aerosol particles move beyond the reference origin, indicating the importance of this new configuration. When flow is reversed (leftward), the velocity profile (aerosol particles) this time travels a distance to the left.

The shifting of the velocity profile represents a net rightward displacement of the aerosol particles near the center of the lumen and a net leftward displacement for those near the wall. The final position of the aerosol particles (bottom portion of the diagram) illustrates

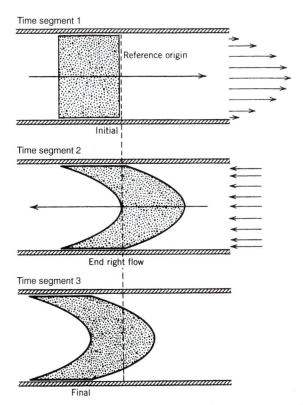

Figure 4-38 *Bulk flow or convective gas movement model. The same point in a conduction system at three different time segments is shown having a bolus of aerosol particles (dots). The vertical dotted line extending across all three time segments is the reference point (origin). From Haselton, F. R. and Scherer, P. W.: "Bronchial Bifurcation & Respiratory Mass Transport," Science, Vol. 208, pp. 68–70, Fig. 1, © 4 April 1980 by the American Association for the Advancement of Science. Used with permission.*

that a bulk flow or convective movement of aerosol particles has taken place across the reference origin. It is speculated that the variations in the velocity profiles during inspiration and exhalation account for the convective movement of gas during conventional breathing.

It has also been proposed that during high-frequency jet ventilation (HFJV), bursts of gas will jet down the center of the airways on inspiration, while exhaled gas molecules simultaneously swirl around the area adjacent to the wall of the tube in the opposite direction.

Pendelluft, the abnormal to-and-fro movements of gas from one lung to another during ventilation, is yet another mode of gas transport. Pendelluft describes the movement of gas between neighboring lung units during cyclic ventilation. Individual lung units will fill and empty at certain rates, dependent on their time constants (the product of resistance and compliance). If adjacent lung units have different time constants, gas molecules can recirculate between them. This interregional gas mixing is enhanced during high-frequency ventilation and is thought to result in a greater tidal volume delivered to the alveoli than that which originates in the trachea.

The final mechanism of gas transport is Taylor-type dispersion. This mechanism is sometimes referred to as **augmented diffusion.** It is the result of interaction between axial convection and lateral diffusion. In contrast to laminar flow, random convective eddies during turbulent flow provide lateral transport of molecules. These eddies result in faster mixing between the central core of fluid and the periphery than that which occurs in laminar flow. During HFV, turbulent flow is likely to predominate because the **Reynold's number** in the trachea has been shown experimentally to be as high as 20,000. The Reynold's number is a value used to indicate whether flow through a tube is laminar or turbulent. This dimensionless number is derived from the Reynold's equation, which incorporates gas velocity, density, viscosity, and tube diameter. A Reynold's number greater than 2,000 denotes the presence of turbulent flow.

Unsteadiness of oscillatory flow is quantified by a ratio known as a **Wormersley number.** For a specific fluid in a specific tube, a large Wormersley number indicates a high frequency, in which viscosity dominates. Under such circumstances, inertia strongly influences the process of acceleration and deceleration. During oscillation, the driving pressure must reverse direction twice in each cycle. Momentum within the central core of the fluid prevents acceleration/deceleration in phase with the pressure gradient. Oscillatory dispersion, therefore, depends on both the speed of flow and the unsteadiness of flow.

Figure 4-39 is a representation of the different modes of gas transport in their suggested zones of dominance within the lung during high-frequency oscillation. In Zone 1, which is comprised of the large conducting airways, there is turbulent flow. Convection and Taylor-type dispersion predominate. In the lower airways, Zone 2, asymmetric co-axial flow predominates because of the presence of laminar flow (asymmetric velocity profiles). Zone 3 is the actual lung parenchyma. There, Pendelluft, cardiac oscillations, and molecular diffusion predominate.

Overall, efficiency of HFV is a function of the five different modes of gas transport. These modes are not mutually exclusive and, in fact, interact. Given specific geometric and physical conditions within the lung, one mode may dominate in a certain region, as suggested above. It should be noted, however, that theoretical analysis of gas flow in the lung at high frequency has certain limitations. First, it is based on observations of fluid flow through rigid, uniform cylinders. This model may not translate well in the in vitro lung in which the airways are not uniform and change dimension (widen and elongate on inspiration; contract and shorten on exhalation).

The exchange of gases during HFV has clinical implications. HFV appears to be a more efficient mode of ventilation than conventional mechanical ventilation in terms of CO_2 removal. As is the case with conventional mechanical ventilation, oxygenation during HFV is primarily related to the mean airway pressure. It has been discovered that the lack of large phasic swings in pressure during HFV, compared with conventional ventilation, may result in significant atelectasis. Recruitment and maintenance of open alveoli during HFV is critical to clinical success.

Recall that, during the discussion of the law of continuity, it was mentioned that once gas flow reaches the smallest airways (generations 16 through 23) it is no longer under the influence of the transairway pressure gradient, which initiated the breath. Instead, gas movement at that point is accomplished by molecular diffusion, that is, the kinetic energy imparted on the gas molecules by the temperature of the internal environment. The gas

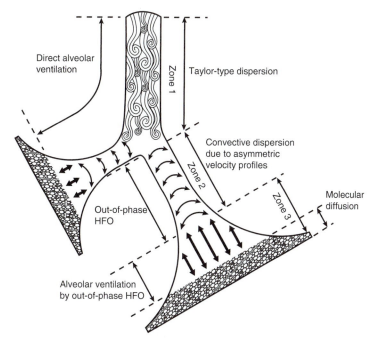

Figure 4-39 *Different modes of gas transport in their suggested zones of dominance in the lungs. Zone 1 (large airways) predominantly accommodates turbulent flow. Zone 2 (small airways) primarily supports laminar flow. Zone 3 essentially experiences Pendelluft, cardiac oscillations, and molecular diffusion. From H. K. Chang, "Mechanisms of gas transport during ventilation by high-frequency oscillation," Journal of Applied Physiology, 56, pp. 553–563, 1984. Reprinted with permission from the American Physiological Society, Bethesda, Maryland.*

flow rate in these airways is essentially zero because the large total cross-sectional area (70 m^2) in this region helps reduce the velocity of flow to that value. Therefore, the gas molecules move via their own kinetic energy.

Resistance to Ventilation

Resistance to ventilation has three components: (1) inertial resistance, (2) elastic or viscous resistance, and (3) airway (airflow) resistance. **Inertial resistance** and **airway (airflow) resistance** are sometimes considered together and are termed **nonelastic resistance.**

A basic attribute of matter is that any object requires a force to act on it in order to change its motion. Therefore, an object at rest tends to remain at rest until an external force sets it in motion. Once in motion, that object tends to remain in motion until acted upon by a force in opposition to its motion.

The inertial resistance to ventilation represents the tendency of the ventilatory system to resist a change in motion. For example, at end-exhalation the ventilatory apparatus is in a motionless state; that is, no airflow occurs at this point during the ventilatory cycle. The inertia of the system tends to maintain this motionless condition. However, the energy expended by the ventilatory muscles performs the mechanical work needed to overcome these inertial forces in order to generate intrathoracic pressure changes to accomplish inspiration. Physiologically, the inertial forces contribute only a small fraction of the total resistance to ventilation and will, therefore, be considered negligible at normal ventilatory frequencies.

The elastic component primarily includes the elastic properties of the lung and the chest wall. Additionally, though, the anatomic structures of the mediastinum and the abdominal viscera contribute to the elastic resistance to ventilation. The elastic resistance represented by these structures is dependent on the volume changes in the ventilatory system. Motion (airflow) within the ventilatory system does not influence the elastic properties, which account for approximately 20% of the total resistance to ventilation in healthy subjects. In fact, the elastic properties of the ventilatory system are studied under static (no airflow) conditions as **compliance** (Δvolume/Δpressure) or as its reciprocal, **elastance** (Δpressure/Δvolume).

The third component of the total resistance to ventilation is airway (airflow) resistance. Airway resistance contributes the remaining 80% of the total ventilatory resistance. As a fluid flows through a conducting system, airway resistance represents (1) the interactions among the fluid molecules and (2) the interactions between the fluid molecules and the walls of the conducting system. These interactions, or internal friction, among fluid molecules can be described as viscosity, which will be discussed later.

As opposed to the elastic resistive forces, airway resistance is measured under dynamic conditions, that is, when air is flowing through the tracheobronchial tree. Flow (volume/time) is, therefore, one of the components of airway resistance. However, before a fluid flow can ever exist, a pressure gradient must be present. During spontaneous breathing, the ventilatory muscles create a pressure gradient between the alveoli (P_{alv}) and the atmosphere (P_{atm}).

$$P_{atm} - P_{alv} = \text{pressure gradient (driving pressure)}$$

As a consequence of the pressure gradient ($P_{atm} - P_{alv}$), air flows from the atmosphere into the person's alveoli. As the air flows through the tracheobronchial tree, airway resistance results.

It was indicated earlier that flow rate is one of the components of airway resistance. Conveniently enough, because the existence of a flow rate necessitates a pressure gradient, the pressure gradient constitutes the other component needed for airway resistance. Therefore, the relationship for airway resistance is

$$\text{airway resistance} = \frac{\text{pressure gradient}}{\text{flow rate}}$$

More specifically, because the pressure gradient describes that which exists across the tracheobronchial tree (i.e., $P_{atm} - P_{alv}$), the expression *transairway pressure* can be used.

Quantitatively, the expression is

$$R = \frac{\Delta P}{\dot{V}}$$

where

R = airway resistance (cm H_2O/liter/sec)

ΔP = transairway pressure gradient (cm H_2O)

$\dot{V}$ = flow rate (liters/sec)

This relationship is analogous to that used to calculate resistance through electrical circuits via **Ohm's law,** which reads

$$R = \frac{V}{I}$$

where

R = electrical resistance (ohms)

I = electrical current (amperes)

V = electromotive force or voltage (volts)

Earlier it was stated that the airway resistance component accounts for approximately 80% of the total ventilatory resistance and the elastic resistance contributes the remaining 20% (inertial resistance is considered negligible). The percentage of the total resistance attributable to airway resistance can be partitioned according to airway generations.

Airway resistance varies throughout the tracheobronchial tree. The irregular dichotomous branching of the airways helps account for the nonuniform distribution of airway resistance. An analogy is sometimes made between the tracheobronchial tree and an inverted funnel (Figure 4-40).

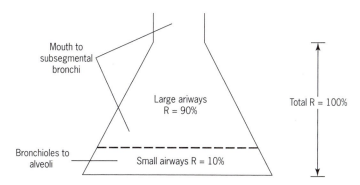

Figure 4-40 *Depiction of the tracheobronchial tree as an inverted funnel indicating the distribution of airway resistance between the large and small airways. Large airways (>2 mm dia.) normally account for 90% of the total airway resistance, while small airways (≤2 mm dia.) ordinarily account for 10%.*

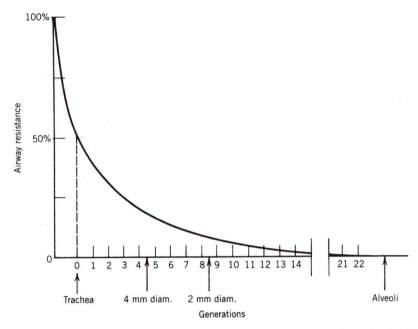

Figure 4-41 *Partitioning of airway resistance from the airway opening (mouth) to the alveoli. Note that 50% of the total airway resistance is encountered as gas flows through the airway opening to the trachea (0) and that the remaining 50% occurs from the trachea to the alveoli. Reproduced with permission from Burrows, B., Knudson, R. J., and Kettel, L. J.:* Respiratory Insufficiency, *copyright © 1975 by Yearbook Medical Publishers, Inc., Chicago.*

The neck (small opening) of the funnel represents generation 0 (trachea) of the tracheobronchial tree. The gradual widening of the funnel depicts successive airway branchings (generations) resulting in an increased cross-sectional area within the lungs. Finally, the wide end of the funnel is analogous to the small airways, or generations 9 through 23.

This funnel model of the tracheobronchial tree shows that, as the number of airways increases (and as cross-sectional area increases) from the trachea to the alveoli, airway resistance steadily decreases. Figure 4-41 further illustrates the partitioning of airway resistance across the entire respiratory system, that is, from the mouth and nose and across all 23 generations.

Airway resistance (*y*-axis) is plotted against airway generations (*x*-axis) 0 through 23, that is, from the trachea to the alveoli. The area between generation 0 (trachea) and the *y*-axis represents the airway resistance in the nose, mouth, pharynx, and larynx. The graph shows that 100% of the airway resistance occurs from the airway openings (nose and mouth) to the alveoli, which, of course, is what is expected. However, note that approximately 90% of the total airway (airflow) resistance (*not* the total resistance to ventilation) takes place in the large airways (≥2 mm diameter), from the airway openings to the segmental bronchi. The remaining 10% of the total airway resistance occurs in the small airways (<2 mm diameter).

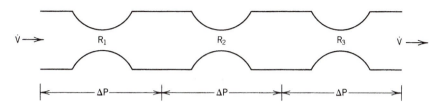

Figure 4-42 *Series resistances. The flow ($\dot{V}$) moving through the system encounters three resistances. The total resistance is the sum of $R_1 + R_2 + R_3$. Therefore, R_{total} will be greater than each individual resistance ($R_1, R_2, \ldots, R_n$) in a series system.*

It will be useful to compare resistances in series and resistances in parallel to quantitatively demonstrate how successive airway branchings contribute to a corresponding decrease in airway resistance.

Let us first observe the resistance to flow through a series circuit. Figure 4-42 depicts a gas flow encountering quantitatively equal resistances at three separate points downstream.

In a series circuit the resistances are additive, for example, $R_1 + R_2 + R_3 = R_{total}$. If the flow rate ($\dot{V}$) through the tube in Figure 4-42 is 2 liters/sec and the driving pressure (ΔP) across each section is 4 cm H_2O, then each resistance would be calculated as

$$R = \frac{\Delta P}{\dot{V}} = \frac{4 \text{ cm } H_2O}{2 \text{ liters/sec}} = 2 \text{ cm } H_2O/\text{liter/sec}$$

The total resistance here would be obtained by adding

$$R_{total} = R_1 + R_2 + R_3$$
$$= 2 \text{ cm } H_2O/\text{liter/sec} + 2 \text{ cm } H_2O/\text{liter/sec} + 2 \text{ cm } H_2O/\text{liter/sec}$$
$$= 6 \text{ cm } H_2O/\text{liter/sec}$$

Figure 4-43 illustrates resistances in a parallel circuit. (See Chapter 2 Algebra, 2-7 Reciprocals.) To obtain the total resistance the reciprocal of each resistance is added;

$$\frac{1}{R_1} + \frac{1}{R_2} + \frac{1}{R_3} = R_{total}$$

If the flow rate ($\dot{V}$) through the parallel circuit in Figure 4-43 is 2 liters/sec and the driving pressure (ΔP) is 4 cm H_2O, then each resistance would be computed

$$R = \frac{\Delta P}{\dot{V}} = \frac{4 \text{ cm } H_2O}{2 \text{ liters/sec}} = 2 \text{ cm } H_2O/\text{liter/sec}$$

The total resistance would be calculated as:

$$\frac{1}{R_{total}} = \frac{1}{R_1} + \frac{1}{R_2} + \frac{1}{R_3}$$

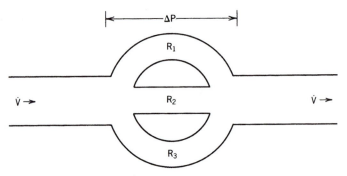

Figure 4-43 *Parallel resistances. The flow ($\dot{V}$) moving through the system encounters three resistances. The total resistance is the sum of the reciprocal of each resistance. Therefore, the total resistance will be less than each individual resistance in a parallel system.*

$$= \frac{1}{2 \text{ cm H}_2\text{O/liter/sec}} + \frac{1}{2 \text{ cm H}_2\text{O/liter/sec}} + \frac{1}{2 \text{ cm H}_2\text{O/liter/sec}}$$

$$= 1.5 \text{ liters/sec/cm H}_2\text{O}$$

Therefore,

$$R_{\text{total}} = \frac{1}{1.5 \text{ liters/sec/cm H}_2\text{O}}$$

$$= 0.67 \text{ cm H}_2\text{O/liter/sec}$$

Notice that R_{total} is 1.5 cm H_2O/liter/sec and that it is less than the individual resistances (R_1, R_2, and R_3) which are 2 cm H_2O/liter/sec. Because the individual resistances in a parallel circuit are added reciprocally, the total resistance in a parallel circuit will always be less than the individual resistances in the circuit.

When comparing the total resistance in each system (series R_{total} = 6 cm H_2O/liter/sec; parallel R_{total} = 0.67 cm H_2O/liter/sec), it can be seen that less driving pressure is needed to generate a flow through the parallel circuit than is required for the series circuit.

In fact, a driving pressure of 0.67 cm H_2O is required to produce a flow rate of 1 liter/sec in the parallel circuit, whereas a pressure gradient of 6 cm H_2O is needed to generate the same flow rate in the series circuit. The pressure gradient required to establish a 1 liter/sec flow rate through the series circuit is approximately nine times greater than that needed to produce the same flow rate in the parallel circuit. That is,

$$\frac{\text{series } \Delta P}{\text{parallel } \Delta P} = \frac{6.00 \text{ cm H}_2\text{O}}{0.67 \text{ cm H}_2\text{O}} = 8.95$$

To reiterate, the irregular dichotomous branching of the airways and the inverse relationship between the cross-sectional area and the velocity of flow contribute to the gradual decrease in airway resistance from the airway openings to the alveoli. This distribution of airway resistance has clinical significance. Large changes can occur in the caliber of the small airways without producing an appreciable change in the total airway resistance because the small airways (<2 mm diameter) account for only 10% of the total airway resistance. On the other hand, small changes in the caliber of the large airways drastically affect total airway resistance.

It is noteworthy to mention that because the small airways contribute such a small percentage to the total airway resistance, early small airway disease is difficult to diagnose. Airway resistance in the peripheral airways must increase substantially before it can be detected. Conversely, large airway disease is more readily detectable because large airways provide the major contribution to the total airway resistance.

It should also be noted that the magnitude of airway resistance is influenced by the flow pattern, that is, laminar or turbulent. Laminar flow is associated with less airway resistance than is turbulent flow.

Figure 4-44 is a diagrammatic representation of how the airway resistance in the small airways compares with that of the large airways. The thrust of this discussion is to impress upon the reader the difficulty of detecting early small airway disease. The tracheobronchial tree is depicted as a combination of series and parallel resistances. The symbol RL_{aw} signifies the airway resistance encountered through the large airways, whereas Rp_{aw} indicates the airway resistance developed throughout the small, or peripheral, airways.

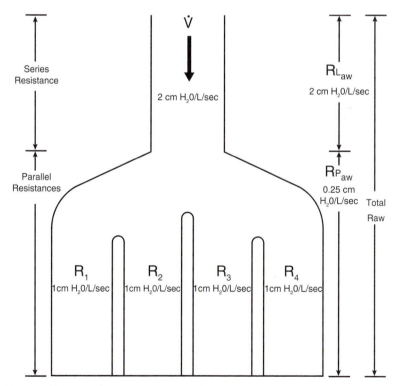

Figure 4-44 *Combination of series resistance (RL_{aw} = large airway resistance) and parallel resistances (Rp_{aw} = small airways resistance) across an entire lung model (Total R_{aw}).*

The value assigned to $R_{L_{aw}}$ in Figure 4-44 is 2 cm H_2O/liter/sec, and the value assigned to the four parallel resistances (R_1, R_2, R_3, and R_4), representing the small airways, is 1 cm H_2O/liter/sec. To obtain the total resistance in this lung model, the total $R_{L_{aw}}$ will be added to the total $R_{P_{aw}}$. Because $R_{L_{aw}}$ represents one resistance, the total $R_{L_{aw}}$ is 2 cm H_2O/liter/sec.

The total $R_{P_{aw}}$ can be computed as follows:

$$\frac{1}{\text{Total } R_{P_{aw}}} = \frac{1}{R_{P_{aw_1}}} + \frac{1}{R_{P_{aw_2}}} + \frac{1}{R_{P_{aw_3}}} + \frac{1}{R_{P_{aw_4}}}$$

$$\frac{1}{\text{Total } R_{P_{aw}}} = \frac{1}{1 \text{ cm } H_2O/\text{liter/sec}} + \frac{1}{1 \text{ cm } H_2O/\text{liter/sec}} + \frac{1}{1 \text{ cm } H_2O/\text{liter/sec}}$$
$$+ \frac{1}{1 \text{ cm } H_2O/\text{liter/sec}}$$

$$\frac{1}{\text{Total } R_{P_{aw}}} = \frac{1 \text{ liter/sec/cm } H_2O + 1 \text{ liter/sec/cm } H_2O + 1 \text{ liter/sec/cm } H_2O}{+ 1 \text{ liter/sec/cm } H_2O}$$

$$\frac{1}{\text{Total } R_{P_{aw}}} = 4.00 \text{ liter/sec/cm } H_2O$$

$$\text{Total } R_{P_{aw}} = \frac{1}{4 \text{ liter/sec/cm } H_2O}$$

$$= 0.25 \text{ cm } H_2O/\text{liter/sec}$$

The total resistance across this lung model now becomes

$$\text{Total Lung Model } R_{aw} = \text{Total } R_{L_{aw}} + \text{Total } R_{P_{aw}}$$

$$= 2 \text{ cm } H_2O/\text{liter/sec } + 0.25 \text{ cm } H_2O/\text{liter/sec}$$

$$= 2.25 \text{ cm } H_2O/\text{liter/sec}$$

Let's examine how the large airways resistance ($R_{L_{aw}}$) and the small airways resistance ($R_{P_{aw}}$) contribute to the total airway resistance in Figure 4-44. The $R_{L_{aw}}$ is 2 cm H_2O/liter/sec. Comparing that value to the total resistance across the lung model, the large airways contribute 89% to the total airway resistance. The small airways resistance, on the other hand, is 0.25 cm H_2O/liter/sec. The $R_{P_{aw}}$ contributes 11% to the total airway resistance. Mathematically, these percentages are calculated below.

CONTRIBUTION OF LARGE AIRWAYS RESISTANCE ($R_{L_{aw}}$) TO THE TOTAL

1) $$\frac{R_{L_{aw}}}{\text{Total } R_{aw}} \times 100 = \% \text{ of contribution}$$

2) $$\frac{2 \text{ cm } H_2O/\text{liter/sec}}{2.25 \text{ cm } H_2O/\text{liter/sec}} \times 100 = 89\%$$

CONTRIBUTION OF SMALL AIRWAYS RESISTANCE (RP$_{aw}$) TO THE TOTAL

1) $\dfrac{R_{Paw}}{\text{Total } R_{aw}} \times 100 = \%$ of contribution

2) $\dfrac{0.25 \text{ cm } H_2O/\text{liter/sec}}{2.25 \text{ cm } H_2O/\text{liter/sec}} \times 100 = 11\%$

Now let's observe the effect on the total resistance across the lung model if two of the four small airway resistances are doubled. Therefore, R_1 and R_2 will equal 2 cm H_2O/liter/sec, while R_3 and R_4 will remain at 1 cm H_2O/liter/sec. The total RP$_{aw}$ would become

$$\frac{1}{\text{Total } RP_{aw}} = \frac{1}{2 \text{ cm } H_2O/\text{liter/sec}} + \frac{1}{2 \text{ cm } H_2O/\text{liter/sec}}$$

$$+ \frac{1}{1 \text{ cm } H_2O/\text{liter/sec}} + \frac{1}{1 \text{ cm } H_2O/\text{liter/sec}}$$

$$\frac{1}{\text{Total } RP_{aw}} = \frac{0.5 \text{ liter/sec/cm } H_2O + 0.5 \text{ liter/sec/cm } H_2O}{+ 1 \text{ liter/sec/cm } H_2O + 1 \text{ liter/sec/cm } H_2O}$$

$$\frac{1}{\text{Total } RP_{aw}} = 3 \text{ liters/sec/cm } H_2O$$

$$\text{Total } RP_{aw} = \frac{1}{3 \text{ liters/sec/cm } H_2O}$$

$$= 0.33 \text{ cm } H_2O/\text{liter/sec}$$

In response to the increased total RP$_{aw}$, the total resistance is

$$\text{Total Lung Model } R_{aw} = 2 \text{ cm } H_2O/\text{liter/sec} + 0.33 \text{ cm } H_2O/\text{liter/sec}$$

$$= 2.33 \text{ cm } H_2O/\text{liter/sec}$$

Despite a 32% airway resistance increase in the small airways, the total airway resistance across the lung model increased only from 2.25 to 2.33 cm H_2O/liter/sec. That increase corresponds with a 3.5% change.

The following calculations illustrate how these percentages were obtained.

SMALL AIRWAYS RESISTANCE (RP$_{aw}$) INCREASE

1) 0.33 cm H_2O/liter/sec (RPaw increased)

   −0.25 cm H_2O/liter/sec (RPaw original)

   0.08 cm H_2O/liter/sec (RPaw difference)

2) $\dfrac{0.08 \text{ cm } H_2O/\text{liter/sec}}{0.25 \text{ cm } H_2O/\text{liter/sec}} \times 100 = 32\%$ change

TOTAL AIRWAY RESISTANCE (R_{aw}) INCREASE

1)
$$2.33 \text{ cm } H_2O/\text{liter/sec (Total } R_{aw} \text{ increased)}$$
$$\underline{-2.25 \text{ cm } H_2O/\text{liter/sec (Total } R_{aw} \text{ original)}}$$
$$0.08 \text{ cm } H_2O/\text{liter/sec (Total } R_{aw} \text{ difference)}$$

2)
$$\frac{0.08 \text{ cm } H_2O/\text{liter/sec}}{2.25 \text{ cm } H_2O/\text{liter/sec}} \times 100 = 3.5\% \text{ change}$$

The point of this discussion again is to quantitatively illustrate how a significant increase (32%) in small airways resistance is difficult to detect because the impact on the total airway resistance is slight (3.5%) in comparison. What accounts for this phenomenon is the vastly greater cross-sectional area in the small airways compared with that in the large airways.

EXAMPLE 1:

Calculate the total airway resistance across the tracheobronchial tree when the pressure at the mouth is one atmosphere and the intra-alveolar pressure is -6 cm H_2O. Assume a constant inspiratory flow rate of 0.5 liter/sec.

Step 1: Convert 1 atmosphere to its equivalent in cm H_2O.

$$1 \text{ atm} = 1{,}034 \text{ cm } H_2O$$

Step 2: Calculate the pressure change, or ΔP (driving pressure).

A. ΔP = the pressure difference (gradient) between the mouth and the alveoli

$$= P_m - P_{alv}$$

B. Mouth pressure is the same as atmospheric pressure; therefore

$$P_m = 1 \text{ atm} = 1{,}034 \text{ cm } H_2O$$

C. Alveolar pressure was stated to be -6 cm H_2O; therefore

$$P_{alv} = 1{,}034 \text{ cm } H_2O + (-6 \text{ cm } H_2O)$$
$$= 1{,}034 \text{ cm } H_2O - 6 \text{ cm } H_2O$$
$$= 1{,}028 \text{ cm } H_2O$$

D.
$$\Delta P = P_m - P_{alv}$$
$$= 1{,}034 \text{ cm } H_2O - 1{,}028 \text{ cm } H_2O$$
$$= 6 \text{ cm } H_2O$$

Step 3: Apply the formula for determining airway resistance.

$$R = \frac{\Delta P}{\dot{V}}$$

where

R = unknown

$\Delta P = 6$ cm H_2O

$\dot{V} = 0.5$ liter/sec

$$R = \frac{6 \text{ cm } H_2O}{0.5 \text{ liter/sec}}$$

$$= 12 \text{ cm } H_2O/\text{liter/sec}$$

EXAMPLE 2:

Compute the total airway resistance for a subject breathing a 500 cc V_T at a rate of 12 breaths per minute with an inspiratory time (T_I) of 2 seconds. Mouth pressure is 1,034 cm H_2O, and intra-alveolar pressure is 1,029 cm H_2O. Assume a constant flow rate.

Step 1: Determine the pressure gradient (ΔP).

$$\Delta P = P_m - P_{alv}$$

$$= 1,034 \text{ cm } H_2O - 1,029 \text{ cm } H_2O$$

$$= 5 \text{ cm } H_2O$$

Step 2: Calculate the flow rate ($\dot{V}$), and assume it to be constant.

A. Convert the 500-cc V_T to liters.

$$500 \text{ cc} = 0.5 \text{ liter}$$

B. The flow rate can be obtained by dividing the tidal volume by the inspiratory time.

$$\dot{V} = \frac{V_T}{T_I}$$

where

$\dot{V}$ = unknown

$V_T = 0.5$ liter

$T_I = 2$ sec

$$\dot{V} = \frac{0.5 \text{ liter}}{2 \text{ sec}}$$

$$= 0.25 \text{ liter/sec}$$

Step 3: Apply the formula for determining airway resistance.

$$R = \frac{\Delta P}{\dot{V}}$$

where

R = unknown

ΔP = 5 cm H_2O

$\dot{V}$ = 0.25 liter/sec

$$R = \frac{5 \text{ cm } H_2O}{0.25 \text{ liter/sec}}$$

$$= 20 \text{ cm } H_2O/\text{liter/sec}$$

PRACTICE PROBLEMS

Refer to Appendix A (pages 607-609) for the solutions and answers to the practice problems.

Solve the following resistance problems.

52. Calculate each individual resistance and the total resistance resistance encountered by a fluid moving through a series of three resistances. The ΔP and flow rate for each respective resistance are shown below.

	ΔP	$\dot{V}$
resistance$_1$	4 torr	2 liters/sec
resistance$_2$	5 torr	2 liters/sec
resistance$_3$	6 torr	2 liters/sec

R_1 _____; R_2 _____; R_3 _____; R_{total} _____

53. Determine each individual resistance and the total resistance encountered by a fluid moving through three parallel resistances. The ΔP and $\dot{V}$ for each respective resistance are given below.

	ΔP	$\dot{V}$
resistance$_1$	9 cm H_2O	3 liters/sec
resistance$_2$	12 cm H_2O	3 liters/sec
resistance$_3$	15 cm H_2O	3 liters/sec

R_1 _____; R_2 _____; R_3 _____; R_{total} _____

54. Determine the airway resistance across the tracheobronchial tree when the pressure at the mouth is 760 mm Hg and the intraalveolar pressure is −5 cm H_2O. Assume a constant flow rate of 3.5 liters/sec. _____

55. Calculate the airway resistance for an individual who has a V_T of 800 cc, a respiratory rate of 12 breaths per minute, and an inspiratory time of 2.0 seconds. Pressure at the mouth is 759 torr; the intra-alveolar pressure is 754 mm Hg. Assume that the flow rate is constant. _____

56. Calculate the total resistance in a conducting system that has both series and parallel resistances. The flow rate through the entire system is 2 L/sec. The resistances are listed below.

Series Resistances		Parallel Resistances	
ΔP		ΔP	
R_1	4 cm H_2O	R_3	10 cm H_2O
R_2	6 cm H_2O	R_4	8 cm H_2O
		R_5	6 cm H_2O
		R_6	4 cm H_2O

R_{total}: _____

Viscosity

The flow of any fluid through a conduit is opposed by the interactions among its molecules. This molecular interaction, or internal friction, is called **viscosity.** Viscosity can also be described as a fluid's resistance to deformity. Because viscosity incorporates the element of time within its units (i.e., CGS = dyne-second/cm², or **poise;** MKS = newton-second/m²; SI* = pascal-second [Pas]), it refers to the relationship between the force applied to a fluid and the rate of deformation.

The property of viscosity manifests itself somewhat differently in liquids than it does in gases. The viscosity of liquids is influenced by the cohesive forces (**van der Waals forces[†]**) among the liquid molecules, whereas gas viscosity results from the collisions among the rapidly moving gas molecules.

Viscosity is temperature dependent. In liquids, for example, the viscosity decreases with increasing temperature. However, gas viscosity increases with increasing temperature. This seeming paradox can be explained on the basis of the kinetic theory of matter. As the temperature of a liquid rises, the kinetic energy ($\frac{1}{2}mv^2$ or $\frac{1}{2}Dv^2$) of the liquid molecules increases, and the cohesive forces among the liquid molecules weaken. The viscosity of the liquid, therefore, decreases because the cohesive forces among liquid molecules determine the viscosity of the liquid.

On the other hand, increasing the temperature of a gas increases the kinetic energy of the gas molecules further. The number of collisions among the gas molecules consequently increases, resulting in a greater internal friction. Because the degree of molecular bombardment determines the viscosity of a gas, gas viscosity increases with increasing temperature.

Consider a gas flowing through a tube in laminar fashion where concentric gas layers are moving parallel to one another. Gaseous diffusion implies that gas molecules will transfer from layer to layer causing molecular collisions and resulting in internal friction. Elevating the temperature of this gas increases the molecular activity; that is, more and more gas molecules will move from one layer to another. This heightened molecular activity manifests itself as increased viscosity (increased internal friction). Eventually, if the temperature is elevated enough, gas molecules will achieve **critical velocity,** and laminar flow will disrupt into a turbulent pattern.

---

*The official abbreviation *SI* refers to the International System of Units, which is from the French *Le système internationale d'unités.*

[†]Van der Waals forces are intermolecular forces resulting from dipole-induced dipole bonds.

Poiseuille's Law of Laminar Flow

Poiseuille's law of laminar flow describes in mathematical language the factors influencing the movement of fluid. The relationship of the factors in Poiseuille's equation below applies specifically to the following conditions: (1) fluid flow must be nonpulsatile and laminar, (2) the single conducting tube must be rigid and cylindrical, and (3) the fluid must be homogeneous and **Newtonian.***

Certainly, neither the tracheobronchial tree nor the cardiovascular network meets these requirements. The ventilatory conduits, however, favor laminar flow by virtue of the tremendous increase in cross-sectional area and the air velocity decrease occurring from the trachea to the alveoli.[†] However, the airways are neither rigid nor cylindrical. They also form a parallel circuit of branchings, hence are not a single tube. During inspiration the airways elongate and widen; during exhalation they shorten and narrow. We often (conveniently so) conceptualize the airways as perfectly cylindrical. The fact is that the dynamics of the internal thoracic environment contribute to the distortion of airway caliber and geometry. For example, such influences as (1) extraluminal pressure applied by surrounding tissues, (2) intrathoracic pressure changes, (3) bronchial wall smooth muscle contraction and relaxation, and (4) mucous gland and goblet cell secretions all influence airway configuration.

Finally, the fluid we breathe, air, is indeed a homogeneous, Newtonian fluid. (At last, a degree of compliance with specifications set forth by Poiseuille's law.)

Despite these obvious incongruities, Poiseuille's law nonetheless provides useful approximations and knowledge concerning in vivo airflow.

Quantitatively, Poiseuille's law of laminar flow is shown as

$$\dot{V} = \frac{\Delta P r^4 \pi}{\eta 8 L} \tag{1}$$

where

$\dot{V}$ = fluid flow rate

ΔP = driving pressure

r = radius of the tube

$\pi/8$ = mathematical constant (the Greek letter pi has the value of 3.14)

η = viscosity of the fluid (represented by the Greek letter eta)

L = length of the conducting tube

According to Poiseuille's equation, the flow rate ($\dot{V}$) is directly proportional to the pressure gradient (ΔP) and the tube radius raised to the fourth power (r^4), and inversely

---

*Newtonian fluids maintain a constant viscosity at all flow rates; non-Newtonian fluids vary in viscosity as flow conditions change.

[†]It is interesting to note that some physiologists believe that laminar flow does not occur anywhere in the tracheobronchial tree. They theorize that airway length is insufficient from division to division for the distorted flow at each branching to convert to laminar flow.

proportional to the viscosity of the fluid (η) and the length of the tube (L) and the mathematical constant ($\pi/8$).

This equation is often rearranged and expressed in terms of either the pressure gradient (ΔP) or in terms of airway resistance ($\Delta P/\dot{V}$). Expressed in terms of ΔP the equation becomes

$$\Delta P = \frac{8L\eta\dot{V}}{\pi r^4} \qquad (2)$$

In terms of $\Delta P/\dot{V}$, it is

$$\frac{\Delta P}{\dot{V}} = \frac{8L\eta}{\pi r^4} \qquad (3)$$

As previously mentioned, this seemingly formidable equation can be conveniently manipulated and thus simplified when certain assumptions are made.

One manipulation of Poiseuille's law attempts to elucidate how the equation incorporates the concept of airway resistance ($R = \Delta P/\dot{V}$). Both mathematical constants, π and 8, can be eliminated because they are constants. Therefore, equation 3 becomes

$$\frac{\Delta P}{\dot{V}} \propto \frac{L\eta}{r^4} \qquad (4)$$

Equation 3 expresses that $\Delta P/\dot{V}$, which represents airway resistance, is proportional to $8L\eta/r^4\pi$. Recall that any time a fluid flows through a conducting system resistive forces are encountered. These impediments to flow result from tube and fluid characteristics. Here the tube resistance factor are length and radius, manifested as L/r^4, whereas the fluid resistance factor is the viscosity η. Therefore, $8L\eta/\pi r^4$ represents the total, or overall, resistance to flow, that is,

$$R = \frac{8L\eta}{\pi r^4} \qquad (5)$$

Because $R = 8L\eta/\pi r^4$, R can replace the fraction representing the overall resistance to flow ($8L\eta/\pi r^4$) in equation 3. The expression now becomes

$$\frac{\Delta P}{\dot{V}} = R \qquad (6)$$

Poiseuille's law can be manipulated in another manner, that is, to eliminate all the factors except ΔP, $\dot{V}$, and r^4. The purpose of this manipulation is to study these three important components involving airflow through the airways. Equation 3 can be rewritten as

$$\Delta P = \frac{8L\eta}{\pi} \times \frac{\dot{V}}{r^4} \qquad (7)$$

If L and η are constant, the factor $8L\eta/\pi$ can equal k. Therefore,

$$k = \frac{8L\eta}{\pi} \qquad (8)$$

Thus, equation 7 becomes

$$\Delta P = k \times \frac{\dot{V}}{r^4} \tag{9}$$

Equation 9 indicates that, for a constant pressure, the rate of flow is directly proportional to the airway radius raised to the fourth power. Therefore, if the ventilating pressure (transairway pressure) is to remain constant, a reduction in airway radius (e.g., bronchospasm) will greatly reduce the flow of gas entering the alveoli.

Equation 9 can be rearranged as

$$\dot{V} = \frac{1}{k} \times \Delta P r^4 \tag{10}$$

Equation 10 now illustrates that, for a constant rate of flow, the pressure gradient is inversely proportional to the airway radius raised to the fourth power. Consequently, if the inspiratory flow (volume/time) is to remain constant, a decrease in airway caliber, again due to bronchospasm, for example, will result in a greatly increased transairway pressure (ΔP).

Reworking Poiseuille's law once again to demonstrate the relationship between airway resistance and airway radius, the factors L and η in equation 5 can be considered constant; thus, $k = 8L\eta/\pi$.

Equation 5 can then be rewritten as

$$R = \frac{k}{r^4} \tag{11}$$

Equation 11 indicates that if all the factors in Poiseuille's law remain constant except the radius and the airway resistance, the airway resistance is inversely proportional to the radius raised to the fourth power.

Equation 11 can be rearranged as

$$R \times r^4 = k \tag{12}$$

Table 4-12 summarizes the steps utilized here in simplifying Poiseuille's law of laminar flow.

We can thus show that if the airway radius is halved, the airway resistance increases 16-fold. For example, utilizing equation 12, let $k = 16$ and r = 1. (For the sake of simplicity, units will be omitted.) Then, solve for R.

$$R \times r^4 = k \tag{12}$$
$$R \times 1^4 = 16$$
$$R = \frac{16}{1}$$
$$R = 16$$

TABLE 4-12 Summary of Equations Relating to Poiseuille's Law of Laminar Flow

---

Step 1: $\dot{V} = \dfrac{\Delta P r^4 \pi}{\eta 8L}$

Step 2: $\Delta P = \left(\dfrac{8L\eta}{\pi}\right)\left(\dfrac{\dot{V}}{r^4}\right)$

Step 3: $\Delta P = k\left(\dfrac{\dot{V}}{r^4}\right)$

Step 4: $\dfrac{\Delta P}{\dot{V}} = \dfrac{k}{r^4}$

Step 5: $R = \dfrac{k}{r^4}$ or $R \times r^4 = k$

If the airway radius is halved and becomes 0.5, and k remains 16, then the quantitative effect on airway resistance can be observed.

$$R \times 0.5^4 = 16$$

$$R = \frac{16}{0.5^4} = \frac{16}{0.0625}$$

$$R = 256$$

The square of 16 (i.e., the original value of airway resistance) is 256. Therefore, the original R increased 16-fold in response to halving the radius.

Conversely, if the radius doubles, airway resistance will decrease by a factor of 16 when all the other factors remain constant.

Table 4-13 summarizes the relationship between airway resistance and airway radius according to equation 12.

TABLE 4-13 Data Relating R and r^4

---

	r	r^4	*k*	R
Original situation	1	1	16	16
Radius halved	0.5	0.0625	16	256
Radius doubled	2	16	16	1

Reynold's Number

In the nineteenth century Osborn Reynolds, an English physicist, derived an equation that expresses the relationship between certain kinetic forces and the frictional force viscosity for flowing fluids. This equation is a ratio in the strict sense of the term; all the units cancel and only a dimensionless value remains.

This dimensionless number, called Reynold's number (R_N), reflects the flow pattern present. For homogeneous fluids, a Reynold's number less than 2,000 indicates the presence of laminar flow, whereas a Reynold's number exceeding 2,000 is indicative of turbulent flow.

Quantitatively, Reynold's equation is written as

$$R_N = \frac{v \times D \times d}{\eta}$$

where

R_N = dimensionless (Reynold's) number indicating the nature of flow

v = velocity of the fluid flowing through the tube

D = fluid density

d = tube diameter

η = fluid viscosity (*eta*)

On inspection of the equation one should note that an increase in any or all of the factors in the numerator, while the viscosity remains constant, will increase R_N and tend to promote turbulent flow. On the other hand, if fluid viscosity increases disproportionately in response to any increases in the numerator, R_N will decrease and laminar flow will be supported.

Reynold's equation should also provide further insight into the rationale for using less dense gases when ventilation is difficult because of obstructions. In Section 4-6, "Fluid Dynamics," the practice of substituting a He-O_2 gas mixture for an air-O_2 mixture was discussed. The theoretical basis for this substitution, you will recall, is that the less dense He-O_2 mixture effects a lesser pressure change across the obstruction than does the more dense air-O_2 mixture. The quantitative basis for this practice is expressed in equation 6 in the discussion of the Bernoulli principle.

So, according to the ratio here, a decreased density factor in the numerator will lower the Reynold's number and favor laminar flow. Conversely, a larger density gas will raise R_N and favor turbulent flow.

The dimensional analysis of Reynold's equation demonstrated below will illustrate that R_N is a dimensionless number. The units for the factors comprising the equation are as follows:

velocity (v) = cm/sec (linear distance per time)

density (D) = kg/cm^3 (mass per unit volume)

diameter (d) = cm (linear distance)

viscosity (η) = $\dfrac{kg \times cm \times sec}{sec^2 \times cm^2}$

Therefore

$$R_N = \frac{\dfrac{cm}{sec} \times \dfrac{kg}{cm^3} \times cm}{\dfrac{kg \times cm \times sec}{sec^2 \times cm^2}} = \frac{\dfrac{kg}{sec \times cm}}{\dfrac{kg}{sec \times cm}}$$

In summary, according to the Reynold's equation, a large R_N (> 2,000) indicates that momentum forces (kinetic energy) predominate and that flow will be turbulent. A small R_N (< 2,000) implies that viscous forces prevail and that the flow pattern will be laminar. A small R_N results by lowering (1) the density of a gas, (2) the diameter of an opening, or (3) the velocity of a gas. R_N also decreases when gas viscosity increases.

4-7 MECHANICS OF VENTILATION

In the previous section it was mentioned that three forms of resistance are encountered during ventilation: (1) inertial resistance, (2) elastic resistance, and (3) airway resistance. At that point, **elastic resistance** was excluded from the discussion because fluid dynamics was being presented. Elastic resistance measurements are valid only when they are obtained during periods of no airflow. Therefore, pressures required to overcome airway resistance do not enter into consideration.

This section will concern itself with the mechanical or static properties of breathing, namely, compliance and elastance. Hooke's law will serve as foundation for the development of these concepts. Consideration will be given to ventilation time constants to demonstrate the interaction of airway resistance (dynamic component) and compliance (static component) with the mechanics of ventilation. Lastly, the influence of surface tension forces, governed by the law of LaPlace, will also be presented.

Hooke's Law

Hooke's law can be applied to solid materials that are elastic. A solid is said to be elastic if it can regain its original length or shape following the removal of the force responsible for stretching or deforming it. This property is known as **elastic recoil.** For example, let a spring suspended from a crossbeam represent an elastic material (Figure 4-45). According to Hooke's law, the spring will stretch equal units of length for each unit of weight or force applied to the bottom of the spring. Part A of Figure 4-45 represents the spring's resting position. The pointer attached to the spring indicates that the spring is not stretched. In part B, a unit of force is applied to the spring, causing the spring to stretch a certain length, as indicated by the pointer's position in reference to the scale. The addition of another (identical) unit of force results in doubling the stretching of the spring. This relationship will remain true until the **elastic limit** of the spring is achieved. At that point, the spring will no longer increase its length proportional to the force added. In fact, additional force will cause the spring to permanently distort.

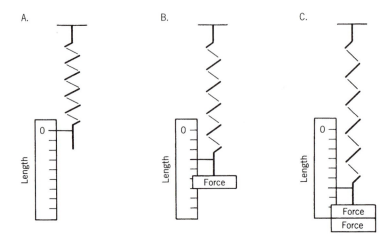

Figure 4-45 *Hooke's law. Part A depicts a spring at rest (reference point). In part B, 1 unit of force is applied, causing 3 units of stretch. In part C, 2 units of force are applied, causing 6 units of stretch. This linear relationship will continue until the spring's elastic limit is exceeded.*

The relationship between length and force as described above is graphically illustrated in Figure 4-46.

The dark line demonstrates that each unit of force applied to the spring corresponds with an equivalent increase in its length. The linear (direct) relationship between these two factors is maintained until the elastic limit of the spring is reached. The elastic limit is represented by the point where the dark line and the dashed line meet. If the stretching force is removed prior to the spring's elastic limit, the spring will return to its resting position as shown in part A of Figure 4-45. If, on the other hand, the stretching force is removed after the elastic limit is reached, the spring will remain stretched or distorted. In other words, the spring will not recoil to its resting position after its elastic limit has been exceeded.

Quantitatively, Hooke's law for a spring can be expressed as

$$k = \frac{\text{force}}{\text{extension}}$$

where k is the spring constant for a given spring.

Lung and chestwall (thorax) tissues are elastic. Therefore, they obey Hooke's law. Lung tissue has natural tendency to collapse or contract, and chest wall tissue has an inclination to bow out or expand. That is to say, the lungs collapse below residual volume (but not to a completely airless state) when they are excised from the intact thorax, and the chest wall, if unopposed by the lungs, would occupy a volume approximately 70% of the total lung capacity (TLC). Therefore, in the intact thorax the forces of contraction (lung tissue) and expansion (chest wall) differ in magnitude and direction throughout most of the ventilatory cycle.

Figure 4-47 schematically illustrates this concept using two springs. The coiled spring represents the natural tendency of the lung tissue to collapse. The bowed springs depict the thorax tending to expand. The arrows indicate the direction in which each of these tissues seeks to move.

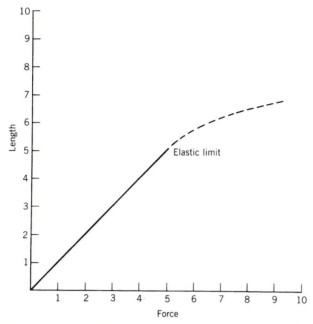

Figure 4-46 *Graphic representation of Hooke's law showing linear relationship between force and length (stretch) until elastic limit is exceeded.*

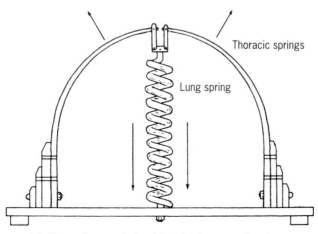

Figure 4-47 *Spring model of lung-thorax relationship. The thorax tends to bow out as the lungs tend to collapse. The arrows indicate the direction of movement. From Spearman, Charles B., and Sheldon, Richard L., editors:* Egan's Fundamentals of Respiratory Therapy, *6th ed., 1995. Mosby-Year Book, Inc., St. Louis.*

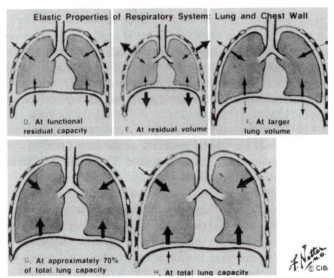

Figure 4-48 *Opposing interaction of the lung and thorax at five different lung volumes: D, functional residual capacity where forces (arrows) are equal in magnitude but opposite in direction; E, residual volume where tendency for thorax expansion is greatest and that for lung collapse is least; F, large lung volume; G, 70% of TLC is the resting point of thorax; and H, at TLC the chest wall and lungs both tend to move in the same direction. © Copyright 1979, CIBA Pharmaceutical Company, Division of CIBA-GEIGY Corporation. Reprinted with permission from* The CIBA Collection of Medical Illustrations, *illustrated by Frank H. Netter, M.D. All rights reserved.*

We will examine the interaction of these two opposing forces at five different ventilatory positions. We will begin by viewing their relationship at functional residual capacity (FRC). In Figure 4-48D the arrows depicting the recoil (contractile) forces of the lung parenchymal tissue are equal in magnitude, but opposite in direction, to those representing the forces of the chest wall expansion. At this particular point in the ventilatory cycle, which can also be termed *normal end-exhalation,* these two opposing forces are in equilibrium.

Figure 4-48E represents residual volume (RV). At this ventilatory position the contractile forces of the lung tissue are less than the expansile forces of the chest wall. Consequently, the tendency of the lung-chest wall system at this point favors lung filling (inspiration).

At a large lung volume, as shown in Figure 4-48F, the contractile forces of the lung tissue are greater than those tending to expand the chest wall. Therefore, at this lung volume the tendency of the lung-chest wall system is to favor lung emptying (exhalation).

At an even larger lung volume, for example, 70% of the total lung capacity (TLC), chest wall elastic recoil is zero (Figure 4-48G). Consequently, the contractile forces of the lung tissue act unopposed and promote exhalation.

Finally, at total lung capacity (Figure 4-48H) both forces, lung and chest wall elastic recoil, act in the same direction. However, the magnitude of the lung parenchymal recoil forces exceeds that of the forces contributed by the chest wall.

During the inspiratory phase of the ventilatory cycle the muscles of inspiration do the work required to produce a pressure change, which, in turn, results in a lung volume change. Normal exhalation requires no muscle effort because the elastic recoil of the lung tissue accomplishes exhalation to the FRC level. To achieve RV, active contraction of certain abdominal and thoracic muscles is required. The normal expansile tendency of the chest wall prevents the passive accomplishment of this act.

Because lung and chest wall tissues are elastic materials, Hooke's law has physiologic applications. However, because of the complexity of the respiratory apparatus, the application of Hooke's law to this physiologic model is not as straightforward as the spring-weight (length-force) system previously described. If we substitute pressure for force and volume for length, a pressure-volume curve can be plotted. This pressure-volume curve is actually a compliance curve. Compliance is defined as a unit of volume change per unit of pressure change and represents the elastic behavior of the respiratory apparatus.

$$\text{Compliance} = \frac{\text{volume change (liter)}}{\text{pressure change (cm } H_2O)} = \frac{\Delta V}{\Delta P}$$

Three types of compliance exist within the respiratory system. They are (1) lung or pulmonary compliance, (2) chest wall or thoracic compliance, and (3) lung-chest wall or total compliance. Each type of compliance can be obtained quantitatively from the expression

$$\frac{1}{C_L} + \frac{1}{C_{CW}} = \frac{1}{C_T}$$

where

$\dfrac{1}{C_L}$ = the reciprocal of the compliance of the lung tissue

$\dfrac{1}{C_{CW}}$ = the reciprocal of the compliance of the chest wall

$\dfrac{1}{C_T}$ = the reciprocal of the compliance of the total respiratory apparatus (i.e., the lungs and chest wall combined)

It should be noted from the equation above that the total compliance will always be less than the compliance of either the lungs or the chest wall.

Lung compliance and total compliance can be directly measured. Lung compliance can be obtained by passing a balloon into the esophagus to the midthoracic level (intra-esophageal pressure is approximately equal to intrapleural pressure). Pressure changes are monitored at different lung volumes during static (no airflow) conditions. Total compliance can be determined by recording pressure changes at lung volumes beyond the end-expiratory level in an anesthetized mechanically ventilated subject.

Chest wall compliance on the other hand, cannot be directly measured. It can only be calculated from the compliance formula after both the lung and total comtliance measurements have been made. For example, experimentation has shown that normal adult male lung compliance is 0.2 liter/cm H_2O and that for the total system is 0.1 liter/cm H_2O. Chest wall compliance can be calculated as follows:

Step 1:
$$\frac{1}{C_L} + \frac{1}{C_{CW}} = \frac{1}{C_T}$$

Step 2:
$$\frac{1}{C_T} - \frac{1}{C_L} = \frac{1}{C_{CW}}$$

Step 3:
$$\frac{1}{0.1 \text{ liter/cm } H_2O} - \frac{1}{0.2 \text{ liter/cm } H_2O} = \frac{1}{C_{CW}}$$

Step 4:
$$10 \text{ cm } H_2O/\text{liter} - 5 \text{ cm } H_2O/\text{liter} = \frac{1}{C_{CW}}$$

Step 5:
$$5 \text{ cm } H_2O/\text{liter} = \frac{1}{C_{CW}}$$

Step 6:
$$C_{CW} = \frac{1}{5 \text{ cm } H_2O/\text{liter}}$$

Step 7:
$$C_{CW} = 0.2 \text{ liter/cm } H_2O$$

Note, once again, that the value for the total compliance is less than that of either the lungs or the chest wall alone.

The compliance curve obtained by plotting lung pressure versus lung volume is not as simple as plotting force versus length for a spring-weight system. The compliance curve shown in Figure 4-49 indicates two plottings, inspiration (lower tracing) and exhalation (upper tracing), between functional residual capacity (FRC) and total lung capacity (TLC). The shape of the curve is sigmoid and the overall shape of the curve exhibits the phenomenon described as **hysteresis,** which refers to a structure whose graphic configuration during deformation (inspiration) differs from that during recoil (exhalation). On inspection one can readily see that the relationship between lung volume and lung pressure changes throughout the ventilatory cycle is not linear.

Because of the nonlinear nature of the lung pressure-volume curve, it should be evident that a single measurement derived from the curve will not accurately reflect the elastic properties of the lungs. The reason is that a given volume change (ΔV) on the steep portion of the curve requires a smaller pressure change (ΔP) than that required for the same volume change on the flat segment of the curve.

Figure 4-50 on page 318 illustrates the lung compliance curve. (If necessary, review Chapter 1 Mathematics, 1-9 Graphs, Sigmoid Curve.) On the x-axis, ΔP-B represents the pressure change in the lung bases during normal resting ventilation, while ΔV-B (y-axis) refers to the corresponding volume change in the bases. The designation ΔP-A signifies the pressure change in the apices during normal tidal breathing, and ΔV-A represents the volume change in the apices caused by the ΔP-A.

Note that ΔP-B equals ΔP-A; however, the corresponding volume change for each pressure change is not equal. The ΔV-A is less than ΔV-B for the same pressure change because the apices are situated close to the flat portion of the compliance curve, whereas the bases are located on the steep portion.

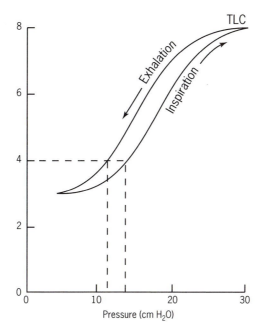

Figure 4-49 *Hysteresis curve caused by the fact that the pressure-volume relationships differ during inspiration and exhalation. A larger pressure gradient is required to cause a volume change during inspiration than during exhalation.*

Another reason why a single compliance measurement obtained from the compliance curve is not quite reliable is that the compliance value changes with lung volume. For instance, a person with a small lung volume will have a lower compliance than someone with a high lung volume, despite the fact that both lungs may have identical elastic and distensible qualities. Consequently, the term **specific compliance,** which represents the elastic behavior of the materials (anatomic structures) comprising the respiratory apparatus, is used to indicate the volume at which the compliance measurement was made. Compliance measurements are often made at functional residual capacity, and the units for specific compliance are liter/cm H_2O/liter. It should be readily apparent that lung compliance is volume specific.

Recall that there are three types of compliance in reference to the respiratory apparatus: (1) lung or pulmonary compliance, (2) chest wall or thoracic compliance, and (3) lung-chest wall or total compliance. Therefore, a pressure-volume curve or compliance curve can be developed for each of these three components.

The reciprocal of compliance is elastance:

$$\frac{1}{C} = E$$

or

$$\text{Elastance} = \frac{\text{pressure change (cm } H_2O)}{\text{volume change (liter)}} = \frac{\Delta P}{\Delta V}$$

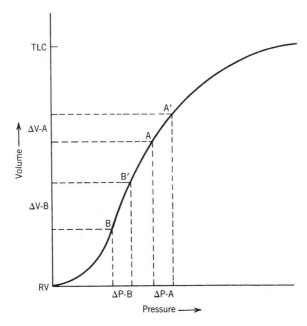

Figure 4-50 *Lung compliance curve illustrating the relationship between pressure-volume changes in the lung bases and apices during a normal ventilatory cycle. The labels B and A signify normal, end-exhalation (FRC) in the bases and apices, respectively; B' and A' indicate normal end-inspiration in the bases and apices, respectively. Note that for the same ΔP (i.e., ΔP-B = ΔP-A), a greater ΔV develops in the bases compared with that experienced by the apices because the bases are lower on the compliance curve. From Kacmarek, R. M., Dimes, S., Mack, C.:* The Essentials of Respiratory Therapy, *3rd ed., 1990, Mosby-Year Book, Inc., Chicago. Used with permission.*

The mathematical relationship between these two physical entities indicates that as lung compliance increases lung elastance decreases. The converse is also true.

The utility of the concept of elastance can be understood when examining two disease conditions, pulmonary emphysema (obstruction) and pulmonary fibrosis (restriction), in the context of Figure 4-51.

The diagram shows three compliance curves. The normal compliance curve is positioned between the two disease conditions used here to demonstrate the mechanical ramifications that changes in elastance have on the respiratory apparatus.

The compliance curve associated with pulmonary emphysema is shifted to the left of normal. In this particular disease condition, lung tissue is lost or destroyed at the acinar level. As lung tissue destruction progresses, the lung becomes flaccid, or more distensible (compliance increases) and alveolar interdependence decreases. At the same time, the lung's elastic recoil or elastance diminishes. The increased compliance and decreased elastance account for the leftward shift of the compliance curve as indicated in Figure 4-51.

The compliance curve representing pulmonary fibrosis is located to the right of the normal compliance curve. This disease entity is characterized by fibrosis or scarring throughout the lungs. As a consequence, the lungs become stiffer and more difficult to

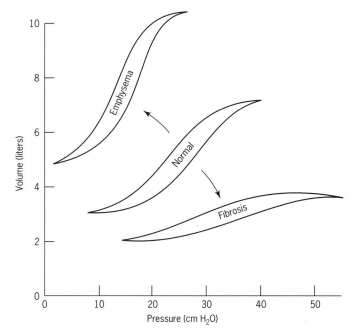

Figure 4-51 *Three compliance (hysteresis) curves. The middle curve represents a normal pressure-volume relationship, the emphysema (obstructive disease) curve displays an increased compliance, and the fibrosis (restrictive disease) curve shows a decreased compliance. From Tisi, Gennaro M.:* Pulmonary Physiology in Clinical Medicine, *© 1980, Williams & Wilkins Co., Baltimore. Used with permission.*

inflate, that is, their compliance decreases. However, the elastic recoil or elastance of the lungs increases. The decreased compliance and increased elastance are responsible for the pulmonary fibrosis compliance curve's movement to the right of normal.

PRACTICE PROBLEMS

Refer to Appendix A (pages 609-610) for the solutions and answers to the practice problems.

Solve the following compliance and elastance problems:

57. Calculate chest wall compliance when the lung-thorax compliance is 0.1 liters/cm H_2O and the pulmonary compliance is 0.2 liters/cm H_2O.

58. A subject with an intraesophageal balloon in place exhibits an intrapleural pressure of −4 cm H_2O at normal end-expiration. The pressure manometer indicates an intrapleural pressure of −6.5 cm H_2O after the subject inhales 500 cc of air. Calculate this person's pulmonary compliance. _____

59. Calculate the value for pulmonary elastance using the data in the previous question. _____

60. Calculate the thoracic compliance when the total elastance measures 13.9 cm H_2O/L and the lung compliance measures 0.12 liter/cm H_2O.

61. Calculate the total elastance of the system in question 60. _____

Ventilation Time Constant

The ventilation time constant, which is the product of airway resistance and pulmonary compliance, establishes the rate of volume and pressure changes in the lungs. The quantitative expression illustrating the relationship between airway resistance and pulmonary compliance is as follows:

$$\text{time constant} = R_{aw} \times C_L$$

where

R_{aw} = airway resistance (cm $H_2O/L/sec$)

C_L = pulmonary compliance (L/cm H_2O)

If, for example, the R_{aw} was 2.5 cm $H_2O/L/sec$ and the C_L was 0.2 L/cm H_2O, the ventilation time constant would be

$$\text{time constant} = (2.5 \ \cancel{cm \ H_2O}/\cancel{L}/sec)(0.2 \ \cancel{L}/\cancel{cm \ H_2O})$$

$$= 0.5 \text{ second}$$

What does this time constant value mean? This time interval determines the rate of pressure and volume changes in the lungs. The instant that we begin to inspire (spontaneous breath), the pressure gradient between the mouth (atmosphere) and the alveoli is at its widest point. As inspiration proceeds, pressure in the alveoli progressively rises because the lungs are continuously filling. At the same time, the inspiratory flow rate steadily diminishes. This drop in the flow rate occurs exponentially (Figure 4-52A), rather than linearly, as the alveolar pressure rises (mouth-alveoli pressure gradient narrows).

Similarly, the rise in alveolar pressure also takes place exponentially (Figure 4-52B). Notice how these two exponential curves relate to each other. After one time constant, i.e., a specific time interval, the inspiratory flow rate has decreased to 37% of its initial value (100%), and the alveolar pressure has increased 63% above its original value (0%). At two time constants, the flow rate has decayed to 13.5%, and the alveolar pressure has risen to 86.5%. At the point of three time constants, the flow rate has diminished to 5% of its original value, while the alveolar pressure achieved 95% over its initial value. Finally, after four time constants the inspiratory flow rate has fallen to 3% of the flow rate at the outset of inspiration. At the same time, the alveolar pressure has achieved 97% of its capacity. Based on this relationship, lung filling will be virtually complete over the span of four time constants.

A time constant can also be described as the time it takes for the flow rate to diminish to 37% of its original value (100%), or the time elapsed in which the alveolar pressure has risen 63% above its initial value (0%). In either case, the time constant is equal to the product of the lung's airway resistance and compliance components.

Let us return to the time constant that we calculated at the beginning of this discussion (i.e., 0.5 sec) to determine specifically what that value represents. Alveolar filling, as well as emptying, can be thought of as occurring over segments of time—1 time constant, 2 time

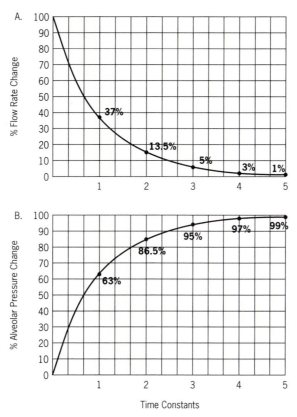

Figure 4-52 *Exponential curves. Graph A shows exponential decay of inspiratory flow rate. The flow rate diminishes to 37%, 13.5%, 5%, 3%, and 1% after 1, 2, 3, 4, and 5 time constants, respectively. Graph B illustrates the exponential increase in alveolar pressure (or volume) during inspiration. The alveolar pressure increases to 63%, 86.5%, 95%, 97%, and 99%. At 1, 2, 3, 4, and 5 time constants, respectively.*

constants, and so on. For the lung which had airway resistance and compliance values of 2.5 cm H_2O/liter/sec and 0.2 liter/cm H_2O, respectively, the lungs will be 63% filled in 0.5 second (1 time constant), 86.5% filled in 1.0 second (2 time constants), 95% filled in 1.5 seconds (3 time constants), and 97% filled in 2.0 seconds (4 time constants). For all practical purposes, equilibrium between the pressure at the mouth and the alveoli is reached after four time constants.

What happens to the time constant when the airway resistance remains the same but the lung compliance changes? The following calculation demonstrates how the time constant is affected when the airway resistance remains 2.5 cm H_2O/liter/sec and the lung compliance decreases to 0.1 liter/cm H_2O (half the initial compliance value). That is,

COMPLIANCE REDUCED 50% TO 0.1 LITER/cm H_2O

time constant = (2.5 cm H_2O/liter/sec)(0.1 liter/cm H_2O)

= 0.25 sec

The new time constant is half the value of the original one. Therefore, lungs having these resistance and compliance values will equilibrate in 1.0 second (4 time constants), or

$$4 \times 0.25 \text{ second} = 1.0 \text{ second}$$

Consider the impact of airway resistance changes on the time constant. Assume that the airway resistance increases to 5 cm H_2O/liter/sec (doubles) and that the lung compliance maintains its original value of 0.2 liter/cm H_2O. The time constant will be

AIRWAY RESISTANCE DOUBLES TO 5 cm H_2O/L/sec

$$\text{time constant} = (5 \text{ cm } H_2O/\text{liter}/\text{sec})(0.2 \text{ liter}/\text{cm } H_2O)$$

$$= 1 \text{ second}$$

Because equilibrium becomes established after four time constants have elapsed, a lung with these resistance and compliance characteristics will achieve equilibrium in 4 seconds. That is,

$$4 \times 1 \text{ second} = 4 \text{ seconds}$$

In general, time constant values increase as airway resistance and/or lung compliance increase. Conversely, time constant values decrease when airway resistance and/or lung compliance decrease.

The foregoing discussion related time constants to the lung as a whole. The same concept applies to individual lung units. Therefore, the time it takes for an individual lung unit to fill or empty is dependent on the compliance and resistance characteristics of that lung unit. For example, if two adjacent lung units have the same compliance and resistance, they will inflate or deflate within the same time because they have the same time constant.

In reality, the lungs are comprised of lung units with differing time constants. Consider the neighboring lung units depicted in Figure 4-53.

Table 4-14 illustrates the time constants and the equilibrium time for alveolus A and alveolus B, depicted in Figure 4-53.

Aveolus A has a smaller time constant (TC) than alveolus B. Therefore, alveolus A has a shorter equilibration time than alveolus B. Alveolus A has an equilibration time (4 time constants) of 0.8 second, and alveolus B has an equilibration time of 3.2 seconds. These equilibration times are determined as follows.

$$\text{number of time constants} \times TC = \text{equilibration time}$$

ALVEOLUS A: $4 \times 0.2 \text{ second} = 0.8 \text{ second}$

ALVEOLUS B: $4 \times 0.8 \text{ second} = 3.2 \text{ seconds}$

If the inspiratory time were 1 second, the alveolar pressure in alveolus A would be 99% above its original value (0%) because it would experience 5 time constants during inspiration (1 second ÷ 0.2 second = 5 TCs).

On the other hand, alveolus B, during the same inspiratory time of 1 second, would achieve only slightly more than 63% of its initial pressure because it would be exposed to only somewhat more than one time constant (1 second ÷ 0.8 second = 1.25 TCs).

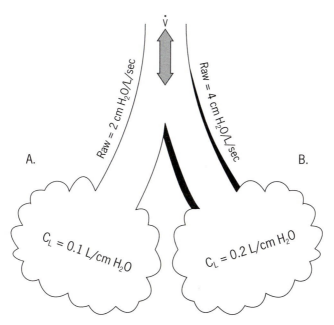

Figure 4-53 *Two neighboring alveolar units. Alveolus A will achieve equilibrium after 4 time constants. Alveolus B will achieve equilibrium in 1 time constant.*

TABLE 4-14 Data for Figure 4-53

	$R_{aw} \times C_L = TC$	Equilibration Time (4 × TC)
Alveolus A	0.2 sec	0.8 sec
Alveolus B	0.8 sec	3.2 sec

Note that these two alveoli will experience nonuniform ventilation and that aveolus B will likely fill less than alveolus A under these conditions. Therefore, when regions of the lungs become pathologic (e.g., emphysema, pneumonia, and chronic bronchitis), the distribution of ventilation is adversely affected by altered local time constants.

The clinical implications of differing time constants throughout the lungs is often significant, especially in the area of mechanical ventilation. The nature of a patient's time constant can influence tidal volume, ventilatory rate, and inspiratory and expiratory time selection.

EXAMPLE:

Calculate the ventilation time constant for a patient whose airway resistance and pulmonary compliance are 3.5 cm H_2O/L/sec and 150 ml/cm H_2O, respectively.

Step 1: Convert 150 ml/cm H_2O to L/cm H_2O.

$$\frac{150 \text{ ml}}{1{,}000 \text{ ml/L}} = 0.15 \text{ L}$$

Therefore, 150 ml/cm H_2O = 0.15 L/cm H_2O.

Step 2: Calculate the ventilation time constant.

$$\text{time constant} = R_{aw} \times C_L$$

$$= (3.5 \text{ cm } H_2O/L/\text{sec})(0.15 \text{ L/cm } H_2O)$$

$$= 0.53 \text{ sec}$$

PRACTICE PROBLEMS

Refer to Appendix A (pages 610-611) for the solutions and answers to the practice problems.

Solve the following ventilation time constant problems:

62. Calculate the time constant for lungs that have an airway resistance of 4 cm $H_2O/L/\text{sec}$ and an elastance of 1.5 cm H_2O/L. _____

63. If an alveolar unit has a time constant of 0.75 second, determine the time elapsed for (a) 1 time constant, (b) 2 time constants, and (c) 3 time constants.

    (a) _____; (b) _____; (c) _____

64. Assume that a lung unit has a time constant of 0.5 second. If it achieves 98% of its volume, how many time constants have elapsed? _____

65. Consider two adjacent alveoli. Alveolus A has a R_{aw} value of 2 cm $H_2O/L/\text{sec}$ and a C_L of 0.05 L/cm H_2O; alveolus B has a R_{aw} and C_L of 4 cm $H_2O/L/\text{sec}$ and 0.125 L/cm H_2O, respectively. Calculate the time constant for each alveolus.

    alveolus A _____; alveolus B _____

66. Assume that alveoli A and B were subjected to an inspiratory time of 0.5 second. Determine (a) the number of time constants experienced by each alveolus and (b) the percent of alveolar filling occurring in each alveolus.

    alveolus A: (a) _____; (b) _____
    alveolus B: (a) _____; (b) _____

Law of LaPlace

Up to this point we have been concerned with the elastic properties of the lung parenchyma and the chest wall only. There is, however, another component of the elastic recoil of the respiratory apparatus yet to be considered. That component is the physical phenomenon known as **surface tension,** which manifests itself at the air-liquid interface in the alveoli.

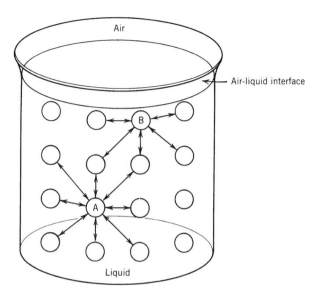

Figure 4-54 *An imbalance of intermolecular interaction at an air-liquid interface accounts for the development of surface tension. Liquid molecule A experiences equal intermolecular forces in all directions. Liquid molecule B at the surface of the liquid, however, is exposed to an imbalance of intermolecular forces because of the lack of liquid molecules above the liquid's surface. Surface tension thus develops.*

Surface tension results from an imbalance of intermolecular forces existing at any gas-liquid interface. Surface tension forces can also be regarded as cohesive forces among the liquid molecules, as is shown in Figure 4-54.

Molecule A in the diagram is experiencing equal intermolecular forces in all directions (above, below, laterally, and obliquely). Molecule B, meanwhile, as a result of being situated near the air-liquid interface, is acted upon by unequal forces. It experiences intermolecular forces laterally, downward, and obliquely, but not upward. Molecule B, therefore, has a net tendency to move downward because of the imbalance of forces acting on it. Likewise, all the molecules located at the air-liquid interface will display this same tendency. Consequently, surface tension forces tend to reduce the area of the liquid surface.

The LaPlace relationship refers to spherical structures that demonstrate the interaction between distending pressure and surface tension forces as the sphere's radius of curvature varies. This mathematical expression is shown as

$$P = \frac{2ST}{r}$$

where

P = the pressure (dynes/cm^2) within the sphere acting against the surface tension forces

ST = the surface tension forces (dynes/cm)

r = the radius (cm) of the sphere

EXAMPLE:

Calculate the pressure within a drop of mercury which has a surface tension of 465.0 dynes/cm and a diameter of 5 mm.

Step 1: Convert the diameter in mm to radius in cm.

$$\frac{\text{diameter}}{2} = \text{radius}$$

$$\frac{5 \text{ mm}}{2} = 2.5 \text{ mm}$$

$$\frac{2.5 \text{ mm}}{10 \text{ mm/cm}} = 0.25 \text{ mm}$$

Step 2: Insert the known values into the LaPlace equation.

$$P = \frac{465 \text{ dynes/cm}}{0.25 \text{ cm}}$$

$$= 1,860 \text{ dynes/cm}^2$$

The intermolecular forces within a drop of water may be depicted as shown in Figure 4-55.

Again, the intermolecular forces among the surface liquid molecules are away from the gas-liquid interface, that is, toward the center of the drop. However, the imbalance of

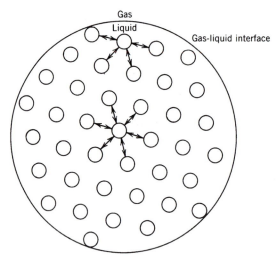

Figure 4-55 *Intermolecular forces among molecules within a drop of water. Molecules away from the surface of the drop are exposed to uniform interaction, whereas those on the drop's surface tend to be pulled inward by adjacent water molecules.*

intermolecular (attractive) forces that exists for molecules adjacent to the gas-liquid interface causes the drop to confine itself to the smallest surface area possible.

Traditionally, the lungs' 300 million alveoli are considered as tiny spheres independently expanding and contracting equally in all directions of their curvature. Based on this model of alveolar mechanics, the alveolar inflation pressure increases as the radius of alveolar curvature decreases when pulmonary surfactant is absent from the alveolar liquid lining layer. This relationship is governed by LaPlace's law. However, the presence of pulmonary surfactant, a physiologic detergent or wetting agent, reduces surface tension as alveolar radius decreases, thereby minimizing alveolar inflation pressure. Therefore, under normal physiologic conditions, when surface tension varies directly with alveolar size, the law of LaPlace does not apply to alveolar mechanics.

In the case of infant respiratory distress syndrome, which is caused by pulmonary prematurity (i.e., surfactant deficiency), the law of LaPlace does apply. When pulmonary surfactant is lacking, surface tension remains constant. Therefore, when the alveolar radius decreases, the inflation pressure rises.

Current research has presented evidence that traditional alveolar depictions, such as tiny spheres, balloons, and soap bubbles, might be incorrect. Rather than being spherical, the alveoli appear to be polyhedral. If this configuration is indeed accurate, pulmonary surfactant would not be uniformly distributed throughout each alveolus, as is presumed to be the case in a spherical alveolus. Instead, pulmonary surfactant would be disproportionately distributed throughout the gas-exchange units, perhaps accumulating in the corners and angles of the polyhedron-shaped alveoli. Nonetheless, it seems as though the proposed polyhedron-shaped alveoli would assume a more rounded or spherical configuration as inspiration proceeds, thus allowing for a more uniform distribution of pulmonary surfactant. In that case, as the alveolar radius increases, pulmonary surfactant in the alveolar lining layer is spread more thinly and surface tension forces become greater, favoring exhalation.

Regardless of alveolar morphology, the presence of pulmonary surfactant within the liquid lining layer of the alveoli alters the surface tension forces as alveolar size fluctuates during ventilation. During lung expansion alveolar size (radius) increases. However, during that time the surface tension forces also increase because the concentration of pulmonary surfactant is distributed over a larger alveolar area and becomes less effective in reducing the surface tension of the liquid lining layer. As exhalation proceeds, alveolar size (radius) diminishes and surface tension forces decrease. At this time, pulmonary surfactant is confined to a smaller area; therefore, its concentration within each alveolus increases and its effect on surface tension forces is heightened.

It is indisputable that the existence of pulmonary surfactant in the alveoli prevents alveolar collapse at low lung volumes. However, another factor known as **alveolar interdependence** also contributes to alveolar stability as alveolar volume decreases. Alveolar interdependence refers to the structural or mechanical phenomenon resulting from the fact that each alveolus relies on surrounding or adjacent alveoli for its patency. Figure 4-56 illustrates a number of polyhedral alveoli.

Note that an individual alveolus shares a number of walls with adjacent alveoli. This structural arrangement creates a mechanical interdependence among the alveoli, thus opposing any tendency for an isolated alveolus to collapse.

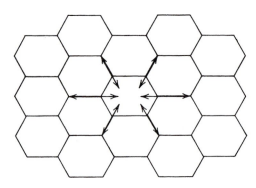

Figure 4-56 *The patency of alveoli is accomplished by alveolar interdependence, which refers to the sharing of structures common to neighboring alveoli. From Levitzky, M.: Pulmonary Physiology, 1982, McGraw-Hill Book Co. Used with permission.*

PRACTICE PROBLEMS

Refer to Appendix A (page 611) for the solutions and answers to the practice problems.

Solve the following problems using the law of LaPlace:

67. Find the surface tension in a sphere that requires an inflation pressure of 1.014×10^4 dynes/cm² and a diameter of 2 mm. _____

68. Compute the pressure needed to inflate a sphere that has a radius of 0.35 cm and a surface tension of 35 dynes/cm. _____

69. Which of the following two spheres requires the greater inflation pressure?

Sphere X	*Sphere Y*
ST = 12 dynes/cm	ST = 12 dynes/cm
r = 0.005 cm	r = 0.0025 cm

Sphere X: _____; Sphere Y: _____

If Sphere X and Sphere Y were in communication with each other, what would be the consequence?

4-8 STARLING'S LAW OF THE CAPILLARIES

Starling's law of the capillaries manifests itself in both the systemic and pulmonary capillary networks. It describes the relationship among the various pressures interacting at the capillary level and explains how fluid movement there is influenced.

This section will describe how the interaction between the hydrostatic and colloid osmotic pressures in the capillary networks helps maintain the normal dynamic equilibrium between the intravascular and interstitial spaces in terms of fluid volume. In addition to the normal physiology, the pathophysiology of peripheral and pulmonary edema, as manifested at the capillary level, will also be explored.

Hydrostatic Pressure

When a liquid occupies a container, it exerts a pressure against the walls of the container. This pressure is called the **hydrostatic pressure**. The hydrostatic pressure of any liquid depends on two factors. One is the density (mass/volume) of the liquid; the other is the height of the liquid in the container.

Blood, a liquid, is contained within the body's vasculature. All the body's blood vessels serve as the blood's container. Therefore, the blood exerts a pressure against the walls of the blood vessels. Clinically, the pressure in the vasculature is referred to as *blood pressure* and is expressed in mm Hg. However, the term that will be used here is *hydrostatic pressure*.

Osmotic Pressure

Before actually describing colloid osmotic pressure, a discussion on **osmosis** in general is in order. By definition, osmosis is the movement of a solvent (e.g., water) through a semipermeable, or a selectively permeable, membrane from a solution of lesser concentration (fewer solutes) to one of higher concentration (more solutes). A semipermeable membrane is one that is completely permeable to the solvent but completely impermeable to the solutes on either side of the membrane. A selectively permeable membrane is freely permeable to the solvent and to some of the solutes. Biological membranes, such as the capillary endothelium and cell walls, are selectively permeable membranes.

Let us first consider molecular movement (diffusion) across a membrane permeable to all species present in two solutions. If the U-shaped tube in Figure 4-57 contained a 20% NaCl solution on the left side, separated from a 40% NaCl solution on the right by a

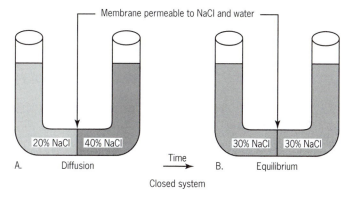

Figure 4-57 *Diffusion across a totally permeable membrane. (A) A U-shaped tube containing two NaCl solutions of differing concentrations (20% and 40%) separated by a membrane permeable to H_2O and NaCl. (B) In time, H_2O and NaCl molecules will diffuse across the membrane, and the two solutions will equilibrate (30% and 30%). Note that the volume of fluid in both limbs of the U-tube in part B is equal.*

membrane permeable to all species, water molecules, NaCl molecules, and Na$^+$ and Cl$^-$ ions would move freely through the membrane in both directions.

Initially, Na$^+$ and Cl$^-$ ions would diffuse to the left side more than to the right. Similarly, more water molecules would initially diffuse from the 20% NaCl solution to the 40% NaCl solution than would diffuse from the 40% NaCl solution to the 20% NaCl solution. As time progressed, the two compartments on both sides of the U-tube would gradually approach the same concentration. Eventually, at equilibrium, both solutions would have equal concentrations, that is, 30% NaCl. At that particular point, equal numbers of Na$^+$ and Cl$^-$ ions would diffuse in both directions. Likewise, equal numbers of water molecules would diffuse in both directions.

In this example, net diffusion of NaCl will occur down the concentration gradient, that is, from the 40% solution to the 20% solution. Simultaneously, the net diffusion of water molecules will take place down its concentration gradient. That is, more water molecules will move from the 20% solution to the 40% solution. Keep in mind that the 20% NaCl solution contains more water molecules than the 40% NaCl solution. Another important point to make here is that at equilibrium the two 30% NaCl solutions will be equal in volume since the membrane is permeable to the solvent and all the solutes.

Now, consider the U-shaped tubes in Figure 4-58. Again, at the onset the first U-tube contains a 20% NaCl solution on the left and a 40% NaCl solution on the right. However, in this instance the two solutions are separated by a semipermeable membrane. This membrane is permeable only to water molecules. Na$^+$ and Cl$^-$ ions cannot diffuse across.

At the onset, more water molecules osmose (move) from the 20% NaCl solution to the 40% NaCl solution than osmose in the reverse direction. In other words, water molecules migrate in both directions, but the net direction of osmosis is toward the 40% NaCl solution.

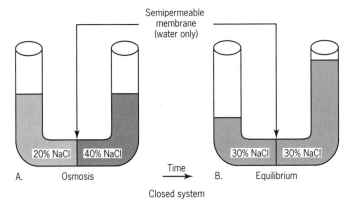

Figure 4-58 *Diffusion across a semipermeable membrane. (A) A U-shaped tube containing two NaCl solutions of differing concentrations (20% and 40%) separated by a membrane permeable only to H$_2$O. (B) In time, H$_2$O will osmose from the 20% NaCl solution to the 40% NaCl solution, causing both solutions to achieve equilibrium (30% and 30%). However, note the increased fluid volume of the 30% NaCl solution in the right limb in part B and the decreased fluid volume of the limb on the left.*

As time elapses, a number of physical events occur. First, the two solutions equilibrate. Both solutions achieve a concentration of 30%. Second, the initially more highly concentrated solution takes on a larger volume than the originally more diluted solution. Net osmosis of water occurs from the 20% NaCl solution into the 40% NaCl solution. Third, by virtue of possessing a greater volume of water at equilibrium, the solution in the right arm exerts a greater hydrostatic pressure.

What has been described in these two illustrations thus far is the distinction between diffusion and osmosis and some of the physical events associated with solutions separated by different types of membrane. *Diffusion* occurs as a result of a concentration gradient (difference) across a membrane permeable to all species present in solution (solute and solvent). *Osmosis*, on the other hand, applies only to the solvent when two solutions are separated by a semipermeable or selectively permeable membrane. Water will diffuse, not osmose, through a membrane that is permeable to water and to all the solutes in solution. Essentially, water diffuses through membranes (Figure 4-57) that are incapable of maintaining concentration gradients. Therefore, in Figure 4-58 water osmoses across the semipermeable membrane from the onset of the experiment until equilibrium is reached. When equilibrium is reached, no concentration gradient exists across the semipermeable membrane. A 30% NaCl solution exists on either side of the membrane. Hence, water diffuses, not osmoses, at an equal rate across the semipermeable membrane from that point onward.

During the time prior to equilibrium in Figure 4-58 net osmosis occurred from the 20% NaCl solution (less concentrated) to the 40% NaCl solution (more concentrated). That is to say, water osmosed down its concentration gradient. The net osmosis into the initially more concentrated solution increased that solution's volume. Consequently, the volume increased the pressure of the solution.

We are now at the point where the concept of osmotic pressure can be discussed. If in Figure 4-58 additional pressure had been exerted in the direction of the 20% NaCl solution, osmosis of water into the 40% NaCl solution would be reduced or terminated. The amount of pressure needed to completely terminate osmosis is called the *osmotic pressure* of that solution. By definition, *osmotic pressure* is the pressure that results from the net osmosis of fluid into a solution. Therefore, in Figure 4-58 the solution in the right arm of the U-tube initially has a greater osmotic pressure than the one in the left arm. The actual determinant of osmotic pressure is the quantity of solute particles per unit volume of solution. Again, in reference to Figure 4-58, the 40% NaCl solution initially contained more solutes (Na^+ and Cl^- ions) than the 20% NaCl solution. Therefore, net osmosis occurred toward the more concentrated solution. The solutes may be in the form of ions, molecules, or both. In the case of an electrolyte, the degree of dissociation or ionization will determine the amount of solute particles (ions and/or molecules) in solution.*

A quantitative presentation of the concept of osmotic pressure should prove helpful. Based on the fact that a 1 M[†] solution of any nonelectrolyte at body temperature (37°C) will

---

*Whether a molecule dissociates or ionizes is determined by its bonding characteristics. Electrovalent compounds have electrovalent (ionic) bonds; hence, they ionize. Covalent compounds possess covalent bonds; therefore, they dissociate.

[†]Recall that M (molarity) refers to the number of moles (or gram-molecular weights)/liter of solution.

exert an osmotic pressure of 19,304 torr*, the osmotic pressure of any solution can be obtained. This relationship can be shown as

$$(\text{mole/liter}) \times \frac{19{,}304 \text{ torr}}{\text{mole/liter}} = \text{nonelectrolyte osmotic pressure (torr)}$$

or

$$\text{molarity} \times \frac{19{,}304 \text{ torr}}{\text{mole/liter}} = \text{nonelectrolyte osmotic pressure (torr)}$$

Although this expression pertains to nonelectrolytes, it can be modified for application to electrolyte solutions. When the degree of dissociation or ionization is known, the expression becomes

$$(\text{mole/liter}) \times \binom{\text{number of ionic}}{\text{species per molecule}} \times \frac{19{,}304 \text{ torr}}{\text{mole/liter}} = \frac{\text{electrolyte osmotic}}{\text{pressure (torr)}}$$

For example, the potential osmotic pressure for a 0.9% NaCl solution can be calculated as follows:

Step 1: Determine the molecular weight of NaCl.

$$\begin{array}{r} 23 \text{ amu (atomic weight of Na)} \\ + \ 35 \text{ amu (atomic weight of Cl)} \\ \hline 58 \text{ amu (molecular weight of NaCl)} \end{array}$$

Step 2: Determine how the molecule either dissociates or ionizes into its component species. NaCl is an electrovalent compound** that ionizes into one Na^+ ion and one Cl^- ion. Hence, one NaCl molecule produces a total of two ions.

Step 3: Determine the molarity of a 0.9% NaCl solution.
   A. molecular weight of NaCl = 58 amu
   B. 0.9% NaCl solution contains 9.0 g of NaCl per liter
   C. 9.0 g of NaCl = 9.0 g of NaCl ÷ 58 g/mole = 0.16 mole of NaCl
   D. molarity = moles/liter
$$= \frac{0.16 \text{ mole}}{1 \text{ liter}}$$
$$= 0.16 \text{ M}$$

Step 4: Determine the osmotic pressure for a 0.9% NaCl solution using the equation

$$M \times \binom{\text{number of ionic species}}{\text{per molecule}} \times \frac{19{,}304 \text{ torr}}{\text{mole/liter}} = \frac{\text{osmotic pressure}}{\text{of an electrolyte (torr)}}$$

---

*This osmotic pressure (19,304 torr) develops when a 1 M, nonelectrolyte solution is separated from a pure H_2O solution by a membrane.

**Remember that an electrovalent (ionic) compound is held together by an electrovalent (ionic) bond wherein electrons are transferred. It, therefore, ionizes. A covalent compound is formed by the sharing of electrons and it dissociates.

$$0.16 \text{ M} \times 2 \text{ (1 molecule of NaCl yields 1 Na}^+ \text{ ion and 1 Cl}^- \text{ ion)} \times \frac{19{,}304 \text{ torr}}{\text{mole/liter}} = 6{,}177 \text{ torr}$$

Experimentation has also shown that the osmotic pressure is directly proportional to the amount of solute (ions and/or molecules) in a given amount of solution. It has been found that 1 mole of solute dissolved in 22.4 liters of solution exerts an osmotic pressure of 1 atmosphere (760 mm Hg) at 0°C. Recall that 1 mole of a gas occupying 22.4 liters at 0°C exerts a pressure of 1 atmosphere.

The unit **osmol** is used to express the concentration of solute because the osmotic pressure of a solution is directly proportional to the number of solute molecules and/or ions in 1 mole (gram-molecular weight) of solute. Molecular size and molecular weight of the species involved have no bearing on the osmotic pressure. Albumin, for example, has a molecular weight of 69,000 amu. Therefore, since albumin does not dissociate, 69,000 grams of albumin is equivalent to 1 osmol of albumin. Similarly, if a solute dissociates or ionizes into two ions, as in the case of NaCl, which ionizes into Na$^+$ and Cl$^-$ ions, 1 gram-molecular weight of solute equals 2 osmols. Hence, 1 mole of NaCl (1 gram-molecular weight of NaCl = 58 grams) is equivalent to 2 osmols, or 1 osmol = 58 g ÷ 2 = 29 grams.

Physiologically, osmolarity is expressed in terms of milliosmols per liter of solution (1 osmol = 1,000 milliosmols). Therefore, in reference to the two examples cited above, 1 milliosmol of albumin is equivalent to 69 grams (69,000 g/1000), and one milliosmol of NaCl becomes 0.029 gram (29 g/1000).

Blood contains a variety of solutes in various concentrations. A large proportion of the blood's solutes are called **crystalloids** (e.g., electrolytes and gases). These substances have complete and passive access across the capillary endothelium into the interstitium. Only a small proportion of the crystalloids contribute to the osmotic pressure that exists in the intravascular space.

Colloids comprise another type of solute present in the blood. These colloids are essentially the protein molecules albumin, globulin, and fibrinogen. These solutes are ordinarily too large to move across the capillary endothelium. In actuality, some of the lower-molecular-weight blood proteins do enter the interstitium. However, the higher-molecular-weight blood protein molecules, as a result of the relative impermeability of the capillary endothelium to them, remain in the intravascular space and are osmotically active there. They, in fact, are largely responsible for the osmotic pressure that exists in the vasculature. However, some of the crystalloids contribute to the colloid osmotic pressure because the protein molecules, which in this medium act as anions, cause a number of diffusible cations to remain in the intravascular space. (This phenomenon, the Gibbs-Donnan rule, will be discussed in more detail shortly. These cations are actually bound to the electronegative charge carried by the protein molecules in the blood.

Normal Capillary Dynamics

The physiologic model that will be developed here involves the interaction of a number of pressures influencing the exchange of intravascular and interstitial fluid across the capillary endothelium. There are four pressures acting here:

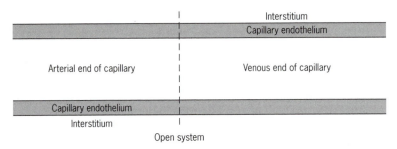

Figure 4-59 *A model of a capillary showing (1) the capillary endothelium, (2) the interstitium, (3) the arterial end of the capillary, and (4) the venous end of the capillary.*

- Capillary hydrostatic pressure
- Capillary colloid osmotic pressure
- Interstitial hydrostatic pressure
- Interstitial colloid osmotic pressure

Before launching into a discussion on capillary dynamics at this point, let us describe the physical relationship of the components that comprise this internal environment. First, the capillary endothelium serves as the selectively permeable membrane between the blood (intravascular fluid) and the interstitial fluid. Basically, this membrane keeps the RBCs, WBCs, platelets, and larger protein molecules within the intravascular space and at the same time allows for the exchange of fluid and smaller molecules in accordance with the relationship of the four pressures listed above.

Second, the capillary endothelium is divided into two segments (Figure 4-59), an arterial end and a venous end. No physical entity serves as this line of demarcation in the body's internal environment at the capillary level; however, distinct physical events take place as capillary blood is transformed from arterial blood to venous blood. For our purposes here, however, we will arbitrarily separate the capillary into these two regions.

Last, the magnitude of the hydrostatic and colloid osmotic pressures acting here determines the direction and quantity of fluid movement across the capillary endothelium.

We will first look at the two hydrostatic pressures, then the two osmotic pressures, and finally the interaction among these four.

The capillary hydrostatic pressure is that pressure exerted by the blood against the capillary endothelium; the interstitial hydrostatic pressure is that pressure exerted by the interstitial fluid against the confines of its compartment, i.e., the interstitium.

The capillary colloid osmotic pressure* arises from the fact that the capillary endothelium is relatively impermeable to the passage of protein molecules out of the vasculature. Proteins are said to remain within the intravascular space because of their large size and high molecular weight. In reality, though, small amounts of the lower-molecular-weight protein molecules filter out of circulation and enter the interstitium. It is this quantity of protein that accounts for the presence of the osmotic pressure in the interstitium.

*Another term used to refer to this pressure is *oncotic pressure*.

Interstitial fluid is often referred to as an **ultrafiltrate** of plasma. As an ultrafiltrate of plasma, interstitial fluid is said to be devoid of thrombocytes (platelets), erythrocytes (RBCs), leukocytes (WBCs), and protein. In reality, however, the interstitium is not completely devoid of protein molecules, but the concentration is low in comparison with that in the vasculature. The ionic components (crystalloids)—for example, Na^+, Cl^-, Mg^{+2}, HCO_3^-, H^+, Ca^{+2}, and K^+—of body fluid permeate freely through the capillary endothelium and contribute little to the osmotic effect at the capillary.

The fact that the intravascular protein concentration is greater than that in the interstitium accounts for a difference in concentration of the diffusible ions in the plasma and the interstitial fluid. The concentration of the diffusible ions (anions and cations) is not equal in these two fluid compartments. This ionic distribution is consistent with the Gibbs-Donnan rule.

The Gibbs-Donnan rule states that, if a nondiffusible species (e.g., protein molecules) is present on one side of a membrane permeable to all the other solutes, the diffusible solutes (anions and cations) will distribute themselves unequally across the membrane according to the following three requirements:

1. The total number of anions must equal the total number of cations on each side of the membrane.

2. On the side of the membrane containing the nondiffusible species (protein molecules), the concentration of the diffusible cations will be greater than, and the concentration of the diffusible anions will be less than, those on the side devoid of the nondiffusible species (protein molecules).

3. The side of the membrane containing the nondiffusible species (protein molecules) will have a greater osmotic pressure than the side devoid of the nondiffusible species (protein molecules).

The Gibbs-Donnan rule can be quantitatively expressed. At equilibrium the product of the concentrations of the total number of diffusible anions and the total number of diffusible cations on one side of the selectively permeable membrane equals the product of the concentrations of the total number of diffusible anions and cations on the other side. The following detailed example will serve to illustrate this concept.

$$[X^-]_1 \times [Y^+]_1 = [X^-]_2 \times [Y^+]_2$$

where

$[X^-]_1$ = total diffusable anion concentration on side one
      of the membrane

$[Y^+]_1$ = total diffusable cation concentration on side one
      of the membrane

$[X^-]_2$ = total diffusable anion concentration on side two
      of the membrane

$[Y^+]_2$ = total diffusable cation concentration on side two
      of the membrane

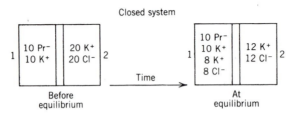

Closed system

Figure 4-60 *Two solutions with differing solute concentrations separated by a selectively permeable membrane (Pr⁻ impermeable). Before equilibrium, the product of the diffusible cations and anions in each compartment is unequal (compartment 1: 10 cations × 10 anions = 100 ions and compartment 2: 20 cations × 20 anions = 400 ions). At equilibrium, the product of the diffusible cations and anions in both compartments is equal (compartment 1: 18 cations × 8 anions = 144 ions and compartment 2: 12 cations × 12 anions = 144 ions).*

Figure 4-60 illustrates the distribution of solutes before equilibrium and at equilibrium in a closed system.

The membrane is permeable to all the species (solutes) in solution except the protein anion (Pr⁻).* At the onset, compartment 1 contains 10 protein ions and 10 K⁺ ions, and compartment 2 contains 20 K⁺ ions and 20 Cl⁻ ions.

The following quantitative relationship for the prediction of the distribution of the solutes at equilibrium is

$$X = \frac{B^2}{A + 2B}$$

where

X = the number of cations and anions lost from compartment 2 to compartment 1 over time

B = the sum of the number of cations and anions originally in compartment 2

A = the sum of the number of cations and protein molecules originally in compartment 1

Therefore,

X = unknown

B = 20 K⁺ + 20 Cl⁻ = 40 ions

A = 10 K⁺ + 10 Pr⁻ = 20 ions

*A protein molecule in a solution with a pH greater than the protein's pK will possess a net negative charge. A protein molecule in a solution with a pH less than the protein's pK will have a net positive charge. A pH at which a protein possesses no net charge is termed its *isoelectric* pH. The protein molecule is a zwitterion (no net charge) at its isoelectric pH.

Hence,

$$X = \frac{(40)^2}{20 + 2(40)}$$

$$= \frac{1600}{100}$$

$$= 16 \text{ ions}$$

Because 16 cations and anions are lost from compartment 2 to compartment 1 at equilibrium, eight cations and eight anions migrate from compartment 2 to compartment 1. Consequently, 12 cations and 12 anions reside in compartment 2 at equilibrium.

As time elapses, equilibrium is reached. At this point, compartment 1 still contains 10 Pr^- ions because the membrane is impermeable to protein. Ten K^+ ions also reside in compartment 1 to electrostatically balance the 10 Pr^- anions. In addition, eight K^+ and eight Cl^- ions diffused from compartment 2 into compartment 1. Meanwhile, compartment 2 houses 12 K^+ ions and 12 Cl^- ions.

From inspection, it can be seen that the diffusible ions are unequally distributed between the two compartments. However, if we review the three Gibbs-Donnan conditions previously addressed, we see that each condition is satisfied. For example, condition one stated that the total number of anions must equal the total number of cations on each side of the membrane. At equilibrium, both compartments are electrostatically balanced as follows:

Compartment 1	Compartment 2
10 Pr^-	
10 K^+	12 K^+
8 Cl^-	12 Cl^-
8 K^+	

The second condition stated that more diffusible cations and fewer diffusible anions migrate to the side containing the nondiffusible species. Again, at equilibrium, compartment 1 contains 18 K^+ cations and 18 anions (8 Cl^- and 10 Pr^-), whereas compartment 2 has 12 K^+ cations and 12 Cl^- anions. There are six more diffusible cations and four less diffusible anions in compartment 1 than in compartment 2.

The third condition addressed the aspect of osmotic pressure. It indicated that the side of the membrane containing the nondiffusible species would develop a greater osmotic pressure than the side devoid of the nondiffusible species. In this example, compartment 1 contains the nondiffusible species and more of the diffusible species (anions + cations). Therefore, because osmotic pressure depends on the amount of solutes/solvent, compartment 1 has a greater osmotic pressure than compartment 2. The osmotic pressure, as it is found in the vasculature, is due primarily to the impermeability of the capillary endothelium to protein molecules and less significantly to the excess of diffusible ions (cations) in that body fluid compartment.

Finally, the equilibrium state also satisfies another quantitative expression associated with the Gibbs-Donnan rule:

$$[K^+]_1 \times [Cl^-]_1 = [K^+]_2 \times [Cl^-]_2$$

$$18 \times 8 = 12 \times 12$$

$$144 = 144$$

The foregoing illustration was presented to demonstrate that the three Gibbs-Donnan requirements can be quantified, thereby exhibiting a more tangible and practical viewpoint of the concepts involved here.

Now, let us discuss the four pressures that determine the magnitude of fluid movement across the systemic capillary endothelium at the arterial end.

1. Capillary hydrostatic pressure (CHP) favors fluid movement out of the vasculature; normal range is 30 to 35 mm Hg.
2. Interstitial hydrostatic pressure (IHP) enhances fluid movement out of the vasculature due to its subatmospheric (negative) nature; approximate range is -2 to -5 mm Hg.
3. Capillary colloid osmotic pressure (COP) tends to cause the retention of vascular fluid by promoting osmosis into the intravascular space; approximate range is 25 to 35 mm Hg.
4. Interstitial colloid osmotic pressure (IOP) favors the movement (osmosis) of fluid out of the vasculature into the interstitium (IOP develops from proteins that have passed through endothelial pores); approximate range is 3 to 5 mm Hg.

Figure 4-61 illustrates how these four pressures interact and determine the net direction and magnitude of fluid movement into and out of the vasculature at the systemic capillary level.

A synopsis of the effects of these pressures on the arterial end of the capillary follows.

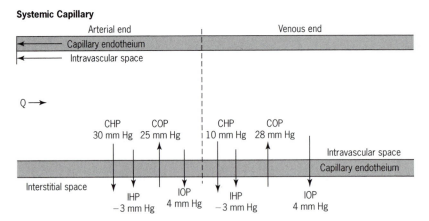

Figure 4-61 *A systemic capillary showing the different pressures (CHP = capillary hydrostatic pressure; IHP = interstitial hydrostatic pressure; COP = capillary oncotic pressure; and IOP = interstitial oncotic pressure) responsible for fluid movement into and out of the vasculature.*

1. The hydrostatic pressure gradient (CHP-IHP) causes the filtration of fluid and certain solutes out of the vasculature and into the interstitium. Because the two hydrostatic pressures involved here are acting in the same direction and augment each other they are additive. Therefore,

    (a) capillary hydrostatic pressure − interstitial hydrostatic pressure = hydrostatic pressure gradient and

    (b) 30 mm Hg CHP − (−3 mm Hg) IHP

    = 30 mm Hg CHP + 3 mm Hg IHP

    = 33 mm Hg hydrostatic pressure gradient

2. The colloid osmotic pressure gradient (COP-IOP) here favors net osmosis of fluid into the intravascular space from the interstitium. Since the two osmotic pressures are in opposition to each other, they are to be subtracted. Therefore,

    (a) capillary colloid osmotic pressure − interstitial colloid osmotic pressure = colloid osmotic pressure gradient and

    (b) 25 mm Hg COP − 4 mm IOP

    = 21 mm Hg colloid osmotic pressure gradient.

3. Subtracting the colloid osmotic pressure gradient from the hydrostatic pressure gradient provides the filtration pressure. Hence,

$$\begin{array}{r} 33 \text{ mm Hg hydrostatic pressure gradient} \\ \underline{-21 \text{ mm Hg colloid osmotic pressure gradient}} \\ 12 \text{ mm Hg filtration pressure} \end{array}$$

Analysis of the pressures interacting at the arterial end of the capillary shows, as is indicated by the filtration pressure (12 mm Hg), that there is a net movement of fluid out of the vasculature into the interstitium. The model, however, is incomplete because, as it stands now, fluid would depart from the vasculature in a relatively short time, leading to hypotension and tissue edema.

As capillary blood flow proceeds toward the venous end of the capillary, the magnitude of the interacting pressures changes. As a consequence, reabsorption occurs.

An outline of the pressures acting at the venous end of the capillary (Figure 4-61) follows.

1. As a consequence of a net loss of fluid at the arterial end of the capillary, the CHP at the venous end decreases. However, the two hydrostatic pressures exerted here continue acting in the same direction and are still additive. The IHP remains basically unchanged because of lymphatic uptake. Therefore, the hydrostatic pressure gradient at the venous end of the capillary is

$$10 \text{ mm Hg CHP} - (-3 \text{ mm Hg}) \text{ IHP}$$
$$= 10 \text{ mm Hg CHP} + 3 \text{ mm Hg IHP}$$
$$= 13 \text{ mm Hg hydrostatic pressure gradient}$$

2. Because osmotic pressure is directly proportional to the concentration of solutes in solution, and because some of the solvent transudated out of the vasculature on the

arterial end, the COP increases slightly on the venous end. The IOP remains essentially the same because the lymphatics take up the excess protein. Therefore, the colloid osmotic pressure at the venous end is

$$28 \text{ mm Hg COP} - 4 \text{ mm Hg IOP}$$

$$= 24 \text{ mm Hg colloid osmotic pressure gradient}$$

3. Subtracting the hydrostatic pressure gradient from the colloid osmotic pressure gradient provides the reabsorption pressure:

$$\begin{array}{r} 24 \text{ mm Hg colloid osmotic pressure gradient} \\ -13 \text{ mm Hg hydrostatic pressure gradient} \\ \hline 11 \text{ mm Hg reabsorption pressure} \end{array}$$

When comparing the filtration pressure at the arterial end of the capillary to the reabsorption pressure at the venous end, the implication is that all the fluid leaving the arterial end does not return to the vasculature at the venous end. This seeming incongruity can be quantitatively shown from the foregoing example. At the arterial end of the capillary the filtration pressure was 12 mm Hg, and at the venous end the reabsorption pressure was 11 mm Hg. Hence,

$$\begin{array}{r} 12 \text{ mm Hg filtration pressure} \\ -11 \text{ mm Hg reabsorption pressure} \\ \hline 1 \text{ mm Hg filtration-reabsorption pressure difference} \end{array}$$

What becomes of the fluid that fails to be reabsorbed? Does it accumulate in the interstitium? The answer to the second question is clearly no. If this fluid did accumulate, the interstitium would soon swell, thus producing an edematous state. The answer to the first question is that the lymphatic system effectively drains the fluid and certain solutes, namely the proteins, from the interstitium and returns them ultimately to the general circulation.

Keep in mind that the physiologic model just described pertains to the capillaries found in systemic circulation. The situation that exists at the capillary level in the pulmonary circulation is somewhat different. The predominant differences are the reduced magnitude of the pulmonary capillary hydrostatic pressure and the increased interstitial osmotic pressure. The mean pulmonary capillary hydrostatic pressure is about 7 mm Hg; the osmotic pressure in the pulmonary interstitium averages about 14 mm Hg.

The lower hydrostatic pressure in the pulmonary circulation results from the lower vascular resistance to blood flow in the pulmonary vasculature compared to the higher systemic vasculature resistance. Two physiologic phenomena peculiar to the pulmonary capillary bed, namely recruitment and distension, promote the low vascular pressures in this system. The term *recruitment* refers to the fact that under normal resting conditions not all pulmonary capillaries are perfused. Such a condition allows for the accommodation of increased blood flow during times of increased cardiac output. What occurs when resting right ventricular output increases is that the ordinarily nonperfused capillaries "open up" and provide additional vessels for pulmonary blood flow. In essence the

Pulmonary Capillary

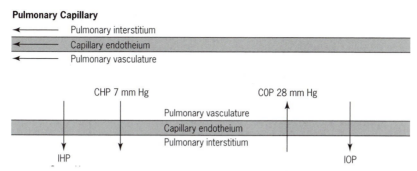

Figure 4-62 *A pulmonary capillary highlighting the different pressures (CHP = capillary hydrostatic pressure; IHP = interstitial hydrostatic pressure; COP = capillary oncotic pressure; and IOP = interstitial oncotic pressure) maintaining fluid balance across the endothelial membrane.*

total cross-sectional area of the pulmonary capillary bed increases. Therefore, the increased pulmonary perfusion can be accepted as more pulmonary capillaries open (are recruited) to permit the passage of blood. At the same time, the increased perfusion does not result in an increased pulmonary capillary hydrostatic pressure. Rather, it remains quite constant.

A further increase in right ventricular output can still be accommodated, even after most of the pulmonary capillaries have been recruited. The event that follows is called *distention*. The thin structure of the pulmonary vessels allows the capillaries here to increase their caliber; these vessels are quite distensible. This vascular distension is accomplished via passive vessel wall expansion and not through any neural vasodilatory mechanism.

The net direction and magnitude of fluid movement at the pulmonary capillary level can be determined from the pressure values shown in Figure 4-62.

The hydrostatic pressure gradient here is determined in the same manner as at the systemic capillary level.

1. Because the mean pulmonary capillary hydrostatic pressure (CHP 7 mm Hg) and the pulmonary interstitial hydrostatic pressure (IHP −8 mm Hg) both enhance the movement of fluid out of the vasculature, the two pressures are additive. Consequently, the hydrostatic pressure gradient is

$$7 \text{ mm CHP} - (-8 \text{ mm Hg}) \text{ IHP}$$
$$= 7 \text{ mm CHP} + 8 \text{ mm Hg IHP}$$
$$= 15 \text{ mm Hg hydrostatic pressure gradient}$$

2. Here the colloid osmotic pressure gradient influences the reabsorption of fluid from the pulmonary interstitium into the pulmonary capillary, as was the situation in the systemic capillary network. The two osmotic pressures oppose each other here and are subtracted. Therefore, colloid osmotic pressure gradient is

$$28 \text{ mm Hg COP} - 14 \text{ mm Hg IOP}$$
$$= 14 \text{ mm Hg colloid osmotic pressure gradient}$$

3. The filtration pressure is arrived at by obtaining the difference between the hydrostatic pressure gradient and the colloid osmotic pressure gradient. Hence

$$
\begin{array}{r}
15 \text{ mm Hg hydrostatic pressure gradient} \\
-14 \text{ mm Hg colloid osmotic pressure gradient} \\
\hline
1 \text{ mm Hg filtration pressure}
\end{array}
$$

The lymphatic system drains this transudated fluid and prevents the accumulation of this fluid in the pulmonary interstitium under normal conditions.

Fluid Dynamics of Edema

Before actually discussing pathophysiologic conditions that disrupt the normal dynamics at the systemic and pulmonary capillary networks, let us first investigate the mathematical model that explains the relationship among the factors influencing fluid movement across the capillaries. The mathematical model, known as the Starling equation, is

$$\dot{Q}_f = K_f[(P_c - P_i) - \sigma(\pi_c - \pi_i)]$$

where

$\dot{Q}_f$ = the net flow of fluid out of the capillaries

K_f = the capillary filtration coefficient (represents the permeability characteristics of the membrane to the fluid)

P_c = the capillary hydrostatic pressure

P_i = the interstitial fluid hydrostatic pressure

σ = the reflection coefficient (represents the membrane's ability to prevent the passage of protein molecules)

π_c = the capillary colloid osmotic pressure

π_i = the interstitial fluid colloid osmotic pressure

Analysis of the Starling equation reveals that the hydrostatic pressure gradient (filtration) is represented by $P_c - P_i$, and the osmotic pressure gradient (reabsorption) is indicated by $\pi_c - \pi_i$.

The filtration coefficient, symbolized as K_f, describes the permeability-surface area characteristics of the capillary endothelium in both the systemic and the pulmonary vascular systems. It is dependent on both the nature of the membrane and its surface area. Specifically, the filtration coefficient will increase in value if either the total surface area of the membrane increases or if the membrane's permeability increases. The converse, likewise, is true. Quantitatively, the greater the filtration coefficient, the faster will be the rate of fluid movement across the membrane for a given net pressure difference. For example, the Starling equation can be viewed as

$$K(\Delta P) = [(\text{filtration forces} - \text{reabsorption forces})]$$

where

K = the filtration coefficient incorporating the permeability-surface area characteristics of the membrane

ΔP = the filtration-reabsorption pressure gradient (filtration forces = $P_c - P_i$ and reabsorptive forces = $\sigma[\pi_c - \pi_i]$)

The membrane's ability to prevent the extravasation of protein is termed the *reflection coefficient* and is symbolized as σ. It ranges numerically from 0.00 to 1.00. Solutes that are completely diffusible across a membrane have a reflection coefficient of 0.00 (zero). Those that are totally impermeable are assigned a reflection coefficient of 1.00. Therefore, the greater the reflection coefficient, that is, the closer it is to 1.00, and the greater the difference in $(\pi_c - \pi_i)$, the greater will be the reabsorptive forces.

Let us examine this mathematical model from still another perspective. In previous sections within this chapter, resistance has been shown as

$$R = \frac{\Delta P*}{\dot{V}} \tag{1}$$

We are now in a position to substitute $\dot{V}$ in equation 1 with $\dot{Q}$ (net flow of fluid out of the capillaries) from the Starling equation. Consequently,

$$R = \frac{\Delta P}{\dot{Q}} \tag{2}$$

This discussion requires the introduction of a new term, **conductance**. Conductance (G) is actually the reciprocal of resistance. Thus

$$G = \frac{1}{R} \tag{3}$$

or

$$R = \frac{1}{G} \tag{4}$$

We can now substitute 1/G (the reciprocal of conductance) from equation 4 for R in equation 2. Therefore

$$\frac{1}{G} = \frac{\Delta P}{\dot{Q}} \tag{5}$$

which, after rearranging the terms and solving for $\dot{Q}$, becomes

$$\dot{Q} = G \times \Delta P \tag{6}$$

*This relationship is analogous to Ohm's law, which states $I = V/R$ where I = electric current (amperes), V = potential difference (voltage), and R = resistance (ohms).

Equation 6 quantitatively expresses that the conductance (G) times the pressure gradient (ΔP) across the membrane will determine the magnitude of the net flow of fluid out of the capillaries ($\dot{Q}$).

Investigation of the Starling equation once again reveals that K, the filtration coefficient, is analogous to G (conductance) in equation 6 and represents the permeability-surface area characteristics of the membrane. Also, the expression $[(P_c - P_i) - \sigma(\pi_c - \pi_i)]$ from the Starling model represents ΔP (filtration-reabsorption pressure gradient) from equation 6.

Unfortunately, the clinical utility of this mathematical model is restricted because the values of the factors within the Starling equation cannot be obtained with a high degree of certainty. However, the Starling equation does provide a useful approach for classifying clinical conditions that may produce edema.

When the normal dynamic equilibrium of the systemic and pulmonary capillary networks is disrupted, peripheral (interstitial) edema and pulmonary edema occur, respectively.

First, we will identify the abnormal factors that can lead to the development of peripheral or interstitial edema. Peripheral or interstitial edema can result from one or any combination of the following pathophysiologic conditions:

1. Increased systemic capillary hydrostatic pressure: Such a situation will increase the hydrostatic pressure gradient and cause an increase in the filtration pressure. More fluid than normal will move out of the peripheral vasculature, primarily in gravity-dependent regions, and can overwhelm the lymphatic system, resulting in peripheral edema. Right ventricular failure from any cause tends to elevate systemic capillary hydrostatic pressure and produces peripheral edema.

2. Decreased capillary osmotic pressure: Fewer protein molecules within the vasculature will reduce the capillary osmotic pressure (oncotic pressure). When this condition develops, both the osmotic pressure gradient and the reabsorption pressure gradient decrease. The effect then is that more fluid is allowed to move out of the vasculature. By the same token, less fluid is able to be reabsorbed. The end result, once again, is an excess of transudate in the peripheries. Hypoproteinemia, specifically
hypoalbuminemia, results in a decreased oncotic pressure.

3. Decreased lymphatic drainage: Ordinarily, the lymphatic system removes excess interstitial fluid and returns it to general circulation. Decreased lymph uptake tends to allow fluid to accumulate in the interstitium, thereby promoting an edematous condition.

4. Increased permeability of the systemic capillaries: Certain conditions can compromise the integrity of the capillary endothelium, thereby increasing the permeability of that membrane. Consequently, fluid exudes from the intravascular space into the interstitium. Circulating toxins such as snake venom or drugs such as histamine increase capillary permeability.

Now, let us consider several factors that contribute to the development of pulmonary edema.

1. Increased pulmonary capillary hydrostatic pressure: Ordinarily, pulmonary capillary hydrostatic pressure is quite low (mean value 7 mm Hg). Low pulmonary vascular hydrostatic pressures promote small amounts of fluid transudate in that area. How-

ever, during left ventricular failure or mitral valve stenosis, back pressure develops from the left ventricle to the pulmonary vasculature. When pulmonary capillary hydrostatic pressure approaches the value of the colloid osmotic pressure in the pulmonary capillary bed, fluid leaves the intravascular space and enters the pulmonary interstitium. If the filtration of fluid overwhelms the pulmonary lymphatics and fills the interstitial spaces, fluid then enters the alveoli, thus producing pulmonary edema.

2. Decreased capillary osmotic pressure: If the concentration of protein molecules in the pulmonary capillaries decreases, more fluid will leave the intravascular space and enter the pulmonary interstitium. Again, both the osmotic pressure gradient and the net reabsorption pressure gradient decrease. Hypoproteinemia has not been described as causing pulmonary edema although it would theoretically seem possible.

3. Decreased lymphatic drainage: As was the situation with the systemic circulation, a loss of lymph drainage will cause an accumulation of fluid in the interstitium. This rarely happens because pulmonary lymphatics regenerate so readily.

4. Increased permeability of the pulmonary capillaries: A variety of insults, such as noxious gases, high oxygen concentrations, and gastric fluid aspiration, can compromise the integrity of the alveolar-capillary membrane. Specifically, the pulmonary capillary endothelium becomes "leaky," that is, fluid accumulates in the pulmonary interstitium and then in the intraalveolar spaces. This "leaky" capillary syndrome essentially represents the initial manifestation of the clinical entity adult respiratory distress syndrome (ARDS).

PRACTICE PROBLEMS

Refer to Appendix A (pages 611-614) for the solutions and answers to the practice problems.

Perform the following calculations:

70. Determine the potential osmotic pressure for a 0.45% NaCl solution. _____

71. Calculate the potential osmotic pressure of a 1 liter solution containing 196 grams of H_2SO_4 (sulfuric acid). _____

72. Compound LFW is a nonelectrolyte having a molecular weight of 100 amu. What is the potential osmotic pressure of 33 grams of LFW dissolved in 1 liter of solution? _____

73. Determine the weight of 1 osmol of each of the following substances:
    a. HCl, molecular weight of 36 g/mole _____
    b. H_2SO_4, molecular weight of 98 g/mole _____
    c. $Al_2(SO_4)_3$, molecular weight of 342 g/mole _____
    d. $NaHCO_3$, molecular weight of 84 g/mole _____

74. Convert the weight of each osmol in problem 63 to its equivalent in milliosmols.

    (a) _____; (b) _____;
    (c) _____; (d) _____

75. Two solutions are separated by a semipermeable membrane that prevents the passage of X^-. The two original solutions are of the following compositions:

compartment 1, 15 X^- and 15 Na^+; compartment 2, 30 Na^+ and 30 HCO_3^- Predict the distribution of the solutes at equilibrium.

Compartment 1

$[Na^+]$ = _____

$[HCO_3^-]$ = _____

$[X^-]$ = _____

Compartment 2

$[Na^+]$ = _____

$[HCO_3^-]$ = _____

76. Verify the distribution of the diffusible solutes in problem 65 at equilibrium. _____

77. The following information is given.

Arterial end of capillary

capillary hydrostatic pressure = 36 torr

colloid osmotic pressure = 32 torr

interstitial hydrostatic pressure = 5 torr

interstitial osmotic pressure = 5 torr

Venous end of capillary

capillary hydrostatic pressure = 30 torr

colloid osmotic pressure = 32 torr

interstitial hydrostatic pressure = 5 torr

interstitial osmotic pressure = 5 torr

Determine (1) the hydrostatic pressure gradient, (2) the osmotic pressure gradient on both the arterial and venous ends of this systemic capillary, (3) the filtration pressure, and (4) the reabsorption pressure.

Arterial end

hydrostatic pressure gradient: _____

osmotic pressure gradient: _____

filtration pressure: _____

Venous end

hydrostatic pressure gradient: _____

osmotic pressure gradient: _____

reabsorption pressure: _____

78. Perform the following calculations relating to Starling's law of the capillaries.

Arterial end of capillary

capillary hydrostatic pressure = 40 torr

capillary oncotic pressure = 25 torr

interstitial hydrostatic pressure = −3 torr

interstitial oncotic pressure = 4 torr

Venous end of capillary

capillary hydrostatic pressure = 20 torr

capillary oncotic pressure = 30 torr

interstitial hydrostatic pressure = −3 torr

interstitial oncotic pressure = 4 torr

Arterial end

hydrostatic pressure gradient: _____

oncotic pressure gradient: _____

filtration pressure: _____

Venous end

hydrostatic pressure gradient: _____

oncotic pressure gradient: _____

reabsorption pressure: _____

4-9 PHYSICAL AND ELECTRICAL OXYGEN ANALYZERS

The development of oxygen toxicity is always a potential hazard when oxygen is being delivered by any of the variety of oxygen appliances available for clinical use. Therefore, monitoring the therapeutic administration of oxygen is one of the functions of the respiratory care practitioner.

Oxygen analysis can be accomplished via a number of different oxygen analyzers. This section is intended to address the principles of operation pertaining to oxygen analyzers whose function is based on the physical principles of paramagnetism and thermal conductivity (Chapter 3, Section 3-7, "Electrochemistry").

Paramagnetic Susceptibility

The reader is asked to review the discussion presented in Chapter 3, Section 3-1, "Atomic Structure," concerning the concept of electron configuration; it is this concept that accounts for the paramagnetic property of the oxygen atom and molecule.

Ordinarily, matter is described as being either magnetic or nonmagnetic. However, all matter, if exposed to extremely strong magnetic influences, is to some degree either attracted or repelled by those forces.

Electrons, negatively charged atomic particles, are believed to be responsible for the magnetic properties of matter. Two aspects of an electron's motion need to be considered in order to understand the concept of magnetism. First, electrons, positioned in their electron shells and orbitals, revolve about the atom's nucleus and impart a magnetic quality to the atom. Figure 4-63 illustrates this situation.

Considering only this aspect of an electron's motion, if a magnetic force comes into contact with an atom, the magnetic force opposes the revolution of the electrons about the nucleus of the atom. In effect, the atoms are repelled by the magnetic force. This phenomenon is termed **diamagnetism**.

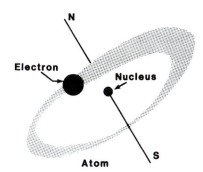

Figure 4-63   *An electron situated in an electron shell rotating about the nucleus of an atom.*

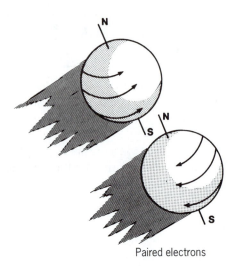

Paired electrons

Figure 4-64 *A pair of electrons spinning in the outermost electron shell of an atom. The paired electrons are spinning in opposite directions of each other; consequently, the atom is diamagnetic.*

The second aspect of an electron's motion to be taken into account here is its rotation or spin about its axis. Each electron, as it rotates on its axis, is actually a permanent magnet. Atoms that have paired electrons in their outermost electron shell exhibit only diamagnetism because paired electrons spin in opposite directions and negate each other's magnetic influence. This situation is shown in Figure 4-64.

The magnetic qualities of these two oppositely spinning electrons cancel. Each individual electron remains a permanent magnet, but the net magnetic characteristics of the atom are lessened. Such atoms display diamagnetism.

On the other hand, atoms such as oxygen, which possess unpaired electrons in their outermost shell, display the property of **paramagnetism**. Figure 4-65 illustrates such an example. The magnetic character of this unpaired electron is unopposed. Therefore, it imparts a net magnetic quality to the atom.

In the case of oxygen, for example, the lone, unpaired electrons in the p_y and p_z orbitals spin about their own axes unopposed. Because neither of these two electrons encounters opposition to its respective spin, the oxygen atom is paramagnetic. As a consequence of this property, oxygen is drawn into, distorts, and actually intensifies a magnetic field.

Figure 4-66 depicts some of the internal structures within the Beckman D-2 oxygen analyzer, which utilizes oxygen's paramagnetic property for measuring the partial pressure and concentration of oxygen in a gas sample.

A hollow glass dumbbell encasing diamagnetic nitrogen gas is suspended by a quartz fiber to which a **torque** has been applied. Each sphere of the dumbbell is positioned within

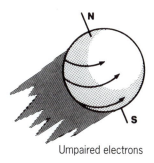

N

S

Umpaired electrons

Figure 4-65 *An unpaired electron spinning in the outermost electron shell of an atom. The magnetic character of this lone electron is unopposed; hence, it imparts a magnetic quality to the atom. An oxygen atom has two such electrons; therefore, oxygen displays paramagnetism.*

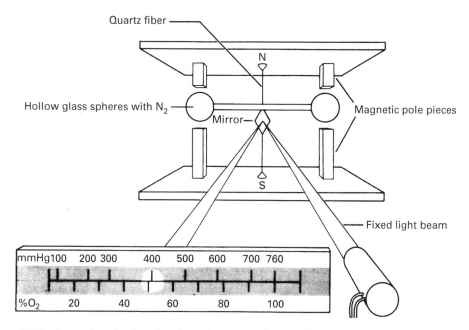

Quartz fiber

N

Hollow glass spheres with N_2

Mirror

Magnetic pole pieces

S

Fixed light beam

mmHg100	200 300	400	500	600	700 760

%O_2	20	40	60	80	100

Figure 4-66 *Internal mechanism of an O_2 analyzer operating according to the paramagnetic principle. From Heironimus, Terring, and Bagaent, Robert:* Mechanical Artificial Ventilation, *3rd ed., 1977. Courtesy of Charles B. Thomas, Publisher, Springfield, IL.*

a magnetic field created by the north and south poles of the permanent magnets. Before reaching the sample chamber, the sample gas is dehumidified by a desiccant located immediately outside the sample chamber.

Once inside the sample chamber, any oxygen in the sample gas distorts the magnetic field, causing the glass dumbbell to rotate a few degrees. As the glass dumbbell rotates, a tiny mirror attached to the quartz fiber reflects a light beam focused on it from the light source inside the analyzer. The light beam reflected from the mirror affixed to the twisted quartz fiber travels to and illuminates a scale calibrated according to *mm Hg* and $\%O_2$.

In essence, as the number of oxygen molecules within the sample chamber increases, the extent of the quartz fiber and mirror rotation increases, causing the light beam to register a larger oxygen partial pressure and oxygen concentration on the scale.

Thermal Conductivity

Certain oxygen analyzers use the physical property of thermal conductivity to measure oxygen concentrations in gas samples. This physical property refers to the ability of a gas to conduct heat. The movement of electrons (electricity or electric current) through a wire causes the wire's temperature and resistance to increase. By virtue of its ability to conduct and dissipate heat, oxygen molecules in the gas sampling chamber reduce the temperature of the conducting wire, thereby allowing more current to flow through the wire (since a direct proportion exists between the temperature of the wire and the resistance through it).

The type of oxygen analyzer to be discussed here is electric and incorporates a Wheatstone bridge, an electronic device used for precise resistance measurements. Figure 4-67 schematically illustrates a Wheatstone bridge.

A Wheatstone bridge consists of a network of four resistors, R_1, R_2, R_3, and R_4. A galvanometer bridges the two parallel electrical circuits ABC and ADC. The galvanometer is used to sense a voltage difference between these two circuits.

Current I is initiated by the battery and travels to point A, where it encounters R_1 and R_4. Assuming that $R_1 + R_2 = R_4 + R_3$, currents I_1 and I_2 will be equal. Furthermore, if

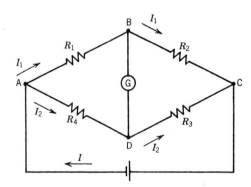

Figure 4-67 *A schematic illustration of a Wheatstone bridge. (R = resistance; I = current; and G = galvanometer.)*

$I_1 = I_2$, no potential difference (voltage) will exist between circuits ABC and ADC, and the galvanometer will indicate zero current between B and D.

With a Wheatstone bridge, if three of the four resistances are known, the fourth can be quickly calculated. For example, because voltage AB equals voltage AD and because voltage BC equals voltage DC the current flowing through circuit ABC equals that moving across ADC. Therefore, from Ohm's law, which states that

$$V = IR \qquad (1)$$

where

V = the potential difference; voltage (volts)

I = the current flowing through the circuit (amperes)

R = the resistance encountered by the current (ohms)

it can be mathematically stated that

$$I_1R_1 = I_2R_4 \qquad (2)$$

and

$$I_1R_2 = I_2R_3 \qquad (3)$$

Dividing equation 2 by equation 3 renders

$$\frac{I_1R_1}{I_1R_2} = \frac{I_2R_4}{I_2R_3} \qquad (4)$$

or

$$\frac{R_1}{R_2} = \frac{R_4}{R_3} \qquad (5)$$

Because equation 5 represents a proportion, any one of the four resistances can be obtained when the remaining three are known.

Figure 4-68 illustrates a skeletal version of an oxygen analyzer that utilizes the principle of thermal conductivity and incorporates a Wheatstone bridge.

The operation of this oxygen analyzer is based on equation 5. When room air is allowed to enter the gas sample chamber (R_4) and the gas cell (R_2), current I will be equal through circuits ABC and ADC. An oxygen reading of 20.93% will be indicated by the galvanometer in this instance, that is, no potential difference between B and D. However, when more oxygen molecules enter the gas sample chamber, the temperature of the resistor wire (R_4) will be reduced and more current will flow through circuit ADC than through ABC. Consequently, a potential difference (voltage) exists across the galvanometer (between B and D) causing the pointer to register an oxygen percentage greater than 20.93% (room air). During oxygen analysis equation 5 becomes

$$R_4 = R_3\left(\frac{R_1}{R_2}\right) \qquad (6)$$

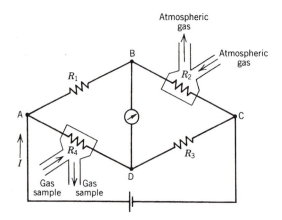

Figure 4-68 *A schematic representation of a Wheatstone bridge found in an O_2 analyzer operating on the principle of thermal conductivity. (R = resistance; I = current.)*

CHAPTER SUMMARY

Work is defined as the product of a force exerted on an object and the distance that object moves in the direction of the applied force. If the force applied to an object does not result in the object's moving in the direction of the force, no work is done. This fact is quantitatively borne out by the formula for work ($W = F \times d$). When the object is not moved by the applied force ($d = 0$), the force will be multiplied by zero.

Power is a rate. Power quantifies the rate at which work is done. The units horsepower, foot-pounds, and watts are used to describe power.

Energy and work are closely related. Energy is the ability of an object to do work. The greater energy an object has, the greater ability the object has to do work. Kinetic and potential energy are forms of mechanical energy. The formulas that define these two forms of energy are derived from the formula that incorporates work.

The kinetic theory of matter states that all forms of matter contain molecules that are in constant motion. The degree of motion is temperature dependent. The temperature affects the state in which matter resides. For example, when water is subjected to a temperature of 32°F (0°C or 273 K) or below, it freezes. Its molecules are still in motion but are only oscillating because intermolecular forces (van der Waals forces) restrict their movement. When the temperature of the ice is raised above 32°F, the intermolecular forces decrease and the molecules move more freely. Finally, as the temperature reaches or exceeds 212°F (100°C or 373 K), the liquid water becomes a gas. Intermolecular attractions are essentially negligible and the molecules are confined only by the walls of their container.

All gases exert a pressure. Pressure is defined as force per unit area. The constant motion of the gas molecules produces the force. The area to which that force is applied is divided into the force to obtain the pressure. Atmospheric pressure results from the force per unit area applied by the constituent gases of the atmosphere. Different units are used to express pressure. They are interconvertible.

Gas behavior can be predicted and explained by certain gas laws based on the relationship among (1) temperature, (2) volume, (3) pressure, and (4) mass. Ideal gas laws are used to characterize gas behavior. The ideal gas laws ignore the van der Waals forces. Therefore, actual gas behavior deviates from predictions based on these gas laws when the pressures are high and the temperatures low.

A number of physiologic and clinical applications are attributed to the ideal gas laws. Boyle's law is the basis for body plethysmography. Charles' law provides the ability to convert ATPS to BTPS conditions. Conversions to STPD and ATPD conditions can also be made using Charles' law. Gay-Lussac's law represents the relationship between gas temperature and volume which applies to a compressed gas cylinder. Avogadro's law compares temperature, pressure, and volume conditions of various molecules. The ideal gas law is a combination of Boyle's, Charles', and Avogadro's laws.

Understanding gas flow through conducting systems is critical in respiratory care. The law of continuity provides the foundation for the Bernoulli principle, which, in turn, helps in understanding the Venturi principle.

Laminar, turbulent, and tracheobronchial flow patterns develop at different points in the tracheobronchial tree. When airway obstruction is present, these gas flows are altered. Frequently, turbulent gas predominates. Turbulent gas flow imparts greater resistance to airflow than laminar flow. Consequently, pressure gradients alter as does the patient's spontaneous breathing patterns.

A significant problem associated with mechanical ventilation is the hemodynamic impact the positive pressure has on the cardiovascular physiology. Positive pressure mechanical ventilation can cause barotrauma and cardiovascular compromise to a patient. Bulk gas flow is a major contributor to some of these adverse effects. Therefore, in some cases positive pressure high frequency ventilation helps reduce the mean intrathoracic pressure and alleviates many of the pulmonary and cardiovascular problems associated with conventional positive pressure ventilation.

The lung is comprised of series and parallel resistances to airflow. Depending on the extent and location of airway obstruction (small or large airways), these resistances to gas flow alter the total airway resistance.

Poiseuille's law of laminar flow describes the relationship among the airway caliber (radius), airway resistance, and a constant depicting a variety of factors. When all the factors in Poiseuille's law are constant except radius and airway resistance, a 16-fold change occurs to the airway resistance when the airway caliber (radius) changes by a factor of one half. Airway length and resistance are inversely related.

Reynold's number summarizes the influence gas flow factors have on laminar and turbulent flow. When Reynold's number exceeds 2,000, laminar flow conditions predominate. A Reynold's number greater than 2,000 indicates the likelihood of turbulent flow. Reynold's number is a dimensionless value.

Hooke's law applies to elastic materials. It relates the force applied to an object and the degree of stretch or distortion experienced by the object. The lung is comprised of elastin which accounts for the organ's stretch and recoil capabilities. Two lung qualities, namely, compliance and elastance, influence lung filling and emptying. Compliance describes the relationship between transpulmonary pressure change and the corresponding lung volume change. Elastance is the reciprocal of compliance. The lung displays different pressure change and volume change values for inspiration and exhalation. This phenomenon is known as hysteresis.

Lung emptying and filling are dependent on the lung's compliance and airway resistance characteristics. The ventilation time constant is the product of compliance and airway resistance. When the lungs become more stiff and the airway resistance remains constant, the ventilation time constant decreases. When the airway resistance increases and the compliance remains constant, the ventilation time constant increases.

Surface tension develops at the air-liquid interface in the alveoli. Pulmonary surfactant reduces the surface tension necessitating less pressure to inflate the alveoli during each inspiration. In certain pathologic conditions, such as with ARDS, pulmonary surfactant becomes inactivated requiring high pressures to inflate the lungs. The result is a tremendous increase in the work of breathing.

The law of La Place does not apply to the lungs when normal physiologic conditions prevail because pulmonary surfactant causes the surface tension to change throughout the ventilatory cycle. However, in the case of infant respiratory distress syndrome, when the surface tension forces remain constant because of surfactant deficiency, the law of La Place applies. Pulmonary surfactant and alveolar interdependence contribute to alveolar stability as alveolar volume changes.

Starling's law of the capillaries quantitatively describes the interaction among the capillary and interstitial hydrostatic pressures and osmotic pressures, which determine fluid movement across the capillary endothelium. The magnitude of the values for these pressures differs at the systemic and pulmonary capillary levels. When the pressure values favor excess fluid movement from the vasculature and/or decreased fluid removal by the lymphatics, or reabsorption of fluid by the venous end of the capillary, edema occurs.

Oxygen's property of paramagnetism is used as the basis for the operation of the paramagnetic O_2 analyzer. The unpaired valence electrons spinning in the outer shell of an oxygen atom account for the molecules' attraction for a magnetic field.

Oxygen also has the ability to conduct heat. The presence of oxygen in an electrical circuit decreases the circuit temperature, allowing for more current to flow at that point. The property of thermal conductivity is incorporated in certain oxygen analyzers.

REVIEW QUESTIONS

4-1 WORK

Questions

1. Define *work*.
2. Express the formula for calculating work.
3. What are the necessary conditions for work to be done?
4. Describe the components of a force that is exerted at an angle to the motion.
5. Write the formula used for calculating work done against the force of gravity.
6. List the different units used to express work.
7. Define *power*.

8. Write the formula used for calculating power.
9. What units are used to express power?
10. Define (a) a watt and (b) a kilowatt.
11. Discuss the relationship between work and time.

4–2 ENERGY

Questions

1. Define *energy*.
2. List the two forms of mechanical energy.
3. List the different units used to express kinetic energy.
4. Write Newton's second law of motion.
5. Define the following terms: (a) *mass*, (b) *acceleration*, (c) *velocity*, and (d) *force*.
6. Derive the formula for kinetic energy.
7. Differentiate between weight and mass.
8. Define *potential energy*.
9. Write the formula used to calculate the potential energy.
10. Derive the formula for potential energy.
11. Define *density*.
12. Explain how density (D) can be incorporated in the formulas for kinetic and potential energy.

4-3 KINETIC THEORY OF MATTER

Questions

1. Describe the kinetic theory of matter.
2. Describe the phenomenon known as Brownian motion.
3. Compare the velocities of the constituent molecules of a solid, liquid, and gas.
4. What are the van der Waals forces and how are they influenced by temperature?
5. Discuss the effect of temperature on the three states of matter.
6. State why ideal gas behavior deviates from real gas behavior.

4-4 PRESSURE

Questions

1. Define *pressure*.
2. Write the formula used to calculate pressure.
3. Explain why it is necessary to use an evacuated tube with one closed end when measuring atmospheric pressure using a liquid in an open reservoir.
4. Why does the height of the liquid remain at the liquid reservoir level when open-ended tubes are immersed in an open reservoir?

5. Write the formula used for calculating the pressure acting on the surface of a liquid in an open reservoir.
6. By employing dimensional analysis, show how multiplying the height of a liquid column by the liquid's density renders the pressure exerted by that liquid.
7. List the equivalent of one atmosphere for the following pressure units: (a) kPa, (b) dynes/cm^2, (c) cm H_2O, and (d) psi.

4-5 GAS LAWS

Questions

1. State the relationship between the variables in Boyle's law.
2. According to Boyle's law, how is the volume affected if the pressure doubles?
3. What factor is constant in Boyle's law?
4. Explain how Boyle's law relates to spontaneous breathing against a closed glottis.
5. Describe how the body plethysmograph applies to Boyle's law.
6. What type of curve results when data from Boyle's law are plotted on a graph?
7. State Charles' law.
8. Describe how the variables relate to each other in Charles' law.
9. What temperature scale must be used when performing Charles' law calculations?
10. When data related to Charles' law are plotted on a graph, what type of curve results?
11. When plotting Charles' law data on a graph relating to the Kelvin temperature scale, at what point does the curve cross the x-axis?
12. How are the variables in Gay-Lussac's law related?
13. Provide a clinical example of Gay-Lussac's law.
14. Write the formula for the combined gas law.
15. What gas laws comprise the combined gas law?
16. What is the utility of the combined gas law?
17. What factor is the constant in the combined gas law equation?
18. What do the following acronyms signify: (1) ATPS, (2) BTPS, and (3) STPD?
19. What mathematical procedure needs to be performed before using the combined gas law when the gases in question are saturated with water vapor?
20. State Dalton's law of partial pressure.
21. When air is moisturized, why must water vapor pressure (P_{H_2O}) be subtracted from the total barometric pressure before the fractional concentration of a gas within the mixture can be calculated?
22. Explain why the individual partial pressures of the constituent gases of inhaled air change as the gas travels from the atmosphere to the trachea and from the trachea to the alveoli.
23. Write the alveolar air equation.
24. In the alveolar air equation, what is the value of $\left(F_{IO_2} + \dfrac{1 - F_{IO_2}}{R}\right)$ when the F_{IO_2} is 1.0?
25. State Avogadro's law.
26. What volume will 1 mole of an ideal gas occupy when it is exposed to standard temperature and pressure?

27. How many molecules of a gas are present in 1 mole at STP?
28. Write the equation for Avogadro's law.
29. Write the ideal gas equation.
30. The ideal gas equation is based on which gas laws?

4-6 FLUID DYNAMICS

Questions

1. Differentiate between the terms *velocity* and *flow*.
2. Upon what physical law is the law of continuity based?
3. For a constant flow system, what happens to the velocity of the flowing fluid when it encounters (a) a decrease in the total cross-sectional area and (b) an increase in the total cross-sectional area?
4. What is the product of the cross-sectional area and the velocity?
5. Describe what happens to the diameter and length of each airway generation proceeding in the direction from the trachea to the alveoli.
6. Distinguish between irregular and regular dichotomous airway branching.
7. What is the approximate total cross-sectional area of the alveoli?
8. Describe the activity at the alveolar level of the gas molecules of an inspired volume.
9. Write the continuity equation as it applies to the entire tracheobronchial tree.
10. Explain why the velocity of blood flow in the pulmonary capillaries decreases as the blood leaves the pulmonary arteries.
11. Explain why the surface area per volume of blood increases at the pulmonary capillary level.
12. Describe the Bernoulli principle.
13. Upon what physical law is the Bernoulli principle based?
14. Quantitatively, express the Bernoulli principle.
15. Why can the expression for potential energy per unit volume be eliminated from the Bernoulli equation as it applies to air flowing through the tracheobronchial tree?
16. Discuss the relationship between lateral wall pressure and fluid velocity as described by Bernoulli.
17. Relate the interaction between lateral wall pressure and fluid velocity to a flowing fluid encountering a partial obstruction.
18. What is the consequence of increasing the flow rate of a gas that encounters a partial obstruction in a conduction system?
19. Name the two gradients produced by a flowing fluid as it encounters a partial obstruction.
20. Draw and label a diagram of a conducting system depicting the Bernoulli principle.
21. What happens to the lateral wall pressure gradient when the density of the gas flowing across a partial obstruction is increased?
22. Describe what happens to the velocity squared gradient $(v_2^2 - v_1^2)$ when a less dense gas passes across a partially obstructed airway.
23. What is the rationale for helium-oxygen therapy in patients with airway obstruction?

24. What are the architectural requirements for a Venturi tube?
25. How do air entrainment devices differ from a true Venturi tube?
26. For a continuously flowing fluid, what is the relationship among the following three factors: (a) the delivered gas flow rate, (b) the source gas flow rate, and (c) the entrained gas flow rate?
27. Draw and label an air entrainment system.
28. List the two flow components that comprise an air:O_2 ratio.
29. List the air:O_2 ratios for an FIO_2 of (a) 0.60, (b) 0.40, and (c) 0.24.
30. List the three types of flow patterns that are said to exist as air travels through the tracheobronchial tree.
31. Describe the characteristics of laminar flow.
32. Define *viscosity*.
33. Define *critical velocity*.
34. Describe the velocity profile associated with laminar flow.
35. Quantitatively, express the pressure gradient needed to produce laminar flow.
36. Describe the characteristics of turbulent flow.
37. Describe the velocity profile associated with turbulent flow.
38. Write the expression showing the pressure gradient required to produce turbulent flow.
39. What is the difference in airway resistance between laminar and turbulent flow?
40. Show the relationship that describes the transairway pressure gradient needed to produce tracheobronchial flow.
41. What form of gas transport predominates in the airways from generations 16 through 23, inclusively, during spontaneous and conventional mechanical ventilation?
42. Describe the influence cardiac oscillations purportedly have on gas diffusion in lung regions so affected.
43. Define *impedance*.
44. What factor opposes air movement at the lungs' resonant frequency?
45. List the five different modes of gas transport identified by H. K. Chang.
46. What is meant by an asymmetric axial velocity profile?
47. Define *Pendelluft*.
48. What is another term that refers to Taylor-type dispersion?
49. How does CO_2 removal associated with HFV compare with that produced by conventional mechanical ventilation?
50. Define *conventional ventilation*.
51. Explain the difference between bulk flow and molecular diffusion.
52. Regarding conventional ventilation, bulk flow and molecular diffusion are said to occur in which lung regions or airway generations?
53. Why does the formula $V_A = V_T - V_D$ not apply to high-frequency ventilation?
54. Differentiate between augmented diffusion and molecular diffusion.
55. Explain the difference between conventional and high-frequency ventilation in terms of gas movement mechanisms.
56. Describe the three components of the total resistance to ventilation.
57. Under what conditions should elastic resistance to ventilation be measured?
58. What two measurements reflect the elastic resistance to ventilation?

59. Under what conditions should airway resistance to ventilation be measured?
60. What is the essential prerequisite for a fluid to flow?
61. What are the components of airway resistance?
62. How does airway resistance differ across the tracheobronchial tree?
63. Why is early small airway disease often difficult to detect?
64. Explain the difference between determining the total resistance in a series circuit and in a parallel circuit.
65. List the CGS, MKS, and SI units for viscosity.
66. Differentiate between the viscosity of liquids and that of gases as changes in temperature occur.
67. What are the conditions that are required for the application of Poiseuille's law?
68. Distinguish between Newtonian and non-Newtonian fluids.
69. Write Poiseuille's law and describe each of the factors comprising it.
70. Which factors in Poiseuille's law can be considered fluid resistance factors?
71. Rewrite Poiseuille's law and show how it can be used to illustrate the relationship among ΔP, $\dot{V}$, and r^4.
72. If all other factors in Poiseuille's law remained constant except radius and airway resistance, what would be the effect on the airway resistance if the radius (a) doubled and (b) decreased by half?
73. Write the Reynold's equation.
74. What influence will changes in (a) the numerator and (b) the denominator have on the Reynold's number?
75. Based on Reynold's equation, what Reynold's number corresponds with (a) laminar flow and (b) turbulent flow?

4-7 MECHANICS OF VENTILATION

Questions

1. Explain Hooke's law and how it applies to a spring-weight system.
2. What happens to a spring if it stretches beyond its elastic limit?
3. Describe the lung-thorax relationship at various lung volumes and how it applies to Hooke's law.
4. Define compliance and its reciprocal.
5. State the three types of compliance that apply to the respiratory system.
6. Explain how total and lung compliance can be measured.
7. Express the compliance equation in terms of chest wall (thorax) compliance.
8. Describe hysteresis and how it applies to the normal lung compliance curve.
9. Discuss the pressure-volume relationship at the (a) steep portion of the compliance curve and (b) at the flat portion of the curve.
10. Why is a single compliance measurement derived from a compliance curve unreliable?
11. What is the usefulness of specific compliance measurements?
12. Explain the compliance and elastance changes during a restrictive and an obstructive process.

13. Describe how the ventilation time constant relates to volume and pressure changes in the lungs.
14. Write the equation used for calculating the ventilation time constant.
15. What does the ventilation time constant value mean?
16. Explain what happens to the pressure gradient ($P_{mouth} - P_{alveoli}$) throughout the inspiratory cycle.
17. Discuss what happens to the inspiratory flow rate throughout the inspiratory cycle.
18. Describe the curve that would be generated if the flow rate throughout inspiration were plotted on a graph.
19. Describe the curve that would be generated if the alveolar pressure or volume throughout inspiration were plotted on a graph.
20. What percentage of the original flow rate would be delivered at (a) 1 time constant, (b) 2 time constants, (c) 3 time constants, (d) 4 time constants, and (e) 5 time constants?
21. What percentage of the alveolar pressure or volume will be present in the lungs at (a) 1 time constant, (b) 2 time constants, (c) 3 time constants, (d) 4 time constants, and (e) 5 time constants?
22. How is the ventilation time constant affected by (a) increased R_{aw}, (b) decreased R_{aw}, (c) increased C_L, and (d) decreased C_L?
23. If a ventilation time constant has a value of 1.5 sec, how many time constants will elapse if the inspiratory time is 2 sec?
24. Generally, how many time constants constitute (a) lung filling and (b) lung emptying?
25. Define *surface tension*.
26. Describe the LaPlace relationship as it refers to a drop of water.
27. Explain how the surface tension in the alveoli changes throughout the ventilatory cycle.
28. How does the law of LaPlace apply (a) to normal lung physiology and (b) to infants born with pulmonary immaturity?
29. Discuss how the presence of pulmonary surfactant alters the LaPlace relationship.
30. Define *alveolar interdependence*.

4-8 STARLING'S LAW OF THE CAPILLARIES

Questions

1. Define the following terms: (a) *hydrostatic pressure*, (b) *osmosis*, (c) *semipermeable membrane*, and (d) *diffusion*.
2. Describe the events that would occur if a totally permeable membrane separated two compartments of which one contained a 25% KCl solution and the other housed a 15% KCl solution.
3. What would occur in time if the membrane in question 2 were semipermeable (permeable only to the water molecules)?
4. Define *osmotic pressure*.
5. A 1 M solution of a nonelectrolyte at 37°C exerts what osmotic pressure?
6. Express the relationship that provides for the calculation of the osmotic pressure of (a) a nonelectrolyte solution and (b) an electrolyte solution.

7. One mole of solute dissolved in 22.4 liters of solution will exert what osmotic pressure at 0°C?
8. What is (a) an osmol and (b) a milliosmol?
9. Differentiate between colloids and crystalloids.
10. List the four pressures that interact and influence the amount of fluid that is exchanged at the capillary level.
11. Explain the events that take place at both the arterial and venous ends of a capillary.
12. What is a synonymous expression for *osmotic pressure*?
13. Describe the Gibbs-Donnan rule.
14. Quantitatively, explain the relationship between the diffusible anions and cations as applied to the Gibbs-Donnan equilibrium.
15. Write the formula that allows for the prediction of the distribution of diffusible anions and cations at Gibbs-Donnan equilibrium.
16. What is the significance of the net filtration pressure and the net reabsorption pressure at the capillary level?
17. Explain the role of the lymph system as it pertains to fluid exchange at the capillary level.
18. Describe the pressure differences at the systemic and pulmonary capillary levels.
19. Write the Starling equation and explain each factor comprising it.
20. What is the significance of the filtration coefficient (K_f) and the reflection coefficient (σ)?
21. Explain how the conductance multiplied by the pressure gradient determines the magnitude of fluid movement out of the capillaries.
22. List and describe various pathophysiologic factors that can result in either interstitial or pulmonary edema.

4-9 PHYSICAL AND ELECTRICAL OXYGEN ANALYZERS

Questions

1. Explain how the motion of an electron is said to account for the magnetic qualities of an atom.
2. Compare the properties *diamagnetism* and *paramagnetism*.
3. Explain the theory that supports the presence of the oxygen atom's paramagnetic property.
4. Describe the interaction between a magnetic field and an oxygen atom.
5. Discuss the physical property of thermal conductivity.
6. Discuss the operation of a Wheatstone bridge incorporated within an oxygen analyzer.
7. Derive the formula that allows for the calculation of an unknown resistance in a Wheatstone bridge.
8. Using an oxygen analyzer as an example, present (a) one explanation whereby no potential difference exists across a galvanometer of a Wheatstone bridge and (b) another situation wherin a potential difference does exist.

Bibliography

Adriani, J. *The Chemistry and Physics of Anesthesia*, 2nd ed. Springfield, IL: Charles C. Thomas, Publishers, 1962.

Briscoe, W.A., Forster, R.E., and Comroe, J.H. Jr. "Alveolar Ventilation at Very Low Tidal Volumes." *Journal of Applied Physiology*, 1954, 7.

Burrows, B., et al. *Respiratory Disorders: A Pathophysiologic Approach*, 2nd ed. Chicago: Year Book Medical Publishers, Inc., 1983.

Burton, G. *Respiratory Care: A Guide to Clinical Practice*, 3rd ed. Philadelphia: J.B. Lippincott Company, 1994.

Cavanagh, K. "High Frequency Ventilation of Infants: An Analysis of the Literature." *Respiratory Care*, 1990, 35:815–830.

Chang, H.K. "Mechanisms of Gas Transport during Ventilation by High-Frequency Oscillation." *Journal of Applied Physiology*, 1984, 56:553–563.

Dantzker, D., et al. *Comprehensive Respiratory Care*. Philadelphia: W.B. Saunders Company, 1995.

Fredberg, J.J. "Augmented Diffusion in the Airways Can Support Pulmonary Gas Exchange." *Journal of the American Physiological Society*, 1980.

Guenter, C., and Welch, M. *Pulmonary Medicine*. Philadelphia: J.B. Lippincott Company, 1977.

Guyton, A. *Basic Human Physiology: Normal Function and Mechanisms of Disease*, 2nd ed. Philadelphia: W.B. Saunders Company, 1977.

Heironimus, T., III, and Bageant, R. *Mechanical Artificial Ventilation: A Manual For Students and Practitioners*. Springfield, IL: Charles C. Thomas, Publishers, 1977.

Henry, J., and Meehan, J. *The Circulation: An Integrative Physiologic Study*. Chicago: Year Book Medical Publishers, Inc., 1971.

Kacmarek, R., et al. *The Essentials of Respiratory Therapy*, 4th ed. St. Louis: Mosby-Year Book, Inc., 1995.

Murray, J. *The Normal Lung*. Philadelphia: W.B. Saunders, 1976.

Netter, F. "Respiratory Systems." *The CIBA Collection of Medical Illustrations*, Vol. 7. Summit, NJ: CIBA Medical Education Division, 1980.

Niemans, G.F. "Mechanism of Lung Expansion: A Review." *Respiratory Care*, 1983, 28(4).

Pitts, R. *Physiology of the Kidney and Body Fluids*, 3rd ed. Chicago: Year Book Medical Publishers, Inc., 1974.

Richardson, D. *Basic Circulatory Physiology*. Boston: Little, Brown and Company, 1976.

Ruppel, G. *Manual of Pulmonary Function Testing*, 7th ed. St. Louis: Mosby-Year Book, Inc., 1998.

Scherer, P.W., Shendalman, L.H., Greene, N.M., et al. "Measurement of Axial Diffusivities in a Model of the Bronchial Airways." *Journal of Applied Physiology*, 1975, 38.

Slutsky, A.S., Brown, R., Lehr, J., et al. "High Frequency Ventilation: A Promising New Approach to Mechanical Ventilation." *Medical Instrumentation*, 1981, 15(4).

Slutsky, A.S., Drazen, J.M., Ingram, R.H. Jr., et al. "Effective Pulmonary Ventilation with Small-Tidal Volume Oscillations at High Frequency." *Science*, 1980, 209.

Smith, J., and Kampine, J. *Circulatory Physiology—The Essentials*. Baltimore: The Williams and Wilkins Company, 1980.

Scanlan, C. *Egan's Fundamentals of Respiratory Care*, 7th ed. St. Louis: Mosby-Year Book, Inc., 1999.

Tisi, G. *Pulmonary Physiology in Clinical Medicine*. Baltimore: The Williams and Wilkins Company, 1980.

West, J. *Pulmonary Pathophysiology—The Essentials*, 2nd ed. Baltimore: The Williams and Wilkins Company, 2000.

Wojciechowski, W. *Advanced Practitioner Exam Review: Guidelines for Success*, 2nd ed., Albany: Delmar Publishers, Inc., 2000.

Wojciechowski, W. *Entry-Level Exam Review: Guidelines for Success*, 2nd ed., Albany: Delmar Publishers, Inc., 2000.

CHAPTER FIVE

STATISTICS

The respiratory care profession frequently provides both the student and the practitioner with clinical situations that either lack a scientific basis or simply pose stimulating questions. To facilitate the research process, as well as to improve the reader's ability to better interpret the literature, a review of some basic statistical concepts have been included in this chapter. For a complete presentation of statistics, the reader is directed to more comprehensive texts dealing with the subject.

CHAPTER OBJECTIVES

Upon completing this chapter, the reader will understand basic statistical concepts that can be applied to research conducted in the respiratory care profession and be able to

5-1 TERMINOLOGY

- Define various statistical terms.
- Describe different study designs.
- Differentiate between quantitative and qualitative data.

5-2 DESCRIPTIVE STATISTICS

- Employ graphical techniques used in statistical analysis.
- Summarize data using measures of central tendency and dispersion.

5-3 PROBABILITY

- Measure the likelihood that a particular event will occur.
- Interpret the meaning of the numerical value of probability.

364

5-4 NORMAL DISTRIBUTION

- Use a normal curve to describe sets of data.
- Understand how different means and standard deviations affect the shape of a normal distribution.
- Compute standard scores for random variables.
- Interpret standard scores for random variables.
- Derive percentile scores from a normal distribution.

5-5 SAMPLING DISTRIBUTION

- Use samples to explain characteristics of a population.
- Account for sampling variability within a population.
- Apply the central limit theorem.
- Understand how changes in the sample size affect how the sample represents the population.

5-6 CONFIDENCE INTERVALS FOR MEAN

- Explain the meaning of the interval estimator.
- Apply the confidence interval formula.

5-7 SAMPLE SIZE DETERMINATION

- Determine the required sample size to obtain an estimate that would meet the margin of error and the confidence level criteria.

5-8 SMALL SAMPLE CONFIDENCE INTERVALS FOR MEAN

- Employ the *t*-distribution.
- Recognize that the *t*-distribution curve is sample-size dependent.
- Use the *t*-distribution to construct confidence intervals.

5-9 RESPIRATORY CARE APPLICATIONS OF DESCRIPTIVE STATISTICS

- Recognize that quality control standards are statistically based.
- Use descriptive statistics to determine bias and precision.
- Employ descriptive statistics to determine normal value ranges.

5-10 TESTING OF HYPOTHESIS FOR MEAN

- Define *null hypothesis* and *alternate hypothesis.*
- Describe Type I and Type II errors.
- Distinguish between statistical significance and clinical significance.
- Apply the six-step method for hypothesis testing.
- Describe the rejection region of a distribution curve.

5-11 COMPARING MEANS OF TWO POPULATIONS (OR GROUPS): INDEPENDENT SAMPLES

- Distinguish between *dependent* and *independent variables.*
- Describe a double-blind study.
- Outline the steps for hypothesis testing concerning treatment versus control groups or two treatment groups.
- Determine confidence intervals for obtaining the difference of means.

5-12 COMPARISON OF MEANS FOR PAIRED (OR DEPENDENT) SAMPLES

- Know when to use a paired-samples *t*-test.
- Treat differences between pairs as a single random sample.

5-13 INFERENCES FOR PROPORTIONS OR PERCENTAGES

- Calculate the point estimate and interval estimates.
- Determine sample size to meet the confidence criteria.

5-14 TWO-SAMPLE INFERENCES FOR PROPORTIONS

- Distinguish between the true proportions and the sample proportions for two populations.
- Calculate the confidence interval for the difference of proportions.

5-15 TESTS FOR MANY POPULATION MEANS

- Write the null and alternative hypothesis for comparing several means.
- Explain the names CRD, *one-way* ANOVA.

5-16 CORRELATION AND REGRESSION

- Measure the strength of the association between a dependent and an independent variable.
- Use regression analysis to predict the effect an independent variable has on a dependent variable.
- Define *simple linear regression.*
- Use the least squares method to estimate (a) the *y*-intercept and (b) the slope of the linear equation.
- Test for the statistical significance of the linear regression model.
- Determine confidence intervals for the slope parameter (β_1).

5-17 CORRELATION

- Interpret the relationship between the dependent and independent variables.
- Calculate the correlation coefficient.

- Calculate the coefficient of determination.
- State the significance of the coefficient of determination value.

FORMULAS USED IN THIS CHAPTER

Mean or average:
$$\bar{x} = \frac{(x_1 + x_2 + x_3 \ldots x_n)}{(n)} = \frac{\Sigma x}{n}$$
(page 373)

Standard deviation:
$$s^2 = \frac{\Sigma(x - \bar{x})^2}{n-1}, \text{ then } s = \sqrt{s^2}$$
(page 375)

Standard score:
$$z = \frac{x - \mu}{\sigma}$$
(page 382)

Confidence interval for mean μ*:
$$\bar{x} \pm \left(t_{\frac{\alpha}{2}}, n-1 \cdot \frac{s}{\sqrt{n}}\right) \text{ or } \bar{x} \pm \left(t_{\frac{\alpha}{2}}, n-1 \cdot \frac{\sigma}{\sqrt{n}}\right)$$
(page 394)

*When σ is known, σ can substitute for s in the equation.

Sample size to infer about μ:
$$n = \left[\frac{z_{\frac{\alpha}{2}} \cdot \sigma}{E}\right]^2$$
(page 391)

Test statistic for testing H_O: $\mu = \mu_o$
$$\frac{\bar{x} - \mu_O}{s/\sqrt{n}}$$
(page 403)

Confidence interval for the difference $\mu_1 - \mu_2$
$$(\bar{x}_1 - \bar{x}_2) \pm t_{\frac{\alpha}{2}}, (n_1 + n_2 - 2)\sqrt{s_P^2\left(\frac{1}{n_1} + \frac{1}{n_2}\right)}$$
(page 406)

Test statistic for testing H_o: $\mu_1 = \mu_2$
$$\frac{\bar{x}_1 - \bar{x}_2}{\sqrt{s_P^2\left(\frac{1}{n_1} + \frac{1}{n_2}\right)}}$$
(page 407)

Confidence interval for proportion P:
$$\hat{P} \pm z_{\frac{a}{2}}\sqrt{\frac{\hat{P}(1 - \hat{P})}{n}}$$
(page 412)

Test statistic for testing H_o: $P = P_o$
$$\frac{\hat{P} - P_O}{\sqrt{\frac{P_O(1 - P_O)}{n}}}$$
(page 413)

Sample size to infer about P:
$$n = \left[\frac{z_{\frac{\alpha}{2}} x\sqrt{P(1 - P)}}{B}\right]^2, \text{ or } n = \left[\frac{z_{\frac{\alpha}{2}} x\sqrt{P(1 - P)}}{E}\right]^2$$
(page 414)

Confidence interval for the difference $P_1 - P_2$:	$\hat{P}_1 - \hat{P}_2 \pm z_{\frac{\alpha}{2}} \sqrt{\dfrac{\hat{P}_1(1 - \hat{P}_1)}{n_1} + \dfrac{\hat{P}_2(1 - \hat{P}_2)}{n_2}}$	(page 416)
Test statistic for testing $H_o: P_1 = P_2$:	$\dfrac{\hat{P}_1 - \hat{P}_2}{\sqrt{\hat{P}(1 - \hat{P})\left(\dfrac{1}{n_1} + \dfrac{1}{n_2}\right)}}$	(page 416)
Simple linear regression:	$y = \beta_0 + \beta_1 x + \text{Error}$	(page 419)
Test statistic for $H_o: \beta_1 = 0$:	$\dfrac{\hat{\beta}_1}{\sqrt{\dfrac{MSE}{SS_{xx}}}}$	(page 421)
Confidence interval for slope parameter β_1:	$\hat{\beta}_1 \pm t_{\frac{\alpha}{2}, n-2} \sqrt{\dfrac{MSE}{SS_{xx}}}$	(page 422)
Estimated mean of y at $x = x_0$:	$\hat{y}_{\text{at } x=x_0} = \hat{\beta}_0 + \hat{\beta}_1 x_0$	(page 423)
Confidence interval for mean of y at $x = x_0$:	$\hat{y}_{\text{at } x=x_0} \pm t_{\frac{\alpha}{2}, n-2} \sqrt{MSE\left(\dfrac{1}{n} + \dfrac{(x_0 - \bar{x})^2}{SS_{xx}}\right)}$	(page 423)
Correlation Coefficient:	$\gamma = \dfrac{SS_{xy}}{\sqrt{SS_{xx} \, SS_{yy}}}$	(page 424)
Coefficient of Determination (R^2):	$R^2 = \gamma^2 = \dfrac{SS_{xy}^2}{SS_{xx} \, SS_{yy}}$	(page 425)

5-1 TERMINOLOGY

Statistics are often considered to be numbers that refer to the batting average of a baseball player or running yards of a football player. However, statistics are equally important in industry and medicine. Statistical analysis is an essential part of the modern research process. This role can be largely attributed to Sir Ronald A. Fisher, a zealous statistician who created the widespread use of statistics to make experiments more efficient, inferences more reliable, and data collection less time-consuming and more cost-effective. It was the use of a simple application of statistical methods that provided the approval for Jonas Salk's polio vaccination in a short period of time.

Analysis of properly designed experiments often yields different results compared with observational experiments. In an experimental study, the investigator controls the specifications of the treatments, assignment of the subjects to each of the treatments, and experimental plan. In contrast, in an observational study the investigator is more like a spectator who just watches what happens and reports the results based on the collected data. The following example illustrates the misleading outcomes of an observational study.

EXAMPLE:

It has become a common practice to view babies in the womb using ultrasound. Originally, one of the concerns had been that ultrasound would cause low birth weight. To investigate this observation, some scientists from Johns Hopkins Hospital in Baltimore conducted an observational study. They found that babies exposed to ultrasound differ in many ways from unexposed babies. They also found a number of confounding variables, like race and smoking status, and adjusted for them. Nonetheless, they found that the babies exposed to ultrasound in the womb had a lower average birth weight than babies not exposed. However, a controlled experiment demonstrated otherwise. The controlled experiment actually showed that ultrasound was more helpful than the observational study indicated. What happened was that obstetricians ordered ultrasound examinations mostly when something "seemed" wrong. As a result of this controlled experiment, ultrasound examinations are done routinely in almost all pregnancies.

The preceding example illustrates the issue of **bias.** Bias refers to the effects of variables other than those considered in a study. Such variables are sometimes called **confounders.** In the preceding example there was a selection bias, in which the method used to select subjects affected the outcome. Other examples of bias are observation bias, measurement bias, and performance bias. Observation bias occurs when observations are interpreted differently. An observation bias might occur, for example, if breath sounds are interpreted inconsistently by researchers. Measurement bias occurs when the wrong measurement is used to assess the response to an intervention. Pulse oximetry is a measurement bias when it would be more appropriate to measure arterial blood gases to assess the results of an experimental maneuver. Performance bias occurs when the subject, or the researcher, applies the experimental maneuver incorrectly. For example, a study might show that a new bronchodilator administered by a metered dose inhaler is ineffective. However, these findings might be the result of a performance bias if the subjects did not use the metered dose inhaler correctly. When designing the experiment, it is important for the researcher to carefully consider the potential effect of bias in the study design.

A cross-sectional study is one in which subjects or treatments are compared with one another at one point in time. A longitudinal study is one in which subjects or treatments are followed over time and compared with themselves at different times. A prospective study is one in which the data are collected after the study is designed. A retrospective study is one that is conducted using data that are already available. Generally, a prospective study design is more useful than a retrospective design because the researcher has more control over the quality of data collection. In biomedical research a control group is usually used. The control group should be as similar as possible to study group except that the control group does not receive the experimental maneuver. This arrangement allows for a comparison of some outcome variable between two (or more) groups. Ideally, subjects should have an equal likelihood of being selected for the study group or the control group. This situation is usually achieved by random sampling of subjects using a list of random numbers. Whenever possible, a blind study design should be used. A single-blind study is one in which either the investigator or the subject does not know whether the subject is in the study group or the control group. A double-blind study is one in which neither the subject nor the investigator knows the group to which the subject was assigned. In some cases, the subject serves as his own control in a crossover design. The ideal study design for medical research is usually a prospective, randomized, double-blind, controlled clinical trial.

Having decided on a type of experiment or study in a particular application, one must collect data. Data are a set of values, observations, or numbers under consideration. The complete set of all observations pertaining to the characteristic of interest is referred to as the *statistical population.* A sample is a subset of the statistical population. As stated previously, subjects should be selected randomly to avoid bias.

All data (the variables measured) are either quantitative or qualitative. Quantitative data are observations measured on a numerical scale. Qualitative data, sometimes called attribute or categorical data, result from information that has been sorted into categories. These categories can be either nominal or ordinal. Nominal data can be grouped, whereas ordinal data can be grouped and placed into an order.

EXAMPLES OF VARIABLES:

- *Quantitative variable:* Number of days that a patient receives mechanical ventilation. This variable is quantitative because it can be measured.
- *Qualitative variable:* Gender of the patient needing mechanical ventilation. This variable is qualitative because it can be classified into only two categories (i.e., male or female). Further, it is nominal because it can be grouped but not ordered.
- *Nominal variable:* Numbers assigned to nonnumerical variables, e.g., 1 = "pure" chronic bronchitis; 2 = "pure" pulmonary emphysema; and 3 = mixed COPD (bronchitis-emphysema).
- *Ordinal variable:* Small, moderate, or large chest expansion in a mechanically ventilated patient. This variable is ordinal because the data can be placed into an order.

A quantitative variable can be discrete or continuous. **Discrete variables** are variables whose values can differ only by fixed amounts. For example, the number of patients admitted to a hospital in a 24-hour period is discrete. Any two 24-hour periods can differ only by integer numbers. The age of patients admitted, however, would be a **continuous variable** because the difference in the age between two patients can be arbitrarily small—a year, a month, a day, an hour, and so on. Generally, variables assuming only integer values are discrete, whereas variables assuming all possible values are continuous.

Once data have been collected, they must be analyzed by graphical methods, mathematical formulations, computational techniques, and finally interpreted in nontechnical terms.

5-2 DESCRIPTIVE STATISTICS

Descriptive statistics are used to provide summary information about groups of data. Descriptive statistics include (1) graphical analysis, (2) measures of central tendency, and (3) measures of dispersion.

The first step in any data analysis involves graphing the data and calculating some statistical measures. There are many graphical techniques used in analysis. However, only the pie chart and the histogram will be discussed here.

PIE CHART

When budgets of a state or country are reported, they are given in the form of a pie with each piece corresponding to a particular expense. Your monthly expenditures can also be depicted using a pie chart. For instance, let us assume that your total expenditure in a month is $2,000, and that you need to keep a record of how much you spend on various expenses. Your expenditures and savings are as shown in Table 5-1.

TABLE 5-1 MONTHLY EXPENSES

Expenditures	Amount In $
Groceries	500
Rent and Utilities	800
Clothes	150
Eating out	200
Transportation	50
Miscellaneous	150
Savings	150
Total	2,000

We would like to depict this distribution of expenses in the form of a pie with each piece representing the percentage of money spent on each type of expenditure. The pie chart would be as follows.

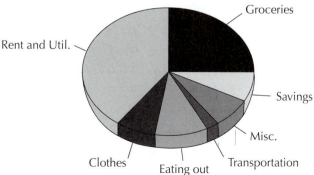

A pie chart is useful in many applications and is easy to understand. However, it is mostly useful for categorical or qualitative data where one is interested in several categories.

HISTOGRAM

A histogram usually represents class intervals or groups of measurements on the horizontal, or x-axis. The vertical, or y-axis, represents the percentage (frequency) contained in each group. To obtain the percentage of each group, the number falling in that interval is divided by the total number and then multiplied by 100.

EXAMPLE:

A respiratory therapist reviews the PEEP levels of 50 patients experiencing acute respiratory failure and finds that 5 patients are receiving 5–7 cm H_2O, 10 are receiving 7–9 cm H_2O, 15 are receiving 9–11 cm H_2O, 12 are receiving 11–13 cm H_2O, and 8 are receiving 13–15 cm H_2O. The resulting frequency histogram is shown in Figure 5-1.

Measures of Central Tendency and Dispersion

Even though a histogram provides a good data summary, data are often summarized by using a measure of central tendency and a measure of dispersion around the central point. The tendency of observations to center around a central point is termed *central tendency.* The measure that represents this center point is termed the *measure of central tendency.*

The most common and best understood measure of central tendency for a quantitative data set is the mean or the average. The average of a data set is the sum of all the

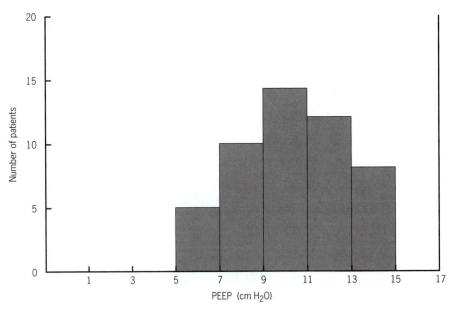

Figure 5-1 *Frequency histogram of acute respiratory failure patients receiving PEEP.*

observations divided by the number of observations in the data set. Another term for average is the **mean.** The average (mean) is obtained by using the following formula:

$$\bar{x} = \frac{(x_1 + x_2 + x_3 + \ldots x_n)}{n} = \frac{\Sigma x}{n}$$

where

$\bar{x}$ = average (mean)

Σ = sum

x = individual observations (measurements)

n = number of observations (measurements)

When the sum of the observations is obtained, that sum is divided by the number of observations to calculate the mean.

Another measure of central tendency is the **median.** The median of a histogram is the value with half (50%) of the area to the left and half to the right. Therefore, the median is the 50th percentile of a data set. The average (mean) and median may not always be the same. If a histogram is symmetrical (or bell-shaped), as shown in Figure 5-2, then the average and median would be about the same. If the histogram has a long right tail (right-skewed), as demonstrated in Figure 5-3, then the mean is affected by the few large numbers

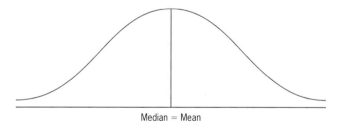

Median = Mean

Figure 5-2 *A symmetric (bell-shaped) distribution. Note that the mean (average) and median are equal.*

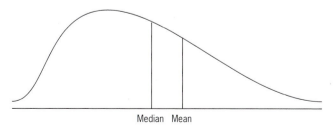

Median   Mean

Figure 5-3 *A right-skewed distribution. Note that the mean (average) is larger than the median.*

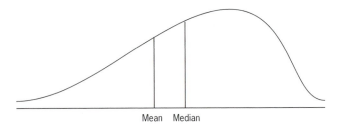

Figure 5-4 *A left-skewed distribution. Note that the mean (average) is smaller than the median.*

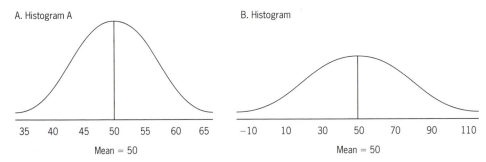

Figure 5-5 *Two symmetric distributions having the same mean (50). However, note that the spread of the observations are different. The observations in A are less spread out from the mean than those in B.*

and will be larger compared with the median. For long left-tailed histograms (left-skewed), as illustrated in Figure 5-4, the mean will be smaller than the median. For long-tailed distributions, the median is used more often than the mean because the mean renders too much importance to a small percentage of the cases in the extreme tail of the distribution. Another indicator of central tendency is the **mode.** The mode is the data point that occurs most frequently in the distribution.

Reporting just the mean or just the median often provides insufficient information because these measurements do not offer information about the shape or the spread of the observations. Two histograms could have the same mean, yet have observations spread out completely differently. Note the histograms in Figure 5-5. Both histograms have an average of 50, but histogram B has observations more spread out (three times as much) from the mean than histogram A. It is not always easy to compare two distributions just by looking at the histograms. The **standard deviation** (SD) is a measure of the spread within a distribution. There are other measures of the spread (e.g., range and coefficient of variation), but the standard deviation is the most useful statistic. The **range** is the difference between the highest and the lowest values (highest − lowest) and the **coefficient of variation** (CV) is the standard deviation divided by the mean (CV = SD ÷ mean).

The standard deviation of a data set measures the average spread of an observation from the mean. The equations for computing the standard deviation are given on the next page.

> ### Formula to Calculate Sample Standard Deviation (s)
>
> $$s^2 = \frac{\Sigma(x - \bar{x})^2}{n - 1} = \text{total of squared deviations of observations}$$
>
> from the mean/(number of observations $- 1$)
>
> where
>
> x = observation
>
> $\bar{x}$ = mean
>
> n = number of observations
>
> Σ = sum
>
> s^2 = sample variance
>
> $s = \sqrt{s^2}$ = sample standard deviation

Because the standard deviation measures the average spread of an observation from the mean, data with a low standard deviation have observations close to the mean. Reliability of results (i.e., consistency) depends on the variation of the data set. Therefore, the smaller the standard deviation the more reliable (consistent) are the results. For most data sets, about 68% of the observations fall within one standard deviation of the mean; 95% of the observations fall within two standard deviations of the mean; and almost all observations fall within three standard deviations of the mean. This relationship is generally known as the Empirical rule. The Empirical rule applies if the distribution (histogram) of the data is bell-shaped. This configuration is described in greater detail later in this chapter as the *normal distribution*.

EXAMPLE 1:

A respiratory therapist measures the tidal volumes of eight mechanically ventilated patients and determines them to be 500, 750, 1,000, 600, 800, 700, 900, and 800 ml. Determine the mean, median, mode, standard deviation, range, and coefficient of variation for these tidal volumes (data set).

a) Determine the mean.

Solution: Use the formula for $\bar{x}$.

$$\bar{x} = \frac{(x_1 + x_2 + x_3 + ...x_n)}{n}$$

$$\bar{x} = \frac{500 \text{ ml} + 750 \text{ ml} + 1,000 \text{ ml} + 600 \text{ ml} + 800 \text{ ml} + 700 \text{ ml} + 900 \text{ ml} + 800 \text{ ml}}{8}$$

$$= 756 \text{ ml}$$

b) Obtain the median.

Solution: Rank the data (tidal volume measurements) from the highest to lowest. The tidal volume in the middle of the distribution is 800 ml. Thus, the median is 800 ml.

c) Find the mode.

Solution: Because there are two tidal volumes of 800 ml and only one each of the other values, the mode is 800 ml.

d) Calculate the standard deviation.

Step 1: Calculate s^2.

$$s^2 = \frac{(x_1 - \bar{x})^2 + (x_2 - \bar{x})^2 + (x_3 - \bar{x})^2 + (x_4 - \bar{x})^2 + (x_5 - \bar{x})^2 + (x_6 - \bar{x})^2 + (x_7 - \bar{x})^2 + (x_8 - \bar{x})^2}{8 - 1}$$

$$= \frac{177,188}{7} = 25,313$$

Step 2: Calculate the standard deviation using the formula for s.

$$s = \sqrt{s^2}$$

$$s = \sqrt{25,313}$$

$$= 159$$

e) Find the range for this data set.

Solution: The range is the difference between the highest and the lowest values. Therefore, subtract 500 ml from 1,000 ml.

$$1,000 \text{ ml} - 500 \text{ ml} = 500 \text{ ml}$$

f) Determine the coefficient of variation.

Solution: The coefficient of variation is the standard deviation divided by the mean. Therefore, divide 159 ml by 756 ml.

$$159 \text{ ml} \div 756 \text{ ml} = 0.210, \text{ or } 21.0\%$$

EXAMPLE 2:

A respiratory therapist is interested in the mean, median, range, and standard deviation for the following data, which represent the days of mechanical ventilation for five patients following thoracic surgery: 3.2, 2.5, 2.1, 3.7, and 2.8 days.

a) Calculate the mean ($\bar{x}$).

Solution: Use the formula below.

$$\bar{x} = (3.2 + 2.5 + 2.1 + 3.7 + 2.8)/5$$

$$= 2.86 \text{ days}$$

b) Obtain the median, i.e., the middle observation (50th percentile).

Solution: To find the median, arrange the data in increasing order: 2.1, 2.5, 2.8, 3.2, 3.7 days. Thus, the median equals 2.8 days. Because the mean (2.86 days) and the median (2.8 days) are close to each other in this data set, the distribution does not appear to be skewed.

c) Determine the range.

Solution: Use the formula

$$\text{range} = \text{largest observation} - \text{smallest observation}$$

$$\text{range} = 3.7 \text{ days} - 2.1 \text{ days}$$

$$= 1.6 \text{ days}$$

d) Calculate the standard deviation (s).

Step 1:   Calculate s^2.

$$s^2 = \Sigma(x - \bar{x})^2/(n - 1)$$

$$s^2 = \frac{(3.2 - 2.86)^2 + (2.5 - 2.86)^2 + (2.1 - 2.86)^2 + (3.7 - 2.86)^2 + (2.8 - 2.86)^2}{5 - 1} = 0.383 \text{ day}$$

Step 2:   Calculate the standard deviation using the formula for s.

$$s = \sqrt{s^2}$$

$$s = \sqrt{0.383}$$

$$= 0.619 \text{ day}$$

EXAMPLE 3:

Describe how the mean compares with the median for a distribution (a) skewed to the left, (b) skewed to the right, and (c) symmetrical.

Solution:

a. A left-skewed distribution indicates that there are only a few extreme or outlying observations compared with the remainder of the observations. The median in this case does not become greatly affected by these outliers. The mean in a left-skewed distribution will be smaller than the median. Consider the data set 0, 31, 32. The mean is 21, i.e., $(0 + 31 + 32)/3$. The median is 31.

b. A right-skewed distribution also indicates that there are only a few outliers compared with the rest of the observations. The median again does not become greatly affected by extreme observations. The mean in a right-skewed distribution will be larger than the median. Consider the data set 31, 32, 63. The mean is 42, i.e., $(31 + 32 + 63)/3$, whereas the median is 32.

c. The mean, median, and mode are equal for a symmetrical distribution. Consider the data set 30, 31, 32. Here the mean and median are both 31. When the distribution is skewed (left or right), the median represents the data better than the mean. Other measures, for example *trimmed mean*, are useful in these cases. A trimmed mean is determined after 5% to 10% of the observations are removed from each tail. The mean calculated from the remaining observations is the trimmed mean.

5-3 PROBABILITY

Probability measures the likelihood that a particular event will occur. Probability, or chance, is measured as a ratio or a percent. The repetition of an experiment is the essence of probability. In this context the repetition of an experiment is a *trial*. Each trial is associated with an outcome. The tossing of a coin will serve as an example experiment here. There are two possible outcomes each time a coin is tossed into the air, i.e., *heads* or *tails*. The probability of tossing heads is 50%, or 1 out of 2 possible outcomes. If the coin is tossed again, the probability of the outcome being heads or tails remains at 50%. No matter how many times in succession the coin is tossed (repetition of the experiment), the probability of either outcome will always be 50% for each toss.

The formula for probability is as follows:

$$\text{probability} = \frac{\text{number of favorable outcomes}}{\text{total number of possible outcomes}}$$

Regarding the coin experiment discussed here, if heads was the favorable outcome, the number of favorable outcomes would be 1, whereas the total number of possible outcomes would be 2 (i.e., heads and tails). Therefore,

$$\text{probability} = \frac{1}{2}$$

or

$$\text{probability} = \left(\frac{1}{2}\right) \cdot 100 = 50\%$$

The numerical value of probability would be zero (0) when an event is impossible. The numerical value of the probability of an event that is certain to occur is 1. Therefore, all other probabilities will range between 0 and 1, or 0% and 100%, respectively.

EXAMPLE:

The letters A, B, C, D, and E are written on five blue and five green tags (one letter on each tag). The ten tags are placed in a box and thoroughly mixed. One tag is randomly selected.

a) Determine the probability for selecting a blue tag.

Step 1:   Determine the number of favorable outcomes.

There are 5 favorable outcomes because there are 5 blue tags in the box.

Step 2:   Determine the total number of possible outcomes.

There is a total number of 10 possible outcomes.

Step 3: Insert the known values into the probability formula to calculate the probability.

$$\text{probability} = \left(\frac{5 \text{ blue tags}}{10 \text{ possible outcomes}}\right) 100 = 50\%$$

b) Determine the probability of selecting a tag labeled A or C.

Step 1: Determine the number of favorable outcomes.

The number of favorable outcomes is 4 (i.e., tag A (blue and green) + tag C (blue and green)).

Step 2: Determine the total number of possible outcomes.

The total number of possible outcomes is 10 (i.e., 5 blue tags + 5 green tags).

Step 3: Insert the known values into the probability formula to calculate the percent probability.

$$\text{probability} = \left(\frac{4 \text{ favorable outcomes}}{10 \text{ possible outcomes}}\right) 100 = 40\%$$

PRACTICE PROBLEMS

Refer to Appendix A (pages 614-615) for the solutions and answers to the practice problems.

1. Consider an experiment of throwing two dice. The following events are of interest:
   a. A = sum of numbers showing is 10.
   b. B = sum of the numbers showing is either 6, 9, or 11.
   Find the probability of events A and B.
2. A popular game called "craps" is played according to the following rules. A player rolls two dice. If the result (sum of the numbers showing) is a 7 or 11, the player wins. For any other sum appearing on the dice, the player continues to roll the dice until that outcome recurs (in which case the player wins) or until a 7 or 11 occurs (in which case the player loses). If the sum is 2 on any roll of the dice, the game is over and the player loses.
   a. Find the chances that a player loses the game on the first roll of the dice.
   b. Find the chances that a player wins the game on the first roll of the dice.
   c. If the player throws a sum of 3 on the first roll, what are the chances that the game ends on the next roll?
3. A box contains 3 blue marbles and 2 red marbles. Two marbles are drawn at random from the box.
   a. What are the chances that both the marbles are blue?
   b. What are the chances that one marble is blue and the other is red?

4. Suppose a particular respiratory care class is historically known to produce the following grade distribution:

Grade	A	B	C	D	F
Chance	30%	20%	20%	15%	15%

For a randomly chosen student who has enrolled in this class,

a. What are the chances that he will get either an A or a B?

b. What are the chances that he will get a grade less than B?

5-4 NORMAL DISTRIBUTION

It was alluded to earlier that a normal curve, or a normal distribution, can be used to describe sets of data. In other words, histograms of many data sets can be approximated by a normal curve. Examples include blood pressure, height, and $PaCO_2$. The characteristic properties of a normal curve are that it is bell-shaped and symmetric about the mean. A normal curve, or a normal distribution, is illustrated in Figure 5-6.

There are many different normal curves (Figure 5-7). Each curve in Figure 5-7 is bell-shaped but differs in the location of the center of the curve and/or in the spread of the curve from its center.

Suppose the heart rate of American adult males follows a normal distribution with a population mean of $\mu = 72$ beats/min and a standard deviation of $\sigma = 9.7$ beats/min. The curve depicting this data is shown in Figure 5-8.

Figure 5-8 indicates that most of the observations fall within 3 standard deviations of the mean. If the standard deviation is 15 beats/min instead of 9.7 beats/min, how will the shape of the curve be affected? Remember that the standard deviation is a measure of the spread

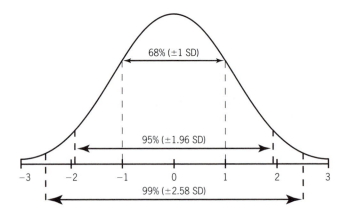

Figure 5-6 *A normal distribution curve. 68% of the observations lie ± 1 SD from the mean; 95% lie ± 1.96 SDs from the mean; 99% lie ± 2.58 SDs from mean.*

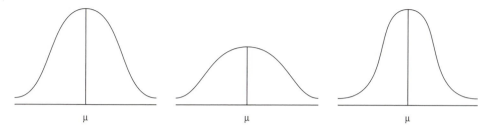

Figure 5-7 *Three normal (bell-shaped) distribution curves differing in the location of the center (mean) of the curve and in the spread of the observations from the mean (μ).*

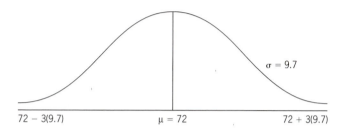

Figure 5-8 *A normal distribution with a mean of 72 beats/min and a standard deviation (σ) of 9.7 beats/min (+3 and −3 = three standard deviations from the mean).*

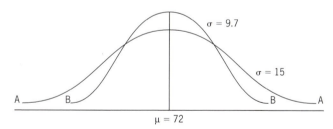

Figure 5-9 *Two superimposed, normal distribution curves having the same mean (72 beats/min) but different standard deviations (A = 15 beats/min; B = 9.7 beats/min). The different standard deviations affect only the shape of the curve.*

from the mean and affects only the shape and not the location. To observe the effect of differing standard deviations in this example, note the two superimposed curves in Figure 5-9. One curve has a standard deviation of 9.7 beats/min, and the other has a standard deviation of 15 beats/min. Observe that the spreads of the two curves differ despite both having a mean of 72 beats/min. However, if the mean were 80 beats/min instead of 72 beats/min with a standard deviation of 9.7 beats/min, the two curves would have the same shape but would differ in their location. This phenomenon is shown by the two curves in Figure 5-10.

An infinite number of normal distributions is possible. The **standard normal distribution** can be used to solve any problem having a normal distribution. If variable *x* has a mean

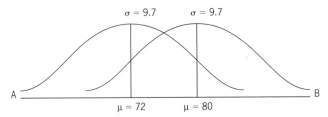

Figure 5-10 *Two superimposed, normal distribution curves having different means (A = 72 beats/min; B = 80 beats/min) but the same standard deviation (9.7 beats/min). Because the means differ, the curves have different locations. Because the standard deviations are equal, the curves have the same shape.*

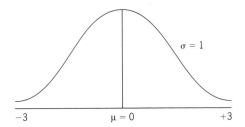

Figure 5-11 *A standard normal curve. Note the mean of 0 and the standard deviation of 1 (+3 and −3 = three standard deviations from the mean).*

(μ) and a standard deviation (σ), then the **standard score** of x can be denoted by z. The standard score is also called the *z-score*. The formula used to determine z-score is

$$z = \frac{x - \mu}{\sigma}$$

where

x = variable

μ = mean

σ = standard deviation

z = standard score, or z-score

For a distribution of x scores, the corresponding distribution of standard scores (z) has a mean of 0 and standard deviation of 1. Therefore, if x has a normal distribution then the standard scores of x will have the standard normal distribution. Any normal curve can be reduced to a standard normal curve by applying this formula. A standard normal curve is a normal curve with mean of 0 and standard deviation of 1. Note Figure 5-11.

The standard score of an observation represents the number of standard deviations from the mean and the direction of the observation. For instance, if the standard score of an observation is +2, that observation is 2 standard deviations above the mean. Similarly, if the standard score is −2, the observation is 2 standard deviations below the mean.

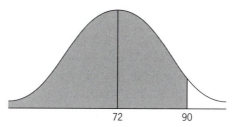

Figure 5-12 *A normal distribution showing a mean of 72 beats/min and the variable 90 beats/min. The percentage of the shaded area below 90 beats/min is sought.*

EXAMPLE 1:

For a hypothetical data set, assume that the mean is 100 and that the standard deviation is 10. Compute and interpret the standard scores for values (random variables) of 90 and 115.

Solution: Use the formula

$$z = \frac{x - \mu}{\sigma}$$

a) For $x = 90$,

$$z = (90 - 100)/10$$
$$= -1$$

The observation 90 is 1 standard deviation below the mean.

b) For $x = 115$,

$$z = (115 - 100)/10$$
$$= 1.5$$

The observation 115 is 1.5 standard deviations above the mean.

EXAMPLE 2:

Consider the heart rate of the population of American adult males to have a normal distribution with a mean of 72 beats/min and a standard deviation of 9 beats/min. If a special military service states that anyone with a heart rate of less than 90 beats/min is eligible for service, what percentage of adult males would qualify? Figure 5-12 illustrates this example.

Solution: What needs to be determined is the percentage of males below 90 beats/min (shaded area). Fifty percent (50%) of the area under the curve is below 72 beats/min. The area that needs to be determined is that which lies between 72 and 90 beats/min. This region can be found using the standard normal distribution. The standard normal distribution will be used to convert variables 72 beats/min and 90 beats/min to z-scores. The graph used in this example can be standardized as follows:

Step 1: Convert 72 beats/min to a z-score using the formula shown below.

$$z = \frac{x - \mu}{\sigma} = \frac{\text{random variable} - \text{mean}}{\text{standard deviation}} = \frac{72\ \text{beats/min} - 72\ \text{beats/min}}{9\ \text{beats/min}} = 0$$

Step 2: Convert 90 beats/min to a z-score.

$$z = \frac{90\ \text{beats/min} - 72\ \text{beats/min}}{9\ \text{beats min}} = 2$$

Step 3: Refer to the portion of the standard normal z-table located alongside the graph with the z line in Figure 5-13 to find the area between 0 and 2. The value associated with a z-score of 2 is 0.4772. Therefore, the shaded area of the curve between 72 beats/min (mean) and 90 beats/min is 0.4772, or 47.72%.

Step 4: Find the area of the curve below 90 beats/min by adding the area below 72 beats/min (mean) to the area between 72 beats/min and 90 beats/min.

$$\binom{\text{area below}}{72\ \text{beats/min}} + \binom{\text{area between}}{72\ \text{and}\ 90\ \text{beats/min}} = \binom{\text{area below}}{90\ \text{beats/min}}$$

$$0.50 \quad + \quad 0.4772 \quad = \quad 0.9772,\ \text{or}\ 97.72\%$$

Therefore, 97.72% of the adult males have a heart rate of less than or equal to 90 beats/min.

Percentile scores can be derived from the foregoing process. For example, a heart rate of 90 beats/min is approximately the 98th percentile because approximately 98% (rounded from 97.72%) of males have a heart rate ≤ 90 beats/minute. Suppose that one wanted to know the 90th percentile heart rate (Figure 5-14). To obtain the percentile score, use the reverse of the process previously illustrated. First, determine the standard score by searching for 0.40 in the body of Table 1, Appendix C, and finding the corresponding standard score. (An abbreviated version of this table is included in Figure 5-14). The number 1.28 is used because the area corresponding to 1.28 is 0.3997, which is close to 0.40. Therefore, the standard score in the graph shown in Figure 5-14 is 1.28. The corresponding 90th percentile heart rate is 1.28 standard deviations above the mean (72 beats/min).

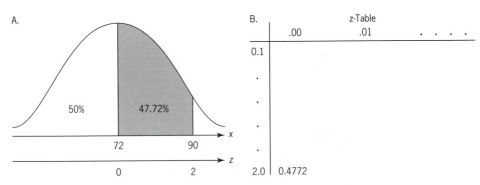

Figure 5-13 *(A) a standard normal curve showing the percentage below 72 beats/min and between 72 and 90 beats/min; (B) a portion of a z-table illustrating z-score of 2 (i.e., 0.4772).*

A.

B.

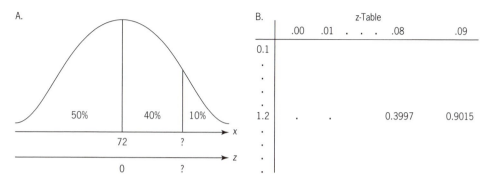

Figure 5-14 *(A) a normal distribution with a mean of 72 beats/min; (B) a portion of a z-table showing z-score (standard score) of 1.28. The heart rate corresponding to the 90th percentile score is sought.*

The 90th percentile heart rate can be determined by multiplying the standard deviation by the standard score and adding the mean, that is,

percentile score = (standard score × standard deviation) + mean

or

90th percentile heart rate = (1.28 × 9 beats/min) + 72 beats/min

= 83.52 beats/min

Therefore, the 90th percentile heart rate is approximately 83 beats/min.

PRACTICE PROBLEMS

Refer to Appendix A (pages 615-616) for the solutions and answers to the practice problems.

5. To find the following areas of the curve, use the normal distribution curve representing the heart rate of American adult males, with mean 72 beats/min and standard deviation 9 beats/min.
   a. The percentage of adult males whose heart rate is less than 95 beats/min.
   b. The percentage of adult males whose heart rate is below 54 beats/min.
   c. The percentage of adult males whose heart rate is between 54 and 90 beats/min.
   d. The percentage of adult males whose heart rate is more than 90 beats/min.
6. Let random variable x denote the hours that a patient is receiving mechanical ventilation. Suppose variable x follows a normal distribution curve with a mean of 12 hours and a standard deviation of 3 hours. Using the normal distribution curve in Figure 5-15,
   a. Compute and interpret the 95th percentile score.
   b. Compute and interpret the 97.5th percentile score.

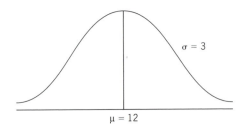

Figure 5-15 *A normal distribution curve with a mean of 12 hours and a standard deviation of 3 hours.*

5-5 SAMPLING DISTRIBUTION

Remember that statistical procedures are applied to explain the population as best as possible with the help of samples. Characteristics of the population (i.e., parameters) such as the mean, standard deviation, median, and mode are of interest. Usually, the corresponding sample characteristic called the *statistic* is used to estimate the parameter. A natural estimate of the population mean is the sample mean. This estimate is termed the **point estimate,** as it provides a single value or number. Although the point estimate provides information about a parameter, it does not explain the degree of proximity to the parameter. The point estimate has this characteristic because it does not take into account sampling variability.

   Sampling distribution provides a study of sampling variability. The sampling distribution of a statistic is the distribution of all values of that statistic when it is computed from all possible random samples of the same size from a population. In real life, only one sample is usually studied. Therefore, how do we determine the sampling variability and the sampling distribution? In most cases these dilemmas are resolved by applying the central limit theorem. The central limit theorem provides information about the sampling distribution of the sample mean without the need for repeated samples.

Central limit theorem: For most data sets with a population mean (μ) and a standard deviation (σ), a random sample size of 30 or more provides a sampling distribution of the sample mean ($\bar{x}$) that approximates a normal curve, with $\mu_{\bar{x}} = \mu$ and

$$\text{standard deviation of the sample mean} = \frac{\text{standard deviation}}{\sqrt{\text{total number of observations}}}$$

$$\sigma_{\bar{x}} = \frac{\sigma}{\sqrt{n}}$$

where

   $\mu_{\bar{x}}$ = the mean of the sample mean $\bar{x}$.
   $\sigma_{\bar{x}}$ = standard deviation of the sample mean $\bar{x}$
   σ = standard deviation
   n = total number of observations

The standard deviation of the sample mean (i.e., $\sigma_{\bar{x}}$) is known also as the *standard error of the mean* (SEM).

As the sample size increases, the sampling variability (or standard deviation) of the sample mean ($\sigma_{\bar{x}}$) gets smaller. Increasing the sample size indicates that the sample more closely represents the population. The standard error provides the rate by which the sampling variability becomes larger or smaller as the sample size varies.

EXAMPLE:

A variable x has a normal distribution with a mean of 25 and a standard deviation of 6. Assume a random sample size of 36 from this distribution.

a) Describe the sampling distribution of the sample mean.

Solution: Because the sample size of 36 ($n = 36$) is large, the central limit theorem is applied. The central limit theorem will cause the distribution of the sample mean to be approximately normal with a mean $\mu_{\bar{x}}$ of 25 and a standard deviation of the sample mean ($\sigma_{\bar{x}}$), or standard error of the sample mean, calculated as follows:

$$\sigma_{\bar{x}} = \frac{\sigma}{\sqrt{n}} = \frac{6}{\sqrt{36}} = 1$$

b) Find and interpret the probability that the sample mean ($\bar{x}$) is less than 26, i.e., $P(\bar{x} < 26)$.

Step 1: Find the z-score of 26.

$$z = \frac{(26 - \mu)}{\sigma_{\bar{x}}} = \frac{(26 - 25)}{1} = 1$$

This value ($z = 1$) indicates that the area below $z = 1$ on the normal curve is sought.

Step 2: Determine the lightly shaded area on the normal distribution curve (Figure 5-16) below $z = 1$ and above $z = 0$.

A z-score of 1 corresponds with 0.3413 (Appendix C, Table 1).

Step 3: Add the percent that corresponds with a z-score of 1 to 0.5 (50%) to obtain the probability that the mean will be less than 26.

$$0.5 + 0.3413 = 0.8413, \text{ or approximately } 84\%$$

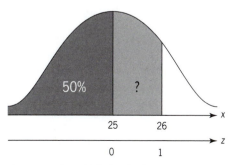

Figure 5-16 *A normal distribution curve for which the shaded area (percent) below a z-score of 1 is sought.*

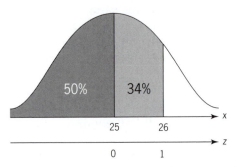

Figure 5-17 *A normal distribution curve showing that 84% of the curve resides below 26.*

There is about an 84% chance that the sample mean of the 36 observations will be below 26 (Figure 5-17).

c) Find and interpret $P(\bar{x} > 27)$.

Step 1: Find the z-score of 27.

$$z = \frac{(27 - \mu)}{\sigma_{\bar{x}}} = \frac{27 - 25}{1} = 2$$

This value ($z = 2$) indicates that the area above $z = 2$ on the normal curve is sought.

Step 2: Determine the area on the normal distribution curve (Figure 5-18) below $z = 2$.

A z-score of 2 corresponds with 0.4772 (Appendix C, Table 1).

Step 3: Subtract the percent that corresponds with a z-score of 2 from 0.5 (50%) to obtain the probability that the mean will be more than 27.

$$0.5 - 0.4772 = 0.0228, \text{ or approximately } 2.3\%$$

There is about a 2.3% chance that the sample mean of the 36 observations will be more than 27 (Figure 5-19).

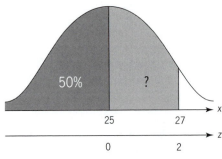

Figure 5-18 *A normal distribution curve for which the lightly shaded area (percent) below a z-score of 2 is sought.*

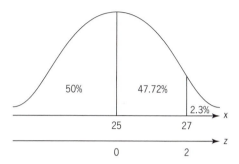

Figure 5-19   *A normal distribution curve showing that 2.3% of the curve resides above 27.*

PRACTICE PROBLEMS

Refer to Appendix A (pages 616-617) for the solutions and answers to the practice problems.

7. Psychomotor retardation scores for a large group of manic-depressive patients were found to be approximately normal with a mean of 930 and a standard deviation of 120. Assume a random sample of 36 manic-depressive patients.

   a. Describe the sampling distribution of the sample mean ($\bar{x}$) retardation score of the 36 patients.

   b. Find the chance that the sample mean retardation score is more than 910.

   c. Find the chance that the sample mean retardation score is between 950 and 970.

5-6 CONFIDENCE INTERVALS FOR THE MEAN

Now that the sampling variability and the sampling distribution of the mean have been explained, an estimate yielding more information about the population mean than the point estimate can be derived. That estimate is called the *interval estimator.* The interval estimator uses an interval instead of a single point. The interval estimator provides an estimate of the population mean ($\bar{x}$) and a margin of error (E) based on the data provided. It also provides a measure of certainty and reliability on the estimate.

$(1 - \alpha)$ 100% Confidence Intervals (C.I.) for Population Mean

$$C.I. = \bar{x} \pm \left(z_{\frac{\alpha}{2}} \cdot \frac{s}{\sqrt{n}} \right)$$

where

$\bar{x}$ = sample mean

$z_{\frac{\alpha}{2}}$ = z-score

s = standard deviation

n = sample size

When σ is known, σ can substitute for s in the equation. Note that $\frac{\sigma}{\sqrt{n}}$ is the standard error of $\bar{x}$.

To construct a confidence interval of 90%, find $z_{0.05}$, which is the 95th percentile of the standard normal distribution. From the body of Table 1 in Appendix C, locate 0.05 and find the corresponding z-score. The z-score is 1.645. Now, substitute this value for z in the confidence interval formula.

EXAMPLE 1:

The director of an intensive care unit wishes to estimate the mean length of stay for patients with ARDS admitted to the ICU. The director randomly selects 49 patients with ARDS and determines the length of stay for each. For this sample $\bar{x} = 19.8$ days and $s = 5$ days. The director wants to be confident about this estimate, so he chooses a 95% confidence interval.

Step 1: Because a 95% confidence interval is sought, α equals 5% and $\frac{\alpha}{2} = 0.025$.

Step 2: Locate the z-score (Appendix C, Table 1) for $z_{0.025}$.

$$z_{0.025} = 1.96$$

Step 3: Calculate the 95% confidence interval.

$$C.I. = \bar{x} \pm \left(z_{\frac{\alpha}{2}} \times \frac{s}{\sqrt{n}} \right)$$

$$\text{upper limit} = 19.8 + \left(1.96 \times \frac{5}{\sqrt{49}} \right) = 21.2 \text{ days}$$

$$\text{lower limit} = 19.8 - \left(1.96 \times \frac{5}{\sqrt{49}} \right) = 18.4 \text{ days}$$

Therefore, the 95% confidence interval is 18.4 to 21.2 days.

These findings can be interpreted three ways: (1) there is 95% certainty that the 18.4–21.2 interval includes the true mean of the length of stay for ARDS patients, (2) with 95% certainty the estimate of the true mean length of stay is 19.8 ± 1.4 days, or (3) the best estimate of the true mean length of stay is 19.8 days, and with 95% certainty this estimate is within ± 1.4 days of the true mean.

EXAMPLE 2:

Note the following steps if a 99% confidence interval is desired.

Step 1: Because a 99% confidence interval is sought, α equals 1% and $\frac{\alpha}{2} = 0.005$.

Step 2: Locate the z-score (Appendix C, Table 1) for $z_{0.005}$.

$$z_{0.005} = 2.575$$

Step 3: Calculate the 99% confidence interval.

$$C.I. = 19.8 \pm \left(2.575 \times \frac{5}{\sqrt{49}}\right) = 18.0–21.6 \text{ days}$$

The 99% confidence interval is 18.0–21.6 days.

PRACTICE PROBLEMS

Refer to Appendix A (page 617) for the solutions and answers to the practice problems.

8. Construct and interpret a 95% confidence interval for the true mean when a random sample of 32 observations yielded an $\bar{x}$ of 12 and an s of 2.5.
9. Construct and interpret a 99% confidence interval for the true mean when a random sample of 32 observations yielded an $\bar{x}$ of 12 and an s of 2.5.

5-7 SAMPLE SIZE DETERMINATION

To determine the required sample size, one must decide how much confidence is required for the estimate and the margin of error (E) that is acceptable. An estimate of the population standard deviation is also needed. From this information the required sample size can be determined.

Sample Size Determination Formula

$$n = \left[\frac{z_{\frac{\alpha}{2}} \cdot \text{standard deviation}}{E}\right]^2$$

where $z_{\frac{\alpha}{2}}$ is determined as with confidence intervals, E is the margin of error, and standard deviation is an estimate (obtained either from past experience, from a pilot study, or using $\hat{\sigma} = \text{range} \div 4$ if the range is known).

EXAMPLE 1:

A practioner wishes to estimate within 2 torr with 95% confidence the true $PaCO_2$ of asthmatic patients admitted from the emergency department. He knows from past experience that the minimum $PaCO_2$ is 35 torr and the maximum is 55 torr.

Solution: Knowing the range, an estimate of the standard deviation can be obtained by dividing the range by 4.

$$\frac{55 \text{ torr} - 35 \text{ torr}}{4} = 5 \text{ torr}$$

The margin of error is 2 because the estimate of the mean sought is within 2 torr. Because α is 5%, or 0.05,

$$\frac{\alpha}{2} = 0.025, \text{ and } z_{0.025} = 1.96$$

Therefore,

$$n = \left[\frac{1.96 \times 5}{2}\right]^2 = 24$$

At least 24 patients ($n = 24$) must be included in the sample to estimate within 2 mm Hg with 95% confidence the true $PaCO_2$ of asthmatic patients admitted from the emergency department.

EXAMPLE 2:

The director of a respiratory care department wants to estimate the average number of mechanical ventilation days for COPD patients. From experience he knows that the minimum and the maximum ventilator days are 2 and 22, respectively. How many random observations are needed in the sample to estimate the average number to within 2 days with 95% confidence?

Because α equals 0.05, $\alpha/2$ equals 0.025 and $z_{0.025}$ equals 1.96. Since the estimate sought is within 2 days of the sample mean, the margin of error (E) is 2. Also, because the possible range of the observations is known, the standard deviation is estimated by dividing the value of the **range** by 4, as follows:

$$\frac{22 \text{ days} - 2 \text{ days}}{4} = 5 \text{ days}$$

Therefore, the sample size (n) required is determined by the formula below.

$$n = \left[\frac{z_{\frac{\alpha}{2}} \cdot \sigma}{E}\right]^2$$

$$n = \left[\frac{1.96 \times 5}{2}\right]^2 = 24$$

At least 24 randomly selected patients ($n = 24$) are needed to estimate the average number of mechanical ventilation days to within 2 days with 95% confidence.

PRACTICE PROBLEMS

Refer to Appendix A (page 617) for the solutions and answers to the practice problems.

10. Medical experiments are often costly because of the involvement of human or animal models. Suppose each observation will cost $10.00 and the experimenter has a budget of $1,800.00.

a. Does the experimenter have enough funds to estimate the mean attribute of interest to within 2 units with a 95% confidence interval? The experimenter knows that the standard deviation will be approximately 15.

b. If a 90% confidence interval is used, will the funds be sufficient?

5-8 SMALL SAMPLE CONFIDENCE INTERVALS FOR MEAN

Federal legislation requires that drug companies conduct extensive tests before marketing a new drug. The testing process is usually conducted on animals before humans. In the case of human testing, the companies are invariably forced to make inferences based on small samples because of risks of unknown side effects. When the sample sizes are small, the central limit theorem may or may not hold true. Therefore, the sampling distribution of the mean may not follow a normal curve. In such cases, the assumption is that the observations in the population follow a normal curve. Under this assumption, another symmetric distribution, called t-distribution, can be used. In practice, the t-distribution can be used even if the distribution of the observations is not very close to normal distribution. The use of the t-distribution under these circumstances is described as the "robustness" property. The curve of the t-distribution is also symmetric about 0 but has thicker tails than the curve of the z-distribution. Figure 5-20 provides t-distributions with different sample sizes.

As the sample size increases, the t-distribution curve approaches that of the z-distribution curve. Thus, the t-distribution curve is sample-size dependent, a property that is due to degrees of freedom. If we have a sample of size n from a single population, then the degrees of freedom is $(n - 1)$. The more parameters that are estimated, the fewer degrees of freedom the distribution will have. Degrees of freedom provides a method of identifying which t-distribution applies to the sample. Tables of the t-distribution are provided in Table II of Appendix C. These tables are limited to the tail probabilities.

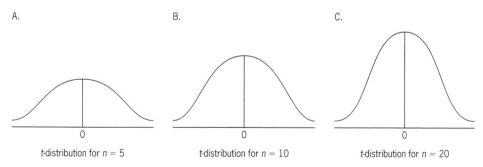

Figure 5-20 *Three* t-*distribution curves with three different sample sizes* (n)*: (A)*n = 5; *(B)*n = 10; *(C)*n = 20.

EXAMPLE 1:

Find and interpret $t_{0.05,n-1}$, or $t_{0.05,9}$, where $n = 10$.

Solution: From Table II in Appendix C, find $t_{0.05}$ in the top row and 9 degrees of freedom (d.f.) in the first column. The number intersecting this row and column is the t-score, or 1.833. This t-score is the 95th percentile of the t-distribution with 9 d.f. Remember that the 95th percentile of z-distribution is 1.645. Also, note that in Table II the numbers decrease down the columns. This trend is caused by the fact that, as the sample size increases, the t-distribution approaches the standard normal distribution. Thus, the last number in the column of $t_{0.05}$ is 1.645, which is also $z_{0.05}$.

EXAMPLE 2:

Dr. Frans van de Werf, et al (*N. Engl. J. Med.*, March 8, 1984) conducted a study on a new drug, t-pA, which may prove to be effective in dissolving blood clots in patients with acute myocardial infarction. One aspect of Dr. van de Werf's research involved measuring the length of time for a heart attack patient's blood clot to dissolve after treatment with t-pA. The times recorded for these seven patients were 50, 75, 0, 35, 38, 35, and 19 minutes. (Statistics by McClave and Dietrich, 1991.) Use these data to construct a 95% confidence interval for the true mean length of time for a blood clot to be dissolved after treatment.

Solution: First, modify the C.I. formula for use with a small sample.

Confidence Interval for μ When n Is Small

$$\bar{x} \pm \left(t_{\frac{\alpha}{2},n-1} \cdot \frac{s}{\sqrt{n}} \right)$$

We have $\alpha = 5\%$, $\alpha/2 = 0.025$, $n = 7$, and $n - 1 = 6$. Then, $t_{0.025,6} = 2.365$ (Appendix C, Table II). Also find $\bar{x}$ and s for the given data. These values are $\bar{x} = 38.43$ minutes and $s = 24.87$ minutes. Substituting these values in the formula yields:

$$38.43 \pm 2.365 \cdot \frac{24.87}{\sqrt{7}} = 38.43 \pm 22.23 \text{ or } (16.2, 60.66)$$

Therefore, with 95% confidence the true mean length of time for the blood clot to be dissolved is between 16.2 minutes and 60.66 minutes.

PRACTICE PROBLEMS

Refer to Appendix A (page 618) for the solutions and answers to the practice problems.

11. The data listed below refer to a study that investigated blood concentrations of growth hormone and glucose levels in 16 low-birth-weight infants 4 days after birth.

	Growth hormone (µg/L)	Glucose (mmol/L)
$\bar{x}$	40.3	6.6
s	16.0	3.2

a. Construct and interpret a 95% confidence interval for the true mean growth hormone level for 4-day-old, low-birth-weight infants.

b. Construct and interpret a 99% confidence interval for the true mean glucose level for 4-day-old, low-birth-weight infants.

12. A study investigating the effect of an anesthetic on the flow rate of aqueous humor (an ocular fluid) yielded the following data:

Anesthetic	n	$\bar{x}$	s
Pentobarbitol	191	0.99	0.235
Urethane	13	1.47	0.314
Ketamine	16	0.99	0.164

a. Construct a 95% confidence interval for the true mean flow rate of aqueous humor for each anesthetic.

b. What will happen to the width of the 95% confidence interval constructed in part (2a) for a sample (n) of 13 for Pentobarbitol instead of an n of 191 which yielded the mean and standard deviation? Explain and verify the answer by constructing the interval with an n of 13.

c. As the sample size increases, explain how the width of the confidence interval will be affected.

5-9 RESPIRATORY CARE APPLICATIONS OF DESCRIPTIVE STATISTICS

Descriptive statistics are frequently applied to many areas of respiratory care. In many instances the clinician may be unaware of these applications. This section will highlight the use of descriptive statistics in specific clinical settings.

Quality Control

Quality control is used in the blood gas laboratory to assure proper function of the blood gas analyzer. A solution with known values for blood gases and pH is introduced into the blood gas analyzer at regular intervals. The known values are compared with the values displayed on the analyzer. Decisions are then made regarding whether the analyzer is operating correctly (*in control*) or incorrectly (*out of control*). It is important to recognize when an analyzer is not in control because results will be erroneous, causing incorrect patient management.

Decisions regarding quality control results are statistically based. Results that are within ±2 SDs are considered *in control*. A variety of sophisticated rules are used to determine if a result greater than 2 SDs requires further action. In general, a single result greater than 2 SDs is considered a wild error and no further action is required (Figure 5-21). However, if a shift in the mean occurs (Figure 5-22) an explanation is required. For example, a shift in quality control may have been the result of electrode maintenance.

Bias and Precision

Descriptive statistics can be used to determine the agreement between a new method and the traditionally accepted method. For example, a respiratory therapy department is considering the purchase of a new brand of pulse oximeter. Before the purchase decision is

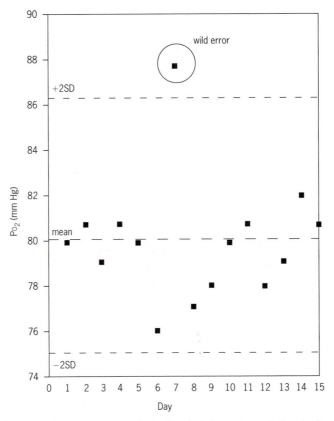

Figure 5-21 *Quality control record for a P_{O_2} electrode highlighting (encircled) a single result greater than 2 SDs from the mean. This single occurrence on day 7 is termed a* wild error, *or random error.*

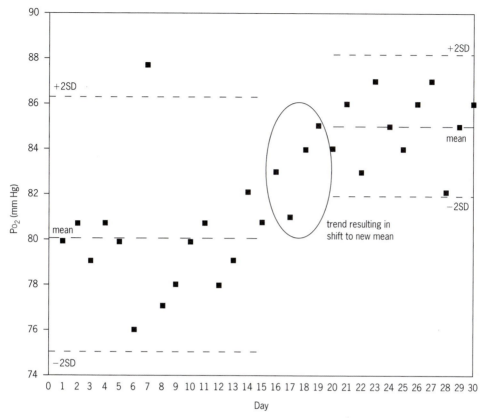

Figure 5-22 *Quality control record for a Po₂ electrode demonstrating a shift in the mean and highlighting (encircled) the trend (days 16 to 19) resulting in the shift to the new mean.*

made, it is important to know that the pulse oximeter saturation (SpO_2) agrees acceptably with the arterial saturation (SaO_2) measured from an arterial blood gas analyzed via a co-oximeter. It is decided to use the pulse oximeter for 50 consecutive patients who have an SpO_2 greater than 80% and who also are having an arterial blood gas determination. The difference between the SpO_2 and the SaO_2 is then determined for each data pair. The mean of these differences is called *bias* and the standard deviation of these differences is called *precision.* Assuming a normal distribution, 95% of the differences will fall within ±2 SDs of the bias. The range of ±2 SDs from the bias is called the *limits of agreement.* The limits of agreement are illustrated in Figure 5-23. The difference between saturations is plotted as a function of the average saturation determined by the two methods. The average is used because the true value is not known.

For this example, the mean difference (bias) is −0.4% and the standard deviation of the differences is 2.4%.

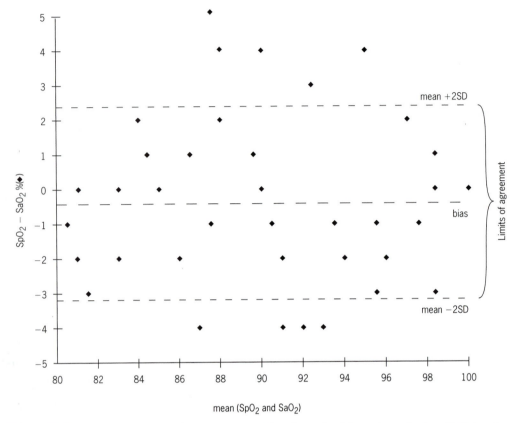

Figure 5-23 *Data representing the average saturation determined by pulse oximetry (SpO_2) and co-oximetry (SaO_2) are plotted against the difference between the saturations obtained by the two methods. The limits of agreement are demonstrated as the range of ± 2 SDs from the bias.*

The limits of agreement are then calculated as

$$-0.004 \pm 2(0.024)$$

$$= (-0.052, 0.044)$$

In other words, 95% of the differences will be between -0.052 and 0.044. The clinician will then need to decide whether or not this level of agreement is acceptable for clinical use of the pulse oximeter.

Normal Value Ranges

Descriptive statistics can be used to determine normal value ranges. Suppose that a respiratory care department wishes to determine the normal value range for the arterial Pco_2 in the community. A sample of 100 normal volunteers (all free of any pulmonary disease) agrees to have an arterial puncture to determine their arterial Pco_2. The mean arterial P_{CO_2} is found to be 40 mm Hg with a standard deviation of 2.5 mm Hg. When the frequency distribution of these arterial P_{CO_2} values is plotted, it appears to be nearly normal. Thus, 95% of the values fall within ±2 standard deviations of the mean, and the normal value range of arterial P_{CO_2} values for this population is 35 to 45 mm Hg (mean ± 2 SD).

Note that, by definition, 2.5% of *normal* persons will have an arterial P_{CO_2} greater than normal (i.e., >45 mm Hg) and another 2.5% of normal persons will have an arterial P_{CO_2} less than normal (i.e., <35 mm Hg). Thus, there is a 5% probability that a *normal* person will have an *abnormal* arterial P_{CO_2}. Also, note that changes within the normal range may be clinically important. For example, an arterial P_{CO_2} that increases from 35 mm Hg to 45 mm Hg in an acute asthmatic patient is clinically important (may indicate fatigue), although both values are within normal limits.

In the previous example, a two-tailed, normal value range was determined. In other words, the middle 95% of the distribution was chosen as normal, and the remaining 5% was chosen as abnormal (i.e., +2.5% and −2.5%). However, there are times when selecting this type of distribution would not make sense. Assume that arterial P_{O_2} values for the 100 normal persons in the previous example produced a mean of 95 mm Hg and a standard deviation of 12 mm Hg. It would not make sense to set the high limit of the range at two standard deviations (12 mm Hg + 12 mm Hg) above the mean because an arterial P_{O_2} of 119 mm Hg is not physiologically possible, breathing room air at sea level. In this case, a one-tailed distribution is used. The bottom 5% of the normal value range is eliminated, and the lower limit of normal is set at 1.64 standard deviations below the mean. With a standard deviation of 1.64 below the mean, the lower limit of normal for the arterial P_{O_2} range for this population becomes approximately 75 mm Hg. That is,

$$\text{\# of S.D.} \times \text{S.D.} = \text{difference between lower limit and mean}$$
$$1.64 \times 12 \text{ mm Hg} = 20 \text{ mm Hg}$$

so

$$95 \text{ mm Hg} - 20 \text{ mm Hg} = 75 \text{ mm Hg (lower limit of range)}$$

The upper limit of normal will be the highest physiologic arterial P_{O_2} value possible, as calculated from the alveolar air equation. In this example, an arterial P_{O_2} less than 75 mm Hg is abnormal (hypoxemia), and an arterial P_{O_2} higher than the upper limit of normal represents a laboratory error.

5-10 TESTING OF HYPOTHESIS FOR MEAN

Suppose that an investigator for the Environmental Protection Agency (EPA) wants to determine whether the mean level of certain types of pollutants released into the atmosphere by a chemical company meets the EPA guidelines. Three parts per million (ppm) is the upper limit allowed by the EPA, and the investigator wants to determine if the chemical company is releasing more than this level. Daily pollution measurements are collected. Since the company knows the EPA guidelines, the investigator assumes that the company is following the guidelines, unless there is evidence to suggest otherwise.

Therefore, the investigator has to assume a population mean (μ) of less than or equal to 3 ppm, unless it can be established that μ is greater than 3 ppm. Thus far, two references about the population mean, namely, a μ of less than or equal to 3 ppm and a μ greater than 3 ppm, have been made. These two references are termed the **null hypothesis** and the **alternate hypothesis,** respectively. An hypothesis is a statement about a parameter or distribution. Generally, data are collected to determine if there is support for a certain hypothesis. That hypothesis is termed the *alternate hypothesis.* The null hypothesis is either the status quo, or just the complement statement of the alternate hypothesis.

A jury trial of an accused murderer is analogous to hypothesis testing. In this example, the status quo in the American system of justice is innocence, which is assumed to be true until proved otherwise. Hence, the null hypothesis, denoted by the symbol H_o, is the assumed innocence of the accused. The alternate hypothesis, or *research hypothesis,* is accepted only when there is sufficient evidence to establish the guilt (i.e., reject the null hypothesis, or the assumed innocence). The alternate hypothesis is represented by the symbol H_a and states that the accused is guilty.

After establishment of the alternate hypothesis, the next step is to collect data to determine if H_o can be negated and H_a supported. For the jury trial example, the evidence in support of guilt is provided by the prosecution, and the jury is supposed to find the accused guilty only if the evidence supports the guilt beyond reasonable doubt. What is meant here is that, if the accused is innocent, then the chance of obtaining evidence to establish guilt must be very small. What is considered a small chance? This consideration depends on the problem. In this example a probability of 0.0001 may be chosen. In other words, there is 1 chance in 10,000 that the accused will be found guilty when in fact he is innocent. This degree of chance is to protect against wrongly convicting an innocent person.

No justice system is free of errors, regardless how small the chance of error may be. In any hypothesis testing, there are two types of errors, *Type I* and *Type II*. The Type I error is to reject H_o in favor of H_a when, in fact, H_o is true. This situation is similar to wrongly convicting an innocent man. The Type II error is to accept H_o when H_a is true. This circumstance is analogous to exonerating a guilty person. Table 5-2 illustrates the concept of correct decision and two types of errors.

TABLE 5-2

		ACTUAL SITUATION	
		PERSON IS NOT GUILTY	PERSON IS GUILTY
Court's Decision	Not Guilty Verdict	Correct Decision	Incorrect Decision: Type II error
	Guilty Verdict	Incorrect Decision: Type I error	Correct Decision

The chance of making a Type I error is represented by α and that of a Type II error is represented by β. Ideally, both α and β should be zero. This possibility exists only if the entire population is considered, in which case hypothesis testing is unnecessary. In reality, only a subset (sample) of the population is tested. Therefore, one can never be 100% certain of the decision that is made regarding the hypothesis. Controlling for Type I and Type II errors is possible. However, as one type of error is decreased, the other will increase unless the sample size is also increased. The only way to minimize both Type I and Type II errors is to increase the sample size. In practice, attempts are usually made to reduce the probability of a Type I error (α). A decision must be made about the value of α to make a decision about the hypothesis. It is required that the person making the decision should have some idea of how much error is allowed. Once the H_o and the H_a have been established and the data collected, evidence to support the H_a is sought.

Suppose that a mechanical ventilator is set to deliver a flow of 40 L/min. To determine if the ventilator is delivering less than 40 L/min, the inspiratory flow is measured for a random sample of 36 cycles with a mean of 39.5 L/min and a standard deviation of 0.9 L/min. In this example the null hypothesis (H_o) states the mean delivered flow (μ) is 40 L/min, and the alternate hypothesis (H_a) is that μ is less than 40 L/min. From these data can a μ of less than 40 L/min be concluded? Note that the sample mean is 39.5 L/min. Is this evidence, indicating that μ is less than 40 L/min, against H_o ($\mu = 40$) and in favor of H_a ($\mu < 40$) beyond reasonable doubt, or is it a result of sampling error (e.g., chance)? One must determine the chance of observing a sample mean of this size or smaller if in fact the population mean is 40 L/min. Remember that the smaller the sample mean, the stronger is the evidence supporting H_a ($\mu < 40$ L/min). According to the null hypothesis, the distribution of $\bar{x}$ is approximately normal (by the Central Limit Theorem, as n is large) with a mean and standard deviation of the distribution of $\bar{x}$ given by

$$\mu_{\bar{x}} = 40 \text{ and } \sigma_{\bar{x}} = \frac{s}{\sqrt{n}} = \frac{0.9}{\sqrt{36}} = 0.15$$

Therefore, the probability is $P(\bar{x} < 39.5) = P(z < -3.33) = 0.5 - 0.499 = 0.001$ (Appendix C, Table I). In other words, there is only a 1 in 1,000 chance of observing a sample mean of 39.5 L/min or less if the ventilator is operating accurately (i.e., delivering 40 L/min). The conclusion then is that the evidence, beyond reasonable doubt, exists supporting H_a, which states that the ventilator is delivering less than 40 L/min. The ventilator is delivering significantly less flow than that for which it is set.

The probability obtained (i.e., 0.001) is the p-value, or observed level of significance. Researchers routinely report p-values for their significant tests. When is it appropriate to state that a result is significant? If the p-value is small, then the evidence is strong against H_o and in favor of H_a. The null hypothesis (H_o) is rejected and, hence, the result is significant. Normally, a p-value of less than 0.05 is considered small enough for a result to be statistically significant. A p-value of less than 0.05 means that there is less than a 5% risk of rejecting H_o if it is true. The smaller the p-value, the stronger statistical significance of the result. The previous discussion should point out that when the p-value is smaller than α, H_o is rejected in favor of H_a. Therefore, the result is statistically significant.

Caution must be applied in distinguishing between statistical significance and clinical (practical) significance. Statistical significance can often be achieved by increasing the sample size, but the result may be insignificant in practice. In the example above, the difference between the measured flow (39.5 L/min) and the set flow on the ventilator (40 L/min) was significantly different (statistical significance). However, this difference probably is not clinically important. If the sample size is small, the t-distribution is used instead of the normal distribution. This substitution is justified by the fact that a t-distribution is almost the same as a z-distribution for a large n. Whenever n is small, the t-distribution is more appropriate than the z-distribution.

EXAMPLE:

The manufacturer of an over-the-counter pain relief medicine claims that its product relieves pain in less than 10 minutes. To make this claim in its advertising, the manufacturer is required by the FDA to show statistical evidence to support the claim. The manufacturer reports that a random sample of 40 people yielded a mean of 9.5 minutes and a standard deviation of 3 minutes. Is this evidence strong enough to allow this advertising claim?

Solution: Unless the manufacturer shows that the drug gives relief in less than 10 minutes, the FDA will assume that it takes at least 10 minutes for the drug to provide relief. Therefore, the status quo is that it takes at least 10 minutes, and the alternative is it takes less than 10 minutes (as the manufacturer has to establish). Thus,

$$H_o: \mu \geq 10 \text{ and } H_a: \mu < 10$$

The distribution of $\bar{x}$ (Figure 5-24) is normal because n is large. The distribution also has a mean ($\mu_{\bar{x}}$) of 10 minutes and an estimated standard error ($s/\sqrt{40}$) of 0.4743 (assuming that the null hypothesis is true). The shaded area in Figure 5-24 indicates the area (p-value) being determined. By using appropriate tables (Appendix C, Table I), the shaded area has a p-value equal to $0.5 - 0.3531$, or 0.1469 ($\approx 15\%$). If the drug takes a minimum of 10 minutes to give relief, there is about a 15% chance of observing a sample mean of 9.5 minutes or less. Therefore, the evidence against H_o is not overwhelming. Hence, there is insufficient evidence to believe the manufacturer's claim.

Traditionally, a decision about the level of significance (α) is made before conducting the experiment. In such cases, the following six-step procedure is used. However, both approaches yield the same decision and conclusions.

Steps for Testing of an Hypothesis	
Step 1	Set up H_o and H_a.
Step 2	Decide on an α.
Step 3	Obtain a test statistic.
Step 4	Define the rejection region via critical value based on α.
Step 5	Decide whether or not to reject H_o.
Step 6	State the conclusion.

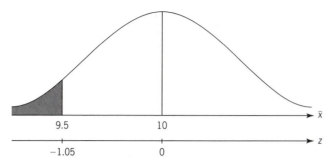

Figure 5-24 *A normal distribution curve with the shaded area representing the* p-value.

Steps 3 through 6 will be discussed for testing for the mean. The *test statistic* is the z-score of $\bar{x}$:

$$\text{test statistic} = \frac{\bar{x} - \mu_\text{o}}{s/\sqrt{n}}$$

The μ_o is the value of the parameter defined by H_o. To obtain μ_o among all the possible values of μ allowed under H_o, the closest value of μ allowed under H_a is chosen. For example, if $H_\text{o}: \mu \leq 6$ and $H_\text{a}: \mu > 6$, then under H_o the values of μ allowed are less than or equal to 6, and the values allowed under H_a are larger than 6. The closest value of μ is 6. Therefore, μ_o equals 6. The reason for choosing this value is that by rejecting H_o for this value of μ, H_o can be rejected for any value of μ that is further away (in this case, any value less than 6).

The rejection region is that part of the distribution curve where H_o is rejected when the observed mean resides in that region. Once again, consider $H_\text{o}: \mu \leq 6$ and $H_\text{a}: \mu > 6$. Here, the values of $\bar{x}$ that would contradict H_o and support H_a are the values that are larger than 6. How much larger depends on the amount of error allowed (i.e., α). The rejection region in this example is the hatched area in Figure 5-25. If α equals 0.05, the $z_{0.05}$ equals 1.645 (Figure 5-26). The rejection region is reject H_o if $\bar{x} > 6 + 1.645 \cdot s/\sqrt{n}$ or if the test statistic exceeds 1.645.

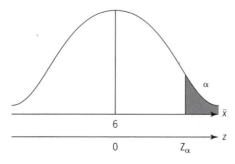

Figure 5-25 *Shaded area under the normal distribution curve represents the rejection region based on the value of* α.

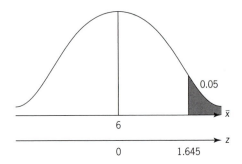

Figure 5-26 *Shaded area under the normal distribution curve has an α value of 0.05, which corresponds with a z-score of 1.645. H_o rejected if $\bar{x} > 6 + 1.645 \cdot \dfrac{s}{\sqrt{n}}$.*

Rejection Region for Large n

(i) $H_o: \mu \leq \mu_o$ versus $H_a: \mu > \mu_o$

Reject H_o if $\bar{x} > \mu_o + z_\alpha\left(\dfrac{s}{\sqrt{n}}\right)$

or, equivalently, if test statistics $> z_\alpha$

(ii) $H_o: \mu \geq \mu_o$ versus $H_a: \mu < \mu_o$

Reject H_o if $\bar{x} < \mu_o - z_{\frac{\alpha}{2}}\left(\dfrac{s}{\sqrt{n}}\right)$

or, equivalently, if test stat $< -z_\alpha$

(iii) $H_o: \mu = \mu_o$ versus $H_a: \mu \neq \mu_o$

Reject H_o if $\bar{x} > \mu_o + z_{\frac{\alpha}{2}}\left(\dfrac{s}{\sqrt{n}}\right)$

or if $\bar{x} < \mu_o - z_{\frac{\alpha}{2}}\left(\dfrac{s}{\sqrt{n}}\right)$

Equivalently, reject H_o if test stat $> +z_{\frac{\alpha}{2}}$
or if test stat $< -z_{\frac{\alpha}{2}}$

Rejection Region for Small n

Reject H_o if $\bar{x} > \mu_o + t_{\alpha,n-1}\left(\dfrac{s}{\sqrt{n}}\right)$.

or, equivalently, if test statistic $> t_{\alpha,n-1}$.
For different H_o and H_a the direction of rejection region
changes as in the large sample case above.

Note that t can be used for almost any sample size as long as the distribution of the observations is not too skewed. Because of the limitation of the availability of t-tables for all sample sizes, z is used if n is large. If you are using statistical software, this concern is meaningless because most types of software automatically use the t-distribution.

Two approaches to hypothesis testing have been provided here. Most researchers simply report the p-value, which is basically the least amount of α required to reject H_o. By reporting the p-value, the reader is given an opportunity to decide about the statistical significance of the result. If the p-value is relatively small (< 0.05), the result is usually reported as statistically significant.

PRACTICE PROBLEMS

Refer to Appendix A (pages 618-619) for the solutions and answers to the practice problems.

13. Studies at a hospital have indicated that the average number of hours of staff time spent per day performing non-emergency chores is 16 person-hours. It is suspected that the time spent on emergency-related chores has increased significantly because of the increase in the crime rate. To determine support for this suspicion, hospital management selected a random sample of 40 days and determined that the mean and standard deviation were 18 person-hours per day and 6 person-hours per day, respectively.

    a. Do the data support the suspicion? Test using an α of 0.01.

    b. Find and interpret the p-value.

14. Because of the development of new techniques and the increase in cost, the average stay in the hospital by a lung cancer patient is believed to be significantly less than three months. To determine if this notion is true, a survey was conducted. A random sample of 26 lung cancer patients was selected. The mean ($\bar{x}$) and standard deviation (s) were 2.1 months and 1.5 months, respectively.

    a. Using an α of 0.001, conduct a test of the hypothesis to determine if the data support the claim.

    b. Find and interpret the approximate p-value. (Note: You will only be able to give limits for the p-value.)

15. A psychologist interested in determining whether male heroin addicts' assessment of self-worth differs from that of the general male population conducted an experiment using 25 randomly selected heroin addicts. The mean and standard deviation for this sample were found to be 44 and 8, respectively. Do these data support the assertion that male heroin addicts' self-worth assessment mean score is different from that of the general male population mean score of 48.6? Use an α of 0.05.

5-11 COMPARING MEANS OF TWO POPULATIONS (OR GROUPS): INDEPENDENT SAMPLES

It is often necessary to conduct a controlled study to decide whether a treatment is effective. Subjects in a control group do not receive the treatment. Subjects in the treatment, or experimental, group receive the treatment. It is often advisable to conduct a double-blind experiment where neither the subjects nor the investigators know which group is the treatment or the control. A double-blind experiment protects against bias. One important aspect in such studies is that the control group should be as similar as possible to the treatment group except for the treatment itself. This aspect ensures that differences in response are likely to be the effect of the treatment and not the result of any other confounding variable.

Sometimes two treatments need to be compared. In such a case, patients are assigned to two treatment groups. These patients are studied and their responses to the treatment recorded. The quantitative bases for "treatment versus control" and for comparing "two treatments" is the same, but they differ in design and interpretation.

Confidence Intervals for the Difference of Means

$$(\bar{x}_1 - \bar{x}_2) \pm t_{\frac{\alpha}{2},(n_1+n_2-2)}\sqrt{s_p^2\left(\frac{1}{n_1} + \frac{1}{n_2}\right)}$$

The notations here are defined in the next box.

The six-step procedure described earlier is followed, but the formulas for the hypotheses and the test statistic are different and are illustrated in the following box.

Steps for Testing Hypotheses Concerning Treatment Versus Control or Two Treatments

Step 1: $H_o: \mu_1 = \mu_2$, $H_a: \mu_1 \neq \mu_2$

Step 2: Decide on an α.

Step 3: Test statistic: $\dfrac{\bar{x}_1 - \bar{x}_2}{\sqrt{s_p^2\left(\frac{1}{n_1} + \frac{1}{n_2}\right)}}$ where $s_p^2 = \dfrac{(n_1 - 1)s_1^2 + (n_2 - 1)s_2^2}{n_1 + n_2 - 2}$

n_1, $\bar{x}_1$, and s_1^2 are sample size, sample mean, and sample variance, respectively, for the control (or the first treatment) sample and, similarly, n_2, $\bar{x}_2$, and s_2^2 are for the second sample.

Step 4: Rejection Region: Reject H_o if test stat $> t_{\frac{\alpha}{2},(n_1+n_2-2)}$ or if test stat $< -t_{\frac{\alpha}{2},(n_1+n_2-2)}$ where $t_{\frac{\alpha}{2},(n_1+n_2-2)}$ is the upper tail percentile of the t-distribution with $(n_1 + n_2 - 2)$ d.f.

Step 5: Decide whether or not to reject H_o.

Step 6: Write the conclusion.

Note: H_a could be one-sided, then rejection region changes accordingly as before.

Two assumptions are made. First, observations from one population have no effect on the observations from the other population. Second, population variances are equal (i.e., $\sigma_1^2 = \sigma_2^2$). If these assumptions are not satisfied, alternative procedures are used. If the first assumption is not satisfied because of the pairing (or matching) of the observations, a paired t-test can be used. However, if the second assumption is not satisfied, a non-parametric test must be used. Statistical software will report the p-value. In the event an α value is determined, compare it with the p-value to make a decision. Reject H_o if p-value is less than α; otherwise, do not reject H_o.

EXAMPLE 1:

A recent study compared a traditional approach to teaching basic respiratory therapy skills with an innovative approach. Students ($n = 42$) enrolled in a respiratory care program participated in the study. Half of the students weve randomly assigned to labs that used the innovative approach. The scores (10 questions) from the two groups were compared. One of the questions concerned the use of a stethoscope. The mean scores for the two groups were 2.55 (traditional) and 3.60 (innovative). A higher score is an indication of having attained better basic respiratory care skills. Suppose that the sample variances were 1.7230 and 2.22, respectively. Test the hypothesis that the innovative approach helps achieve better basic respiratory care skills. Let μ_1 and μ_2 represent the mean scores of the innovative and traditional approaches, respectively.

Step 1: Set up H_o and H_a.

H_o: $\mu_1 \leq \mu_2$ (innovative approach is as good or worse than the traditional approach).

H_a: $\mu_1 > \mu_2$ (innovative approach is better than the traditional approach).

Step 2: Use an α of 0.05.

Step 3: Since n_1 and n_2 are small (21 each), use the t-test statistic.

$$\text{test statistic} = \frac{\bar{x}_1 - \bar{x}_2}{\sqrt{s_p^2\left(\frac{1}{n_1} + \frac{1}{n_2}\right)}}$$

Determine s_p^2.

$$s_p^2 = \frac{(n_1 - 1)s_1^2 + (n_2 - 1)s_2^2}{n_1 + n_2 - 2} = \frac{(20 \times 1.7230) + (20 \times 2.22)}{21 + 21 - 2} = 1.9715$$

Thus,

$$\text{test statistic} = \frac{3.60 - 2.55}{\sqrt{1.9715\left(\frac{1}{21} + \frac{1}{21}\right)}} = 2.423$$

Step 4: Define the rejection region via critical value based on α of 0.05.

The d.f. $= n_1 + n_2 - 2 = 21 + 21 - 2 = 40$. If the decision is to use an α of 0.05, the rejection region is reject H_o if test stat $> t_{\alpha,n_1+n_2-2} = 1.684$.

Step 5: Because the test statistic is larger than 1.684, reject H_o in favor of H_a.

Step 6: The *p*-value is 0.01. Therefore, an α value as low as 0.01 can be used and still be in agreement with the conclusion that the innovative approach is better than the traditional approach.

EXAMPLE 2:

Suppose $n_1 = 15$, $\bar{x}_1 = 19.2$, $s_1 = 1.7$, $n_2 = 20$, $\bar{x}_2 = 18.5$, and $s_2 = 1.2$.

a) Test H_o: $\mu_1 = \mu_2$ versus H_a: $\mu_1 > \mu_2$

Step 1: Use an α of 0.05.

Use the *t*-distribution because sample size is small (most types of statistical software use *t*-distribution regardless of the sample size).

Step 2: Calculate the test statistic.

$$\text{test statistic} = \frac{\bar{x}_1 - \bar{x}_2}{\sqrt{s_p^2\left(\frac{1}{n_1} + \frac{1}{n_2}\right)}}$$

$$\bar{x}_1 - \bar{x}_2 = 19.2 - 18.5 = 0.7$$

$$\text{d.f.} = n_1 + n_2 - 2 = 33.$$

$$s_p^2 = \text{pooled variance estimate} = \frac{(n_1 - 1)s_1^2 + (n_2 - 1)s_2^2}{n_1 + n_2 - 2} = \frac{(15 - 1)1.7^2 + (20 - 1)1.2^2}{15 + 20 - 2} = 2.055$$

$$\text{test statistic} = 1.43$$

Step 3: Define the rejection region.

Rejection region: Reject H_o if test stat $> t_{0.05,33} = 1.310$ (approximately).

Step 4: Because the test statistic is larger than 1.310, reject H_o in favor of H_a.

Step 5: Conclusion: Sufficient evidence exists to conclude that the population mean μ_1 is significantly larger than the population mean μ_2.

b) Construct a 90% confidence interval for $\mu_1 - \mu_2$.

Solution: Use the formula

$$(\bar{x}_1 - \bar{x}_2) \pm t_{\frac{\alpha}{2}, n_1 + n_2 - 2}\sqrt{s_p^2\left(\frac{1}{n_1} + \frac{1}{n_2}\right)}$$

Substitute: $0.7 \pm 1.310 \times 0.4896 = 0.7 \pm 0.6414 = (0.0586, 1.3414)$.

Interpretation: There is 95% confidence that the true mean difference between μ_1 and μ_2 is included in the interval (0.059, 1.34). Because the interval is only on the positive side, the conclusion is that μ_1 is significantly larger than μ_2.

PRACTICE PROBLEMS

Refer to Appendix A (pages 619-621) for the solutions and answers to the practice problems.

16. To examine the relationship between the intensity of parental punishment practices and various demographic characteristics of mothers, researchers selected a random sample of mothers and studied their punishment practices. One of the characteristics studied was marital status, i.e., single mothers versus separated mothers. The following data were obtained on parental punishment (higher score indicates greater intensity of punishment).

	Single mothers	Separated mothers
n	8	6
$\bar{x}$	70.75	77.33
s	14.80	13.69

   a. Using a 90% confidence interval for the difference between the mean intensity of parental punishments for the single and separated mothers, indicate whether there is a statistically significant difference between the two.

   b. Conduct a test H_o: $\mu_1 = \mu_2$ versus H_a: $\mu_1 \neq \mu_2$. Use an α of 0.10 and interpret the findings.

   c. Will the conclusions of (a) and (b) be the same? Explain.

17. In a heart surgery study, an investigational issue was the effect of drugs called beta-blockers on the pulse rate of patients during surgery. Researchers selected 42 patients and divided them into two groups of 21. One group received a beta-blocker, the other a placebo. The pulse rate of each patient at a critical point during the surgery was recorded. The treatment group had a mean of 65.2 beats per minute and a standard deviation of 7.8 beats per minute. The control group had a mean and standard deviation of 70.3 beats/minute and 8.3 beats/minute, respectively.

   a. Is there sufficient evidence to conclude that beta-blockers reduce the pulse rate during surgery? Use an α of 0.05.

   b. Construct a 95% confidence interval for the difference in the mean heart rates and interpret the findings.

18. An experiment was conducted to compare the mean number of study hours expended per week by students in a respiratory care program to that of students in a physical therapy program. A random sample of 25 students from each group yielded the following data:

	Respiratory care	Physical therapy
$\bar{x}$	25.5 hr/wk	24.2 hr/wk
s	4.5 hr/wk	5.3 hr/wk
n	25	25

a. Construct and interpret a 95% confidence interval for the difference between the mean number of study hours.

b. Is there enough evidence to conclude that students in the respiratory care program study significantly more than those in the physical therapy program? Use an α of 0.01.

5-12 COMPARISON OF MEANS FOR PAIRED (OR DEPENDENT) SAMPLES

An experiment was conducted to study the efficacy of normal saline instillation of endotracheal suctioning. Ten (10) ICU patients were selected. Each patient was suctioned either with or without saline instillation. At least 90 minutes elapsed between suctioning events. To eliminate any effect caused by the sequence of the type of suctioning performed, five randomly selected patients were suctioned with saline instillation first, and then at least 90 minutes later these five were suctioned without saline instillation. The remaining five patients were suctioned with no saline instillation first, followed 90 minutes later by suctioning with saline instillation. The purpose of the study was to compare the amount of secretions obtained from the two suctioning methods. Data are presented below for mass (grams) obtained with both methods.

Patient (n)	1	2	3	4	5	6	7	8	9	10
saline instillation (grams)	5.0	5.0	3.5	3.0	4.0	6.0	3.5	5.0	4.0	3.0
no saline instillation (grams)	0.5	1.0	2.0	1.5	2.0	4.0	1.0	1.5	0.5	1.0

A two-sample t-test should not be used. One of the assumptions for using the two-sample t-test is that the observations from one sample (or population) should have no effect on the observations from the other. Here this assumption is not satisfied because the observations are patient dependent. Each pair of observations (with and without saline instillation) is based on a particular patient. Hence, the observations (in a particular pair) are dependent on each other. This type of study is described as a *paired difference experiment*. The amount of secretions suctioned by a particular method is not a concern; rather the difference in the amount of secretions suctioned is the issue. If a patient has copious secretions, both suctioning methods will yield high values. Similarly, both methods will produce low values if a patient has few secretions.

Because only the difference between the pairs is of interest, the differences are calculated.

Patient (n)	1	2	3	4	5	6	7	8	9	10
Difference between saline and no saline instillation (grams)	4.5	4.0	1.5	1.5	2.0	2.0	2.5	3.5	3.5	2.0

These differences are treated as a random sample. The hypotheses are $H_o: \mu_D = 0.0$ (there is no difference between the two suctioning methods) and $H_a: \mu_D > 0.0$ (suctioning with saline instillation results in the removal of more secretions). If the differences were obtained in the reverse order, then the hypotheses would have to be adjusted accordingly. Thus, $H_o: \mu_D = 0$ and $H_a: \mu_D < 0$. However, reversing the order will not change the conclusion.

The first step in testing the hypothesis is to calculate the mean of the differences ($\bar{x}_D = 2.8$ grams) and the standard deviation of the differences ($s_D = 1.0593$ grams). Then perform a one-sample t-test:

$$\text{test statistic} = \frac{\bar{x}_D}{s_D/\sqrt{n}} = \frac{2.8}{1.0593/\sqrt{10}} = 8.36$$

Reject H_o if test statistic $> t_{\alpha,n-1} = t_{0.05,9} = 1.833$. Therefore, H_o is rejected and the conclusion is that the amount of secretions is significantly higher with saline instillation. A standard α of 0.05 is used. It is appropriate to report the exact p-value as it will demonstrate the strength of the significance. In this case the p-value is 0.000008. Also, confidence intervals for μ_D can be constructed using the formula

$$\bar{x}_D \pm t_{\frac{\alpha}{2},n-1} \times \frac{s_D}{\sqrt{n}}$$

For the example above, a 95% confidence interval for μ_D is given by first calculating

$$t_{0.025,9} = 2.262 \text{ (Table II, Appendix C)}$$

and

$$\frac{s_D}{\sqrt{n}} = \frac{1.0593}{\sqrt{10}} = 0.335$$

The confidence interval, therefore, is

$$2.8 \pm 2.262 \times 0.335 = 2.8 \pm 0.7578 = (2.0422, 3.5578)$$

Interpretation: We are 95% confident that the true mean difference in the amount of secretions with and without saline instillation is included in the interval (2.04 g, 3.56 g). More secretions, 3.56 grams, are suctioned with saline instillation than without saline instillation.

PRACTICE PROBLEMS

Refer to Appendix A (pages 621-622) for the solutions and answers to the practice problems.

19. The forced expiratory volume in one second (FEV_1) is a standard pulmonary function measurement obtained from spirometry. It is expected that after 20 years of age pulmonary function measurements reflect a decline in a person's pulmonary function performance. To test this hypothesis, 10 nonsmoking females ranging in age from 35–40 years, with heights 64–68 inches were selected. Their FEV_1 values (liter) were measured and then obtained again two years later. The data are given below.

Person (n)	1	2	3	4	5	6	7	8	9	10
FEV_1 (initial)	3.22	4.06	3.85	3.50	2.80	3.25	4.20	3.05	2.86	3.50
FEV_1 (after 2 yrs)	2.95	4.75	4.00	3.42	2.77	3.20	3.90	2.76	2.75	3.32

a. Test the hypothesis that the true mean FEV_1 decreases for the females in the age and height group considered. Use an α of 0.05.

    b. Using a 95% confidence interval, estimate the true mean decrease in the FEV_1 after two years.

20. A hospital is testing the effectiveness of a new drug that is purported to reduce serum cholesterol. A random sample of people identified as having a high serum cholesterol level is selected. After their cholesterol levels are measured, they are prescribed the new drug for three months. The serum cholesterol level is measured at the end of the third month. The data are as follows:

Patient (n)	1	2	3	4	5	6	7	8
Serum cholesterol level before drug (mg/dl)	255	290	281	269	310	291	276	289
Serum cholesterol level after drug (mg/dl)	232	245	276	270	250	241	210	262

    a. Do the data support the theory that the new drug reduces the mean cholesterol level? Test using an α of 0.01.

    b. Construct a 95% confidence interval for the true mean difference in the serum cholesterol level before and after the drug was administered.

5-13 INFERENCES FOR PROPORTIONS OR PERCENTAGES

Sometimes what is of interest is the proportion of success or the chance of an event happening. The following problem concerning the funding of student loan programs will exemplify this concept. Although there are many student loan programs, funds for these programs are being depleted. This situation is caused by a substantially declining return rate (i.e., proportion of students returning the money). This problem has adversely affected banks and the government. Approximately 50% of student loans guaranteed by the government are in default. A random sample of 400 student loans were selected from a particular region of the country. Of these, 232 loans were in default. What inferences can be drawn from these data? What do these data reflect concerning the true rate of defaults (P)?

A point estimate of P can be obtained by calculating the sample default rate ($\hat{P}$) as follows:

$$\left(\begin{array}{c} \text{number of} \\ \text{loans defaulted} \end{array} \right) \div \left(\begin{array}{c} \text{number of} \\ \text{loans selected} \end{array} \right) = \left(\begin{array}{c} \text{sample proportion of} \\ \text{the loans that are defaulted} \end{array} \right)$$

$$232 \text{ loans} \quad \div \quad 400 \text{ loans} \quad = \quad 0.58, \text{ or } 58\%$$

Using the formula below, confidence intervals for P can be constructed to obtain information about the accuracy of the estimate:

$$\text{confidence interval for } P: \hat{P} \pm z_{\frac{\alpha}{2}} \sqrt{\frac{\hat{P}(1 - \hat{P})}{n}}$$

A test conducted to make a decision about the true proportion P is shown below. Notice that the steps are similar to those used for testing the mean.

Step 1: Write the hypotheses (one- or two-sided). For example, $H_o: P = P_o$ versus $H_a: P > P_o$.

Step 2: Calculate the test statistic.

$$\frac{\hat{P} - P_o}{\sqrt{\dfrac{P_o(1 - P_o)}{n}}}$$

Step 3: Write the rejection region exactly as in the case of the mean. For example, reject H_o if the test statistic $> z_\alpha$ (for the one-sided, upper tail test).

Step 4: Decide to reject or not to reject H_o.

Step 5: Write the conclusion in terms of the problem.

Step 6: Report and interpret the *p*-value.

The steps given here are for the purpose of performing the calculations and understanding the principles. The hypotheses and the *p*-value are generally reported and followed by comments regrading the statistical significance of the results.

Example 1:

Consider the student loan problem discussed above.

a) Construct a 95% confidence interval for the true rate of defaults.

Solution: As calculated earlier, $\hat{P} = 0.58$. Also, $z_{0.025} = 1.96$.

$$0.58 \pm 1.96 \sqrt{\frac{0.58(1 - 0.58)}{400}} = 0.58 \pm 0.048$$

The true rate of college student loan defaults is estimated to be 58%. With 95% confidence this estimate has a margin of error of $\pm 4.8\%$. In other words, there is 95% confidence that the true rate of defaults is between 53.2% and 62.8%.

b) Test the hypothesis that the true rate of defaults for the considered region is different from the national default rate of 50%. Use a level of significance of 5%.

Solution: Hypotheses: $H_o: P = 50\%$ versus $H_a: P \neq 50\%$.

$$\text{test statistic:} \quad \frac{0.58 - 0.50}{\sqrt{\dfrac{0.5(1 - 0.5)}{400}}} = 3.2$$

Rejection region: Reject H_o either if test statistic < -1.96 (i.e., $z_{0.025}$) or if test statistic > -1.96. Decision: Reject H_o in favor of H_a and conclude that the true rate of defaults for this region of the country is significantly different from the national default rate at an α of 0.5. The *p*-value is < 0.002. At a level of significance of 0.002, it can be concluded that this region of the country has a significantly different rate of defaults than the national rate. Note that the smaller the *p*-value, the more statistically significant is the result. A statistically significant result usually means rejecting H_o and accepting H_a.

For the example above, before selecting the sample of loans, suppose one wanted to know how many loans must be selected with 95% certainty that the error of estimation does not exceed a certain amount, e.g., 3%. This problem is a sample size determination problem similar to the one discussed for the case of estimating the mean. The formula used is

$$n = \left[\frac{z_{\frac{\alpha}{2}} \times \sqrt{P(1-P)}}{B} \right]^2$$

where

B = the error (or bound) of estimation by confidence interval*

P = the true proportion.

*E = margin of error (E can be used in place of β.)

The formula would therefore be:

$$n = \left[\frac{z_{\frac{\alpha}{2}} \times \sqrt{P(1-P)}}{E} \right]^2$$

If there is some knowledge of an approximate value of P from the previous studies, then use that value of P in the formula. In the absence of this knowledge, a P of 0.5 can be used to provide a conservative estimate of n. A P of 0.5 provides the largest possible sample size required to meet the conditions of confidence and the error. If the true value of P is different from 0.5, many more observations than needed will be made, whereas if P is close to 0.5, the sample size will be sufficient.

For the student loan problem, the national default rate is known to be 50%. Therefore, a P of 0.5 is used. If a 95% confidence is sought, $z_{0.025} = 1.96$. Also, if an error of 5% is targeted, then B equals 0.05. Thus,

$$n = \left[\frac{1.96 \sqrt{(0.5(1-0.5))}}{0.05} \right]^2 = 385$$

At least 385 students loans must be selected to estimate the true default rate correct to within 5% with 95% certainty. This number is slightly less than 400 which was selected. This discrepancy occurred because we chose a higher margin of error. If we chose the margin of error to be 4.8%, then the formula above will give $n = 417$, which is larger than 400. This is because the value of $P = 0.5$ used in our formula leads to conservative (larger) values of n. If we had a better idea of the true P, then that should be used instead of the conservative $P = 0.5$. If a sample size cannot be achieved, any or all of the following three manipulations can be applied: (1) choose a lower confidence level, e.g., 90%; (2) select a higher error rate, e.g., 6% or 7%; or (3) conduct a pilot study to get an idea about the true P. These efforts will reduce the sample size required.

EXAMPLE 2:

It is hypothesized that regular aerobic exercise is an effective preventative measure against cardiovascular fatalities. To substantiate this claim, a sample of 1,260 males, age 40 to 60 years, who jog at least 10 miles per week are selected in the study. It is found that after 3 years 80 of them had died because of cardiovascular disease. It is known that the death rate for the general male population in the age group 40 to 60 years is 9.5%.

a) Construct and interpret a 99% confidence interval for the death rate for 40- to 60-year-old males who jog at least 10 miles per week. Use the formula

$$\hat{P} \pm z_{\frac{\alpha}{2}} \sqrt{\frac{\hat{P}(1 - \hat{P})}{n}}$$

Solution: Here, $\hat{P}$ is the sample death rate (or proportion) of the 40- to 60-year-old male population who jog at least 10 miles per week. It also represents the number of males who died divided by the total number of males selected. That is,

$$80 \div 1,260 = 0.064, \text{ or } 6.4\%$$

Also, when α equals 0.01, $\alpha/2$ is 0.005. Therefore, $z_{0.005} = 2.575$.
Substitute these values into the formula.

$$0.064 \pm 2.575 \sqrt{\frac{0.064(1 - 0.064)}{1260}} = 0.064 \pm 0.018 = (0.046, 0.082)$$

The true death rate for male 10-mile/week joggers in the age group of 40 to 60 years is estimated at 6.4%. This estimate has a margin of error of ±1.8%. In other words, it is with 99% confidence that the true death rate is between 4.6% to 8.2%.

b) By constructing an appropriate hypothesis, indicate whether the data provide sufficient support to substantiate the claim. Use an α of 0.005. Hypotheses: $H_o: P \geq 0.095$ (death rate is the same or worse for males who jog compared to the general male population in the age group 40–60) versus $H_a: P < 0.095$ (death rate is smaller for the males who jog).

$$\text{test statistic: } \frac{\hat{P} - P_o}{\sqrt{\frac{P_o(1 - P_o)}{n}}} = \frac{0.064 - 0.095}{\sqrt{\frac{0.095(1 - 0.095)}{1,260}}} = -3.75$$

Rejection region: Reject H_o if test statistic $< -z_{0.005} = -2.575$. Because the test statistic falls in the rejection region, H_o is rejected in favor of H_a. The data provide sufficient evidence to believe that jogging at least 10 miles per week does reduce the death rate from cardiovascular disease in the male population between 40 and 60 years of age.

PRACTICE PROBLEMS

Refer to Appendix A (pages 622-623) for the solutions and answers to the practice problems.

21. Smokers recognized as being at risk for heart disease are persuaded to quit smoking. In this study, 62 smokers were persuaded to quit. After one year, 29 of them had started smoking again. The proportion of ex-smokers who start smoking again is termed the *recidivism rate*.

    a. Construct a 95% confidence interval for the recidivism rate. Interpret the findings.

    b. This part of the program will receive continued funding only if the program is able to demonstrate that the recidivism rate is significantly less than 50%. Is there sufficient evidence for continued funding? Conduct a test using an α of 0.05.

22. Researchers in cancer therapy often report only the number of patients who survive for a specified time after treatment rather than the patients' actual survival times. Suppose that 25% of the patients who undergo the standard treatment are known to survive five years. Doctors claim that a new therapy will significantly increase the proportion of people surviving five years. To substantiate this claim, they administered the new treatment to 162 patients and found that 56 of them are still alive after a period of five years.

    a. Do the data provide sufficient evidence for the doctors' claim? Use an α of 0.001.

    b. Find and interpret the *p*-value.

5-14 TWO-SAMPLE INFERENCES FOR PROPORTIONS

Let P_1 and P_2 denote the true proportions for the two populations of interest, and let $\hat{P}_1$ and $\hat{P}_2$ denote the corresponding sample proportions. The confidence intervals for the difference of proportions is

$$\hat{P}_1 - \hat{P}_2 \pm z_{\frac{\alpha}{2}}\sqrt{\frac{\hat{P}_1(1 - \hat{P}_1)}{n_1} + \frac{\hat{P}_2(1 - \hat{P}_2)}{n_2}}$$

A test of the hypotheses for the difference of the proportions can be conducted. The steps involved are outlined below.

Step 1: Write the hypotheses (one-sided or two-sided). For example, H_o: $P_1 = P_2$ versus H_a: $P_1 > P_2$.

Step 2: Calculate the test statistic.

$$\frac{\hat{P}_1 - \hat{P}_2}{\sqrt{\hat{P}(1 - \hat{P})\left(\frac{1}{n_1} + \frac{1}{n_2}\right)}}$$

where $\hat{P}$ = overall sample proportion = $(x_1 + x_2)/(n_1 + n_2)$.

Step 3: Write the rejection region exactly as in the mean case. For example, reject H_o if the test statistic $>z_\alpha$ (for the one-sided, upper tail test).

Step 4: Make the decision about the rejection or non-rejection of H_o.

Step 5: Write the conclusion in terms of the problem.

Step 6: Report and interpret the *p*-value.

EXAMPLE:

Is cocaine deadlier than heroin? To answer this question, a study was conducted on rats. It was found that rats with unlimited access to cocaine had poorer health, had more behavior disturbances, and died at a higher rate than did a corresponding group of rats given unlimited access to heroin. The death rates after 30 days were as follows:

	# of rats in study	# of dead rats at 30 days
Cocaine-fed rats	100	90
Heroin-fed rats	100	36

a) Construct and interpret a 95% confidence interval for the difference in the death rates.

Solution: $\hat{P}_1 = 0.90$ and $\hat{P}_2 = 0.36$ and $z_{0.025} = 1.96$.

Substitute values into the appropriate C.I. formula.

$$(0.90 - 0.36) \pm 1.96\sqrt{\frac{0.9(1 - 0.9)}{100} + \frac{0.36(1 - 0.36)}{100}} = 0.54 \pm 0.1109$$

Interpretation: We estimate that the true death rate for cocaine-fed rats is 54% higher than that for the heroin-fed rats. With 95% certainty this estimate has a margin of error of $\pm 11.09\%$.

b) Do the data provide sufficient evidence to believe that cocaine is more deadly? Use an α of 0.025. Hypotheses: H_o: $P_1 = P_2$ versus H_a: $P_1 > P_2$.

Solution: Calculate the overall sample proportion and the test statistic.

$$\hat{P} = (90 + 36)/(100 + 100) = 0.63$$

$$\text{test statistic:} \quad \frac{0.9 - 0.36}{\sqrt{0.63(1 - 0.63)\left(\frac{1}{100} + \frac{1}{100}\right)}} = 7.9$$

Because the test statistic is large, the conclusion is that there is highly significant evidence to believe that the cocaine is far more deadly than the heroin. The *p*-value for this will be almost zero.

PRACTICE PROBLEMS

Refer to Appendix A (pages 623-624) for the solutions and answers to the practice problems.

23. An article entitled "New Stance Taken on Blood Cholesterol" stated that 10,000 patients have been treated surgically and 10,000 comparable patients have been treated medically. Five years later, 91% of the surgical patients are alive and 90% of the medical patients are alive.

    a. Construct a 95% confidence interval for the difference in the proportions and interpret your findings.

    b. Do the data provide enough evidence to suggest that the two methods are different? Use an α of 0.05. Interpret the findings based on the difference between statistical and practical significance. (This is an example where the difference between statistical significance and practical significance may become apparent. It should be noted that by taking large sample sizes one can make the smallest differences appear statistically significant; however, those differences may not have a practical significance.)

5-15 TESTS FOR MANY POPULATION MEANS

When there are more than two independent treatment (or population) means to be compared, the concepts above can be extended, but the mathematical formulas become more complicated. The hypotheses to be tested would be

$$H_o: \text{all means are equal}$$
$$H_a: \text{at least two means are different.}$$

A procedure called Analysis of Variance (ANOVA) is used to test such hypotheses. Most statistical software packages are capable of performing ANOVA and reporting a *p*-value. The decision and interpretation of the *p*-value are similar to the ones explained in the previous sections. This design, where there are several independent population means to be compared, is termed a *one-way* ANOVA, or Completely Randomized Design (CRD).

5-16 CORRELATION AND REGRESSION

Suppose the relationship between smoking and lung capacity is to be studied. Lung capacity is the dependent variable of interest. Generally, the variable of interest is termed the *response variable,* or *dependent variable.* Lung capacity may depend on smoking, which is the *independent variable.* If the purpose of the study is to determine the effect smoking has on lung capacity and to measure the strength of the association between the two variables, then the correlation (defined later in this chapter) between the two variables needs to be calculated. On the other hand, if the lung capacity of a person is to be predicted, based on the length of time a person has been smoking, then a mathematical relationship between the two variables via regression analysis will be established. Regression analysis is used to establish the relationship between the dependent and independent variables.

The discussion of regression analysis will be limited here to involve only the study of a linear relationship between one dependent and a single independent variable. This type of regression analysis is termed *simple linear regression*. A simple linear regression model is given by the formula

$$y = \beta_0 + \beta_1 x + \text{Error}$$

where

y = dependent variable

x = independent variable

Error = chance variable

β_0 = y-intercept

β_1 = slope of the linear equation

If length of time a person has been smoking (x) exactly determines the lung capacity (y), then the model above would not have the Error term. Also, β_0 and β_1 would be exactly determined. However, even though x may play a significant role in determining y, there are other variables, such as genetics, which cannot be accounted for. Therefore, a chance variable (Error) is needed to represent such unaccountable variables. For the model above, there are observations (data) on y for various values of x, for which the parameters β_0 and β_1 are sought (estimated) to predict a value of y (or mean of y) for a given value of x with a certain degree of accuracy.

Least Squares Estimators of β_0 and β_1

$$\hat{\beta}_1 = \frac{SS_{xy}}{SS_{xx}}, \qquad \hat{\beta}_0 = \bar{y} - \hat{\beta}_1 \bar{x}$$

where

$$SS_{xy} = \Sigma xy - \frac{(\Sigma x)(\Sigma y)}{n}$$

$$SS_{xx} = \Sigma x^2 - \frac{(\Sigma x)^2}{n}$$

$$\bar{y} = \frac{\Sigma y}{n}$$

$$\bar{x} = \frac{\Sigma x}{n}$$

n = number of observations

SS = sum of squares

SS_{xx} = sum of squares of x

SS_{xy} = sum of squares of xy product

Least squares model: $\hat{y} = \hat{\beta}_0 + \hat{\beta}_1 x$

The *least squares method* is used to estimate the parameters β_0 and β_1 such that the error sum of squares (i.e., the sum of squared differences between the actual values of y and the predicted values of y) is minimum. The least squares estimators are obtained by the formulas in the box above.

EXAMPLE 1:

Consider the lung capacity example discussed above. Suppose the independent variable is the number of years a person has smoked and the dependent variable is the patient's lung capacity measured on a scale of 0% to 100%. Data for five randomly selected patients are listed below.

Patients (n)	Number of years of smoking (x)	Lung capacity (y)
1	10	75
2	25	30
3	17	45
4	12	58
5	16	47

Obtain the least squares estimates, write the least squares model, and interpret the parameter estimates.

Step 1: Calculate SS_{xy} and SS_{xx}.

$$\Sigma x = 10 + 25 + 17 + 12 + 16 = 80$$

$$\Sigma y = 75 + 30 + 45 + 58 + 47 = 255$$

$$\Sigma xy = (10 \times 75) + (25 \times 30) + (17 \times 45) + (12 \times 58) + (16 \times 47) = 3{,}713$$

$$\Sigma x^2 = 10^2 + 25^2 + 17^2 + 12^2 + 16^2 = 1{,}414$$

$$SS_{xy} = \Sigma xy - \frac{(\Sigma x)(\Sigma y)}{n} = 3713 - \frac{(80)(255)}{5} = -367$$

$$SS_{xx} = \Sigma x^2 - \frac{(\Sigma x)^2}{n} = 1{,}414 - \frac{(80)^2}{5} = 134$$

$$\bar{y} = \frac{\Sigma y}{n} = \frac{75 + 30 + 45 + 58 + 47}{5} = 51$$

$$\bar{x} = \frac{\Sigma x}{n} = \frac{10 + 25 + 17 + 12 + 16}{5} = 16$$

Step 2: Calculate the estimators.

$$\hat{\beta}_1 = \frac{SS_{xy}}{SS_{xx}} = \frac{-367}{134} = -2.74$$

$$\hat{\beta}_0 = \bar{y} - \hat{\beta}_1\bar{x} = 51.0 - (-2.74) \times 16.0 = 94.84$$

Step 3: Write the model.

$$y = \hat{\beta}_0 + \hat{\beta}_1 x = 94.84 - 2.74x$$

Step 4: Interpret the estimates $\hat{\beta}_0$ and $\hat{\beta}_1$.

$\hat{\beta}_0 = 94.84$: If the person has not smoked (i.e., $x = 0$), then the estimated average lung capacity is 95%.

$\hat{\beta}_1 = -2.74$: For every year increase in the number of years smoked, the estimated average lung capacity decreases by 2.7%.

A statistical test can be conducted to determine if the years of smoking have had a significant effect on the lung capacity. In other words, this test can be conducted as follows:

Test for the Adequacy (or Significance) of the Linear Regression Model

$H_o: \beta_1 = 0$ versus $H_a: \beta_1 \neq 0$

$$\text{Test statistic} = \frac{\hat{\beta}_1}{SE(\hat{\beta}_1)} = \frac{\hat{\beta}_1}{\sqrt{\dfrac{MSE}{SS_{xx}}}}$$

$$\text{Critical value} = \pm t_{\frac{\alpha}{2}, n-2}$$

Decision: Reject H_o either if test statistic $> t_{\frac{\alpha}{2}, n-2}$ or if test statistic $< -t_{\frac{\alpha}{2}, n-2}$

Note: $\hat{\beta}_1$ is calculated as before, $SE(\hat{\beta}_1)$ is the standard error of $\hat{\beta}_1 = \sqrt{\dfrac{MSE}{SS_{xx}}}$, and

$$MSE = \frac{\text{Error sum of squares}}{n-2} = \frac{[SS_{yy} - \hat{\beta}_1 \times SS_{xy}]}{n-2}$$

and

$$SS_{yy} = \Sigma y^2 - \frac{(\Sigma y)^2}{n}$$

Note: *MSE* is the mean square error, which is used as an estimate of the variance.

Example 2:

Test the adequacy of the model obtained earlier. Use an α of 0.05.

Step 1: Calculate mean square error (*MSE*).

$$\Sigma y^2 = 75^2 + 30^2 + 45^2 + 58^2 + 47^2 = 14{,}123$$

$$SS_{yy} = \Sigma y^2 - \frac{(\Sigma y)^2}{n} = 14{,}123 - \frac{(255)^2}{5} = 1{,}118$$

$$MSE = \frac{[SS_{yy} - \hat{\beta}_1 \times SS_{xy}]}{n-2} = \frac{[1{,}118 - (-2.74)(-367)]}{3} = 37.47$$

Step 2: Calculate the standard error of $\hat{\beta}_1$.

$$SE(\hat{\beta}_1) = \sqrt{\frac{MSE}{SS_{xx}}} = \sqrt{\frac{37.47}{134}} = 0.529$$

Step 3: Set the hypothesis.

$$H_o: \beta_1 = 0 \qquad \text{versus} \qquad H_a: \beta_1 \neq 0$$

Step 4: Calculate the test statistic.

$$\text{test statistic} = \frac{\hat{\beta}_1}{SE(\hat{\beta}_1)} = \frac{-2.74}{0.529} = -5.2$$

Step 5: Obtain the critical value (C.V.).

$$\text{C.V.} = \pm t_{\frac{\alpha}{2}, n-2} = \pm t_{0.025,3} = \pm 3.182 \text{ (Appendix C, Table II)}$$

Compare the test statistic with the C.V. and make a decision. Since the test statistic (-5.2) is less than -3.182, H_o is rejected in favor of H_a.

Step 6: Write the conclusion.

Based on the information provided, sufficient evidence exists to conclude that the number of years a person smoked contributes significantly in predicting the variation in lung capacity, at a level of significance $\alpha = 0.05$.

Confidence intervals for β_1 can be constructed to determine the variation in the lung capacity for a year increase in the number of years smoked.

C.I. for β_1
$$\hat{\beta}_1 \pm t_{\frac{\alpha}{2}, n-2} \times SE(\hat{\beta}_1)$$
where
$SE(\hat{\beta}_1) = \sqrt{\dfrac{MSE}{SS_{xx}}}$ is the stand error of $\hat{\beta}_1$

EXAMPLE 3:

Construct a 95% confidence interval for the slope parameter and interpret the interval.

Step 1: Calculate SE ($\hat{\beta}_1$).

$$SE(\hat{\beta}_1) = \sqrt{\frac{MSE}{SS_{xx}}} = 0.529$$

Step 2: Obtain $t_{\frac{\alpha}{2}, n-2}$

$$t_{\frac{\alpha}{2}, n-2} = t_{0.025, 3} = 3.182$$

Step 3: Substitute values into the equation $\hat{\beta}_1 \pm t_{\frac{\alpha}{2}, n-2} \, SE(\hat{\beta}_1)$

upper limit: $-2.74 + 3.182 \times 0.529 = -1.06$

lower limit: $-2.74 - 3.182 \times 0.529 = -4.42$

Therefore, the 95% confidence interval is -4.42 to -1.06.

Step 4: Interpret the interval. With 95% certainty, it is estimated that for every year increase in the number of years smoked, the average lung capacity decreases from 1.06% to 4.4%.

To predict the lung capacity of patients who have smoked for 18 years, the least squares model can be used. Here $x_0 = 18$ years.

$$\hat{y} = \hat{\beta}_0 + \hat{\beta}_1 x_0 = 94.84 - 2.74 \times 18 = 45.52$$

Therefore, for patients with an 18-year smoking history, the average lung capacity is estimated to be about 46%. This is a point estimator of the mean of y. An interval estimate of the mean of y can also be provided.

Confidence Interval for the Mean of y at $x = x_0$.

$$\hat{y}_{\text{at } x=x_0} \pm t_{\frac{\alpha}{2}, n-2} \sqrt{MSE\left(\frac{1}{n} + \frac{(x_0 - \bar{x})^2}{SS_{xx}}\right)}$$

where

$\hat{y}_{\text{at } x=x_0} = \hat{\beta}_0 + \hat{\beta}_1 x_0$ is the point estimator of the mean of y at $x = x_0$,

and

x_0 is the value of x for which estimation of the mean of y is desired

---

EXAMPLE 4:

Construct a 99% confidence interval for the average lung capacity of patients who have been smoking for 18 years. Here, $x_0 = 18$ years. Therefore, the point estimator of the mean of y when x equals 18 years is

$$\hat{y}_{\text{at } x=18} = \hat{\beta}_0 + \hat{\beta}_1 \times 18 = 45.52$$

Step 1: Calculate $MSE\left(\frac{1}{n} + \frac{(x_0 - \bar{x})^2}{SS_{xx}}\right)$

$$MSE\left(\frac{1}{n} + \frac{(x_0 - \bar{x})^2}{SS_{xx}}\right), \text{ or } 37.47\left(\frac{1}{5} + \frac{(18 - 16)^2}{134}\right) = 8.6$$

Step 2: Take the square root of 8.6.

$$\sqrt{8.6} = 2.93$$

Step 3: Obtain $t_{\frac{\alpha}{2}, n-2}$

$$t_{\frac{\alpha}{2}, n-2} = t_{0.005,3} = 5.841$$

Step 4: Substitute these values into the C.I. formula.

lower limit: $45.52 - 5.841 \times 2.93 = 28.4$

upper limit: $45.52 + 5.841 \times 2.93 = 62.6$

Therefore, the 99% confidence interval is 28.4 to 62.6.

Step 5: Interpret the interval.

If patients have been smoking for 18 years, their average lung capacity can be estimated with 99% confidence to be between 28% and 63%.

5-17 CORRELATION

The sign (positive or negative) of the slope estimate (β_1) indicates the positive or negative relationship between x and y. Also, the rejection of the hypothesis "slope equals zero" (i.e., H_o: $\beta_1 = 0$) results in the conclusion that x contributes significantly in predicting y. However, it is not known how strongly the two variables (x and y) are related. A measure of the strength of the "linear relationship" between two variables (x and y) is termed the *correlation coefficient*. For a given set of sample data, one can obtain the sample *correlation coefficient* (γ) by the formula given below.

Correlation Coefficient

$$\gamma = \frac{SS_{xy}}{\sqrt{SS_{xx}SS_{yy}}}$$

SS_{xx}, SS_{yy}, and SS_{xy} are as calculated before.

Note: γ is always between -1 and $+1$, inclusively.

$\gamma = 0$ implies no correlation.

$\gamma = 1$ implies perfect positive correlation.

$\gamma = -1$ implies perfect negative correlation.

Also, the coefficient of determination γ^2 (usually denoted by R^2) represents the proportion of the total variability of the y-values that is accounted for by the linear relationship between x and y values. R^2 is a very useful measure because of its understandable interpretation. The higher the value of R^2 (R^2 is always between 0 and 1, inclusively), the higher the proportion of variation in y-values is explained by the variable x. So, it is natural to expect a higher value of R^2 for a good model.

Coefficient of Determination (R^2)

$$R^2 = \gamma^2 = \frac{SS_{xy}^2}{SS_{xx}SS_{yy}}$$

Example:

Calculate γ and R^2 for the previous linear model of lung capacity and interpret R^2.

Step 1: Calculate γ.

$$\gamma = \frac{SS_{xy}}{\sqrt{SS_{xx}SS_{yy}}} = \frac{-367}{\sqrt{134 \times 1,118}} = -0.9482$$

Step 2: Calculate R^2.

$$R^2 = \gamma^2 = 0.8991 \approx 90\%$$

Step 3: Interpret $R^2 = 90\%$.

Ninety percent of the variation in the lung capacity values is explained (or accounted for) by the linear relationship between the years of smoking and lung capacity. Caution: The discussion of correlation and regression here is provided to introduce the concepts and is not meant as a complete coverage of this topic.

PRACTICE PROBLEMS

Refer to Appendix A (pages 624-625) for the solutions and answers to the practice problems.

24. A study was conducted to investigate the relationship between age (years) and blood alcohol concentration (BAC) measured when drivers were arrested for driving under the influence (DUI). Data on eight drivers arrested for DUI in a certain region of the country are as follows:

Driver (n)	1	2	3	4	5	6	7	8
Age (yr)	17.2	43.5	30.7	53.1	37.2	21.0	27.6	46.3
BAC	0.19	0.20	0.26	0.16	0.24	0.20	0.18	0.23

a. Fit a linear regression model to establish the relationship between age and BAC. (Estimate the parameters using the least squares method and interpret the values).

b. Test if the model obtained in part (a) is useful in predicting the BAC based on the age.

c. Construct a 90% confidence interval for the slope parameter. Interpret the interval.

   d. Construct a 95% confidence interval for the mean BAC for people who are 20 years old.

   e. Find the correlation coefficient (γ) and coefficient of determination R^2. Interpret R^2.

CHAPTER SUMMARY

This chapter provided various basic statistical concepts and has discussed their usefulness in respiratory care sciences.

In many applications simple descriptives of the data are needed. Descriptions can be in the form of graphic summary statistics. For such purposes, we have described two graphical procedures known as the pie chart and the histogram. For summary statistics, we have discussed measures of central tendency (namely mean, median and mode) and measures of dispersion (standard deviation). In many situations one requires to know the likelihood of certain events of interest. Therefore, the calculation of probability of events can be used. Most continuous data usually tend to follow a bell-shaped curve, i.e., the histogram of the data tends to be bell-shaped. We discussed a bell-shaped distribution known as normal distribution. Since there can be an infinite number of normal distributions, we provide a standardization technique by which any normal distribution can be transformed to the unit-free standard normal distribution. In most situations the statistical population is too large. However, information regarding population characteristics (termed as parameters) is needed. Usually, a random sample is taken from the population of interest to infer about the population characteristics. To study the accuracy of such inferences (or estimation), one must study the sampling variability. Study of the sampling validity is accomplished by studying the sampling distribution of the sample characteristics (termed statistics). Using the sampling distribution of the sample mean, we have provided inferential techniques such as confidence interval estimation and hypothesis testing. These techniques are discussed for cases when there are either one or more groups of comparison. Sample size determination techniques are also discussed. In medical and political applications it is common to estimate the chances of events. Inferential techniques, similar to the mean example, allow for making inferences about the population proportions or percentages. In many situations one is interested in studying the relationship (or correlation) between variables. The simple linear regression techniques can be used to predict the value of the dependent variable using the information on an independent variable.

REVIEW QUESTIONS

5-1 TERMINOLOGY

Questions

   1. Contrast a designed experimental study with an observational study.

   2. What types of variables are called confounders?

   3. Define the following types of bias: (a) observation bias, (b) measurement bias, and (c) performance bias.

4. Describe the following study designs: (a) cross-sectional study, (b) longitudinal study, (c) prospective study, and (d) retrospective study.
5. Differentiate a control group from a study group.
6. How do the following types of studies differ from each other: (a) single-blind study, (b) double-blind study, and (c) a cross-over study.
7. What is a statistical population?
8. How does a sample relate to a statistical population?
9. How do quantitative data differ from qualitative data?
10. What other terms are used to describe qualitative data?
11. Provide examples of nominal and ordinal qualitative data.
12. Provide examples of discrete and continuous quantitative data.

5-2 DESCRIPTIVE STATISTICS

Questions

1. What is the purpose for using descriptive statistics?
2. Give three examples of descriptive statistics.
3. Describe the x- and y-axes of a histogram.
4. Define *central tendency*.
5. What term is used to describe the measure that represents this central point?
6. Define (a) *mean*, (b) *median*, and (c) *mode*.
7. Write the formula for determining the mean.
8. Describe how the (a) median and (b) mode are determined.
9. How would the mean and median compare on a (a) bell-shaped histogram, (b) right-skewed histogram, and (c) left-skewed histogram?
10. Why does using only the mean or only the median often provide insufficient information?
11. What is the standard deviation?
12. Describe the range and coefficient of variation.
13. Write the formula used to calculate the standard deviation and define the variables used in the formula.
14. How does the size of the standard deviation relate to the reliability of the results?
15. For a data set that produces a bell-shaped distribution curve, what percentage of observations fall within (a) one standard deviation of the mean, (b) two standard deviations of the mean, and (c) three standard deviations of the mean?
16. Describe the Empirical rule.

5-3 PROBABILITY

Questions

1. What does probability measure?
2. What symbol is used to represent probability?

3. Write the formula for probability.
4. What would be the numerical value of probability when the occurrence of an event is (a) impossible or (b) certain?

5-4 NORMAL DISTRIBUTION

Questions

1. List the two characteristic properties of a normal curve.
2. How would two distribution curves compare if they had different means but the same standard deviation?
3. What is another name for the standard score?
4. Write the formula for the z-score.
5. For a distribution of x scores, what would be the value of the mean and standard deviation for the distribution of standard scores (z).
6. What will be the values of the mean and standard deviation for a standard normal curve?
7. What does the standard score of an observation represent?

5-5 SAMPLING DISTRIBUTION

Questions

1. What is a parameter?
2. What type of information does the central limit theorem provide?
3. What is a natural estimate of the population mean?
4. What is the point estimate?
5. Why doesn't the point estimate explain the degree of proximity to the parameter that it estimates?
6. What is the utility of the sampling distribution?
7. How are sampling variability and sampling distribution determined?
8. What is the standard error of the sample mean?
9. What is the effect on the sampling variability of the sample mean as the sample size increases?
10. What is the relationship between the sample and the population as the sample size increases?
11. What information is provided by the standard error?

5-6 CONFIDENCE INTERVALS FOR THE MEAN

Questions

1. Define the *interval estimator*.
2. Describe how to construct a confidence interval.
3. List three interpretations of a 95% confidence interval of 25 to 30 hours.

5-7 SAMPLE SIZE DETERMINATION

Questions

1. What must be known to determine the required sample size?
2. Describe how knowing the range can provide an estimate of the standard deviation.

5-8 SMALL SAMPLE CONFIDENCE INTERVALS FOR MEAN

Questions

1. How do small sample sizes affect the central limit theorem?
2. If the sampling distribution of the mean does not follow a normal curve, what assumption is made?
3. What is the t-distribution?
4. How does the t-distribution compare with the z-distribution for (a) small sample sizes and (b) large sample sizes?
5. If the sample size is n, then what is the degrees of freedom?
6. How does the number of estimated parameters affect the degrees of freedom a distribution will have?

5-9 RESPIRATORY CARE APPLICATIONS OF DESCRIPTIVE STATISTICS

Questions

1. How are decisions related to quality control of a variety of respiratory care equipment made?
2. How can descriptive statistics be used?
3. Define (a) *bias* and (b) *precision*.
4. Assuming a normal distribution, what percentage of the differences between data pairs will fall within ± 2 SDs of the bias?
5. What are limits of agreement?
6. Assume that the mean $PaCO_2$ is 40 torr with a 2.5 torr SD and that the frequency of distribution is relatively normal. Therefore, 95% of the values fall within ±2 SDs of the mean. What is (a) the normal $PaCO_2$ range for this data set and (b) the probability that a normal person will have an abnormal $PaCO_2$?
7. Give an example of when a one-tailed distribution should be used.
8. Write the formula for calculating the lower limit of normal for a one-tailed distribution.

5-10 TESTING OF HYPOTHESIS FOR MEAN

Questions

1. Define the term *hypothesis.*
2. Define (a) *null hypothesis* and (b) *alternate hypothesis.*
3. What is another name for the alternate hypothesis?
4. What symbol is used to denote the (a) null hypothesis and (b) alternate hypothesis?
5. List the two types of errors that are associated with hypothesis testing.
6. What type of error occurs when H_o is rejected in favor of H_a when H_o is actually true?
7. What type of error exists when H_o is accepted when H_a is actually correct?
8. Define the use of α and β in the context of errors associated with hypothesis testing.
9. Under what conditions would α and β equal 0?
10. How can one type of error be decreased?
11. List the six steps for testing an hypothesis.
12. What is a test statistic?
13. Define the rejection region.
14. What is the meaning of a small *p*-value?

5-11 COMPARING MEANS OF TWO POPULATIONS (OR GROUPS): INDEPENDENT SAMPLES

Questions

1. Differentiate between a control group and an experimental group.
2. List two advantages of a double-blind experiment.
3. What two assumptions are made when testing hypotheses concerning experimental versus control groups or two treatment groups?

5-12 COMPARISON OF MEANS FOR PAIRED (OR DEPENDENT) SAMPLES

Questions

1. Describe a paired difference experiment.
2. Should a two-sample *t*-test not be used in a paired difference experiment?

5-13 INFERENCES FOR PROPORTIONS OR PERCENTAGES

Questions

1. How are the hypotheses and *p*-values usually expressed?
2. What is a confidence level?

5-14 TWO-SAMPLE INFERENCES FOR PROPORTIONS

Questions

1. What is the significance of a high test statistic value?
2. Provide an example of a test of the hypotheses for the difference of proportions.

5-15 TESTS FOR MANY POPULATION MEANS

Questions

1. When is analysis of variance (ANOVA) used?
2. What is another name for a one-way ANOVA design?

5-16 CORRELATION AND REGRESSION

Questions

1. Define the terms (a) *dependent variable* and (b) *independent variable*.
2. Differentiate correlation from regression.
3. What statistical method is used to establish the relationship between the dependent and independent variables?
4. What is a simple linear regression?
5. Write the formula that describes a simple linear regression model.
6. What factor in the simple linear regression formula represents (a) the y-intercept and (b) the slope of the linear equation?
7. In the simple linear regression model, what factor represents unaccountable variables?
8. What is the least squares method?

5-17 CORRELATION

Questions

1. What does the sign of the slope estimate signify?
2. What is the interpretation in terms of the interaction between x and y if the slope equals zero?
3. What does the correlation coefficient measure?
4. Write the formula for calculating the correlation coefficient.
5. What is the implication when γ equals (a) 0, (b) +1, (c) −1?
6. What is represented by the symbol γ^2?
7. What other symbol can substitute for γ^2?
8. What is the numerical range for γ^2?
9. What is the meaning of a high γ^2 value?
10. Write the formula for calculating γ^2.

Bibliography

Baily, D. *Research for the Health Professional: A Practical Guide.* Philadelphia: F. A. Davis Company, 1991.

Chatburn, R., and Craig, K. *Fundamentals of Respiratory Care Research.* East Norwalk: Appleton & Lange, 1988.

Dantzker, D., et al. *Comprehensive Respiratory Care.* Philadelphia: W. B. Saunders Company, 1995.

CHAPTER SIX

PHYSIOLOGIC CHEMISTRY

Both the respiratory care student and the respiratory care practitioner continue to achieve higher levels of academic and clinical sophistication. For this reason it is appropriate that we discuss basic aspects of biochemistry in order to relate certain biochemical principles to select concepts of cardiopulmonary physiology and therapeutic intervention.

CHAPTER OBJECTIVES

Upon completing this chapter, the reader will understand certain fundamental elements of biochemistry and their application to certain clinical practices and physiologic concepts. Additionally, the reader will be able to

6-1 THE FUNCTIONAL ANATOMY AND CHEMISTRY OF THE LIVING CELL

- Describe the structural similarities of a typical living cell.
- Discuss the chemistry associated with a typical living cell.
- State the anatomic and chemical dissimilarities among different types of cells.

6-2 BASIC PRINCIPLES OF ORGANIC CHEMISTRY

- Explain basic principles of organic chemistry.
- Discuss the bonding capabilities of hydrogen, oxygen, nitrogen, and carbon.
- Write the structural formulas of various functional groups.

6-3 CARBOHYDRATES

- Discuss biochemical roles of carbohydrates.

William Bradshaw Davis, Ph.D. compiled the organic chemistry review found in Sections 6–1 through 6–6. Alan Jobe, M.D., Ph.D., developed the topic of pulmonary surfactant in Section 6–5 Lipids. Dean Hess, PhD., RRT, wrote Section 6–9, Biochemistry and Clinical Applications of Inhaled Nitric Oxide. Ronald Allison, M.D., Ph.D., wrote Section 6–10 Biochemical Etiology of Adult Respiratory Distress Syndrome, and Lawrence Sindell, M.D., contributed Section 6–11 Biochemical Mechanisms of Bronchospasm.

- Differentiate among monosaccharides, disaccharides, and polysaccharides.
- Distinguish between aerobic and anaerobic respiration.

6-4 PROTEINS

- Describe biochemical roles of proteins.
- State the basic structure of an amino acid.
- Explain why proteins have physiologic buffering capabilities.
- Classify certain biologically important proteins according to their components and their configurations.

6-5 LIPIDS

- Explain biochemical roles of lipids.
- Discuss the role of lipids as major components of cell membranes.
- Relate the significance of the lecithin/sphingomyelin ratio as it pertains to lung maturity.
- List the components of pulmonary surfactant.
- Discuss aspects regarding the release of pulmonary surfactant.
- Describe some differences between synthetic and animal lung source surfactants.
- Describe the postulated orientation of pulmonary surfactant at the air-liquid interface.
- State the relationship between alveolar surface tension and the alveolar concentration of pulmonary surfactant.

6-6 NUCLEIC ACIDS

- Relate biochemical roles of nucleic acids.
- Indicate the structure of the cyclic nucleotide 3′,5′-adenosine monophosphate (cyclic AMP).
- Differentiate between deoxyribonucleic acid (DNA) and ribonucleic acid (RNA).

6-7 HEMOGLOBIN BIOCHEMISTRY

- Discuss the biochemistry of the hemoglobin molecule.
- Describe the structure of hemoglobin.
- Explain the relationship among the normal hemoglobin variants.
- Discuss mutant hemoglobins.
- Relate the function of the hemoglobin molecule in terms of (1) oxygen transport, (2) carbon dioxide transport, and (3) physiologic buffering.
- State the degradation process of the hemoglobin molecule.

6-8 BIOCHEMICAL ASPECTS OF OXYGEN TOXICITY

- Discuss the biochemical aspects of oxygen toxicity.
- State the origin and activity of free radicals.
- Discuss the process of lipid peroxidation.

- Describe the role of endogenous antioxidants.
- Distinguish between systemic and pulmonary oxygen toxicity.

6-9 BIOCHEMISTRY AND CLINICAL APPLICATIONS OF INHALED NITRIC OXIDE

- Explain the biochemistry and clinical applications of inhaled nitric oxide.
- Trace both the endogenous and exogenous pathways regarding NO· activity.
- List factors that influence the amount of a person's exhaled NO·.
- State the purpose of inhaling NO·.
- List diseases for which NO· inhalation is used as a treatment.
- Describe the pulmonary and systemic effects of inhaled NO·.

6-10 BIOCHEMICAL ETIOLOGY OF ADULT RESPIRATORY DISTRESS SYNDROME

- Discuss the biochemical etiology of adult respiratory distress syndrome (ARDS).
- Explain the hypotheses concerning the mechanisms of acute lung injury.
- Describe the role of inflammatory mediators in the pathogenesis of ARDS.
- State the pathophysiology of ARDS.

6-11 BIOCHEMICAL MECHANISMS OF BRONCHOSPASM

- Explain biochemical mechanisms associated with bronchospasm.
- Relate events responsible for bronchial smooth muscle tone.
- Discuss the biochemistry of bronchospasm due to immediate hypersensitivity reactions.
- Describe the rationale for certain pharmacologic agents administered to prevent or to reverse bronchospasm.

6-1 THE FUNCTIONAL ANATOMY AND CHEMISTRY OF THE LIVING CELL

The living cell is the fundamental unit comprising all living organisms including plants, animals, and fungi as well as microbes (bacteria and protozoa), which exist as a single cell. However, no such entity as a "typical" cell exists. Single-cell organisms such as bacteria and amoeba differ from one another, as do the cells of the brain, muscle, and connective tissue.

Despite their functional differences, they are all cells and have certain structural similarities. For example, they all possess a cell membrane, cytoplasm, organelles, a nuclear region, and, with the exception of bacteria, a nuclear membrane. (See the discussion on the cell envelope in Section 7-3, "Bacterial Ultrastructure.")

The animal cell prototype contains within its nucleus a vast network of genetic material called **chromatin**, which consists of deoxyribonucleic acid (DNA) and protein (nucleoprotein). Immediately outside the nucleus, in the cytoplasm, animal cells have a centrosome, which is a small granule involved in mitosis (cell division). During mitosis the centrosome divides and each resulting component moves apart to form poles to which spindle fibers become attached. These spindle fibers are involved in pulling chromatin material apart during cell division. These cell structures are seen in Figure 6-1.

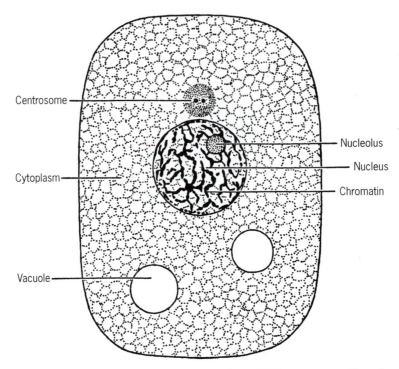

Centrosome

Nucleolus

Nucleus

Cytoplasm

Chromatin

Vacuole

Figure 6-1 *Prototypical animal cell illustrating common characteristic components. From Brachet, J.: "The Living Cell,"* Scientific American, *September 1961, page 54, W.H. Freeman & Co., New York. Used with permission.*

Scattered in the cytoplasm are mitochondria, which often appear as long or short rods, or as small granules. The Golgi apparatus is particularly prominent in nervous and secretory cells of animals and seems to be closely associated with secretory activity. However, its true structure and function are yet to be resolved.

Some cells have vacuoles, which appear as "holes" in the cytoplasm. These structures seem to be important in the storage of nutrients for the cell and a place for subsequent nutrient digestion by the cell. Some cells also contain compartments of digestive enzymes. These compartments appear as dense bodies in the cytoplasm and are referred to as **lysosomes.** Lysosomes frequently fuse with vacuoles, releasing enzymes into the vacuoles, which can in turn act upon any matter present in the vacuoles. The resulting structure is called a **phagolysosome.**

When a cell is cleared of viable granules by centrifugation, a clear ground substance remains that is thought to represent the fundamental architecture of the cell. Electron microscopy has revealed that this substance is a continuous network of the outer membrane and nuclear membrane. This cytoskeleton or continuous invagination and convolution is called the **endoplasmic reticulum.** The Golgi apparatus appears to be an extra-tight network of the endoplasmic reticulum. Figure 6-2 is a schematic representation of a cell emphasizing the endoplasmic reticulum, Golgi body, and mitochondria. Attached all along the

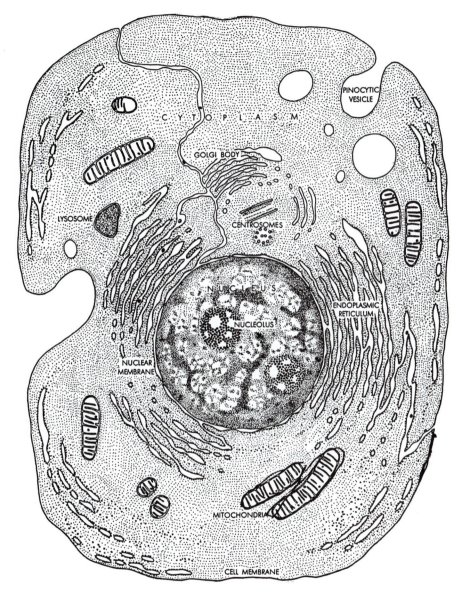

Figure 6-2 *A typical animal cell featuring numerous organelles. From Brachet, J.: "The Living Cell,"* Scientific American, *September 1961, page 55, W.H. Freeman & Co., New York. Used with permission.*

"cytoplasmic side" of the endoplasmic reticulum are dense particles or granules. These granules are exceedingly rich in ribonucleic acid (RNA) and are called **ribosomes.** These structures serve as the principal site for protein synthesis.

The ultrastructures of the cell that have been most extensively studied include the nucleus, the cell membrane, and the mitochondria.

A cell can survive for a short time without a nucleus (enucleated); however, for the cell to function normally and undergo division, the nucleus is essential. The nucleus contains chromosomes, which consist of deoxyribonucleic acid (DNA) and are responsible for directing all synthetic activities of the cell. In addition, RNA also can be found in the nucleus along with lipids, proteins, enzymes, phosphorous-containing organic compounds, and various inorganic compounds (mostly salts). In the nucleus, the nucleolus serves as the storage site for RNA, which functions in guiding protein synthesis.

The cytoplasmic membrane provides an osmotic barrier traversed at intervals by specific transport systems. The barrier is very efficient in retaining metabolites as well as in excluding certain external compounds. All ions and molecules penetrate very slowly, except those that traverse by active transport. The membrane, in essence, is a two-dimensional fluid made up of phospholipid molecules with a polar water-soluble (hydrophilic) end and a long lipid-soluble (hydrophobic) end. The molecules orient themselves to form a bilayer structure with the lipid-soluble ends directed toward the inside and the water-soluble aspects directed to the outside (Figure 6-3).

The zigzag lines represent the lipid-soluble part of the phospholipid molecules, and the solid circles are the polar water-soluble ends. The shaded bodies are the protein molecules interspersed throughout the phospholipid molecules. The proteins serve as transport systems called **permeases.** These permeases transport nutrients and other substances essential for cellular survival.

The transport of nutrients and other substances across the membrane requires energy in the form of adenosine triphosphate (ATP) and is referred to as **active transport.**

The mitochondrion is frequently called the *powerhouse* of the cell because it is the principal site for the generation of ATP (see Section 6-3, "Carbohydrates"). Depending on the type of cell, there are usually several hundred mitochondria. An average mitochondrion is cylinder-shaped. Its architecture resembles that of a Thermos bottle; it has a two-layered wrapping, an outer membrane and an inner membrane with an aqueous fluid filling the space between them. Invaginations of the inner membrane project into the interior portion of the mitochondrion. These projections are called **cristae.**

The internal surfaces of the cristae are lined with smaller particles called **elementary units.** It is in these bodies that the chemical activities necessary for ATP synthesis occur. Figure 6-4 depicts a cutaway drawing of a typical mitochondrion.

The primary classes of compounds in the cell qualitatively consist of water, proteins, lipids, carbohydrates, nucleic acids, and salts. Quantitatively, the cytoplasm of any plant or

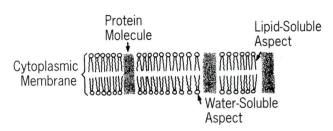

Figure 6-3 *Cytoplasmic membrane illustrating phospholipid bilayer with lipid- and water-soluble aspects and interspersed protein molecules.*

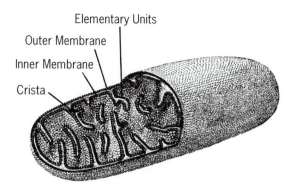

Outer Membrane
Elementary Units
Inner Membrane
Crista

Figure 6-4 *Drawing of mitochondrion demonstrating its internal structures. From Green, D.: "The Mitochondrion,"* Scientific American, *January 1964, page 64, W.H. Freeman & Co., New York. Used with permission.*

animal cell is lioely to be 75 to 85% water, 10 to 20% protein, 2 to 3% lipid, 1% carbohydrate, 1% nucleic acid, and 2% salts and miscellaneous substances. Although the predominant constituent is water, the substances that contribute most significantly to the cellular structure are the proteins, lipids, and carbohydrates.

Cellular water occurs in two forms—free and bound. Free water is available for metabolic processes, whereas bound water is loosely combined to protein by hydrogen bonds. Thus bound water can be considered a part of the cytoplasmic structure.

Proteins, which are chains of amino acids, not only provide structure to the cell but also participate as enzymes and conjugate to substances such as heme and nucleic acids.

Lipids make up a wide variety of molecules, including fats, phospholipids, and sterols. Lipids are essential for the integrity of the cell membrane and have an important role in numerous cellular metabolic functions.

Carbohydrates are sugars referred to as **monosaccharides, disaccharides,** and **polysaccharides,** depending on the number of a particular carbohydrate molecule present. Glucose, a monosaccharide, is important in cell metabolism and serves as the basic nutrient for energy production. Disaccharides, such as sucrose and maltose, contain glucose and are important dietary sources for the molecule. Polysaccharides are important skeletal material in cells, especially of plants, as is the case with cellulose. In addition, polysaccharides such as starch serve as a major source of dietary glucose.

Two main forms of nucleic acids have been identified, DNA and RNA. DNA is predominantly found in the nucleus, and RNA is located mainly in the cytoplasm. Differences between these nucleic acids exist in conjugated sugars (deoxyribose in DNA versus ribose in RNA), pyrimidine bases (uracil in RNA versus guanine in DNA), and molecular size. Functionally, DNA serves as the basis for the genetic material, and RNA provides the messenger molecules for the genetic code.

Salts are present in all cells and are necessary as osmotic regulators. They participate in numerous chemical reactions.

Cationic salts are present usually in the form of potassium (K^+), magnesium (Mg^{2+}), sodium (Na^+), and calcium (Ca^{2+}). The dominant anion of the cell is phosphate (PO_4^{3-}). Other important anions include bicarbonate (HCO_3^-) and chloride (Cl^-). Salts of a large number of other elements are also present, for example, iron, manganese, copper, zinc, nickel, vanadium, molybdenum, and tin. Some of these ions are necessary for the function of certain enzymes.

Vitamins are a diverse group of compounds required in various quantities for the growth and normal function of cells. They are sometimes referred to as *growth factors*. Vitamins play an important part in cellular metabolism, acting chiefly as cofactors for enzymes or as biological catalysts.

6-2 BASIC PRINCIPLES OF ORGANIC CHEMISTRY

From a chemistry standpoint, physiologic chemistry is an offshoot of inorganic and organic chemistry as related to the living cell. In short, physiologic chemistry is the interaction of molecules that results in the life process. Most of our considerations will focus on a basic understanding of the chemistry of hydrogen (H), oxygen (O), nitrogen (N), and particularly carbon (C). Let us now review some basic chemical concepts concerning these elements.

Hydrogen

Hydrogen is always monovalent; that is, each hydrogen atom has only one bond. For example, each of the four hydrogen atoms shown below can form only a single bond between itself and the carbon atom or any other atom.

$$H{-}\underset{\displaystyle C}{\overset{\displaystyle H}{C}}{-}H \qquad \text{(one single bond)}$$

Oxygen

Oxygen is usually divalent; that is, each oxygen atom has two bonds. Note the two examples that follow:

$$-\overset{|}{\underset{|}{C}}{-}O{-}H \qquad \text{(two single bonds)}$$

$$\overset{|}{\underset{|}{C}}{=}O \qquad \text{(one double bond)}$$

Nitrogen

Nitrogen is usually trivalent. Each nitrogen atom has three bonds. Typically, nitrogen exists with an extra pair of electrons. Examples include the following:

$$-\overset{|}{\underset{|}{N}}: \qquad \text{(three single bonds)}$$

$$-\ddot{N}=C \qquad \text{(one single bond and one double bond)}$$

$$-C\equiv N: \qquad \text{(one triple bond)}$$

When nitrogen occurs in a tetravalent form (four bonds), it acquires a positive charge (see Section 6-4, "Proteins").

Carbon

The building block of biochemistry is the carbon atom. Carbon–carbon bonds are strong covalent bonds that are conducive to forming long-chained molecules. Carbon is always tetravalent; that is, each carbon atom has four covalent bonds. The following examples serve to illustrate the different carbon bonds:

$$-\overset{|}{\underset{|}{C}}- \qquad \text{(four single bonds)}$$

$$\overset{|}{\underset{|}{C}}=\overset{|}{\underset{|}{C}} \qquad \text{(one double bond and two single bonds)}$$

$$-C\equiv C- \qquad \text{(one single bond and one triple bond)}$$

Although single bonds are more frequent, double and triple bonds sometimes occur between atoms.

Functional Groups

Functional groups are atoms, radicals, or groups of atoms that are largely responsible for the properties of a compound. Commonly encountered functional groups include the following:

$-OH$	(alcohol)	$-\overset{O}{\overset{\|}{C}}-O-R$	(ester)
$-\overset{O}{\overset{\|}{C}}-H$	(aldehyde)	$-NH_3^+$	(amine)
		$-CO_3^{2-}$	(carbonate)
$-\overset{O}{\overset{\|}{C}}-$	(ketone)	$-NO_3^-$	(nitrate)
$-\overset{O}{\overset{\|}{C}}-OH$	(carboxylic acid)	$-\overset{O}{\underset{OH}{\overset{\|}{P}}}-OH$	(phosphate)

The presence of certain functional groups in compounds can be used to explain and/or predict certain characteristics and properties of compounds. For example, compounds with amines (NH_3^+) can occur in various ionized states as a result of their ability to accept or release hydrogen ions into the environment. Of course, compounds with COOH groups may behave as acids as a result of their ability to donate electrons. Consider the following example:

$$\underset{\text{—C—OH}}{\overset{\overset{\textstyle O}{\|}}{}} \rightarrow \underset{\text{—C—O}^- + H^+}{\overset{\overset{\textstyle O}{\|}}{}}$$

The designation R will appear throughout this chapter. It is used for writing shortened versions of molecules that have long or complex structural formulas. Essentially, R can signify any atom, group of atoms or functional group. For example, acetic acid

$$(CH_3 \overset{\overset{\textstyle O}{\|}}{—C} —OH)$$

can be shown as

$$R \overset{\overset{\textstyle O}{\|}}{—C} —OH$$

where R substitutes for CH_3. Again, R can represent any chemical moiety.

6-3 CARBOHYDRATES

The terms *carbohydrate* and *sugar* are often used interchangeably. As a class of compounds, carbohydrates include simple sugars (glucose) and large complex compounds (starch and cellulose).

The functional group of a carbohydrate can be an aldehyde or alcohol. Broadly, carbohydrates are defined as polyhydroxylated molecules with at least three carbons, one of which is a ketone or an aldehyde.

The basic molecular unit of a simple carbohydrate is called a *monosaccharide*. Monosaccharides are often named based on the length of the carbon chains that comprise them. A sugar with three carbons in its chain is called a *triose*. Likewise, sugars with four carbons are *tetroses*, five carbons *pentoses*, and six carbons *hexoses*. The suffix *-ose* is applied to all simple sugars. Figure 6-5 provides a depiction of two structural configurations which may occur with a very important monosaccharide, glucose. Glucose can exist in the straight-chain aldehyde form shown on the left or as a ring structure, shown on the right.

The most important monosaccharides from a physiologic standpoint are the hexoses. In addition to glucose, they include galactose and fructose; each of these is biochemically significant.

Glucose, often referred to as *dextrose,* is the normal blood sugar occurring in man and is utilized in man as the main source of energy for the production of ATP; it also provides precursors often used in the synthesis of proteins and lipids.

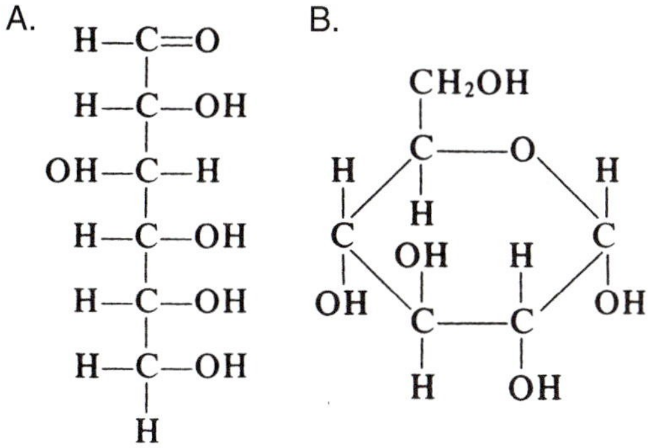

A.

$$H-C=O$$
$$H-C-OH$$
$$OH-C-H$$
$$H-C-OH$$
$$H-C-OH$$
$$H-C-OH$$
$$H$$

B.

Figure 6-5 *Two structural configurations of glucose. (A) straight-chain aldehyde; (B) ring structure.*

Glucose serves as the initial substrate for a process known as *glycolysis,* a metabolic process that occurs in the cytoplasm of most cells. During glycolysis one molecule of glucose is broken down to form two three-carbon compounds called *metabolic intermediates.* The end-product of glycolysis can be lactic acid or pyruvic acid, depending on the availability of oxygen. In the absence of sufficient oxygen the glycolytic pathway results in the formation of lactic acid from pyruvate. However, in the presence of oxygen, pyruvate is utilized further by being converted to acetyl CoA in the mitochondrion.

Metabolism of glucose occurring in the presence of oxygen is known as *aerobic metabolism,* whereas in the absence of oxygen it is known as *anaerobic metabolism.* The aerobic conversion of glucose to pyruvic acid results in the extraction of chemical energy contained in the bonds of the glucose molecule. This energy is stored metabolically in high-energy phosphate bonds of ATP. In mammalian cells the quantity of ATP generated by the breakdown of glucose to pyruvate represents only a minor amount of the total ATP that can be formed during the breakdown of glucose. The majority of ATP is generated by the conversion of pyruvate to acetyl CoA, which is the first substrate in a cyclic metabolic pathway known as the *tricarboxylic acid cycle* (Krebs cycle). During the tricarboxylic acid cycle the coenzymes NAD^+ and FAD^+ are reduced to NADH and $FADH_2$, respectively. These reduced coenzymes, in turn, donate their electrons to components of the electron transport system that are located on the inner membrane of the mitochondrion. In terms of energy production, electrons will flow from a more negative to a less negative, or oxidized, component. Because NADH and $FADH_2$ are more negative than oxygen, electrons will flow from NADH or $FADH_2$ to oxygen. Thus, electrons are sequentially passed through the electron transport components with oxygen acting as the final electron acceptor. The end result is the reduction of oxygen to form water.

During sequential oxidation and reduction of the electron transport components, ATP is generated. The overall process of generating ATP by electron transport is called *oxidative phosphorylation.* The majority of ATP is generated during the breakdown of glucose and can occur only under aerobic conditions, that is, when oxygen is present.

In short, it is well established that a total of 38 moles of ATP are formed per mole of aerobically metabolized glucose. Two of these ATP molecules are generated for metabolic use during the glycolytic breakdown of glucose to pyruvate. Two more ATP molecules are

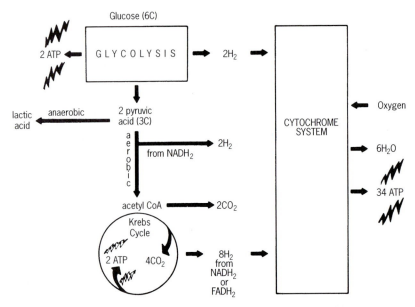

Figure 6-6   *Aerobic breakdown of a glucose molecule through numerous biochemical pathways resulting in the generation of 38 ATP molecules.*

directly generated by reactions in the tricarboxylic acid, or Krebs, cycle, with the remaining 34 ATPs resulting from oxidative phosphorylation. The overall process of the aerobic breakdown of glucose with the generation of ATP is schematically shown in Figure 6-6.

When two monosaccharides are linked together, the resulting compound is a disaccharide. Disaccharides include sucrose (glucose + fructose), maltose (glucose + glucose), and lactose (glucose + galactose). Each of these disaccharides, upon digestion, can serve as a source of glucose. The structure of maltose, as an example, is shown in Figure 6-7.

Sucrose is commonly called *cane sugar* and is the sugar used as common table sugar for sweetening. It occurs naturally in beets and sugar cane. Lactose is a disaccharide present in milk, whereas maltose is present in grain.

Polysaccharides are large molecules consisting of chains of individual units of monosaccharide molecules. The most important polysaccharides are composed of repeating units of the hexose sugars. From a nutritional standpoint, the most important polysaccharide is starch, which is made up of repeating units of maltose. A representation of starch is shown in Figure 6-8.

Glycogen is a polysaccharide consisting of repeating units of glucose, which occur in branched chains. Glycogen is formed metabolically in man by a process known as *glycogenesis*. Glycogenesis occurs in the liver and serves as a mechanism by which glucose can be stored. The glycogen reserves provide a readily available source of glucose when dietary glucose is unavailable and energy is required.

This conversion of glycogen back to glucose occurs during a fasting state and is referred to as *glycogenolysis*. When glycogen is depleted, noncarbohydrate precursors can also be

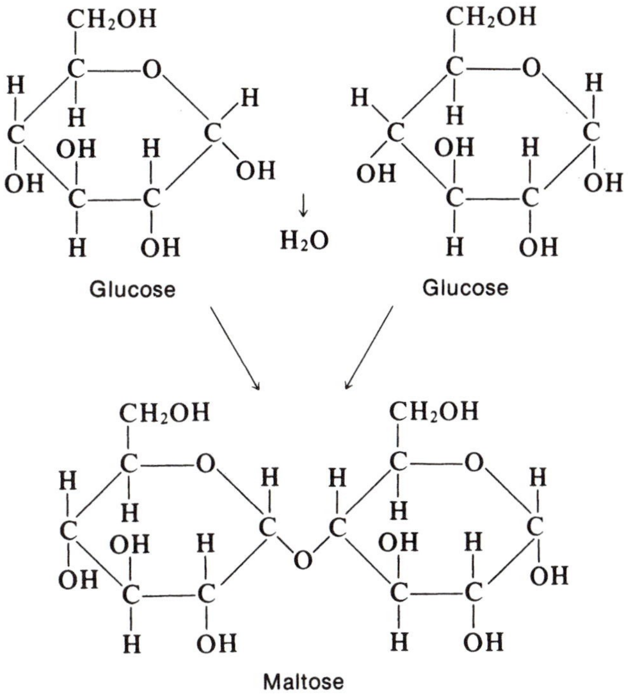

Figure 6-7 *Two glucose molecules (monosaccharides) linking to form maltose (disaccharide).*

converted into glucose by the process known as *gluconeogenesis.* Among these precursors are certain amino acids, which are derived from proteins (see Section 6-4, "Proteins").

From a physiologic viewpoint, it is safe to say that carbohydrate metabolism centers on the utilization of glucose and that this utilization, in many ways, is the center of metabolism; it provides the necessary energy and molecular building blocks for the cell.

Figure 6-9 provides a highly simplified depiction of the position of glucose metabolism in the overall anabolic and catabolic processes that occur in mammalian cells.

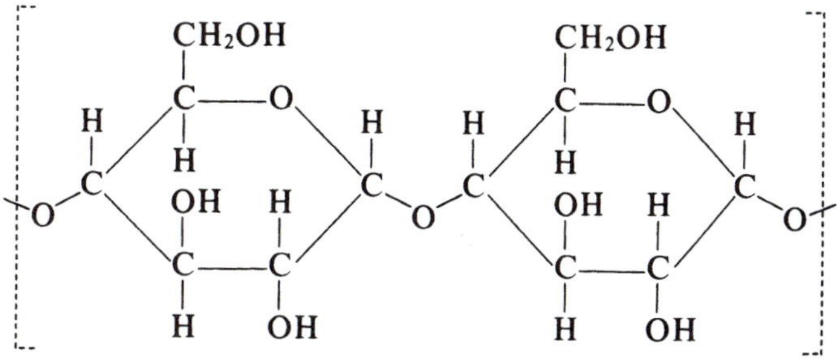

Figure 6-8 *Repeating maltose unit of starch (polysaccharide).*

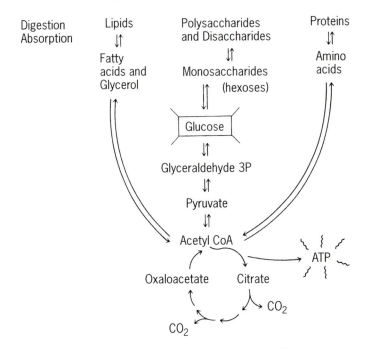

Figure 6-9 *Simplified schematic of glucose metabolism in mammalian cells.*

6-4 PROTEINS

Proteins are large molecules that consist of repeating units of amino acids. Proteins have a wide role in cellular metabolism ranging from structural molecules for tissues, such as cartilage, skin, hair, nails, and other connective tissues, to functional roles, as with enzymes, hormones, antibodies, and muscle contraction.

Proteins are an important dietary constituent. In fagt, the primary source of nitrogen and sulfur for the body comes from dietary protein. The nitrogen and sulfur derive mainly from the presence of amino acids.

To understand proteins, it is first important to understand the chemistry of amino acids. The physiologic role of a protein molecule is determined by (1) the total number of constituent amino acids, (2) the sequence of the amino acids, and (3) the kind of amino acids.

There are 20 known amino acids that serve as building blocks for protein molecules. Considering the vast number of proteins that each species of animal can synthesize, it seems phenomenal that such a task can be accomplished with the availability of only 20 different kinds of amino acids. However, if one considers that any three different entities—for example, *A, B,* and *C*—can be arranged in six different ways and that mathematically ten such entities can have up to four million variations, it is possible to understand the diversity that can occur among protein molecules when there are only 20 different ones from which to choose. Further, the same amino acid can be present more than once in a given protein molecule. In

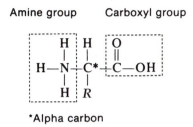

Amine group   Carboxyl group

*Alpha carbon

Figure 6-10 *A typical amino acid structure. A common (alpha) carbon atom combines with an amine (NH_2) group and a carboxyl (COOH) group.*

fact, it is common to have many of the various 20 amino acids occurring in a protein repetitiously or repeatedly. As a result of its containing hundreds of amino acid residues, the molecular weight of a protein usually varies from around 10,000 to many million daltons.

Amino acids are molecules characterized by having at least one amine (NH_2) and one carboxyl (COOH) group attached to the same carbon atom, which is known as the *alpha carbon.* Figure 6-10 depicts the basic structure of a typical amino acid. However, there are two exceptions, proline and hydroxyproline.

Amino acids are commonly grouped according to the nature of their constituents. Neutral or aliphatic amino acids contain one carboxyl group to one amine group. Acidic amino acids consist of two carboxyl groups and one amine group, whereas basic amino acids have a ratio of one carboxyl group to two amine groups.

Amino acids such as cysteine, cystine, and methionine have sulfur atoms within their structure; thus they are called the *sulfur-containing amino acids.* Aromatic amino acids consist of carbon-containing, ring-shaped molecules. Examples include phenylalanine and tyrosine. Heterocyclic amino acids contain one or more elements other than carbon in their rings and include histidine, tryptophan, proline, and hydroxyproline. Table 6-1 presents the structures of the various amino acids within their respective groups. See if you can identify those with alpha carbons.

Because they have at least one amine group and one carboxyl group, amino acids can have a positive or negative charge, depending on the ionization state of the molecule. There is a pH for each amino acid at which the molecule is electrically neutral, that is, the number of positive charges equals the number of negative charges. This pH value is called the *isoelectric point* for that particular amino acid. Figure 6-11 depicts a typical amino acid as it would occur at its isoelectric point.

It is important to recognize that, when an amino acid is in a solution acidic to its isoelectric point, the carboxyl group loses its negative charge as a result of taking on a

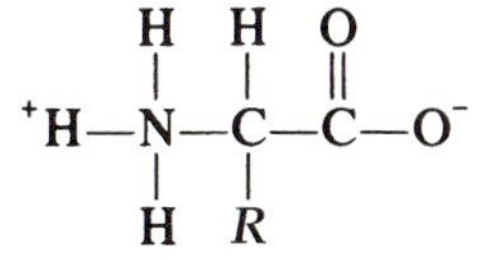

$$
\begin{array}{c}
\quad \text{H} \quad\ \text{H} \quad\ \text{O} \\
\quad\ |\qquad |\qquad || \\
^{+}\text{H—N—C—C—O}^{-} \\
\quad\ |\qquad | \\
\quad\ \text{H} \quad\ R
\end{array}
$$

Figure 6-11 *A typical amino acid at its isoelectric point. Note that the number of positive and negative charges are equal.*

TABLE 6-1 Amino Acids

Amino Acid	Structure	Amino Acid	Structure
Glycine	$H-\underset{NH_2}{\overset{H}{C}}-C\overset{O}{\underset{OH}{}}$	Aspartic acid	$\underset{HO}{\overset{O}{}}C-CH_2-\underset{NH_2}{\overset{H}{C}}-C\overset{O}{\underset{OH}{}}$
Alanine	$CH_3-\underset{NH_2}{\overset{H}{C}}-C\overset{O}{\underset{OH}{}}$	Asparagine	$\underset{NH_2}{\overset{O}{}}C-CH_2-\underset{NH_2}{\overset{H}{C}}-C\overset{O}{\underset{OH}{}}$
Valine	$\underset{CH_3}{\overset{CH_3}{}}CH-\underset{NH_2}{\overset{H}{C}}-C\overset{O}{\underset{OH}{}}$	Glutamic acid	$\underset{HO}{\overset{O}{}}C-CH_2-CH_2-\underset{NH_2}{\overset{H}{C}}-C\overset{O}{\underset{OH}{}}$
Leucine	$\underset{CH_3}{\overset{CH_3}{}}CH-CH_2-\underset{NH_2}{\overset{H}{C}}-C\overset{O}{\underset{OH}{}}$	Glutamine	$\underset{NH_2}{\overset{O}{}}C-CH_2-CH_2-\underset{NH_2}{\overset{H}{C}}-C\overset{O}{\underset{OH}{}}$
Isoleucine	$CH_3-CH_2-\underset{CH_3}{\overset{}{C}}H-\underset{NH_2}{\overset{H}{C}}-C\overset{O}{\underset{OH}{}}$	Phenylalanine	(benzene ring)$-CH-\underset{NH_2}{\overset{H}{C}}-C\overset{O}{\underset{OH}{}}$
Serine	$HO-CH_2-\underset{NH_2}{\overset{H}{C}}-C\overset{O}{\underset{OH}{}}$	Tyrosine	$HO-$(benzene ring)$-CH_2-\underset{NH_2}{\overset{H}{C}}-C\overset{O}{\underset{OH}{}}$
Threonine	$CH_3-\underset{OH}{\overset{H}{C}}-\underset{NH_2}{\overset{H}{C}}-C\overset{O}{\underset{OH}{}}$	Tryptophan	(indole ring)$-C-CH_2-\underset{NH_2}{\overset{H}{C}}-C\overset{O}{\underset{OH}{}}$
Cysteine	$HS-CH_2-\underset{NH_2}{\overset{H}{C}}-C\overset{O}{\underset{OH}{}}$	Histidine	$HC=\underset{N}{\overset{}{C}}-CH_2-\underset{NH_2}{\overset{H}{C}}-C\overset{O}{\underset{OH}{}}$
Methionine	$CH_3-S-CH_2-CH_2-\underset{NH_2}{\overset{H}{C}}-C\overset{O}{\underset{OH}{}}$		
Lysine	$NH_2-CH_2-CH_2-CH_2-CH_2-\underset{NH_2}{\overset{H}{C}}-C\overset{O}{\underset{OH}{}}$	Proline	(pyrrolidine ring)$CH-C\overset{O}{\underset{OH}{}}$
Arginine	$NH_2-\underset{\overset{\|\|}{NH}}{C}-NH-CH_2-CH_2-CH_2-\underset{NH_2}{\overset{H}{C}}-C\overset{O}{\underset{OH}{}}$		

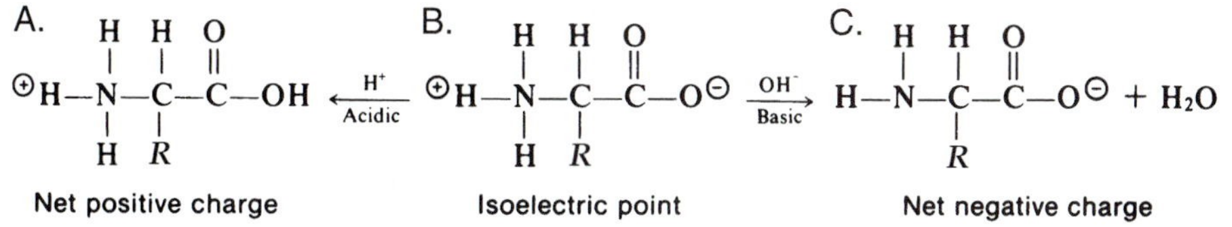

Figure 6-12 *An amino acid as it would exist at an acidic, at an alkalotic pH, and at its isoelectric point. (A) At an acid pH, the amino acid has a net positive charge; (B) At a neutral pH, the molecule has a balance of charges; (C) At a basic pH, it has a net negative charge.*

hydrogen ion. The net result is that the molecule assumes an overall positive charge by virtue of the amine group. Conversely, in a solution alkaline to the isoelectric point the amine group gives up a hydrogen ion, thus losing its positive charge. In this situation the net effect is that the molecule assumes an overall negative charge as a result of the carboxyl group. It is this ability of constituent amino acids to remove or contribute hydrogen ions to their environment that endows proteins with a physiologic buffering capacity. Figure 6-12 provides a schematic representation of an amino acid as it would appear acidic and basic to its isoelectric point.

In considering that proteins are made up of amino acids, proteins will also exhibit an isoelectric point at a given pH depending on the overall number of positive charges as compared to the overall number of negative charges on the amino acid residues that comprise the protein.

Amino acids are joined together in a protein by a chemical bond known as a *peptide bond.* Amino acids are coupled by peptide bonds as a result of the loss of water between the amine on one amino acid and the carboxyl on another. The reaction (glycine + alanine → glycyl-alanine) shown in Figure 6-13 provides an example of the formation of a peptide bond between two amino acids.

When two amino acids are joined by a peptide linkage, they are referred to as a *dipeptide.* Three amino acids are called a *tripeptide,* and so forth. Many amino acids linked by peptide bonds are referred to as *polypeptides* or *proteins.*

Proteins are classified into two major classes depending on the nature of their amino acid chains. Those proteins that consist solely of pure amino acid chains are referred to as *simple proteins,* and those linked to another type of biomolecule (e.g., sugars and lipids) are referred to as *conjugated proteins.* Table 6-2 lists some biologically important proteins, which are classified as either simple proteins or conjugated proteins.

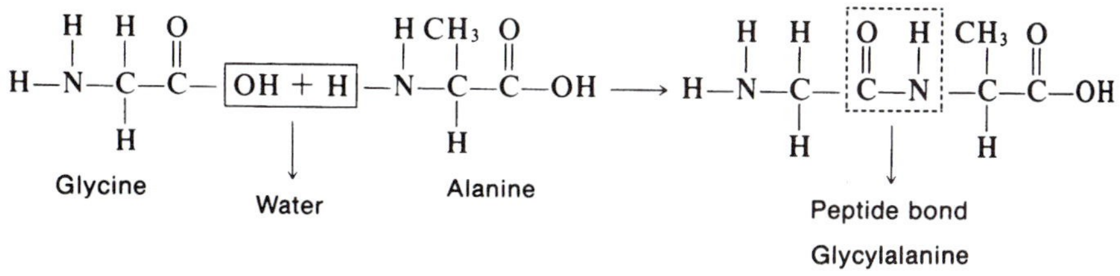

Figure 6-13 *A reaction between the amino acids glycine and alanine to form the dipeptide glycylalanine. Note the formation of a peptide bond when the amino group of alanine reacts with the carboxyl group of glycine.*

TABLE 6-2   Major Classes of Proteins

Simple Proteins	Conjugated Proteins
Albumins (serum, egg whites)	Nucleoproteins (DNA and protein)
Globulins (antibodies, fibrinogen, enzymes)	Hemoglobin (globin and heme)
	Glycoprotein (mucin of saliva)
Glutelins (wheat, corn, barley)	Phosphoprotein (casein of milk)
	Lipoprotein (protein linked to cholesterol or other fats)

X-ray analysis has shown that proteins have a three-dimensional structure. Fundamentally, there are four different levels of protein structure. The most basic level is the primary structure. The **primary structure** of a protein simply relates to the linear sequence of amino acids that comprises the polypeptide chain.

Most other proteins occur in a secondary, tertiary, or quaternary structure. **Secondary structure** refers to a single polypeptide chain that is twisted or coiled, often in a helical form. **Tertiary structure** occurs when a polypeptide that is in the secondary level of structure becomes folded and convoluted about itself, resulting in a globular-shaped molecule. **Quaternary structure** refers to the interaction between two or more polypeptides in the tertiary structure, resulting in the formation of a multichained protein. An example of a protein molecule with a quaternary structure is hemoglobin, which consists of four interconnected polypeptide chains (see Section 6-7, "Hemoglobin Biochemistry"). Table 6-3 lists the four different levels of protein structures and their respective configurations.

TABLE 6-3

Protein Structure		
Level or Structure	Description	Configuration
primary	straight chain sequence of amino acids	
secondary	coiled or helical	
tertiary	convolution of secondary level	
quaternary	linkage	

The bonds responsible for the secondary and tertiary structures occur from intra-molecular interactions between groups associated with constituent amino acids. Examples of these bonds are hydrogen bonds, disulfide bonds, and ionic bonds. Where these bonds are broken by heat, chemical agents, and so on, the protein unfolds. This process is known as *denaturation.*

6-5 LIPIDS

Lipids play the following physiologic roles: They are (1) integral structural components in cell membranes, (2) metabolic energy sources from dietary supply and fat storage, (3) thermal and electrochemical insulators, and, in some cases, (4) essential nutrients in the form of vitamins.

Lipids are categorized into five major classes: (1) fatty acids, (2) fats, (3) phospholipids, (4) sphingolipids, and (5) steroids.

Fatty acids are the integral components of many other lipids and provide the metabolic energy harbored within their own carbon–carbon bonds. The two main functional groups comprising fatty acids are a carboxylic acid group and a hydrocarbon chain. The hydrocarbon chain varies in length depending on the type of fatty acid. Fatty acids that are biologically important have 16, 18, or 20 carbons in the hydrocarbon chain. The hydrocarbon chain is a nonpolar moiety that imparts the insolubility characteristics that lipids have in water and in other polar solvents.

Fatty acids are either saturated or unsaturated. In saturated fatty acids all the carbons are singly bonded to one another and have at least two hydrogen bonds. Unsaturated fatty acids have at least one carbon–carbon double bond in the hydrocarbon chain. Figure 6-14 depicts examples of a saturated fatty acid (A) and an unsaturated fatty acid (B).

When the carboxyl group of a fatty acid reacts with the alcohol glycerol, the result is the formation of a molecule referred to as a *fat.* The fatty acid can react with any one of the three

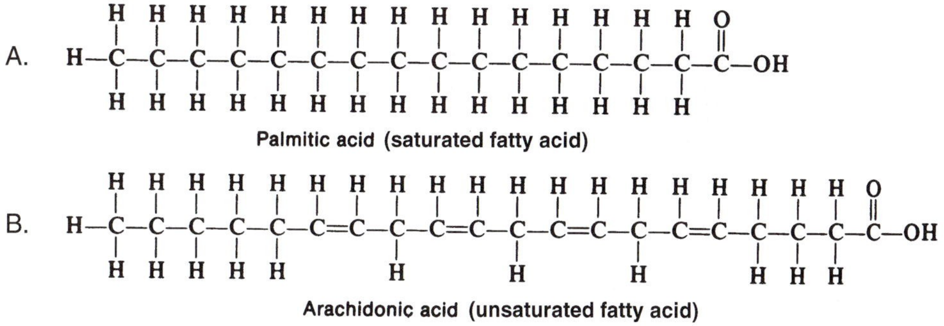

Figure 6-14 *Two fatty acid molecules. (A) 16-carbon, saturated fatty acid (palmitic acid) with a single-bonded carbon chain and each carbon having at least two hydrogen bonds; (B) 20-carbon, unsaturated fatty acid (arachidonic acid) with double-bonded carbon linkages in the chain. Some carbon atoms in the chain have only one hydrogen bond.*

hydroxyl groups present on a glycerol molecule, thus allowing a variety of products to form. One such product, commonly known as *triglyceride*, plays a very important role in the human body. It is from triglyceride that the metabolic energy contained in the fatty acids can be stored and utilized when carbohydrate stores become depleted.

Phospholipids are important molecules that make up the main structure of membranes by acting as a bilayer. (Refer to Sections 6-1 and 7-3 for a depiction of a typical cell membrane.)

Lecithin, a physiologically important phospholipid, plays an essential role in reducing the surface tension in the alveoli as it is the major component of pulmonary surfactant. Pulmonary surfactant is actively produced and secreted by the lung itself. Specifically, the Type II alveolar cells perform this function. (Section 4-7, "Mechanics of Ventilation," under the subheading Law of LaPlace, discusses the physical events associated with lung mechanics and pulmonary surfactant.)

Despite the previous discussion of the surface properties of pulmonary surfactant and the LaPlace relationship, the salient biochemical aspects of this surface-active material will be presented. Surfactant can be recovered from lungs by bronchoalveolar lavage using a saline solution. Surfactant is a multicomponent mixture (Figure 6-15) of phospholipids, neutral lipids, and surfactant-specific proteins referred to as SP-A, SP-B, and SP-C. The major component of pulmonary surfactant by weight is saturated phosphatidylcholine (PC), which is the primary surface-active lipid in the molecule. Most of the saturated phosphatidylcholine has two palmitic acids esterified to the glycerol backbone of the surfactant molecule (Figure 6-16). Most of the unsaturated phosphatidylcholine contains one palmitic acid and one long chain mono-unsaturated fatty acid (Figure 6-17). Phosphatidylglycerol (PG) is the other phospholipid that is important for surfactant function. There are small amounts of phosphatidylethanolamine, sphingomyelin, phosphatidylinositol, and phos-

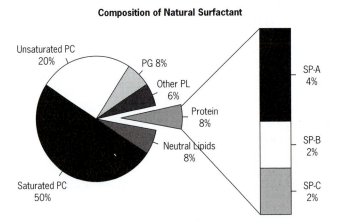

Figure 6-15 *Composition of natural surfactant. Natural surfactant is comprised of 84% phospholipids, 8% proteins, and 8% neutral lipids. The major phospholipid by weight is PC (70%). The surfactant-specific proteins are SP-A (4%), SP-B (2%), and SP-C (2%). (PC = phosphatidylcholine; PG = phosphatidylglycerol; PL = phospholipids; SP-A = surfactant protein A; SP-B = surfactant protein B; and SP-C = surfactant protein C.)*

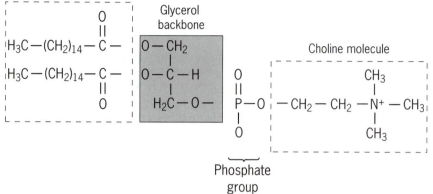

Palmitic acid molecules (saturated)

Figure 6-16 *Saturated phosphatidylcholine molecule constituents. Two palmitic acid molecules (dotted box on left) esterified to glycerol (shaded box) which connects phosphate group (bracket) and choline molecule (dotted box on right).*

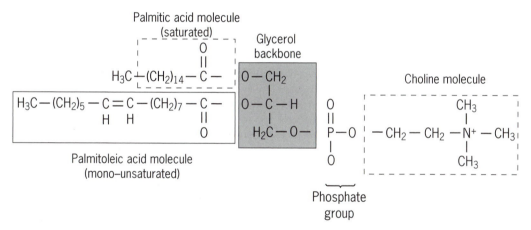

Figure 6-17 *Unsaturated phosphatidylcholine molecule constituents. Palmitic acid molecule (dotted box on upper left) and mono-unsaturated palmitoleic acid molecule (heavy line clear box on lower left) esterified to glycerol molecule (shaded box) which bonds with phosphate group (bracket) and choline molecule (dotted box on right).*

phatidylserine in surfactant. These constituents contribute very little to the surface-active properties of pulmonary surfactant. The major neutral lipid in surfactant is cholesterol. This lipid mixture does not have the biophysical properties of surfactant.

In addition to being comprised of 92% phospholipids, surfactant contains at least three surfactant-specific proteins (SP-A, SP-B, and SP-C) that are present in low concentration (8%). The sequences for these proteins are highly conserved across mammalian species. SP-A is a complex, multimeric protein containing eighteen 26-kilodalton (kD) proteins that are each glycosylated to yield monomer molecular weights of 32 to 36 kD. Therefore, the native form of this protein has a multimer molecular weight of about 650 kD. This protein binds and aggregates the surfactant phospholipids in the presence of calcium ions. Although SP-A alone has only modest effects on the surface properties of the surfactant lipids, it acts cooperatively with SP-B and SP-C to augment surface activity. It also regulates the secretion and reuptake of the surfactant lipids. The carbohydrate on the molecule can function as a lectin (a plant protein with a high affinity for specific sugar residues) and bind to microorganisms to assist with host defense of the alveoli. SP-B and SP-C proteins, 8 kD and 4 kD, respectively, are unusual in that they extract into lipid solvents and behave as lipids. These lipid-like proteins associate with surfactant lipids and enhance biophysical activity. SP-B enhances absorption of the phospholipids to the interface between air and water and acts cooperatively with SP-A to form tubular myelin.

The cellular metabolism of the multicomponent surfactant system also is complex (Figure 6-18). The phospholipids and proteins are synthesized in the endoplasmic reticulum of the type II alveolar cell. The lipophilic proteins, SP-B and SP-C, coalesce with the surfactant lipids to form a stacked lipid-protein array within a storage-secretory granule called the lamellar body. If SP-B is absent, as in congenital SP-B deficiency, lamellar bodies do not form. The lamellar bodies are secreted by exocytosis to yield an alveolar pool of surfactant in reserve for the formation of the surface film. The lamellar bodies unravel to become tubular myelin and loose lipid arrays which absorb to the surface as the film. Small vesicles are not surface-active and are utilized for the recycling of surfactant phospholipids. The proteins also are recycled although the pathways have not been identified. In preterm and newborn infants, the surfactant components are efficiently recycled, whereas recycling is less efficient in adults.

Surfactant synthesis and storage begins in the human fetus after about 20 weeks' gestation. The lungs of most human infants are sufficiently mature to support normal ventilation after 36 weeks' gestation. Surfactant composition changes as the lung develops *in utero.* In preterm infants at risk for developing respiratory distress syndrome (1) the amount of surfactant is decreased, (2) the relative amount of saturated phosphatidylcholine is decreased, (3) phosphatidylglycerol is absent, and (4) phosphatidylinositol is increased. The relative amounts of the surfactant proteins also are decreased. The immaturity of the surfactant system can be evaluated clinically by measuring the ratio of lecithin (phosphatidylcholine) to sphingomyelin (L/S ratio), or the amount of phosphatidylglycerol, in an amniotic fluid sample. As the human fetus matures, the amniotic fluid phospholipid composition changes to become similar to that of the adult lung. Amniotic fluid measurements reflect the maturational status of the fetal lung because the fetal lung secretes fluid continually. Some of this fetal lung fluid, together with any surfactant that has been secreted, mixes with the amniotic fluid.

Production of pulmonary surfactant begins during intrauterine life at approximately 22 to 24 weeks' gestation. The biochemical synthesis of this phospholipid molecule relies on the presence of two different metabolic pathways—the methyl transferase system (22 to 24 weeks) and the phosphocholine transferase system (35 weeks).

Assessing the lecithin/sphingomyelin (L/S) ratio via amniocentesis provides a measure of lung maturity. Prior to 35 weeks' gestation, sphingomyelin (another phospholipid) predominates, thus rendering an L/S ratio less than 2. At approximately 35 weeks' gestation, lecithin production increases and its concentration in the amniotic fluid begins to

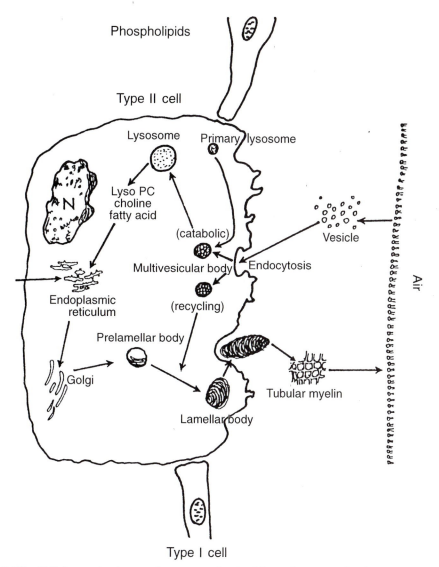

Phospholipids

Type II cell

Lysosome   Primary lysosome

N

Lyso PC
choline
fatty acid

(catabolic)

Vesicle

Multivesicular body   Endocytosis

Endoplasmic
reticulum

(recycling)

Air

Prelamellar body

Golgi

Tubular myelin

Lamellar body

Type I cell

Figure 6-18 *Cellular mechanisms and structures involved in surfactant production in a Type II alveolar cell.*

exceed that of sphingomyelin. An L/S ratio of 2:1 or greater reflects lung maturation sufficient to support extrauterine life. Such an L/S ratio indicates less than a 5% risk for the development of respiratory distress syndrome (RDS), whereas a ratio of 1:1 or less is associated with a greater than 90% risk. A transitional L/S ratio (1.5:1) indicates a 50% probability of risk.

Like other phospholipids, lecithin has a **hydrophobic** and a **hydrophilic** aspect. The postulated alignment of the lecithin molecule within the alveolar lining layer is that the

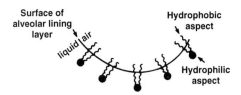

Figure 6-19 *Depiction of orientation of phospholipid molecules in pulmonary surfactant. Hydrophobic aspect projects toward alveolus (air), and hydrophilic aspect extends toward alveolar lining layer.*

hydrophilic portion actually penetrates the liquid phase, and the hydrophobic region protrudes into the air above the liquid phase. Figure 6-19 illustrates the suggested orientation of lecithin molecules (pulmonary surfactant) within the alveolar lining layer at the air-liquid interface.

Unlike most other liquids, the surface tension of the alveolar lining layer is area dependent; that is, alveolar surface tension and alveolar radius are directly proportional. Measurements have shown that the maximum surface tension of the alveolar lining layer is 45 dynes/cm (water surface tension = 75 dynes/cm; saline surface tension = 70 dynes/cm), whereas at relatively low surface areas it exhibits a surface tension near 0 dynes/cm.

Figure 6-20 demonstrates the proposed alignment of pulmonary surfactant molecules at the air-liquid interface at a high lung volume (A) and at a low volume (B).

At high lung volumes, the surfactant molecules are farther apart from one another. Consequently, surface tension of the alveolar lining layer increases (lung compliance decreases). Portion B of Figure 6-20 shows the relationships among the pulmonary surfactant molecules at a lower lung volume. At this point, the surfactant molecules are much closer together; thus, alveolar surface tension is effectively reduced (lung compliance increases). Essentially, pulmonary surfactant (1) reduces alveolar surface tension and (2) helps maintain alveolar stability.

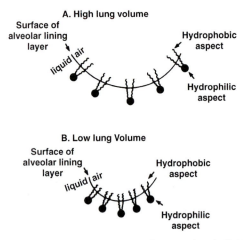

Figure 6-20 *Depiction of alignment of pulmonary surfactant phospholipid molecules at the air-liquid interface at (A) a high lung volume and (B) a low lung volume.*

Because phospholipids can contain both saturated and unsaturated fatty acids, one could speculate about the influences of hyperoxia directly on pulmonary surfactant. As a point of conjecture, would oxygen, or any of its free radical derivatives, interact with the unsaturated fatty acid portion of the lecithin molecule? (See Section 6-8.)

Surfactant was approved for the treatment of RDS in the United States in 1990 after extensive clinical trials demonstrated decreased pneumothorax and death. The surfactants used clinically are of two types: a mixture of synthetic lipids (Exosurf®) and organic solvent extracts of animal lung source surfactant (Survanta®). The animal lung source surfactant contains the lipophilic proteins SP-B and SP-C together with the surfactant lipids. Animal lung derived surfactants cause more rapid improvements in oxygenation than do the synthetic lipid surfactants because animal lung derived surfactants cause a more rapid increase in lung gas volumes. Surfactant treatments can be given in the delivery room during intubation and resuscitation to preterm infants who are at high risk for developing RDS. Surfactant can also be administered to infants via direct instillation through an endotracheal tube after initial stabilization and diagnosis of RDS. The rationale for surfactant treatments is that the primary abnormality in RDS is surfactant deficiency. Surfactant treatments replace this lack of surfactant and facilitate the respiratory support of the infant until the lungs mature and manufacture enough surfactant. The treatment strategy is biochemically favorable because surfactant phospholipids are not catabolized rapidly in preterm infants. The surfactant used for treatment enters the metabolic pathways in the lungs by recycling and acts as a substrate for the preterm lungs.

6-6 NUCLEIC ACIDS

The two principal nucleic acids of a cell are deoxyribonucleic acid (DNA) and ribonucleic acid (RNA). The DNA of a cell carries the genetic information necessary for synthesis of proteins specific for a species, whereas RNA participates as the machinery for the process.

Just as proteins are chains of amino acids, nucleic acids are chains of basic molecular units referred to as **nucleotides.** Nucleotides consist of a nitrogenous ring-structured molecule, a five-carbon sugar, and a phosphoric acid. There are five different nitrogenous bases. Three are categorized as **pyrimidine** bases and the remaining two as **purine** bases. The pyrimidine bases are uracil, thymine, and cytosine. The purines are guanine and adenine. Figure 6-21 shows the structure of the nucleotide adenosine monophosphate (AMP). Nucleotides for the remaining bases also exist.

In addition to their presence in DNA and RNA, nucleotides also function biologically as free molecules. Most notable in this regard is the high-energy-containing triphosphate, adenosine triphosphate (ATP), depicted in Figure 6-22. Although ATP is the principal molecule serving as a storage source of energy, triphosphates for the other nucleotides occur also and, like ATP, have high-energy bonds. Another group of nucleotides are the cyclic nucleotides, which participate in numerous biochemical reactions. The structure for the cyclic nucleotide 3',5'-AMP is shown in Figure 6-23.

Important distinctions need to be made regarding the nucleotides that comprise DNA versus those of RNA. First, the five-carbon sugar of DNA nucleotides is always deoxyribose, whereas that for RNA nucleotides is ribose. Second, the base thymine is found only

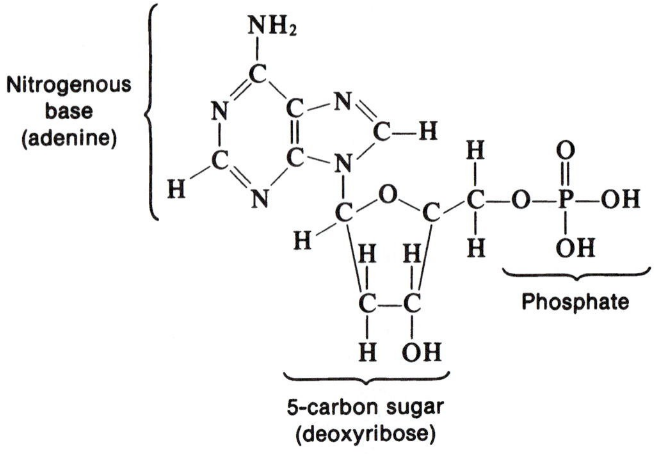

Figure 6-21 *Adenosine monophosphate (AMP) molecule.*

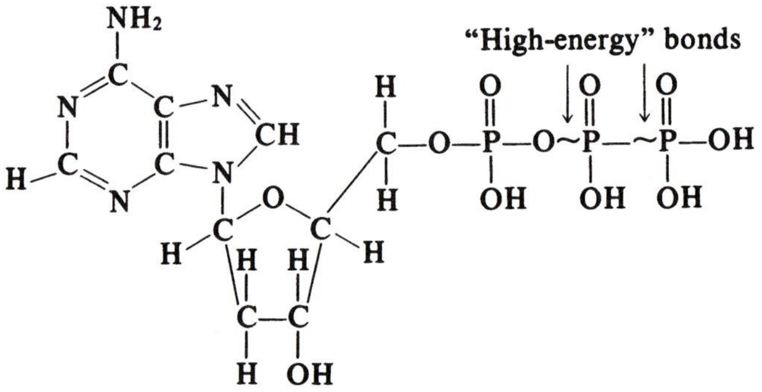

Figure 6-22 *Adenosine triphosphate (ATP) showing "high energy" bonds between the phosphate groups.*

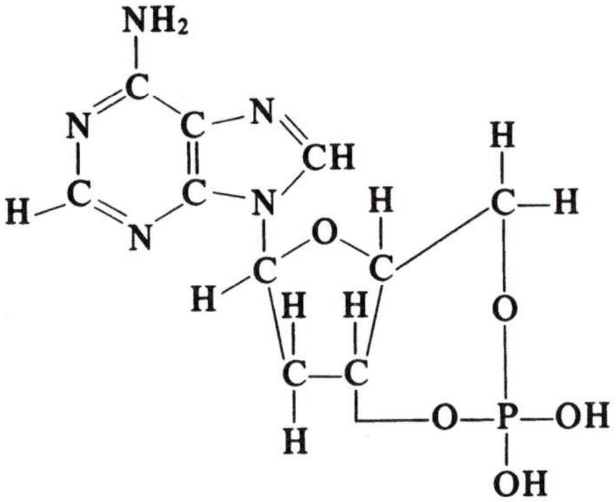

Figure 6-23 *3′,5′-adenosine monophosphate (cyclic AMP); a cyclic nucleotide found in cells such as the bronchial smooth muscle cells and mast cells.*

TABLE 6-4   DNA-RNA Compositional Comparison

DNA	Components	RNA
Adenine		Adenine
Guanine		Guanine
Cytosine	Nitrogenous bases	Cytosine
Thymine[a]		Uracil[b]
Deoxyribose[a]	Sugar	Ribose[b]
Phosphate	Phosphate	Phosphate

[a]present in DNA, but not in RNA.
[b]present in RNA, but not in DNA.

in DNA, whereas the base uracil occurs only in RNA. Table 6-4 summarizes the similarities and differences between DNA and RNA nucleotides.

As mentioned above, nucleic acids are actually polynucleotides, that is, chains of nucleotides. The nucleotides are linked together by phosphate groups between the sugar molecules, as is shown in Figure 6-24.

DNA is a double-stranded molecule that occurs in the shape of a double helix. In short, DNA consists of two strands of polynucleotides wrapped around each other. Each strand is attracted to the other by hydrogen bonds, which occur between certain complimentary bases. In complimentary DNA strands, adenine always pairs with the thymine and guanine always pairs with cytosine, as is hypothetically depicted in Figure 6-25.

RNA occurs in three basic forms, all of which consist of a single strand of a polynucleotide. The three basic forms are messenger RNA (mRNA), transfer RNA (tRNA), and ribosomal RNA (rRNA). It is primarily important here to recognize that RNA is synthesized using DNA as the template. Cellular enzymes link RNA nucleotides by using the DNA nucleotide sequence as a pattern. However, when adenine appears in the DNA template,

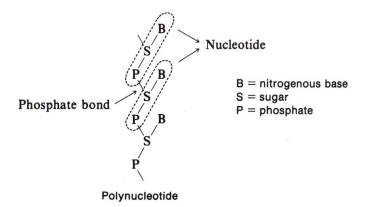

Figure 6-24   *A phosphate bond between the phosphate group of one nucleotide and the sugar component of another nucleotide. This bonding between nucleotide molecules forms polynucleotides.*

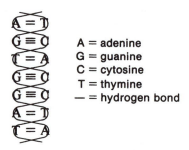

Figure 6-25 *Hypothetical DNA molecule illustrating a double helix formed by two strands of polynucleotides wrapped around each other. Hydrogen bonds hold the strands together.*

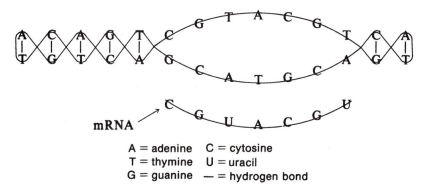

Figure 6-26 *Hypothetical DNA molecule and DNA template. Whenever adenine appears in the DNA template, uracil matches with the new RNA molecule formed.*

uracil rather than thymine is matched in the new RNA molecule synthesized. This process is illustrated in Figure 6-26.

Knowing the process whereby RNA is made from DNA is important in understanding how cells can direct their destiny by synthesizing proteins. It is the DNA nucleotide sequence that comprises a gene. The amino acid sequence in a protein is, in turn, determined by the nucleotide sequence in a gene. Thus, the sequence of nucleotides formed by synthesis of RNA provides a transcription of the coded information in DNA for a sequence of amino acids in a given protein. This transcribed code is subsequently translated into a protein when amino acids are aligned with the respective nucleotide bases in RNA on the ribosomes. Peptide bonds are formed between the amino acids, thus creating a protein.

Because the details of protein synthesis are beyond the focus intended for this text, the reader is referred to the bibliography.

6-7 HEMOGLOBIN BIOCHEMISTRY

The respiratory care practitioner is frequently concerned with the oxygenation and acid-base status of his patients. The hemoglobin molecule is involved in the homeostasis of both of these physiologic processes and is often overlooked or given only slight consideration by the practitioner.

The purpose of this section is to elucidate the physiologic activities of hemoglobin by presenting some biochemical concepts associated with the molecule. Included here are the following aspects of hemoglobin biochemistry: (1) structure, (2) variants, (3) function, and (4) degradation.

Structure

The hemoglobin molecule is a large protein structure (molecular weight of approximately 66,700 daltons) consisting of a **globin** portion and four **heme** units. The globin portion is a protein molecule comprised of four polypeptide chains. There are two alpha (α) polypeptide chains, each with 141 amino acids, and two beta (β) polypeptide chains, each having 146 amino acids.

Each polypeptide chain binds to an iron atom that is in the center of the heme molecule. A histidine residue in both the alpha and beta chains is the site for attachment to heme.

Ordinarily, most protein molecules have a low helix content; however, hemoglobin possesses a high helix content. The alpha and beta polypeptide chains of adult hemoglobin exhibit helical segments interrupted by nonhelical regions. Each polypeptide chain folds and bends into a tertiary structure. Because the globin portion of the hemoglobin molecule exists as a multichained protein complex (two or more polypeptide chains), hemoglobin is described as having a quaternary structure (Table 6-3).

Figure 6-27 illustrates the hemoglobin tetramer (four shapes) that occurs as a consequence of the three-dimensional (tertiary) structure of the globin molecule. Note the elliptical (shaded) structure overlapping a portion of the alpha and beta chains. It represents a heme molecule. The four polypeptide chains are arranged into one unit such that the heme moieties are far apart. Simplistically, the stereochemistry of the hemoglobin molecule is presented in Figure 6-28.

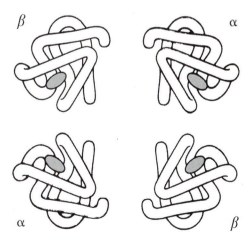

Figure 6-27 *Hemoglobin tetramer (four shapes) comprised of alpha and beta polypeptide chains with heme molecule highlighted.*

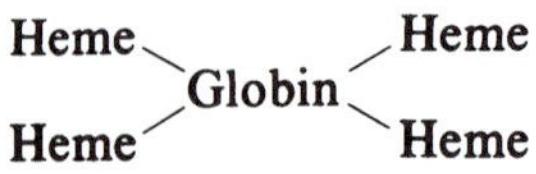

Figure 6-28 *Simplified depiction of orientation among the globin and four heme portions of a hemoglobin molecule.*

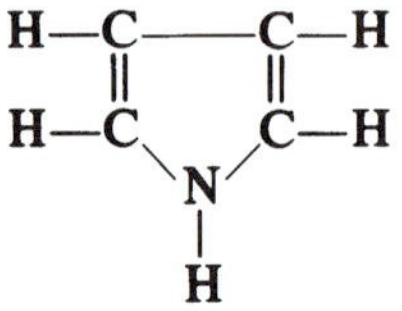

Figure 6-29 *Pyrrole molecule. Heme contains four pyrrole molecules cyclically arranged.*

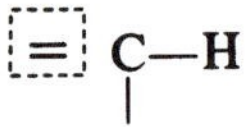

Figure 6-30 *Methylene bridge. The four pyrrole molecules cyclically arranged in heme are linked by methylene bridges.*

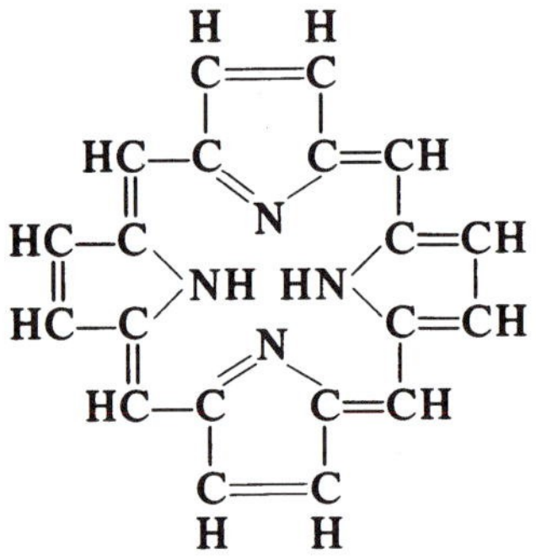

Figure 6-31 *Porphyrin. The linkage of four pyrrole molecules via methylene bridges produces a porphyrin. Porphyrins often combine with metals forming metalloporphyrins.*

Heme is a nonprotein, organic, ring-shaped molecule. The ring-shaped configuration arises from the fact that heme contains four pyrrole groups. Figure 6-29 shows the structure of a pyrrole group.

Pyrrole groups are linked to one another by **methylene bridges.** The structural components of a methylene bridge are illustrated in Figure 6-30.

The structure resulting from the linkage of the four pyrroles by the methylene bridges is called a **porphyrin.** The porphyrin structure is depicted in Figure 6-31.

Porphyrins are nitrogen-containing compounds that occur in nature as free porphyrins or as **metalloporphyrins** (porphyrins combined with a metal). Hemoglobin is an important

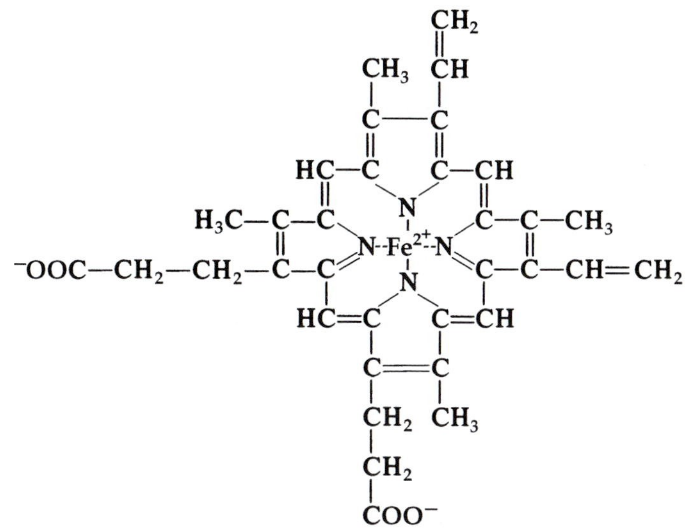

Figure 6-32   *Heme portion of hemoglobin molecule. The metalloporphyrin comprising heme normally contains a ferrous state (Fe^{2+}) atom in its center.*

metalloprotein. The metalloporphyrin contained in the heme portion of the hemoglobin molecule has an iron (Fe^{2+}, ferrous state) atom in its center. The molecular structure of heme is illustrated below in Figure 6-32.

Another familiar protein possessing a metalloporphyrin structure with an iron (ferrous state) atom is the **myoglobin** molecule contained in muscle tissue. Myoglobin temporarily stores oxygen that awaits cellular respiration. More will be said about myoglobin later in this chapter.

The iron atom that occupies the center of the porphyrin ring in the hemoglobin molecule has six bonds available. Four are utilized by the nitrogen atoms in each of the four pyrrole molecules. Another bond, the fifth, binds the porphyrin to the globin. Specifically, this linkage is between the iron atom and the nitrogen atom of the imidazole group of the histidine residue on the globin molecule. Figure 6-33 shows the imidazole group of the histidine residue (R) on the globin chain bonded to the iron atom of the heme group.

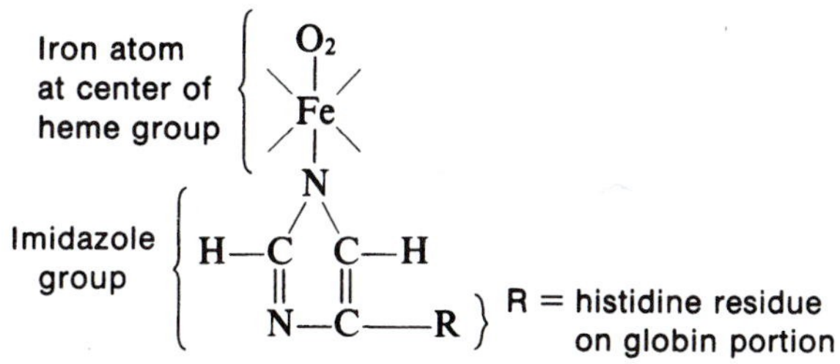

Figure 6-33   *Imidazole group bonded to heme. A side chain (imidazole group) of the amino acid histidine links heme to globin portion of hemoglobin molecule.*

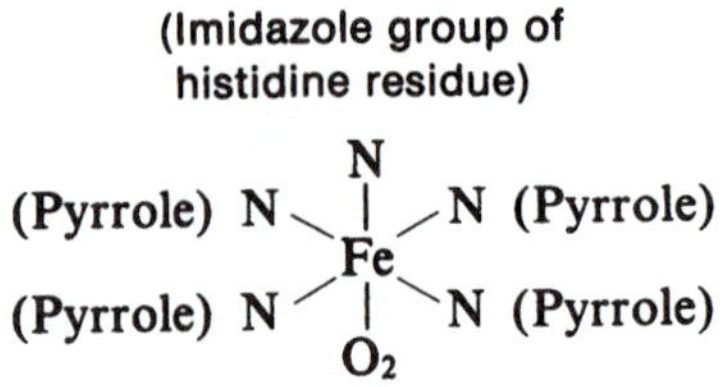

(Imidazole group of
histidine residue)

N

(Pyrrole) N   N (Pyrrole)

Fe

(Pyrrole) N   N (Pyrrole)

O_2

Figure 6-34 *Ferrous ion (Fe^{2+}) in center of heme forming six bonds. Four bonds formed with the pyrroles, one with the imidazole group of histidine, and one with oxygen.*

The sixth bond is available for the reversible attachment of oxygen. When hemoglobin is deoxygenated, the sixth bond of iron is empty.

A schematic depiction of an iron atom with its six available bonds, as it functions in heme, is shown in Figure 6-34.

Variants

Throughout the course of a human life, a person will have synthesized four hemoglobin variants as a result of forming five different globin chains. These chains include

- alpha chains (α)
- beta chains (β)
- gamma chains (γ)
- delta chains (δ)
- epsilon chains (ϵ)

The hemoglobin variants resulting from different combinations of these chains include

- embryonic hemoglobin (two α chains and two ϵ chains)
- fetal hemoglobin or HbF (two α chains and two γ chains)
- normal adult hemoglobin or HbA (two α chains and two β chains)
- adult variant hemoglobin or HbA_2 (two α chains and two δ chains)

Each of the hemoglobin variants identified here always has two normal alpha chains.

The type of the globin chain synthesized changes throughout life as the source of oxygen changes. Figure 6-35 depicts the percentage of the type of polypeptide chains present in the globin molecule versus chronological age.

During embryonic life oxygenation needs are fulfilled via the interstitial fluid of the mother. At this time the embryo has two types of hemoglobin in circulation. One type consists of two alpha chains and two epsilon chains; the other type contains two alpha chains and two gamma chains.

As gestation proceeds, the epsilon polypeptide chains disappear (circa 12 weeks), thus allowing fetal hemoglobin (HbF), which has two alpha chains and two gamma chains, to be the sole form of hemoglobin during this period. However, about six weeks preceding birth, adult hemoglobin (HbA) with two alpha and two beta chains begins to develop. At

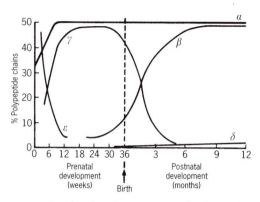

Figure 6-35 *A graphic representation showing the percentage of polypeptide chains comprising the globin portion of the hemoglobin molecule during prenatal and postnatal life (α = alpha; β = beta; ε = epsilon; γ = gamma; δ = delta).*

birth, the neonate possesses both HbF and HbA. HbF remains in circulation until about six months following birth.

Just prior to birth another form of hemoglobin begins to develop. Its globin portion contains two alpha and two delta chains. It is a variant of adult hemoglobin, designated as HbA_2, which constitutes about 2–3% of the total amount of hemoglobin in adult circulation and persists throughout the remainder of life.

Mutant Hemoglobins

Numerous mutant, or abnormal, hemoglobins have been described in the literature. Many hemoglobin mutations result from erroneous amino acid sequencing within either the alpha or beta polypeptide chains in the globin portion of the molecule. These mutations can occur during hemoglobin synthesis or after the hemoglobin molecule is formed. In other words, alteration in hemoglobin's molecular structure can be inherited or acquired.

Methemoglobinemia, for example, occurs when the ferrous ion (Fe^{2+}) in the heme portion of the hemoglobin molecule becomes oxidized to the ferric state (Fe^{3+}). This oxidation takes place when the amino acid tyrosine substitutes for a histidine in either the α or β chain in the globin portion of the hemoglobin molecule. The tyrosine side chain causes the ferrous ion to oxidize to the ferric state.

When the heme's iron atom is oxidized to Fe^{3+}, heme can no longer transport oxygen because the ferric ion can form only five bonds compared to the six formed by Fe^{2+}. The ferric ion forms four bonds with the four nitrogen atoms of the pyrrole molecules in the porphyrin ring and one bond with the globin portion of the hemoglobin molecule. No bond is available for binding chemically and reversibly with oxygen. Table 6-5 outlines the binding capabilities of both the ferric and ferrous ions associated with the heme portion of the hemoglobin molecule. When the blood contains an excess of methemoglobin, the condition is described as methemoglobinemia.

Sickle cell hemoglobin (HbS) is caused by the replacement of the amino acid glutamine on the β polypeptide chains with valine at position 6 in the amino acid sequence. Note the

TABLE 6-5   Bonds Formed by Ferric and Ferrous Ions in Hemoglobin

Ferric (Fe^{2+}) Ion (Normal Hemoglobin)	Ferrous (Fe^{3+}) Ion (Methemoglobin)
• 4 bonds with 4 N atoms of pyrroles in prophyrin ring • 1 bond with globin • 1 bond with O_2	• 4 bonds with 4 N atoms of pyrroles in porphyrin ring • 1 bond with globin

TABLE 6-6   Abbreviated β-chain Amino Acid Sequence for HbA and HbS

β-chain Position	Hemoglobin A	Hemoglobin S
1	valine	valine
2	histidine	histidine
3	leucine	leucine
4	threonine	threonine
5	proline	proline
6	**glutamine**	**valine**
7	glutamine	glutamine
8	lysine	lysine

sequence of the first eight amino acids in the β chain in normal adult hemoglobin (HbA) compared with the amino acid sequence in hemoglobin S (Table 6-6).

Function

Hemoglobin performs a vital function in both the delivery of oxygen to the tissues and the removal of carbon dioxide from the tissues. In addition to its role in gas transport, hemoglobin also is an effective buffer in the red blood cell.

As a vehicle for oxygen transport, hemoglobin has more than one active site. Each hemoglobin molecule contains four hemes. Because each heme group is capable of binding one molecule of oxygen, each hemoglobin molecule has the capacity to carry four oxygen molecules.

The binding of a molecule of oxygen at one site affects the activity of the other three sites. In other words, when unsaturated (deoxygenated) hemoglobin molecules enter the pulmonary capillary system, the combination of one oxygen molecule with one of the heme groups increases the affinity of the remaining three sites for oxygen. The addition of a second molecule of oxygen enhances the binding potential for the third, and so on. This phenomenon is termed **cooperativity** or *cooperative binding.*

Conversely, at the tissue level the unloading of one oxygen molecule facilitates the release of oxygen at the other sites. The release of a second one further reduces the oxygen-hemoglobin affinity. Oxygen's affinity for hemoglobin decreases with the release of each successive oxygen molecule. Hemoglobin is thus capable of delivering a larger load of oxygen to the tissues than it could without cooperativity.

Other factors influence oxyhemoglobin affinity. These factors include body temperature, arterial blood P_{CO_2}, arterial blood pH, and 2,3-diphosphoglycerate (2,3-DPG) levels in the erythrocyte. Low temperature, low arterial P_{CO_2}, high pH, and low 2,3-DPG levels all cause the oxyhemoglobin dissociation curve to shift leftward. Such conditions increase oxyhemoglobin affinity, thus reducing the release of oxygen to the tissues. The regulatory activities of these specific molecules (H^+, CO_2, and 2,3-DPG) greatly influence oxyhemoglobin binding despite the large distance between the heme and where H^+, CO_2, and 2,3-DPG bind on the hemoglobin molecule. The interactions between these spatially distinct sites are called *allosteric interactions.*

Conversely, high temperature, high P_{CO_2}, low pH, and high levels of 2,3-DPG cause the oxyhemoglobin dissociation curve to shift to the right. These physiologic factors facilitate the release of oxygen to the tissues by lessening the oxyhemoglobin affinity. None of these factors negates cooperativity. Each merely restricts or enhances oxygen loading and unloading.

The cooperative binding and releasing of oxygen by hemoglobin is responsible for the sigmoid shape of the oxyhemoglobin dissociation curve, which plots the partial pressure of oxygen (*x*-axis) versus the saturation of hemoglobin (*y*-axis), as shown in Figure 6-36.

The concept of cooperativity with respect to the hemoglobin molecule can further be appreciated when one compares the dissociation curve of myoglobin to that of hemoglobin. First of all, myoglobin is a hemoprotein consisting of one polypeptide chain attached to one heme. This molecular arrangement is structurally similar to a subunit of hemoglobin; that is, a heme molecule bound to a polypeptide chain. Consequently, myoglobin possesses the capability of reversibly combining with one molecule of oxygen. Since myoglobin has only a single polypeptide chain and one heme group, the shape of the oxymyoglobin dissociation curve is hyperbolic (Figure 6-37).

The advantages of cooperativity can be observed when the two dissociation curves are superimposed (Figure 6-38).

The oxymyoglobin curve lies far to the left of the hemoglobin curve. This situation indicates that myoglobin does not significantly reduce its affinity for oxygen until the P_{O_2} falls below 10 mm Hg. Hemoglobin, on the other hand, by virtue of its four oxygen-combining

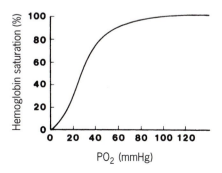

Figure 6-36 *Sigmoid-shaped oxyhemoglobin dissociation curve. P_{O_2} is plotted on the x-axis and S_{O_2} is plotted on the y-axis.*

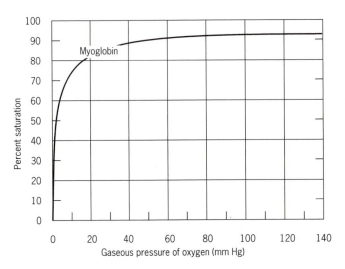

Figure 6-37 *Hyperbolic, oxymyoglobin dissociation curve. Po_2 is plotted on the x-axis and myoglobin saturation is plotted on the y-axis.*

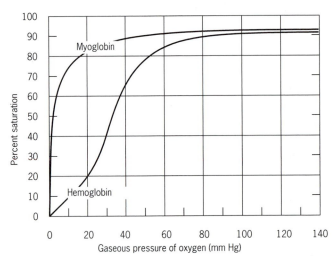

Figure 6-38 *Superimposed oxyhemoglobin and oxymyoglobin dissociation curves demonstrating the advantage of cooperativity regarding the oxyhemoglobin curve. Myoglobin reduces its affinity for oxygen at a Po_2 of about 10 torr; oxyhemoglobin reduces its oxygen affinity at a Po_2 of around 50 torr.*

sites exhibiting cooperativity, releases its oxygen at comparatively much higher Po_2s (less than 50 mm Hg).

The hemoglobin molecule interacts differently with carbon dioxide than it does with oxygen. Heme is not the site of carbon dioxide attachment; globin is. At the tissue level carbon dioxide affixes to the terminal amine groups of the polypeptide chains of the globin.

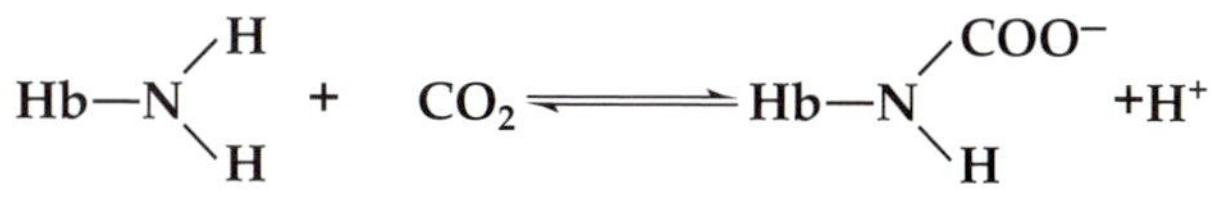

Figure 6-39 *Carbon dioxide affixes to hemoglobin by combining with a terminal amine group on the globin portion of the hemoglobin molecule.*

The reaction is rapid and reversible, as is the interaction between heme and oxygen. Carbaminohemoglobin ($HbCO_2$) represents approximately 10% of the total amount of carbon dioxide carried in the blood. An increase in the arterial Pco_2 increases carbaminohemoglobin formation, thereby reducing hemoglobin's affinity for oxygen. The relationship between carbaminohemoglobin and oxyhemoglobin, measured as the So_2, describes the Haldane effect. The chemical combination of carbon dioxide and a terminal amine group on one of the globin polypeptide chains is represented in Figure 6-39.

The hemoglobin molecule also functions as an effective blood buffer by accepting free protons (H^+) present in the erythrocyte. The fact that hemoglobin is a conjugated protein (i.e., it contains a nonprotein portion, heme, and a protein portion, globin) accounts for its buffering ability. Proteins have the capacity to act as both acids and bases because they contain at least one carboxyl group and an amine group. The carboxyl group buffers by releasing H^+ in alkaline solutions; the amine group behaves as a buffer by accepting hydrogen ions in acid solutions. (It might be useful for the reader to review the definition of a *zwitterion* presented in Section 4–8 and Section 6-4.)

The release of oxygen to the tissues, that is, the transformation of oxyhemoglobin to deoxyhemoglobin, increases the pK of hemoglobin from 6.2 to 7.7. This event, therefore, changes the range within which this buffer is most effective (i.e., from 5.2–7.2 at a pK of 6.2 to 6.7–8.7 at a pK of 7.7).

Most of hemoglobin's buffering activity at physiologic pH is accomplished by the imidazole group of the amino acid histidine in the polypeptide chains (globin portion). The imidazole group itself has a pK of about 7.0. Therefore, its effective range is 6.0 to 8.0—a range that is certainly within the physiologic range for blood. (Reviewing Section 3–4, "Law of Mass Action and Henderson-Hasselbalch Equation," under the subheadings of "pH Concepts" and "Buffer Solutions" might prove helpful to the reader.) Figure 6-40 depicts the imidazole group of the amino acid histidine for both deoxygenated (HHb) hemoglobin and oxygenated (HbO$_2$) hemoglobin.

Figure 6-41 presents a schematic overview of the series of reactions occurring both in the tissues and in the lungs and summarizes the reversible reactions between hemoglobin and oxygen and carbon dioxide and between hemoglobin and hydrogen ions.

Degradation

The average life span of an erythrocyte is about 120 days. During the course of its normal existence, the erythrocyte undergoes an aging process due to metabolic change. In time, the ferrous ion is oxidized to the ferric state.

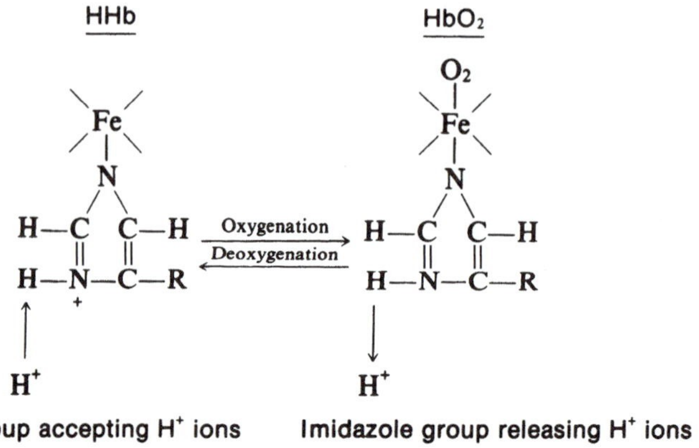

Figure 6-40 *The accepting and releasing of H⁺ ions occurs when hemoglobin is deoxygenated and oxygenated, respectively. HHb forms when O_2 is released from hemoglobin. H⁺ ions are released from HHb when HbO_2 forms.*

$$Fe^{2+} \xrightarrow{\quad e^- \text{ (electron)} \quad} Fe^{3+}$$

As a result, the heme portion becomes incapable of combining with oxygen. As hemoglobin degradation proceeds, red blood cells are removed from circulation and taken up by the liver, spleen, and bone marrow. Hemoglobin is eventually degraded into three components: protoporphyrin IX, iron, and globin.

The porphyrin ring opens as one of the methylene bridges splits. An open heme ring complexed to the polypeptide chains (globins) results. This molecule is called *verdohemoglobin*. The iron atom is removed and enters the liver, where it is stored as ferritin and made available for the synthesis of new heme molecules. Globin molecules undergo a breakdown of their polypeptide chains into their constituent amino acids. These amino acids enter the amino acid pool and are reused for future protein synthesis. What remains now is an open porphyrin compound called *biliverdin*. Eventually, biliverdin is reduced to form bilirubin. Bilirubin is transported to the liver and excreted in the bile. If the liver cannot process the bilirubin properly, jaundice results.

6-8 BIOCHEMICAL ASPECTS OF OXYGEN TOXICITY

The therapeutic administration of oxygen can be considered life-saving when it ameliorates hypoxemia and hypoxia. However, it becomes life-threatening when given in excessive amounts. Joseph Priestly, who is credited with having discovered oxygen, perhaps sensed this dual nature of oxygen when he said in 1775, " . . . it [oxygen] might be peculiarly salutary to the lungs in certain morbid cases . . . " and " . . . oxygen might burn the candle of life too quickly, and too soon exhaust the animal powers within. . . . "

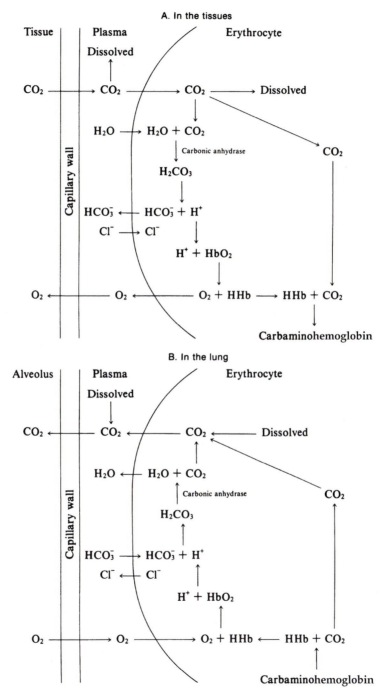

Figure 6-41 *(A) CO$_2$ uptake and O$_2$ release at the tissue level; (B) O$_2$ uptake and CO$_2$ release at the lung level. From Levitzky, Michael G.:* Pulmonary Physiology, *1982, McGraw-Hill Book Co. Used with permission.*

The purposes of this section are (1) to present an overview of some of the biochemical processes involved in the normal cellular utilization of oxygen, (2) to discuss the implications of these processes in the context of hyperoxia, (3) to explain the biochemical role of antioxidants as a protective mechanism, preventive against the cytotoxic effects of free radicals, and (4) to describe briefly the salient pathophysiologic aspects of pulmonary oxygen toxicity.

Oxygen Radicals

After air is inspired into the lungs from the environment, oxygen passively diffuses across the alveolar-capillary membrane, physically dissolves in the plasma, passively enters the red blood cells, and reversibly and chemically binds to hemoglobin. Both the plasma and hemoglobin oxygen transport mechanisms deliver this vital nutrient to the cells of the body. Aerobic organisms use oxygen as an electron acceptor (oxidation) in mitrochondrial electron transport systems. It is at the cellular level that the cytotoxic effects of free radicals can become manifest. Paradoxically, oxygen from the atmospheric air is necessary for aerobic metabolism to occur. Fortunately, endogenous antioxidant defense mechanisms normally exist to counteract the potentially harmful effects of the oxygen metabolites generated during cellular respiration.

As discussed in Section 3–1, "Atomic Structure and Electron Configuration," each oxygen molecule possesses two unpaired electrons spinning in the same direction in the molecule's outermost electron shell. As reduction proceeds during cellular metabolism, some oxygen can undergo univalent reduction. The expression **univalent reduction** refers to the acceptance by oxygen of one electron at a time as oxygen proceeds through its metabolic pathways. The metabolic pathway of interest here is located intracellularly, specifically within mitochondria. These organelles contain a series of catalysts known as the *electron transport chain*, or *respiratory chain*. At the end of this metabolic pathway, oxygen undergoes univalent reduction four times. The final (fourth) reduction produces a molecule of water. The overall reduction (gain of electrons) reaction for oxygen by the electron transport chain in mitochondria is expressed as

$$O_2 + 4H^+ + 4e^- \rightarrow 2H_2O$$

Partial reduction to $O_2^-\cdot$ occurs at several points, but full reduction to H_2O happens only at the end of the pathway. Consequently, biochemical units having an unpaired electron in their outermost shell are formed. These units are called *oxygen free radicals.*

These free radicals, intermediates of oxygen metabolism, are responsible for compromising the integrity of cell membranes. An interesting point to make here is that the life span of these free radicals is extraordinarily brief. Their existence is usually expressed in terms of milliseconds. However, despite their transient nature, the oxygen free radicals are cytotoxic if present in large quantities and if the organism lacks biochemical mechanisms (antioxidants) to protect itself from their lethal activity.

As oxygen is utilized by the cells, it can yield four metabolic byproducts that are classified as *reactive oxygen species*. These cytotoxic metabolites are

- $O_2^-\cdot$ (superoxide anion)
- H_2O_2 (hydrogen peroxide)

- HO· (hydroxyl radical)
- OH_2· (perhydroxyl radical)

During respiratory metabolism a series of oxidation-reduction reactions occurs. In the process, oxygen gains electrons and is, therefore, reduced. The following products are the result of oxygen reduction at the cellular level:

- Superoxide radical (O_2^-·)
- Hydrogen peroxide (H_2O_2)
- Water (H_2O)

The respective equations yielding these end-products are shown below.

- $O_2 + e^- \rightarrow O_2^-$·
- $O_2 + 2H^+ + 2e^- \rightarrow H_2O_2$
- $O_2 + 3H^+ + 3e^- \rightarrow H_2O_2 + HO$·
- $O_2 + 4H^+ + 4e^- \rightarrow 2H_2O$

The overall reaction that takes place via the mitochrondrial cytochromes where a molecule of oxygen is reduced to water is as follows:

$$O_2 \xrightarrow{e^-} O_2^- \cdot \xrightarrow{e^- + 2H^+} H_2O_2 \xrightarrow{e^- + H^+} HO \cdot \xrightarrow{e^- + H^+} H_2O$$
$$\downarrow$$
$$H_2O$$

The end-product (i.e., water) is obviously totally innocuous to the cell and the respiring organism *in toto*. In fact, most (98%) of the oxygen that we normally consume is reduced by cytochrome oxidase in the mitochondria without the production of any detectable free radicals. Hydrogen peroxide is, however, cytotoxic because it is a moderate oxidative agent. Furthermore, under excessive respiratory conditions hydrogen peroxide can be transformed to the highly destructive hydroxyl radical (HO·) by certain metallic ions.

Hydrogen peroxide also reacts with the superoxide anion (O_2^-·) in the presence of an iron catalyst to form the hydroxyl radical and singlet oxygen ($^1O_2$), as shown here.

$$H_2O_2 + O_2^- \cdot \xrightarrow{Fe^{2+}} HO \cdot + {}^1O_2 + OH^-$$

The resulting HO· radical and singlet oxygen are more biologically active, and potentially more destructive, than either hydrogen peroxide or the superoxide anion.

Similarly, any organic hydroperoxide, symbolized as ROOH, can react with the superoxide anion according to the following reaction:

$$ROOH + O_2^- \cdot \longrightarrow RO \cdot + OH^- + O_2$$

The result of this oxidative event is an organic alkoxyl radical (RO·), which serves to perpetuate the oxidative chain reaction at the cell level.

The paradox is that aerobically respiring species demand the presence of oxygen to propagate. But, at the same time, the presence of these oxygen free radicals has a cytotoxic effect. It is, therefore, reasonable to assume the existence of other biochemical mechanisms that counteract the deleterious effects of the free radicals since the oxidative process normally does not proceed in an uncontrolled fashion.

Lipid Peroxidation

Before we discuss the topic of lipid peroxidation, a few aspects of the molecular structure of cell membranes will be presented. Currently, cell membranes are described as fluid mosaics consisting primarily of phospholipid bilayers interspersed with protein molecules, as shown in Figure 6-42. (Section 6-1, "The Functional Anatomy and Chemistry of the Living Cell," and Section 7-3, "Bacterial Ultrastructure," provide additional information about cell membranes.) The cell membrane is composed of phospholipid-protein complexes and other membrane-bound components.

The highly reactive intermediates of oxygen reduction (i.e., the oxygen free radicals) cause lipid peroxidation of cell membrane phospholipids containing unsaturated fatty acids. Saturated fatty acids are less susceptible to lipid peroxidation.

Recall the distinction between saturated fatty acids and unsaturated fatty acids discussed in Section 6-5, "Lipids." Saturated fatty acids are characterized by the presence of chains of singly bonded, evenly numbered carbon atoms with hydrogen atoms occupying the remaining carbon-bonding sites, except for the carboxyl group at the end of the molecular structure. For example, the structural formula for the fatty acid palmitic acid is given below.

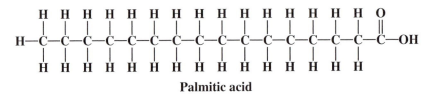

Palmitic acid

Unsaturated fatty acids, on the other hand, are comprised of chains of singly bonded carbon atoms containing one or more pairs of doubly bonded carbon atoms, for example, palmitoleic acid.

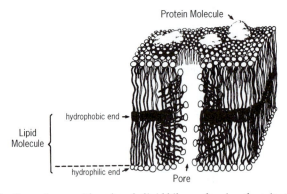

Figure 6-42 *A typical cell membrane with a phospholipid bilayer showing the orientation of the hydrophobic and hydrophilic ends of the phospholipid molecules and proteins interspersed throughout the membrane.*

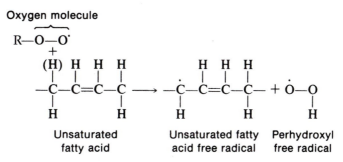

Figure 6-43 *Hydrogen abstraction from an unsaturated fatty acid by an O_2 molecule yielding an unsaturated fatty acid free radical and a perhydroxy free radical.*

| 16 | 15 | 14 | 13 | 12 | 11 | 10 | 9 | 8 | 7 | 6 | 5 | 4 | 3 | 2 | 1 |

$$H-\overset{\overset{\displaystyle H}{|}}{\underset{\underset{\displaystyle H}{|}}{C}}-\overset{\overset{\displaystyle H}{|}}{\underset{\underset{\displaystyle H}{|}}{C}}-\overset{\overset{\displaystyle H}{|}}{\underset{\underset{\displaystyle H}{|}}{C}}-\overset{\overset{\displaystyle H}{|}}{\underset{\underset{\displaystyle H}{|}}{C}}-\overset{\overset{\displaystyle H}{|}}{\underset{\underset{\displaystyle H}{|}}{C}}-\overset{\overset{\displaystyle H}{|}}{\underset{\underset{\displaystyle H}{|}}{C}}-\overset{\overset{\displaystyle H}{|}}{C}=\overset{\overset{\displaystyle H}{|}}{C}-\overset{\overset{\displaystyle H}{|}}{\underset{\underset{\displaystyle H}{|}}{C}}-\overset{\overset{\displaystyle H}{|}}{\underset{\underset{\displaystyle H}{|}}{C}}-\overset{\overset{\displaystyle H}{|}}{\underset{\underset{\displaystyle H}{|}}{C}}-\overset{\overset{\displaystyle H}{|}}{\underset{\underset{\displaystyle H}{|}}{C}}-\overset{\overset{\displaystyle H}{|}}{\underset{\underset{\displaystyle H}{|}}{C}}-\overset{\overset{\displaystyle H}{|}}{\underset{\underset{\displaystyle H}{|}}{C}}-\overset{\overset{\displaystyle O}{||}}{C}-OH$$

Palmitoleic acid

Note that a double bond exists between carbon atoms 9 and 10. The hydrogen atoms bound to carbon atoms immediately adjacent to the doubly bonded carbon atoms are the sites in unsaturated fatty acids that are highly susceptible to abstraction by free radicals.

Figure 6-43 illustrates hydrogen abstraction from an unsaturated fatty acid by a hydroxyl or peroxyl radical during lipid peroxidation resulting in an unsaturated fatty acid free radical and a perhydroxyl free radical.

Cell membranes that contain considerable quantities of unsaturated fatty acids are extremely vulnerable to lipid peroxidation because those fatty acids have doubly bonded carbon atoms. As the number of doubly bonded carbon atoms in an unsaturated fatty acid increases, the likelihood of membrane damage by free radicals also increases. It is hypothesized that the oxygen free radicals initiate chain reactions along the unsaturated fatty acids, thus producing an organic hydroperoxide radical (ROOH·) and a peroxide (ROO·) free radical. These biochemical units then, in turn, attack other unsaturated fatty acids in the membrane and abstract more hydrogen atoms. The result, of course, is the creation of more hydroperoxides and peroxides to perpetuate this chain reaction.

Lipid peroxidation per se is not a pathophysiologic phenomenon. In fact, it is an indispensable aerobic cellular mechanism associated with a number of normal physiologic events, including aging and leukocytic phagocytosis. The point to be made here is that under hyperoxic conditions lipid peroxidation can occur on a large scale; therefore, it is potentially deleterious to the cells and ultimately to the organism.

Antioxidant Defense Mechanisms

It would seem that, in the presence of such potentially toxic products (i.e., reactive oxygen species and free radicals), the tissues should become irreversibly damaged. What exists,

TABLE 6-7   Enzymatic and Nonenzymatic Antioxidant Defense Mechanisms

Enzyme	Protective Action
Superoxide dismutase (SOD)*	Catalyzes the reaction of two superoxide anion molecules to H_2O_2 and oxygen.
Catalase*	Catalyzes the reaction of two H_2O_2 molecules to water and oxygen.
Glutathione peroxidase*	Converts H_2O_2 and other peroxides produced during oxidative stress to water and alcohols.
Vitamin E (α-tocopherol)**	Terminates free-radical reactions.
Vitamin C (ascorbic acid)**	Works synergistically with Vitamin E to terminate oxidative reactions.

*enzymatic mechanism; **nonenzymatic mechanism*

however, are biochemical mechanisms that restrain free radical activity at the cellular level from pursuing a potentially lethal course. Antioxidants provide protection to the respiring cells by neutralizing the activity of the free radicals. An endogenous antioxidant defense system is critical to the normal health of the cell and the entire organism because it prevents the cytotoxic effects that can be caused by reactive oxygen species and free radicals.

Antioxidant defense mechanisms can be placed into two categories—enzymatic and nonenzymatic. These antioxidants and their protective actions are listed in Table 6-7.

Among aerobic organisms, superoxide dismutase (SOD) is the primary means by which the superoxide anion is cleared. This enzyme catalyzes the dismutation of $O_2^- \cdot$ into H_2O_2 and O_2 according to the reaction that follows:

$$2O_2^- \cdot + 2H^+ \xrightarrow{\text{SOD}} H_2O_2 + O_2$$

SOD provides protection to all aerobic cells from the potential cytotoxic effects of $O_2^- \cdot$.

Intracellular peroxisomes (other organelles) and the cytosol contain the protective enzyme catalase. Catalase prevents the accumulation of H_2O_2 by decomposing H_2O_2 into $H_2O + O_2$, as shown in the following reaction:

$$2H_2O_2 \xrightarrow{\text{catalase}} 2H_2O + O_2$$

Glutathione peroxidase is another enzyme present in significant concentrations in cellular cytoplasm and mitochondria. This enzyme converts H_2O_2 to H_2O. Glutathione peroxidase is also responsible for metabolizing lipid hydroperoxide (ROOH·) to virtually unreactive hydroxy-fatty alcohols (ROH), as shown below.

$$H_2O_2 + 2GSH \xrightarrow[\text{peroxidase}]{\text{glutathione}} 2H_2O + GSSG$$

Superoxide dismutase, catalase, and glutathione peroxidase are intracellular, free-radical scavenging enzymes. They reside throughout the cell's cytoplasm and inactivate free radicals present in that compartment.

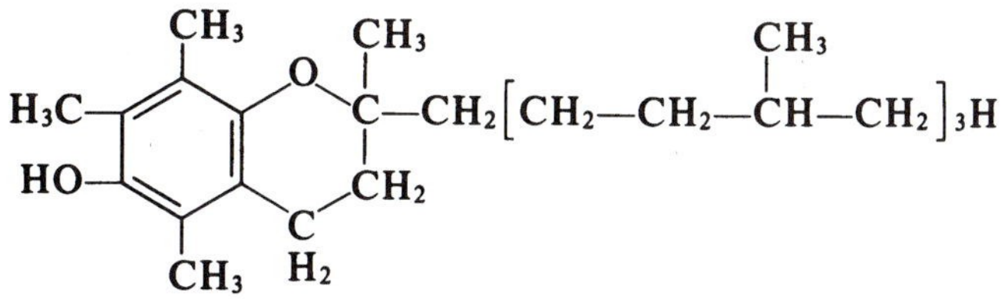

Figure 6-44 *Vitamin E (alpha tocopherol), a membrane-bound antioxidant.*

Vitamin C and vitamin E (nonenzymatic mechanisms) are membrane-bound antioxidants; vitamin E is an actual component of the cell membrane structure, and vitamin C gains access to the milieu by virtue of its water solubility.

Membrane-bound antioxidants react with free radicals in a similar manner. For example, vitamin E (alpha tocopherol) possesses a saturated hydrocarbon side chain, allowing the molecule to be lipid soluble. At the same time, it also has a phenolic group that affords reactivity with free radicals. These structural characteristics allow vitamin E to stop the propagation of lipid peroxidation. The molecular structure of vitamin E is shown in Figure 6-44.

Vitamin E is not synthesized by the organism as are many of the intracellular antioxidants. Therefore, its presence is entirely reliant upon diet and the organism's ability to digest and absorb fat. Assuming both adequate dietary intake and normal intestinal absorption, vitamin E will function in the role of a membrane-bound antioxidant. Its function as a free-radical scavenger depends on a daily replenishment from the diet because it is destroyed during its antioxidant role.

Vitamin E terminates the chain reaction of lipid peroxidation of unsaturated fatty acids in the phospholipids of the cell membrane by inactivating free radicals. A vitamin E free radical (vit E·) results from the reaction between vitamin E and a lipid free radical (lipid $-O-O\cdot$). Vit E· is essentially unreactive; therefore, the propagation of lipid peroxidation is terminated. The overall reaction is shown below.

$$\text{lipid } -O-O\cdot + \text{vit E} \rightarrow \text{lipid } -O-O-H + \text{vit E}\cdot$$

Vitamin C has the ability of reducing vit E· back to vit E and forming the very unstable free-radical semihydroascorbate, according to the following reaction:

$$\text{vit E}\cdot + \text{vit C} \rightarrow \text{vit E} + \text{semihydroascorbate}$$

Figure 6-45 schematically shows the biochemical pathways associated with free-radical activity, lipid peroxidation, and free-radical inactivation.

Phagocytic Cells and Oxygen Radicals

Polymorphonuclear leukocytes (PMNs) and macrophages produce large quantities of bactericidal oxidizing agents, such as the superoxide anion and its subsequent metabolites. When bacterial cells are present, **chemotaxis** takes place summoning phagocytic cells to the

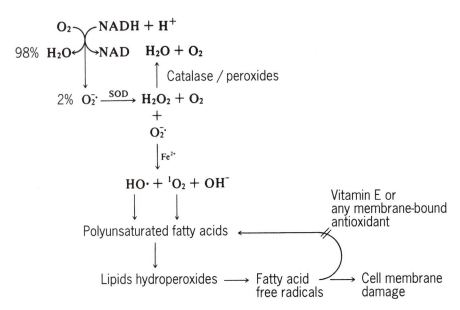

Figure 6-45 *Different biochemical pathways showing free-radical activity, lipid peroxidation, and free-radical inactivation.*

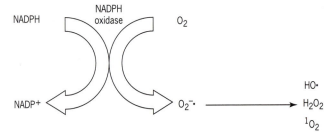

Figure 6-46 *The NADPH-oxidase system. Membrane-bound NADPH oxidase causes the univalent reduction of oxygen at the expense of NADPH, producing $NADP^+$ and $O_2^-\cdot$. The $O_2^-\cdot$ leads to the formation of $HO\cdot$, H_2O_2, and $^1O_2$. Other microbicidal products can also form.*

site of infection. As the PMNs phagocytize bacteria, $O_2^-\cdot$ and its subsequent metabolites (H_2O_2, $^1O_2$, and $HO\cdot$) are formed via the membrane oxidase system shown in Figure 6-46.

Concurrently, another membrane-oxidase system is activated to produce more microbicidal agents. As phagocytosis proceeds, myeloperoxidase (MPO) interacts with H_2O_2 and a halide (Cl^-, Br^-, or I^-). The most likely product of this reaction (below) is hypochlorous acid (HOCl).

$$H_2O_2 + Cl^- \xrightarrow{\text{MPO}} HOCl + OH^-$$

The abundance of these bactericides causes the destruction of the bacterial cell membrane and the ultimate demise of the bacterium. The stimulation of these membrane-bound oxidase systems is termed the *respiratory burst*.

Interestingly, children afflicted with chronic granulomatous disease possess neutrophils capable of phagocytosis but incapable of exhibiting a respiratory burst. Therefore, these PMNs cannot kill invading bacteria. Unfortunately, these patients experience frequent, severe infections.

The accumulation of phagocytizing cells at an infection site not only results in the killing of invading microorganisms, but also induces a chemotaxis that summons more phagocytic cells. As the population of these phagocytizing cells increases at the infection site, the increase of reactive oxygen species and free radicals at this locale produces an inflammatory response. The consequence is the spread of injury to adjacent tissue. An almost endless cascade of inflammation is propagated as stimulated phagocytes gather.

Systemic and Pulmonary Oxygen Toxicity

Oxygen toxicity can be classified as either systemic or pulmonary. *Systemic oxygen toxicity* refers to the effects of oxygen administration on organ systems separate from the lungs (e.g., the eyes with respect to retinopathy of prematurity and the central nervous system with respect to disorders including convulsions, paresthesia, and reduced mucociliary activity).

Pulmonary oxygen toxicity, on the other hand, manifests itself at the alveolar-capillary membrane. During hyperoxic exposure the pathophysiologic changes associated with pulmonary oxygen toxicity usually proceed along a predictable pathway. First, there is an exudative phase. This phase is of acute onset and is characterized by destruction of the capillary endothelium, perivascular and interstitial edema, and hemorrhage. The acute stage is followed by a proliferative phase. This phase is marked by further outpouring of exudates from the vasculature and a thickening, or fibrosing, of the alveolar interstitium. Hyperplasia of the Type II alveolar cells also occurs. These alveolar cells, in terms of their ability to replicate, are relatively resistant to the cytotoxic effects associated with oxygen therapy. In fact, they eventually differentiate to Type I alveolar cells to replace those Type I cells destroyed by the effects of hyperoxia. Figure 6-47 schematically depicts the sequence of events commonly associated with pulmonary oxygen toxicity.

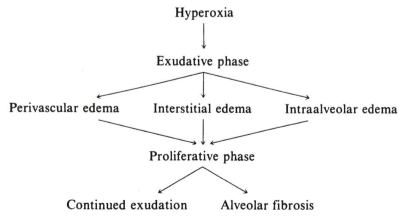

Figure 6-47 *A schematic depiction of three phases associated with pulmonary oxygen toxicity. Phase one = exudative phase; phase two = proliferative phase; phase three = fibrotic phase.*

6-9 BIOCHEMISTRY AND CLINICAL APPLICATIONS OF INHALED NITRIC OXIDE

It has been known for some time that endothelial cells produce a substance that stimulates relaxation of nearby vascular smooth muscle cells. This endothelium derived relaxation factor (EDRF) is now known to be the highly reactive nitric oxide free radical (NO·). The NO· is an ideal local transcellular messenger molecule because it is small, lipophilic, and has a short duration of action. In fact, the biological half-life of NO• is only 0.1 second to 5 seconds because it is quickly inactivated once it combines with hemoglobin. The diverse physiologic functions of NO· include (1) smooth muscle relaxation, (2) neurotransmission, (3) immunoregulation, and (4) inhibition of platelet aggregation. Nitrosovasodilators, such as nitroprusside and nitroglycerin, function by releasing NO·.

Table 6-8 demonstrates the relationship among ppm, ppb, and percent. Concentrations of NO· are expressed as parts per million (ppm) or parts per billion (ppb). The nitric oxide free radial is a common environmental pollutant and exists in the atmosphere at about 10 ppb. It is present in cigarette smoke at concentrations of 400 to 1000 ppm. The Occupational Safety and Health Administration (OSHA) has set NO· exposure limits at 25 ppm when breathed for 8 hours per day in the workplace.

Figure 6-48 illustrates endogenous and exogenous pathways regarding NO· activity. In endothelial cells, NO· is synthesized from L-arginine in the presence of nitric oxide synthase (NOS).

Subsequently, NO· diffuses into local pulmonary vascular smooth muscle cells where it binds to soluble guanyl cyclase, stimulating the production of cyclic guanosine monophosphate (cGMP) and causing the relaxation of pulmonary vascular smooth muscle. Along the exogenous pathway, inhaled NO· passively diffuses from the alveoli to the pulmonary vascular smooth muscle cells ultimately eliciting pulmonary vasodilation. There are at least six isozymes of NOS. These isozymes have been grouped as constitutive Ca^{2+}-dependent NOS (vascular endothelium, cerebellum, adrenal tissue, and platelets) and inducible Ca^{2+}-independent NOS (lung, hepatic Kupffer cells, and macrophages). The inducible NOS is stimulated by endotoxin and inhibited by glucocorticoids. Inhibitors of NOS decrease NO· production; inhibitors of guanyl cyclase, e.g., methylene blue, inhibit the action of NO·; and cGMP-specific phosphodiesterase inhibitors potentiate the actions of NO·.

Analysis of normal human and experimental animal expirate indicates a NO· concentration of less than 50 ppb. Substances that release NO·, such as nitroprusside and nitroglycerin, increase the person's exhaled NO· concentration. Exhaled NO· is decreased in cigarette smokers, increased in asthmatics, and increased with exercise. There is significant

---

TABLE 6-8 Relationship Among Parts per Million (ppm), Parts per Billion (ppb), and Percent

---

1% = 1 part per 100 = 10,000 ppm = 10,000,000 ppb
0.0001% = 1 ppm = 1,000 ppb
0.0000001% = 1 ppb

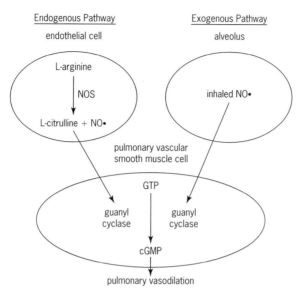

Figure 6-48 *Endogenous and exogenous NO· pathways. Endogenously, NO· forms from L-arginine and causes pulmonary vasodilatation. Exogenous NO· accomplishes the same end, but enters the pulmonary system via the alveoli.*

NO· production (greater than 100 ppb) in the nasopharynx from the normal bacterial flora, which may result in normal auto-inhalation of NO·.

An important role may be played by NO· in sepsis. Endotoxin activation of NOS may result in increased NO· release, the physiologic consequence of which is vasodilation and hypotension. In experimental animal models of sepsis, increased NO· is present in the exhaled gas. This finding raises the possibility of clinically using NOS inhibition in the treatment of sepsis. However, this hypothesis has not yet been subjected to clinical trials to establish efficacy and safety.

There is considerable clinical interest in the use of inhaled NO·. Inhaled NO· is a selective pulmonary vasodilator. Being a selective pulmonary vasodilator means that NO· produces vasodilation only for those areas of the lung that are ventilated. Systemic vasodilation does not occur because NO· is rapidly inactivated by hemoglobin. Unlike nitrosovasodilators (nitroprusside and nitroglycerin), inhaled NO· produces pulmonary vasodilation without systemic hypotension. This effect raises the clinical possibility for the use of inhaled NO· to treat diseases characterized by pulmonary hypertension, such as primary pulmonary hypertension (PPH) and persistent pulmonary hypertension of the newborn (PPHN). Inhaled NO· is currently receiving considerable clinical investigation in the treatment of PPHN.

Inhaled nitric oxide is also receiving much attention as a selective pulmonary vasodilator in the treatment of the adult respiratory distress syndrome (ARDS). ARDS is associated with $\dot{V}/\dot{Q}$ mismatch, hypoxemia, and pulmonary hypertension. Nitrosovasodilators lower the pulmonary artery pressure but worsen the hypoxemia by increasing blood flow to poorly ventilated alveoli. As a selective pulmonary vasodilator, inhaled NO· increases blood flow to ventilated alveoli. The results include (1) an improved $\dot{V}/\dot{Q}$, (2) an improved

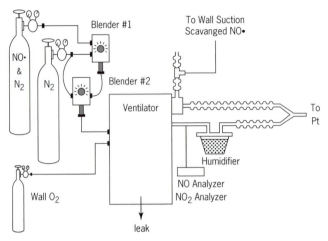

Figure 6-49 *Inhaled NO· gas delivery system for mechanically ventilated patients.*

arterial oxygenation, and (3) a lower pulmonary artery pressure. Inhaled NO· is currently not FDA approved, but many clinical investigations (including a large, randomized, placebo-controlled, double-blind study) are underway to determine the utility of inhaled NO· in the treatment of ARDS. Inhaled NO· is also a bronchodilator, but its bronchodilating effects in human subjects are less than those of beta-agonists.

Inhaled NO· can be administered to spontaneously breathing or mechanically ventilated patients. In current practice, NO· is usually administered to mechanically ventilated patients (Figure 6-49).

Gaseous NO· is supplied in bulk storage systems (compressed gas cylinders) containing high concentrations of NO·, e.g., 800 ppm, mixed with nitrogen (N_2). The NO· is then diluted in N_2, or air, and mixed with oxygen for patient administration at the desired concentration. For ARDS patients, doses less than or equal to 20 ppm are typically used. Higher doses may be necessary to treat pulmonary hypertension, but doses greater than 80 ppm are rarely, if ever, indicated. To avoid atmospheric pollution of the workplace, NO· released from the gas administration system is usually scavenged from the exhalation port of the ventilator. However, the need for this practice is questionable because the typical administration dose is less than OSHA standards and critical care units are already well ventilated for infection control purposes.

Inhaled NO· does not exhibit systemic effects because it rapidly binds with hemoglobin to produce nitrosyl hemoglobin, which is oxidized to methemoglobin (metHb), according to the following reaction:

$$NO· + Hb \rightarrow \text{nitrosyl Hb} \rightarrow \text{metHb}$$

Methemoglobin is a dysfunctional hemoglobin in which Fe^{2+} in the heme portion of the hemoglobin molecule is oxidized to Fe^{3+}. Methemoglobin decreases the oxygen carrying capacity of the blood and shifts the oxyhemoglobin dissociation curve to the left. Ordinarily, people are able to convert methemoglobin to normal hemoglobin because of the presence of methemoglobin reductase in the red blood cells. Methemoglobin levels greater than 5% are very rare at the inhaled NO· levels typically used (i.e., less than or equal to 20 ppm).

Another complication of inhaled NO· therapy is the production of nitrogen dioxide (NO$_2$). OSHA has set safety limits for NO$_2$ at 5 ppm. Airway reactivity and parenchymal lung injury have been reported with the inhalation of as little as 2 ppm. The conversion of NO· to NO$_2$ is determined by the NO· concentration, oxygen concentration, and the residence time for NO· with oxygen. The second-order kinetics of this relationship are described by the equation

$$-d[NO·]/dt = k \times [NO·]^2 \times [O_2]$$

which can be integrated to

$$1/[NO·]_t - 1/[NO·]_0 = k \times [O_2] \times t$$

where

t = residence time

$[NO·]_t$ = [NO·] after time t

$[NO·]_0$ = initial [NO·]

$k = 1.45 \times 10^9$ (rate constant for conversion of NO· to NO$_2$)

The difference between $[NO·]_0$ and $[NO·]_t$ is the nitrogen dioxide concentration, or [NO$_2$]. For mechanical ventilator administration systems, residence time is determined by the minute ventilation and the volume of the ventilator system. Levels of NO$_2$ are typically greater for higher [NO·], higher FiO$_2$, and longer residence times of NO· and O$_2$ (Figure 6-50).

In aqueous solutions, NO· reacts with the superoxide anion (O$_2^-$·) to produce the highly cytotoxic peroxynitrite radical (OONO$^-$). The actual pulmonary cytotoxic effects of inhaled NO· are currently unknown; however, this species potentially may oxidize sulfhydryl groups in proteins, disrupting their function. The available evidence suggests that inhaled NO· is safe at the doses used clinically for the treatment of ARDS and pulmonary hypertension.

There is no evidence that inhaled NO· produces tachyphylaxis. However, dependence has been observed in which discontinuation of NO· results in rebound hypoxemia and

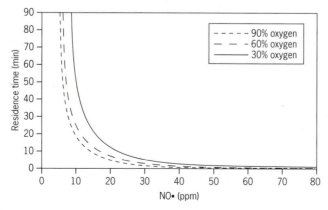

Figure 6-50 *NO· ppm versus residence time (min) at 30%, 50%, and 90% oxygen concentrations.*

pulmonary hypertension. The reason for this effect is not clear. It may result from a decreased NOS activity, or increased cGMP-phosphodiesterase activity, in the presence of inhaled NO·.

Although the theoretical dilutions to achieve desired NO· doses can be calculated, continuous analysis is mandatory because of the potential toxic effects of both NO· and NO_2. The traditional method for NO· and NO_2 analysis is chemiluminescence. This method has been used for many years in industrial and environmental applications and can be adapted to biomedical uses. In this method, the sample gas (NO·) reacts with ozone (O_3) to produce the activated compound NO_2^*.

$$NO· + O_3 \rightarrow NO_2^* + O_2$$

NO_2^* changes back to ground state by emitting electromagnetic radiation, that is,

$$NO_2^* \rightarrow NO_2 + h\nu$$

The radiation emitted has a maximum at 1,200 nm and is detected photoelectrically. To measure NO_2, it is first converted to NO· in a thermal converter (325°C) containing molybdenum (Mo), resulting in the following reaction:

$$3\,NO_2 + Mo \rightarrow 3\,NO· + MoO_3$$

The sum of NO· measured with and without the converter is referred to as NOx ([NOx] = [NO·] + [NO_2]). Most chemiluminescent analyzers measure NO· and NOx simultaneously and display [NO·], [NOx], and [NO_2]. A potential problem with chemiluminescence is quenching. Some of the NO_2^* produced by ozonation of NO· changes to ground state by reacting with other molecules, e.g., O_2, H_2O, CO_2. The greater the concentrations of these quenching molecules, the lower will be the chemiluminescence. Consequently, the NO· and NOx values will be in error. The effects of quenching can be mathematically corrected or avoided by calibrating the analyzer with the same gases that will be present during analysis.

Chemiluminescent analyzers are very accurate and precise. However, they are also typically large, expensive, and cumbersome to use. Electrochemical cells have recently become available to measure both NO· and NO_2. These analyzers are designed specifically for medical applications and are small, portable, rugged, and less expensive than chemiluminescent devices. Evaluations of these devices have found them to be suitably accurate for clinical use. Because electrochemical NO· cells are affected by humidity, they should sample NO· before the gas is humidified. These cells are also pressure sensitive. Pressure sensitivity can be lessened by the use of sidestream sampling techniques.

6-10 BIOCHEMICAL ETIOLOGY OF ADULT RESPIRATORY DISTRESS SYNDROME

The essential feature of the adult respiratory distress syndrome (ARDS) is the decreased barrier function of the alveolar-capillary membrane to fluid and protein movement into the extravascular spaces of the lungs. The consequences of this increased vascular permeability on lung mechanics and gas exchange depends on the amount of edema that accumulates and the severity of the lung injury. Many causes of acute lung injury in humans and experimental animals have been described. The most common causes are infection, sepsis, aspiration, and various forms of trauma. A goal of research has been to identify a final common pathway of lung injury (if it exists) or, at least, common mechanisms that produce the type of lung injury seen in ARDS.

Hypotheses about the mechanisms of acute lung injury have focused on the roles of infection, inflammation, or direct toxicity. Although ARDS appears to develop in 10 to 35% of patients with the sepsis syndrome, the mechanism by which infection and sepsis injure the lungs is not known with certainty. The injury may be related to factors other than direct damage by bacteria because prognosis is not related to the presence of documented bacteremia or pneumonia. Intravenous infusions of gram-negative bacterial endotoxins, or the biologically active lipid portion of endotoxins, have been shown to produce permeability pulmonary edema in some research animals. In sheep, the acute lung injury caused by endotoxin is believed to be an inflammatory response, mediated in part by neutrophils (polymorphonuclear leukocytes) and by tumor necrosis factor.

Substantial evidence has accumulated to implicate inflammatory responses of the host as the underlying mechanism of many forms of acute lung injury. The etiology of inflammation in the development of acute lung injury is prominently focused on the neutrophil, which seems to have two roles: (1) as a component of host defense vitally important to the killing of invading microorganisms and, oppositely, (2) as a potent offender containing humoral mediators which, in themselves, can injure the lungs. The potential role of mediators released from neutrophils and other cells in acute lung injury of ARDS is discussed below.

There is certainly evidence that direct toxicity plays a role in some forms of ARDS. Acute lung injury occurs in neutropenic patients, and animal models exist which demonstrate lung injuries apparently not requiring the presence of neutrophils, e.g., ethchlorvinyl, oleic acid, and paraquat. In humans, agents that seem to directly injure the lung include toxic chemicals and gases (nitrogen dioxide, chlorine, phosgene, high concentrations of oxygen, aspiration of fresh or salt water, and hydrocarbon compounds). Many of these injuries develop rapidly, if not instantaneously, which supports the contention that the injury is caused directly by contact of the agent with the lungs.

Inflammatory Mediators

Inflammation is the response to a variety of insults (i.e., trauma, infection, sepsis, or other etiologies which have been identified with ARDS). Although the lung is the organ primarily involved in gas exchange, it plays a crucial role in host defense as well. Anatomically, the lung is interposed between the environment and the rest of the body. This barrier consists not only of the airways, with their mucociliary clearance mechanisms, but also of immune and nonimmune cells, which are constantly exposed to both inhaled and blood-borne stimuli. The precise mechanisms that govern the initiation or maintenance of an acute inflammatory response are the subject of intense investigation. Because of the interest in the mediators of the inflammatory response associated with ARDS, these mechanisms will be described more fully (Table 6-9).

TABLE 6-9   Inflammatory Mediators

I.   Lipid Mediators
   A.   Arachidonic acid metabolites
      1. cyclooxygenase products—PGD_2, PGE_2, PGI_2, thromboxane A_2, $PGF_{2\alpha}$
      2. lipoxygenase products—LTB_4, LTC_4, LTD_4, LTE_4 (leukotrienes)
   B.   Platelet activating factor (PAF)
II.   Reactive Oxygen Metabolites (Oxygen Radicals)
   Superoxide ion, hydrogen peroxide, hydroxyl free radical, hydroperoxyl
      radicals,
III.   Peptide Mediators of Inflammation
   A.   Neutrophil and macrophage proteases—neutrophil elastase, etc.
   B.   Cytokines
      1.   tumor necrosis factor (TNF)
      2.   interleukin-1 (IL-1)
      3.   IL-1 receptor antagonist protein (IRAP)
      4.   interleukin-8 (IL-8)
IV.   Coagulation and Fibrinolytic System Components
   A.   Intrinsic coagulation cascade
   B.   Extrinsic coagulation cascade
   C.   Fibinolytic cascade
   D.   Complement cascade
V.   Neutrophil-Endothelial Cell Interactions
   A.   Leukocyte adhesion molecules
      1.   beta-2 integrins (CD11/CD18)
      2.   L-selectins
   B.   Endothelial cell adhesion molecules
      1.   E- and P-selectins
      2.   intracellular adhesion molecule

Lipid Mediators

Cell membranes contain phospholipids that can be released in response to certain stimuli. These phospholipids are subsequently metabolized into potent lipid mediators of inflammation via specific enzyme-dependent pathways. Upon cellular activation, intracellular calcium is mobilized and the membrane-associated enzyme, phospholipase A_2, is activated. Phospholipase A_2 results in the release of free fatty acids, including arachidonic acid metabolites and a low molecular weight lipid which may be metabolized to platelet activating factor (PAF). Arachidonic acid can be metabolized via the cyclooxygenase or the lipoxygenase pathway, resulting in the formation of biologically active lipid products, including prostaglandins, prostacyclin, thromboxanes, and leukotrienes (see Section 6-11, "Biochemical Mechanisms of Bronchospasm").

   The cyclooxygenase products PGD_2, PGE_2, and PGI_2 (prostaglandins) decrease vascular tone and pulmonary smooth muscle tone and inhibit inflammatory cell function in general.

Alternatively, thromboxane A_2 and $PGF_2\alpha$ are cyclooxygenase products which increase vascular tone and pulmonary smooth muscle tone. Although $PGF_2\alpha$ has no apparent effect on inflammatory cell function, thromboxane A_2 results in inflammation. Experiments suggest that the lipoxygenase products LTA_4, LTB_4, LTC_4, LTD_4, and LTE_4 (leukotrienes) increase vascular tone, pulmonary smooth muscle tone, and vascular permeability. Lung cells appear to vary in their generation of arachidonic acid metabolites. Specifically, platelets and stimulated mast cells produce chiefly thromboxane A_2, prostaglandins PGD_2 and PGE_2, and leukotrienes LTC_4, LTD_4, and LTE_4. Neutrophils, on the other hand, predominantly produce leukotriene LTB_4. Monocytes and alveolar macrophages produce a variety of arachidonic acid metabolites which are dependent on both the nature of the stimulus and the source of arachidonic acid (exogenously supplied or enzymatically released from membrane phospholipids). Human pulmonary alveolar macrophages produce mainly LTB_4, PGE_2, and thromboxane A_2.

A correlation between circulating levels of arachidonic acid metabolites and mortality in patients in septic shock has been demonstrated. The release of these products may influence several aspects of pulmonary function, including altered pulmonary mechanics, pulmonary artery hypertension, hypoxemia, loss of hypoxic vasoconstriction response, aggregation of leukocytes with enhanced adhesion to the vascular endothelium, and augmented vascular permeability.

The hydrolysis of phosphatidylcholine by phospholipase A_2 and its subsequent acetylation results in the low molecular weight lipid known as platelet activating factor (PAF). PAF may consist of a number of cell membrane acetylated phospholipids with 1-O-hexadecyl-2-acetyl-SN-glycero-3-phosphocholine representing the major metabolically active form. PAF is known for its ability to cause platelet aggregation and degranulation, as well as neutrophil and mononuclear cell chemotaxis and activation. PAF stimulates the release of prostaglandins, thromboxane A_2, and leukotrienes. PAF also augments neutrophil-endothelial cell adhesion, increases vascular permeability, and promotes pulmonary smooth muscle cell contraction. Therefore, many researchers believe PAF production plays a central role in the pathogenesis of acute lung injury. In addition, the use of PAF receptor antagonists have been shown to significantly ameliorate the effects of endotoxin on the lung, resulting in a reduction of pulmonary vascular resistance and permeability.

Reactive Oxygen Species

Activation of neutrophils in animal models leads to pulmonary vascular injury through the release of reactive oxygen species (Section 6-8, "Biochemical Aspects of Oxygen Toxicity"). Animal experiments have also shown that this injury is attenuated by the administration of antioxidants. The role of oxygen products in mediating lung injury is also supported by evidence of oxidant species identified in bronchoalveolar lavage fluids of patients with ARDS.

Not only may the reactive oxygen species cause direct microvascular injury at the lung level, they may also serve to promote neutrophil-dependent microvascular injury. Their formation may shift the balance of proteases versus alpha-1-antiprotease (alpha-1-antitrypsin) to favor that of the neutrophil proteases, since there is evidence that oxygen metabolites may inactivate alpha-1-antiprotease, leading to unopposed tissue injury by the neutrophil proteases.

Peptide Mediators of Inflammation

Human neutrophils and mononuclear cells contain a variety of proteolytic enzymes (proteases) capable of degrading parenchymal lung components. Additionally, these products can recruit and activate more phagocytes, which release more proteases. Neutrophil elastase is the most extensively studied proteolytic enzyme. Neutrophil elastase has the capacity to degrade elastin, collagen, fibrinogen, fibronectin, and proteoglycans and to cleave some complement proteins. When neutrophils are activated, not only are toxic oxygen metabolites produced, but neutrophil elastase and other proteolytic enzymes are released. Under conditions of inflammation the normal balance between the proteolytic activity of elastase and alpha-1-protease inhibitor (alpha-1-antiprotease) is shifted toward the unopposed expression of neutrophil elastase.

Cytokines are a diverse group of biologically active polypeptides that appear to play major roles in the development of an acute inflammatory response. Although a number of cytokines may be important in mediating acute lung injury, the cytokines most studied include tumor necrosis factor (TNF) and interleukin-1 (IL-1), an IL-1 antagonist, and a potent neutrophil activating and chemotactic factor (IL-8). The early response cytokines (TNF and IL-1) have overlapping effects on a variety of cellular functions. At sites of local inflammation, these cytokines are important in regulating early cellular communication and sequential events in the initiation, maintenance, and repair of injury. In contrast, the exaggerated release of TNF and IL-1 can lead to systemic manifestations of inflammation and increased morbidity and mortality. Their role in mediating septic shock in ARDS has been clearly suggested by several studies in which elevated levels of TNF and IL-1 have been detected in the serum of patients with septic shock. In addition, TNF produces pathophysiologic effects that are similar to endotoxin or infusion of gram-negative bacteria when systemically administered. On the other hand, the administration of a monoclonal TNF antibody has a beneficial effect in experimental animals injected with lethal doses of E. coli.

Recent reports of an IL-1 inhibitor have led to the isolation, purification, cloning, and expression of an IL-1 receptor antagonist protein (IRAP). This protein has been shown to be produced from peripheral blood mononuclear cells in response to endotoxin and appears to have inhibitory activity at the level of the IL receptor without agonist activity. In addition, IRAP was found to have a protective role in the lungs of rats receiving either intratracheal endotoxin or IL-1.

A recently isolated and cloned cytokine, interleukin-8, has demonstrated potent activating and chemotactic activity for neutrophils. IL-8 is a potent neutrophil chemotactic factor in nanomolar concentrations, and a potent activating factor at micromolar concentrations. This cytokine has been isolated from several cellular sources, including endothelial cells, fibroblasts, epithelial cells, alveolar macrophages, neutrophils, and peripheral blood monocytes.

Coagulation and Fibrinolytic Cascade

In ARDS a prominent pathologic feature is the presence of intraalveolar fibrin, intravascular platelet aggregates, and alveolar hemorrhage. Thus, components of the coagulation and fibrinolytic pathways are important in the pathogenesis of lung injury and repair. Many proteolytic enzymes are constituents of either the coagulation or the fibrinolytic cascades. Under normal conditions a delicate balance exists between a state of microvascular thrombosis and thrombolysis. Under conditions of acute inflammation, however, this balance shifts in favor of a procoagulant environment. Endothelial cell injury and loss of the endothelial surface initiates thrombosis by exposing an actively charged surface. This condition leads to activation of factor XII and the remaining components of the intrinsic coagulation system. In addition, the extrinsic coagulation pathway is activated, as well as the production of plasminogen activator inhibitor, resulting in the inactivation of the fibrinolytic system. Thus, a cascade of events occurs which leads to direct activation of the intrinsic and extrinsic coagulation pathways and indirect inhibition of the fibrinolytic system, culminating in the full expression of disseminated intravascular coagulation (DIC) and microvascular injury.

Damage to the alveolar-capillary membrane during acute lung injury is associated with intraalveolar fibrin, glycoproteins, and cellular debris—the hallmark of hyaline membrane formation. If the lung injury in ARDS is to improve, the resolution of hyaline membranes appears to be critically dependent on their subsequent resorption; otherwise, pulmonary fibrosis may develop.

Neutrophil-Endothelial Cell Interactions

The interactions of neutrophils and pulmonary capillary endothelial cells are obviously important to the recruitment of neutrophils from blood to sites of acute lung inflammation. Recently, there has been significant progress made regarding the basic mechanisms of neutrophil-endothelial cell interaction. The development of monoclonal antibody technology and the description of inherited leukocyte adhesion deficiency (LAD) patients have provided insights into the molecular mechanisms of neutrophil adhesion. The family of beta-2 leukocyte integrin adhesion molecules consists of a complex group of glycoproteins that are expressed only on the surface of leukocytes. When neutrophils are activated by certain chemotactic factors, a rapid translocation of CD11/CD18 glycoproteins from secondary and tertiary granules to the cell surface occurs. These adhesion molecules bind to several receptors in a calcium-dependent fashion. Some studies demonstrate that anti-CD11/CD18 antibodies are dramatic in attenuating neutrophil accumulation in the lung, as well as neutrophil-dependent vascular permeability. It has also been discovered that there are other adhesion molecules present on neutrophils. Leukocyte-endothelial cell adhesion molecule-1 (LECAM-1 or L-selectin) is a member of a unique family of adhesion molecules referred to as selectins. As it now appears, neutrophil-derived L-selectin adhesion molecule and its interaction with endothelial cells is an early event, producing a margination, or "rolling," of neutrophils along the endothelium. Subsequently, the neutrophil-derived beta-2 integrins are crucial in the arrest of leukocyte movement and their subsequent transmigration between endothelial cells into the lung interstitium.

The full sequence of neutrophil margination, diapedesis (outward passage of neutrophils through intact vessel walls), and migration to sites of inflammation is also dependent on the expression of endothelial cell-derived adhesion molecules. Intercellular adhesion molecule (ICAM-1) is a important ligand/receptor for CD11/CD18 on neutrophils. Both

E-selectin and P-selectin are important endothelial-surface adhesion molecules for the promotion of neutrophil adhesion. E-selectin is synthesized and expressed on the surface of endothelial cells in response to endotoxin, TNF, or IL-1. Whereas E-selectin is expressed over several hours (peaks by 6 hours), P-selectin is more rapidly mobilized to the surface of endothelial cells following exposure to platelet-activating stimuli, including thrombin and histamine.

Pathophysiology of ARDS

The light and electron microscopic appearance of ARDS has been well described. Exudative, proliferative, and fibrotic stages usually appear in sequence following the injury. In the exudative stage, the earliest changes are characterized by interstitial and alveolar edema and the appearance of hyaline membranes. The damage may be more apparent at the alveolar epithelium than at the vascular endothelium, even following a blood-borne insult. Widespread destruction of Type I alveolar epithelial cells (pneumocytes) with denuded basement membranes are early findings. The interstitium is widened by edema and is rich in leukocytes, platelets, and red blood cells. The microvascular endothelium is usually preserved, showing occasional irregular focal thickening resulting from cytoplasmic swelling or vacuoles and greater numbers of luminal leukocytes.

The exudative phase is usually followed by the proliferative phase, during which fluid is resorbed from the air spaces. Fibrin deposition may be prominent along with inflammatory cells and fibroblasts. The alveolar epithelium is made up predominantly of proliferating Type II pneumocytes, and the alveolar-capillary membrane is greatly thickened. Structural alterations in the pulmonary vascular bed are seen. The proliferative phase may be associated with fever, leukocytosis, low systemic vascular resistance, diffuse alveolar infiltrates, and neutrophilia on bronchoalveolar lavage, all in the absence of any infection.

The fibrotic stage occurs about two weeks after the initial insult and is manifest by fibrotic changes in the alveolar ducts, alveoli, and interstitium. Alveoli may be lost, however, and there is a slow recovery toward normal with passage of time. Recovery may be delayed because of the severity of the initial damage or the underlying architecture of the lungs. However, even the severe changes seen at any of these stages may be reversible with a normalization of the chest radiograph and complete or nearly complete return of normal pulmonary function months later.

6-11 BIOCHEMICAL MECHANISMS OF BRONCHOSPASM

The respiratory care practitioner is often confronted with patients experiencing bronchospasm arising from a variety of causes. The intention of this section is to describe the biochemical events responsible for (1) the maintenance of bronchial smooth muscle tone, (2) the production of bronchospasm, and (3) the alleviation of bronchial smooth muscle constriction.

Bronchial Smooth Muscle Tone

Bronchial smooth muscle tone is normally maintained via a variety of influences. The primary responsibility for the maintenance of this state seems to lie with the autonomic nervous system. Despite the absence of sympathetic (adrenergic) nerve fibers in the human tracheobronchial tree, both the sympathetic and parasympathetic divisions of the autonomic nervous system have receptor sites on bronchial smooth muscle cells. The stimulation and inhibition of these receptor sites govern the activity of a series of intracellular biochemical events, which, in turn, influence the net physiologic response.

Two intracellular cyclic nucleotides, namely, 3′,5′-adenosine monophosphate (cyclic AMP) and 3′,5′-guanosine monophosphate (cyclic GMP), presumably are influential in determining the net physiologic bronchial smooth muscle response. The prevailing hypothesis concerning these two biochemical entities is that increased intracellular cyclic AMP levels elicit bronchodilatation, whereas increased intracellular levels of cyclic GMP produce bronchoconstriction.

Based on this premise, bronchodilatation results from the following mechanisms: (1) adenyl cyclase activation, (2) prevention of guanyl cyclase activation, and (3) phosphodiesterase inhibition.

Adenyl cyclase is an enzyme activated when the β_2-adrenergic receptor sites on the bronchial smooth muscle cell surface are stimulated. Adenyl cyclase then, in the presence of magnesium (Mg^{2+}) ions, catalyzes the reaction that converts ATP to cyclic AMP resulting in bronchodilatation.

Guanyl cyclase is also an enzyme activated at the surface of bronchial smooth muscle cells. However, its activity responds to stimulation of α-adrenergic receptor sites. This enzyme then catalyzes the conversion of guanosine triphosphate (GTP) to cyclic GMP. Therefore, effective inhibition of the α-adrenergic receptor sites prevents the activation of guanyl cyclase and the related ensuing biochemical events. Cyclic GMP levels then remain low, promoting bronchodilatation.

Parasympathetic stimulation, that is, stimulation of the cholinergic receptors on the surface of the bronchial smooth muscle cell, likewise activates guanyl cyclase. The same biochemical events associated with α-adrenergic stimulation occur at this juncture, thus ultimately increasing the level of cyclic GMP and producing bronchospasm. Hence, blockade of the cholinergic receptor sites will contribute to the maintenance of decreased intracellular cyclic GMP levels and bronchial smooth muscle relaxation.

Finally, elevated levels of cyclic AMP result from the inhibition of phosphodiesterase, the enzyme responsible for the degradation of cyclic AMP to 5′-AMP. If the degradative activity of phosphodiesterase is retarded or prevented, cyclic AMP concentrations rise. Once again, the physiologic response is bronchial relaxation.

Figure 6-51 represents a bronchial smooth muscle cell and four separate mechanisms by which cyclic 3′,5′-AMP levels are said to increase.*

In addition to this neurologic input, the prevention of mast cell mediator release is critical in the maintenance of normal bronchial smooth muscle tone. Mast cells are ubiquitous;

*For the sake of brevity, other bronchial smooth muscle cell receptor sites, such as those for histamine, serotonin, prostaglandins, leukotrienes, ECF-A, etc., have been omitted. Also, these pathways are not as well understood.

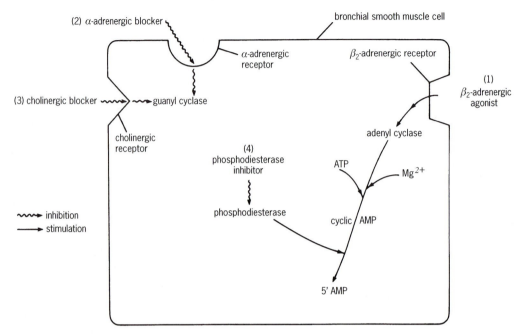

Figure 6-51 *A bronchial smooth muscle cell demonstrating four mechanisms involved with increasing intracellular levels of cyclic 3',5'-AMP.*

they are located in loose connective tissue in all organ systems. In reference to the tracheobronchial tree, mast cells reside near the mucosal surface, in the submucosal layer, and in perivascular regions.

Mast cells play no apparent active role in maintaining normal bronchial smooth muscle tone. They do, however, become influential and alter the normal state during immediate hypersensitivity reactions. The biochemical pathways associated with this event will be considered in the next section.

Mast Cell Degranulation

The mast cell has an important role in medicine. It is a major culprit in asthma and in a multitude of allergic diseases. It is interesting to ask why a component of the immune system that creates disease in about 25% of the human population continues to exist? Not only is the mast cell conserved among the human species, but it is also found in all mammals. What makes the price of having mast cells worth paying?

Parasitic infestations represent the most prevalent infectious agents of humans. The number of parasitic infections far exceeds the total human population. For example, hookworms represent the most significant cause of iron-deficiency anemia in the world. Clearly, the role of the mast cell in fighting parasitic disease has been critical throughout the animal kingdom. In western societies, parasitic disease is less common, and it may appear that mast cells exist only for the mischief they can cause.

A major characteristic of the mast cell is the presence of a high affinity receptor (FcεRI) for immunoglobulin E (IgE). The only other cell of the body to have this high affinity receptor is the basophil. All other cells with IgE receptors have low affinity receptors (FcεRII). The FcεRI is essential to mast cell specificity. Specific IgE antibodies will bind to these receptors (Figure 6-52). When a multivalent antigen is bound simultaneously by two or more mast cell-associated IgE antibodies, the membrane perturbs and mast cell secretion of mediators occurs. Other biologic chemicals can cause mast cell activation. These antigens include complement components C5a and C3a. Cytokines from lymphocytes and mononuclear cells, lymphokines, eosinophil-derived proteins, and neuropeptides can all activate mast cells, also.

Human mast cells can be separated into two distinct groups. These are differentiated from one another by the presence of the enzyme chymase. All human mast cells seem to contain the enzyme tryptase. Hence, the nomenclature MC_T for those with tryptase alone and MC_{TC} for mast cells with both tryptase and chymase. In addition, these types of mast cells tend to localize in different areas of the body. The MC_T cells are the predominant type found in the lungs and in the mucosa of the small intestines. The MC_{TC} type mast cells are found in the intestinal submucosa, skin, and normal synovium. Note that this description refers to the predominant mast cell type in a tissue. Both types are frequently found together, and the relative abundance can change with disease states.

Mast cells produce a series of chemicals important for their effects on the organism. When mast cells are activated, a series of intracellular events leads to the release of preformed mediators and to the production of additional mediators. The earliest event linked

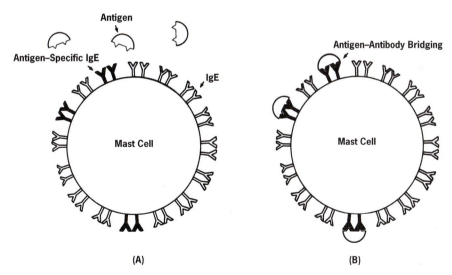

(A)

(B)

Figure 6-52 *Mast cell. (A) Numerous IgE molecules coating the mast cell surface indicating mast cell sensitization to an antigen; (B) antigen-antibody reactions occurring on the mast cell surface initiating mast cell degranulation.*

to mast cell activation is phosphorylation of tyrosine, serine, and threonine residues on the FcεRI. The next steps in activation appear to involve a group of GTP-dependent proteins, kinases, and phosphatases that then regulate adenyl cyclase, phospholipase C, and phospholipase A_2. Other mast cells may use different signal transduction pathways than those used with antigens.

Cyclic AMP (cAMP) appears to be an important second messenger in the mast cell activation process. Treatment of human pulmonary mast cells with a β-agonist before activation inhibits mediator release. A β-agonist causes increased levels of intracellular cAMP. Theophylline blocks adenosine receptors on the mast cell surface and, at 10 to 100 times higher levels, inhibits phosphodiesterase causing an accumulation of cAMP inside the mast cell. The latter effect is of questionable clinical importance because of the high levels of the phosphodiesterase inhibitor required. Timing of these effects is important on the impact of mediator release. Increased levels of cAMP seem to inhibit mediator release if present before activation. When present after activation, cAMP augments mediator release.

Adenosine has shown a variety of effects on mast cell mediator release. As alluded to above, there are adenosine receptors on the mast cell surface. Inhibition of these receptors in rats can reverse histamine release inhibition by adenosine. Not all mast cell mediators respond with the same release of inhibition. In human asthmatics, inhalation of adenosine causes bronchospasm. This bronchospasm is inhibited by antihistamines and disodium cromoglycate. Theophylline, on the other hand, is an adenosine antagonist. Yet theophylline is associated with decreased mast cell mediator release. Thus, it appears that adenosine can both increase and inhibit mediator release.

The widespread distribution of mast cells among bronchial smooth muscle cells highlights the importance of mast cell stabilization in maintaining normal bronchial smooth muscle tone. It is, however, well recognized that sensitized mast cells have antigen-specific immunoglobulin E (IgE) molecules fixed to and circumscribing the cell surface. When exposure to the appropriate antigen occurs, in the form of the bridging of two IgE molecules of the same specificity, the antigen-antibody reaction triggers the biochemical sequence that ultimately leads to mast cell degranulation. Figure 6-52 illustrates a sensitized mast cell (A) and an antigen-antibody reaction (B) occurring on the mast cell surface.

The antigen-antibody reaction increases cell membrane permeability to calcium (Ca^{2+}) ions and activates adenyl cyclase, which catalyzes the conversion of ATP to cyclic AMP within the mast cell. Cyclic AMP then interacts with a protein kinase. Another ATP molecule provides energy for the phosphorylation of an unidentified protein. The phosphorylation process causes the granule to migrate toward the mast cell surface.

Concurrently, the mast cell membrane is the site of biochemical events that eventually allow vasoactive-filled granules to fuse to the inner surface of the mast cell membrane. Increased mast cell permeability allows for the release (secretion) of the stored vasoactive mediators into the pulmonary interstitium.

The mediators of mast cells are of two distinct groups: preformed mediators that are stored ready for release and newly-generated mediators produced after mast cell activation. In human mast cells there are at least a dozen preformed mediators. Histamine is the best known. It has two distinct activities derived from the occupation of either the H_1 or the H_2 receptor on cell surfaces. The H_1 effects include bronchial and intestinal smooth muscle contraction. In asthmatics H_1 effects are associated with the onset of asthma symptoms. The sensitivity of subjects to histamine can differentiate asthmatics from nonasthmatics and suggests the level of airway nonspecific reactivity. Recently-developed specific H_1 antagonists (antihistamines) can ameliorate allergen-induced bronchospasm. However, antihistamines still have little therapeutic role in treating asthma.

The H_2 effect of histamine down regulates cellular immune responses. However, the H_2 effect that has been most important is the stimulation of stomach acid secretion. H_2 antagonists are used to reduce gastric inflammation.

Eosinophil chemotactic factor (ECF) is stored in mast cells. Its release is associated with eosinophil chemotaxis and activation. There is also a neutrophil chemotactic factor. Neutrophil chemotaxis and activation follow release of this mediator. Both neutrophils and eosinophils are important in the chronic inflammation of asthma.

The newly generated mediators of mast cells are derived from the metabolism of arachidonic acid and are called *eicosanoids*. There are two synthetic pathways recognized, the cyclooxygenase pathway and the lipoxygenase pathway. Cyclooxygenase products include prostaglandins (PG) and thromboxane A_2 (TXA_2). Lipoxygenase enzymes generate a group of sulphidopeptides. Known as slow-reacting substances of anaphalaxis (SRS-A) for 41 years after their discovery in 1938, these products now are termed leukotrienes (LT). In addition, a nonsulphated product of this pathway, LTB_4, is produced. LTB_4 is chemotactic for neutrophils and eosinophils and may play a role in the inflammation of asthma. The effects of these mediators are usually local, i.e., the mediators are produced and broken down near the site of their effects.

Activities of the arachidonic acid metabolites are varied. PGD_2, 9α, 11β-PGF_2, $PGF_2\alpha$, LTC_4, LTD_4, and TXA_2 are all powerful bronchial smooth muscle contractile elements. LTC_4 and LTD_4 are the most powerful bronchospastic mediators known. At concentrations of 0.75 to 8 μM (10^{-6}) they reduce air flow significantly. Similar effects require 10 times more PGD_2 and 35 times more $PGF_2\alpha$. Other eicosanoids are 500 to 1,000 times less potent than LTC_4 and LTD_4. In addition to causing bronchospasm, these mediators increase vascular permeability, vasoconstriction, and/or platelet aggregation.

The mediators (histamine, prostaglandins, serotonin, bradykinin, leukotrienes, eosinophil chemotactic factor of anaphylaxis [ECF-A], etc.) stimulate the respective receptor sites located on the bronchial smooth cells and trigger a chain of biochemical events responsible for decreasing their intracellular cyclic AMP levels. The net physiologic response is bronchospasm.

Figure 6-53 illustrates the hypothesized biochemical pathway induced by antigen-antibody reactions on the mast cell.

Rational Basis for Therapeutic Intervention

Understanding certain aspects of the receptor theory allows one to pursue a reasonable therapeutic course. β_2-adrenergic agonists [Figure 6-51(1)] are useful for restoring bronchial smooth muscle tone because they stimulate the activation of adenyl cyclase and thereby increase bronchial smooth muscle levels of cyclic AMP and promote bronchodilatation.

Because guanyl cyclase catalyzes the production of cyclic GMP, the cyclic nucleotide thought to be responsible for bronchospasm, its inhibition by pharmacologic agents

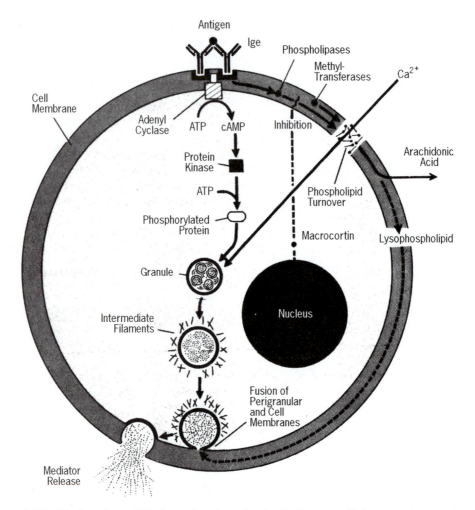

Antigen

Ige

Phospholipases

Methyl-
Transferases

Ca^{2+}

Cell
Membrane

Adenyl
Cyclase

ATP   cAMP

Inhibition

Arachidonic
Acid

Protein
Kinase

ATP

Phospholipid
Turnover

Phosphorylated
Protein

Macrocortin

Lysophospholipid

Granule

Intermediate
Filaments

Nucleus

Fusion of
Perigranular
and Cell
Membranes

Mediator
Release

Figure 6-53 *The hypothesized biochemical pathway involved with mast cell degranulation, starting with the antigen-antibody reaction (top) and ending with mediator release (bottom). From Austen, Frank:* The Biology of Immunologic Disease, *1983, Sinauer Associates, Inc., Sunderland. Drawn by Bunji Tagawa. Used with permission.*

decreases cyclic GMP levels and promotes bronchodilatation [Figure 6-51(2)]. Therefore, α-adrenergic blockers are effective in decreasing intracellular cyclic GMP levels. Likewise, medications that block cholinergic receptor sites [Figure 6-51(3)] inhibit the activity of guanyl cyclase, lessening cyclic GMP levels and eliciting bronchial smooth muscle relaxation. Additionally, medications that directly inhibit the action of phosphodiesterase [Figure 6-51(4)], the enzyme responsible for the degradation of cyclic AMP to 5′-AMP, facilitate the reversal of bronchospasm. Their utility manifests itself in reducing the degradation or inactivation of cyclic AMP to 5′-AMP.

Finally, cromolyn prevents bronchospasm by inhibiting antigen-antibody reactions on the surface of mast cells. The prevention of these reactions stabilizes the mast cell membrane and prevents degranulation and mediator release. The obvious result is the avoidance of bronchospasm. It is important to note that cromolyn is not a bronchodilator, nor does it block receptor sites. Therefore, it is completely ineffective in the treatment of existing bronchospasm.

The use of antihistamines to block the effects of histamine are effective in allergic disease in general. However, antihistamines have only a minor effect on asthma. This lesser influence is most evident in allergen-induced asthma. The effect of antihistamines on the upper airway may be the most important contribution to asthma therapy.

Eicosanoids appear to be the most important mast cell mediators of asthma. There are several ways to modulate the production and release of these factors. Systemic steroids inhibit their production. This effect takes several hours of exposure to demonstrate. The major steroid effect in asthma may not involve the mast cell. Nonsteroidal, anti-inflammatory drugs (NSAIDs) inhibit the cyclooxygenase pathway. This inhibition does not generally have clinical efficacy in asthma except in a subgroup of patients who can experience both increased symptoms with a single use and improvement in chronic symptoms with regular use of NSAIDs.

Table 6-10 lists a number of medications often administered prophylactically to maintain normal bronchial smooth muscle tone or to reverse existing bronchospasm.

TABLE 6-10   Pulmonary Pharmacologic Influences

Medication	Activity	Effect
Isoproterenol	β_2 Stimulation	Adenyl cyclase activation; ↑ cyclic AMP
Terbutaline	β_2 Stimulation	Adenyl cyclase activation; ↑ cyclic AMP
Epinephrine	β_2 Stimulation[a]	Adenyl cyclase activation; ↑ cyclic AMP
Phentolamine	α Blockade[a]	Prevents guanyl cyclase activation; ↓ cyclic GMP
Tolazoline	α Blockade[a]	Prevents guanyl cyclase activation; ↓ cyclic GMP
Methylxanthines	Phosphodiesterase inhibition	Prevents degradation of cyclic AMP to 5'-AMP; ↑ cyclic AMP
Atropine	Cholinergic blockade	Prevents guanyl cyclase activation; ↓ cyclic GMP
Cromolyn	Blocks antigen-antibody reaction	Prevents mast cell degranulation and mediator release

[a]*Because bronchial smooth muscle cells normally possess very few α-adrenergic receptor sites, the α-adrenergic response elicited by these drugs is considered much less significant than the β_2 response. Consequently, these drugs assume more importance in the treatment of cardiovascular disorders, where both α and β effects are notably important.*

CHAPTER SUMMARY

All living organisms are comprised of cells. Living organisms include plants, animals, fungi and microbes. Although a few structures are common to all cells (e.g., cell membrane and cytoplasm), many differences exist among these cells. These differences in structure and organization lead to functional differences.

Cells are comprised of compounds that are used as nutrients or media for transport. These compounds include water, proteins, lipids, carbohydrates, and nucleic acids.

Biochemical molecules are mainly comprised of the following atoms: carbon (C), nitrogen (N), hydrogen (H), oxygen (O), and a variety of functional groups. Some of the common functional groups are:

- alcohols
- aldehydes
- ketones
- carboxylic acid
- esters
- amines
- carbonates
- nitrates
- phosphates

These elements and some of these functional groups comprise the metabolic substrates carbohydrates, proteins, and lipids. These three substrates are catabolized during the body's metabolic process. Carbohydrates includes sugars and complex compounds called starch and cellulose. Glucose is a six-carbon sugar that is the principal energy source in man. Glucose metabolism in the presence of oxygen is called aerobic respiration. In the absence of oxygen glucose can be metabolized via anaerobic metabolism. That is,

aerobic metabolism of glucose $\rightarrow$ CO_2 and H_2O

anaerobic metabolism of glucose $\rightarrow$ pyrurvic acid

Dietary proteins constitute the body's primary source of sulfur and nitrogen. Amino acids are the building blocks of protein molecules. Twenty (20) amino acids exist and are joined together in various combinations held in place by peptide bonds.

Lipids are comprised of fatty acids, and (1) are found extensively in cell membranes, (2) provide a metabolic source of energy, (3) offer thermal and electrochemical insulation, and (4) serve as essential dietary nutrients.

Lipids are categorized as (1) fatty acids, (2) fats, (3) phospholipids, (4) sphingolipids, and (5) steroids.

In addition to the major roles stated above phospholipid molecules function as specialized molecules. For example, pulmonary surfactant (lecithin) is a phospholipid that helps reduce the surface tension of the alveolar-lining fluid at the air liquid interface in the alveoli.

Deoxyribonucleic acid (DNA) and ribonucleic acid (RNA) are nucleic acids performing specialized physiologic functions. DNA carries the organism genetic information. RNA provides the machinery for this process. Nucleic acids are chains of nucleotides. Nucleotides, in turn, are comprised of nitrogenous bases, a five-carbon sugar, and a phosphoric acid. The five nitrogenous bases are classified as pyrimidines (uracil, thymine, and cytosine) and purines (guanine and adenine).

Hemoglobin is a conjugate protein containing a globin portion and four heme molecules. The protein globin is normally made up of 2 alpha and 2 beta polypeptide chains. Heme (non-protein molecule) consists of a porphyrin ring with a ferric ion at its center. Oxygen chemically and reversibly combines with the ferric ion. Oxygen is able to combine with each of the four hemes located on a hemoglobin molecule. Hemoglobin is also an effective buffer and a CO_2 transporter.

Abnormal or mutant hemoglobin molecules have been identified. These molecules tend to be ineffective transporters of oxygen. Some mutant hemoglobin molecules are sickle cell hemoglobin (HbS), and methemoglobin (HbM).

In addition to being an excellent transporter of gas, hemoglobin is an exceptional buffer. Hemoglobin buffers H^+ ions released in the RBC during the reaction between CO_2 and H_2O. The $H+$ ions combine with the imidazole side chain branching off the histidine amino acid.

The oxyhemoglobin dissociation curve describes the relationship between the partial pressure of oxygen dissolved in the plasma (Po_2) and the amount of hemoglobin saturated with oxygen (So_2). The curve is a dynamic one in that it shifts to the left and right of the textbook normal curve.

When hemoglobin is degraded, it is broken down to its basic components, namely protoporphyrin IX, iron, and globin.

As an oxygen molecule moves along the electron transport chain, it undergoes univalent reduction at four sites. Along this metabolic pathway oxygen metabolites are formed. The metabolites are called oxygen free radicals, which include (1) the superoxide anoin, (2) hydrogen perixode, (3) the hydroxyl radical, and the perhydroxyl radical. The overall reduction reaction for oxygen along the electron transport chain is as follows.

$$O_2 + 4H^+ + 4e^- \rightarrow 2\,H_2O$$

Cell membranes that contain significant amounts of unsaturated fatty acids are vulnerable to lipid peroxidation. The toxic end-products of oxygen free radicals are prevented from taking place normally because the body contains an effective endogenous antioxidant defense mechanism. The body's antioxidants include the superoxide anion, catalase, glutathione peroxidase, vitamin E, and vitamin C.

Nitric oxide (NO) is a naturally occurring pulmonary vasodilator. It is released from the pulmonary vascular endothelium, specifically from L-arginine in the presence of nitric oxide synthase (NOS). Inhaled nitric oxide is used to therapeutically cause pulmonary vascular dilatation.

Adult respiratory distress syndrome (ARDS) is the disintegration of the alveolar-capillary membrane. ARDS has numerous etiologies, however, the constellation of signs and symptoms and pathophysiology of the condition are the same.

The onset of ARDS is caused by a variety of inflammatory mediators. The inflammatory mediators include lipids and reactive O_2 species, proteolytic enzymes, coagulation and fibrinolysis. ARDS is characterized by two distinct phases an exudative phase and fibrotic phase.

Bronchospasm can be explained from a biochemical standpoint. The normal bronchial smooth muscle tone is lost when mast cells degranulate, releasing mediators such as, histamine, eosinophil chemotactic factor (ECF), leukotrienes, bradykinin, serotonin. The mediatros stimulate bronchial smooth muscle cell receptors, triggering a series of biochemical events leading to bronchospasm.

The therapeutic approach to counteract bronchospasm is directed to increasing the intracellular level of cyclic 3,5 AMP. Beta-2 agonists, anticholinergic bronchildators (cholinergic blockers), alpha blockade, and phosphodiesterase inhibition are some activities that are deemed useful in overcoming bronchial smooth muscle constriction.

REVIEW QUESTIONS

6-1 THE FUNCTIONAL ANATOMY AND CHEMISTRY OF THE LIVING CELL

Questions

1. List five cytoplasmic structures present in a cell.
2. What is the most abundant substance in a cell?
3. Describe the function of each of the following cellular components: (1) cytoplasmic membrane, (2) centrosome, (3) ribosome, (4) phagolysosome, and (5) mitochondrion.
4. Distinguish between active transport and passive diffusion.
5. What are the anions present in a cell? Cations?
6. Describe the major components of a cell membrane and their orientation.

6-2 BASIC PRINCIPLES OF ORGANIC CHEMISTRY

Questions

1. How many chemical bonds are formed by each of the following atoms: (1) hydrogen, (2) oxygen, (3) carbon, and (4) nitrogen?
2. Draw the structural formula for at least five functional groups.

6-3 CARBOHYDRATES

Questions

1. Name three hexoses that are important in metabolism.
2. What are the functional groups of a carbohydrate molecule?
3. Name the disaccharides that contain glucose.
4. Why is starch a nutritionally useful substance?
5. What are the molecular units that comprise table sugar?
6. How many moles of ATP are generated by the aerobic oxidation of 1 mole of glucose?
7. Diagrammatically summarize the aerobic metabolism of glucose.

6-4 PROTEINS

Questions

1. Define the six different categories of amino acids.

a.
$$H-\overset{\overset{\displaystyle H}{|}}{\underset{\underset{\displaystyle H}{|}}{C}}-\overset{\overset{\displaystyle H}{|}}{\underset{\underset{\displaystyle NH_3}{|}}{C}}-\overset{\overset{\displaystyle O}{\parallel}}{C}-OH$$

b.
$$H-\overset{\overset{\displaystyle CH_3}{|}}{\underset{\underset{\displaystyle CH_3}{|}}{C}}-\overset{\overset{\displaystyle H}{|}}{C}-\overset{\overset{\displaystyle H}{|}}{\underset{\underset{\displaystyle NH_3}{|}}{C}}-\overset{\overset{\displaystyle H}{|}}{C}-\overset{\overset{\displaystyle O}{\parallel}}{C}-OH$$

c.
$$H_2N-\overset{\overset{\displaystyle H}{|}}{\underset{\underset{\displaystyle H}{|}}{C}}-\overset{\overset{\displaystyle H}{|}}{\underset{\underset{\displaystyle H}{|}}{C}}-\overset{\overset{\displaystyle H}{|}}{\underset{\underset{\displaystyle NH_3^+}{|}}{C}}-\overset{\overset{\displaystyle O}{\parallel}}{C}-O^-$$

2. Identify the α carbon for each of the preceding amino acids.
3. Define the *isoelectric point* for an amino acid.
4. Draw the structure of an amino acid as it would occur (1) acidic to its isoelectric point and (2) basic to its isoelectric point.
5. Describe the mechanism by which proteins can be physiologic buffers.
6. Differentiate between simple and conjugated proteins.
7. Describe the four different levels of protein structure.
8. Draw the following amino acids as a dipeptide.

$$H-\overset{\overset{\displaystyle H}{|}}{N}-\overset{\overset{\displaystyle H}{|}}{\underset{\underset{\displaystyle CH_3}{|}}{C}}-\overset{\overset{\displaystyle O}{\parallel}}{C}-OH \qquad H-\overset{\overset{\displaystyle H}{|}}{N}-\overset{\overset{\displaystyle H}{|}}{\underset{\underset{\underset{\underset{\displaystyle CH_3}{|}}{\displaystyle HCH}}{|}}{C}}-\overset{\overset{\displaystyle O}{\parallel}}{C}-OH$$

6-5 LIPIDS

Questions

1. What are the five classes of lipid molecules?
2. What are the basic molecular units of a triglyceride?
3. Describe the role of lecithin in reducing surface tension via pulmonary surfactant.

4. Discuss the utility of measuring the lecithin/sphingomyelin ratio as an evaluation of fetal lung maturity.
5. Describe the difference between the positions of pulmonary surfactant molecules relative to one another at high lung volumes and low lung volumes.
6. List the components of pulmonary surfactant.
7. What is the major component by weight of pulmonary surfactant?
8. What is the primary surface active lipid in pulmonary surfactant?
9. Name the major neutral lipid in pulmonary surfactant?
10. What is the role of SP-A in the pulmonary surfactant molecule?
11. Where are the phospholipids and proteins of pulmonary surfactant synthesized?
12. The formation of lamellar bodies is dependent upon which protein molecule?
13. Explain how lamellar bodies form and release pulmonary surfactant.
14. List four factors responsible for preterm infants developing respiratory distress syndrome.
15. What is the clinical utility for measuring the amount of phosphatidylglycerol in amniotic fluid?
16. What fluid reflects the maturational status of the fetal lung *in utero?*
17. Describe two types of artificial pulmonary surfactant clinically used today.
18. How do animal-lung derived pulmonary surfactants compare with synthetic lipid surfactants?
19. Discuss the clinical role of surfactant therapy.

6-6 NUCLEIC ACIDS

Questions

1. Name the nitrogenous bases found in (1) DNA and (2) RNA.
2. Diagram the linkages that occur between nucleotides to make up a molecule of DNA.
3. What is the complimentary base in DNA for (1) adenine and (2) guanine?
4. What are the complimentary bases for (1) adenine and (2) guanine in RNA?

6-7 HEMOGLOBIN CHEMISTRY

Questions

1. Describe the composition of the hemoglobin molecule.
2. Explain the interaction between globin and heme within a hemoglobin molecule.
3. Describe the composition and structure of heme.
4. Discuss the bonding capabilities of the ferrous ion in heme.
5. List the five different polypeptide chains comprising the normal hemoglobin variants present throughout a normal lifetime.
6. Describe the globin structure of the following hemoglobin variants: (1) embryonic, (2) fetal, (3) adult, and (4) adult variant.

7. Discuss the onset, duration, and termination of the normal hemoglobin variants throughout the course of a lifetime.
8. When can mutant hemoglobins form?
9. Describe how methemoglobin is formed.
10. How does methemoglobin adversely affect tissue oxygenation?
11. How does HbS differ from HbA?
12. Give an example of an allosteric interaction.
13. State the site where (1) oxygen, (2) carbon dioxide, and (3) hydrogen ions combine with the hemoglobin molecule.
14. Discuss how cooperativity enhances the binding of oxygen to hemoglobin at the lungs and how it facilitates the release of oxygen to the cells at the tissues.
15. List four other factors that influence oxygen-hemoglobin affinity.
16. Explain how those factors influence the position of the oxyhemoglobin dissociation curve.
17. Define (a) the Bohr effect and (b) the Haldane effect.
18. What phenomenon is responsible for the shape of the oxyhemoglobin dissociation curve?
19. Describe the composition of the myoglobin molecule.
20. Compare oxygen-hemoglobin affinity to oxygen-myoglobin affinity.
21. Why is deoxyhemoglobin a better buffer than oxyhemoglobin?
22. Diagrammatically summarize the reactions between hemoglobin, oxygen, carbon dioxide, and hydrogen ions occurring (1) at the lungs and (2) at the tissues.
23. What is the average life span of an RBC?
24. Describe the sequence of biochemical events involved in the degradation of hemoglobin.

6-8 BIOCHEMICAL ASPECTS OF OXYGEN TOXICITY

Questions

1. Describe what is meant by *univalent reduction.*
2. Describe oxygen free radicals.
3. List four oxygen free radicals.
4. List the end-products of oxygen reduction at the cell level.
5. Write the equations that indicate how these end-products form.
6. State the two ways that H_2O_2 can lead to the formation of HO·.
7. Discuss the process of lipid peroxidation.
8. Describe the structure of a cell membrane.
9. State where lipid peroxidation is likely to occur on the molecule shown below.

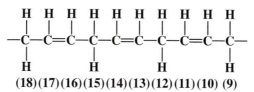

(18)(17)(16)(15)(14)(13)(12)(11)(10) (9)

10. What is an *antioxidant?*
11. What is the potential danger to a cell that has large quantities of polyunsaturated fatty acids comprising its outer membrane and a reduced endogenous antioxidant defense mechanism?
12. How does the presence of hyperoxia increase the potential threat to such a cell as described in question 11?
13. List four intracellular and two membrane-bound antioxidants.
14. What is the biochemical activity of superoxide dismutase as it relates to the super-oxide anion?
15. Which biochemical units act upon H_2O_2?
16. What are the end-products of the removal of H_2O_2?
17. Explain how vitamin E works as an antioxidant.
18. List the two forms of oxygen toxicity.
19. Describe the pathophysiologic events associated with pulmonary oxygen toxicity.

6-9 BIOCHEMISTRY AND CLINICAL APPLICATIONS OF INHALED NITRIC OXIDE

Questions

1. State the former name used to describe the nitric oxide free radical.
2. Write the notation for the nitric oxide free radical.
3. List four physiologic functions of the nitric oxide free radical.
4. Name two nitrosovasodilators that function by releasing $NO\cdot$.
5. State the concentration of $NO\cdot$ in (a) normal atmosphere, (b) cigarette smoke, and (c) workplace as set by OSHA.
6. From which amino acid is $NO\cdot$ synthesized?
7. What enzyme catalyzes the reaction?
8. List the molecule to which $NO\cdot$ binds after diffusing into local smooth muscle cells.
9. State the effect nitric oxide synthase inhibitors have on $NO\cdot$ production.
10. What effect does the inhibition of guanyl cyclase have on $NO\cdot$ action?
11. What is the effect of cGMP-specific phosphodiesterase inhibitors on $NO\cdot$ action?
12. What is the approximate concentration of $NO\cdot$ in normal human expirate?
13. Compared with the normal $NO\cdot$ concentration in exhaled human air, how is the exhaled $NO\cdot$ affected by (a) cigarette smoking, (b) asthma, and (c) exercise?
14. Approximately how much $NO\cdot$ is produced by the normal bacterial flora in the human nasopharynx?
15. Explain why the inhibition of NOS may be clinically useful in the treatment of sepsis.
16. In reference to $NO\cdot$, what is meant by the expression "selective pulmonary vasodilator"?
17. With regard to the systemic vasculature, how does inhaled $NO\cdot$ differ from nitro-prusside and nitroglycerin?
18. Describe the role of inhaled $NO\cdot$ in treating (a) PPHN and (b) ARDS.
19. Explain how $NO\cdot$ can be administered to mechanically ventilated patients.

20. Describe how NO· is inactivated by hemoglobin.
21. What enzyme in the erythrocyte is responsible for converting methemoglobin to normal hemoglobin?
22. What adverse effects can be caused by the production of NO_2 associated with NO· administration?
23. Name the oxidant that forms from the reaction between NO· and O_2^- in aqueous solutions.
24. What problems have sometimes been observed following the discontinuation of NO· inhalation?
25. What method of analysis is used to measure the inhalation of NO· and NO_2?
26. Why is quenching a potential problem associated with the analysis of NO· and NO_2?
27. What two problems can occur when NO· and NO_2 are analyzed via electrochemical cells?
28. What is the purpose of using sidestream sampling techniques when performing electrochemical cell NO· and NO_2 analysis?

6-10 BIOCHEMICAL ETIOLOGY OF ADULT RESPIRATORY DISTRESS SYNDROME

Questions

1. What is the essential feature associated with adult respiratory distress syndrome (ARDS)?
2. What entity is the primary focus of the etiology of inflammation in the development of acute lung injury?
3. What proof is there that direct toxicity plays a role in some forms of ARDS?
4. What role does phospholipase A_2 play in causing inflammation?
5. What two pathways are responsible for the metabolism of arachidonic acid?
6. List four lipid products that result from the metabolism of arachidonic acid.
7. List three cyclooxygenase products that decrease vascular tone and pulmonary smooth muscle tone and inhibit inflammatory cell function.
8. How is thromboxane A_2 formed and what responses does it evoke?
9. List four lipoxygenase products.
10. What effects do lipoxygenase products have on the pulmonary vascular permeability and on smooth and vascular muscle tone?
11. What type of arachidonic acid metabolites do neutrophils predominantly produce?
12. What aspects of lung function are adversely affected by arachidonic acid metabolites?
13. Why is platelet aggregation factor (PAF) thought to play a central role in the pathogenesis of acute lung injury?
14. What is the purported interaction between reactive oxygen species and neutrophil proteases?
15. What component of connective tissue is degraded by neutrophil elastase?
16. Under inflammatory conditions, what is the relationship between proteolytic activity of elastase and alpha-1 protease inhibitor?

17. List four cytokines.
18. What can the exaggerated release of tumor necrosis factor (TNF) and interleukin-1 (IL-1) cause?
19. What is the relationship between patients with septic shock and serum levels of TNF and IL-1?
20. Compare the responses to an increased serum level of TNF and monoclonal TNF antibodies.
21. What is the origin of the IL-1 receptor antagonist protein?
22. Name three cellular sources of interleukin-8.
23. How does endothelial cell injury and loss of endothelial surface initiate thrombosis?
24. How are disseminated intravascular coagulation (DIC) and microvascular injury brought about?
25. If the resolution of the hyaline membrane does not occur, what consequence may result?
26. What factors constitute hyaline membrane formation?
27. What is the significance of neutrophil-endothelial cell interaction?
28. What are selectins?
29. What molecule is crucial in arresting leukocyte movement and its subsequent transmigration between endothelial cells into the lung interstitium?
30. What activities depend on the expression of endothelial cell-derived adhesion molecules?
31. What molecules are important endothelial-surface adhesion molecules promoting neutrophil adhesion?
32. Describe each of the three stages of ARDS.

6-11 BIOCHEMICAL MECHANISMS OF BRONCHOSPASM

Questions

1. State the two cyclic nucleotides that interact within bronchial smooth muscle cells determining the net physiologic effect of bronchial smooth muscle.
2. Explain how (1) α-adrenergic blockade, (2) β_2-adrenergic stimulation, (3) phosphodiesterase inhibition, and (4) cholinergic blockade influence the biochemical events within bronchial smooth muscle cells and the ultimate physiologic response.
3. Discuss the significance of antigen-antibody reactions occurring on the surface of the mast cell.
4. List five vasoactive substances that are released during mast cell degranulation.
5. Describe the rationale for using the following medications for the treatment of bronchospasm: (1) aminophylline, (2) atropine, (3) isoproterenol, (4) terbutaline, and (5) tolazoline.
6. Relate the utility of cromolyn for the treatment of asthma.

Bibliography

Amin, S., Chen, Y., Collipp, P.J., et al. "Selenium in premature infants." *Nutr. Metab.* (1980) 24:331–340.

Austen, F. "Tissue mast cells in immediate hypersensitivity." *Hosp. Pract.* (Nov., 1982).

Balla, G., Makay, A., Pollár, Z., et al. "Damaging effect of free radicals liberated during the reduction of oxygen: Its influencing by drugs." *Acta Paediatr. Acad. Scient. Hung.* (1982) 23(3):319–325.

Barker, R. *Organic Chemistry of Biological Compounds.* Englewood Cliffs, NJ: Prentice-Hall, Inc., 1971.

Berman, B. "Cromolyn: Past, present, and future." *Pediatr. Clin. North Am.* (1983), 30.

Bieri, J.G., Corash, L., and Hubbard, V.S. "Medical uses of vitamin E." *N. Engl. J. Med.* (1983), 308.

Bigatello, L.M., Hurford, W.E., Kacmarek, R.M., Roberts, J.D., Zapol, W.M. "Prolonged inhalation of low concentrations of nitric oxide in patients with severe adult respiratory distress syndrome. *Anesthesiology* (1994) 80:761–770.

Brachet, J., Lehninger, A.L., Alfrey, V.G., et al. "The living cell." *Sci. Am.* (1961) 205.

Burton, G. "Vitamin E: molecule and biological function," *Proceedings of the Nutrition Society* (1994) 53:251–262.

Butler, J., et al. "Increased leukocyte histimine release with elevated cyclic AMP-phosphodiesterase activity in atopic dermatitis." *J. Allerg. Clin. Immunol.* (1983), 71.

Cantarow, A., and Scheparty, B. *Biochemistry.* 4th ed. Philadelphia: W.B. Saunders, 1967.

Comroe, J.C. Jr. *Physiology of Respiration.* 2nd ed. Chicago: Year Book Medical Publishers, Inc., 1975.

Crapo, J., et al. "Mechanism of hyperoxic injury of the pulmonary microcirculation." *Physiologist* (1983), 26.

Demopoulos, H. "Control of free radicals in biologic systems." *Fed. Proc.* (1973), 32.

Dixon, F., and Fisher, D. *The Biology of Immunologic Practice.* Boston: Sinauer Associates, Inc., 1983.

Dyson, R. *Cell Biology: A Molecular Approach.* Boston: Allyn and Bacon, Inc., 1974.

Ehrenkranz, R.A., Ablow, R.C., and Warshaw, J.B. "Prevention of bronchopulmonary dysplasia with vitamin E administration during the acute stages of respiratory distress syndrome." *J. Pediatr.* (1979), 95.

Ehrenkranz, R.A., Borta, B.W., Ablow, R.C., et al. "Amelioration of bronchopulmonary dysplasia after vitamin E administration: A preliminary report." *N. Engl. J. Med.* (1978), 299.

Frank, L., and Massaro, D. The lung and oxygen toxicity. *Arch. Intern. Med.* (1979), 139.

Gutteridge, J. "Lipid peroxidation: some problems and concepts." *Upjohn Symposium/ Oxygen Radicals,* April, 1987.

Ignatowicz, E., and Rybczynska, M. "Some biochemical and pharmacological aspects of free radical-mediated tissue damage." *Polish J. Pharmacol.* (1994) 46:103–114.

Irani, A., and Schwartz, L. Neutral proteases of mast cells. In: Neutral proteases as indicators of human mast cell heterogeneity, Karga, Basel, Monogr. *Allergy,* (1990) 27: 146–462.

Jellnick, P.H. *Biochemistry.* 1st ed. New York: Holt, Rhinehart and Winston, 1963.

Jobe, A.H. "Pulmonary surfactant therapy." *N. Engl. J. Med.* (1993) 328:861–868.

Jobe, A.H. and Ikegami, M. "Surfactant metabolism." *Clin. in Perinatology* 20:683–696, 1993.

Karnovsky, M. "Cytochemistry and reactive oxygen species: a retrospective." *Histochemistry* (1994) 102:15–27.

Mazurek, N., et al. "A binding site on mast cells and basophils for the antiallergic drug disodium cromoglycate." *Nature* (1980) 286:722.

McCord, J. "The biochemistry and pathophysiology of superoxide." *Physiologist* (1983), 26.

McCord, J.M. "Superoxide, superoxide dismutase and oxygen toxicity." *Rev. Biochem. Toxicol.* (1979).

McCord, J.M., and Fridovich, I. "The biology and pathology of oxygen radicals." *Ann. Intern. Med.* (1978), 88.

Middleton, E. Jr., et al. *Allergies: Principles and Practice.* 4th ed., Vol. 1. St. Louis: Mosby-Year Book, Inc., 1993.

Monaco, W. "Ultrastructural evaluation of the retina in retinopathy of prematurity and correlations with vitamin E therapy." *Curr. Eye Res.* (1983), 2.

Murray, J. *The Normal Lung.* Philadelphia: W.B. Saunders Company, 1976.

Nishimura, M., Hess, D., Kacmarek, R.M., Ritz, R., and Hurford, W.E. Nitrogen dioxide production during mechanical ventilation with nitric oxide in adults. Effects of ventilator internal volume, air versus nitrogen dilution, minute ventilation, and inspired oxygen fraction. *Anesthesiology*, (1995) 82: 1246–1254.

Oroszlan, G., Lakatos, L., and Karmazsin, L. "Neonatal oxygen toxicity and its prevention: D-penicillamine offers benefits without harmful side-effects." *Acta Pediatr. Acad. Scient. Hung.* (1982), 23(4):459–471.

Oski, F. "Metabolism and physiologic roles of vitamin E." *Hosp. Pract.* (October, 1977). 12:79.

Phelps, D., and Rosenbaum, A. "Vitamin E in kitten oxygen-induced retinopathy." *Arch. Ophthalmol.* (1979), 97.

Phillips, S.M., and Fox, E.G., "The immunopathology of parasitic disease." *Clinics in Immunology and Allergy,* (1982), 2:667–703.

Priestly, J. "Experiments and observations on different kinds of air." Lond. J. Johnson at St. Paul's Churchyard (1775), 2:101–102.

Repine, J., and Tate, R. "Oxygen radicals and lung edema." *Physiologist* (1983), 26.

Rossaint, R., Falke, K.J., Lopez, F., Slama, K., Pison, U., Zapol, W.M. "Inhaled nitric oxide for the adult respiratory distress syndrome. *N. Engl. J. Med.* (1993), 328:300–405.

Siraganian, R.P., et al. "Specific in vitro histamine release from basophils by bivalent haptens: evidence of activation by simple bridging of membrane bound antibody." *Immunochemistry* (1975), 12:149.

Taylor, A., and Martin, D. "Oxygen radicals and the microcirculation." *Physiologist* (1983), 26.

Thibeault, D., and Gregory, G. *Neonatal Pulmonary Care.* Boston: Addison-Wesley Publishing Company, 1979.

Wessel, D.L., Adatia, I., Thompson, J.E. "Delivery and monitoring of inhaled nitric oxide in patients with pulmonary hypertension." *Crit. Care Med.* (1994), 80:930–938.

White, A., Handler, P., and Smith, E. *Principles of Biochemistry.* 4th ed. New York: McGraw-Hill Book Company, 1968.

Whitsett, J.A. "Composition and structure of pulmonary surfactant." In Boynton, B.R., Carlo, W.A. and Jobe, A.H. Eds. *New Therapies for Neonatal Respiratory Failure.* New York: Cambridge University Press, 1994, pp. 3–15.

Winslow, C., and Austen, F. "Enzymatic regulation of mast cell activation and secretion by adenylate cyclase and cyclic AMP-dependent protein kinases." *Fed. Proc.* (1982), 41.

Zapol, W.M., Hurford, W.E. "Inhaled nitric oxide in the Adult Respiratory Distress Syndrome and other lung diseases." *New Horizons* (1993), 1:638–650.

CHAPTER SEVEN

MICROBIOLOGY

In the respiratory care practitioner's role within the health care team, a basic understanding of microbiology is necessary. Basic skills involved include (1) the collection of sputum samples; (2) the treatment of patients having bacterial, viral, or fungal diseases; (3) the disinfection and sterilization of respiratory care equipment; (4) the adherence to and the utilization of appropriate isolation procedures; and (5) the prevention of nosocomial infections.

CHAPTER OBJECTIVES

Upon completing this chapter, the reader will have a fundamental understanding of certain principles of microbiology as they relate to respiratory care and will be able to

7-1 CLASSIFICATION OF MICROBES

- Classify microbes.
- Differentiate between procaryotes and eucaryotes.
- Identify examples of the different kingdoms of microbes.

7-2 BACTERIAL MORPHOLOGY AND STAINING CHARACTERISTICS

- Define the different morphologies of bacteria.
- Describe the utility of identifying bacterial staining characteristics.
- Explain the Gram stain and acid-fast stain methods.

7-3 BACTERIAL ULTRASTRUCTURE

- State the three anatomic regions of a prototype bacterium.
- Describe the difference between the cell envelope for gram-positive and gram-negative bacteria.

This chapter was written by William Bradshaw Davis.

- Explain the significance of the cell envelope structure.
- Describe the various regions and constituents characteristic of cell cytoplasm.
- Discuss the function of cell appendages.

7-4 BACTERIAL GROWTH REQUIREMENTS

- Describe different bacterial growth requirements.
- Describe the sporulation process.
- Know the chemical constituents of artificial growth media.
- Discuss the four primary environmental requirements for bacterial growth.
- Describe the utility of various types of artificial growth media.

7-5 BACTERIAL GROWTH AND CELL DIVISION

- Define generation time.
- Explain the different stages of bacterial growth.

7-6 CONTROL OF MICROORGANISM GROWTH

- Differentiate among the various methods available for the control of microorganism growth.
- Describe various sterilization methods along with their modes of action.
- Discuss a variety of disinfection and sanitization procedures and their modes of action.
- State the general mechanism by which antimicrobics control the growth of microorganisms.
- Discuss the action of different chemotherapeutic agents.

7-7 NORMAL FLORA AND HOST-PARASITE RELATIONSHIPS

- Discuss the importance of the normal flora.
- Identify microorganisms residing in normal flora at different sites.
- Discuss the potential ability of an organism to cause disease.

7-8 FUNGI

- Differentiate between yeasts (molds) and mycelium.
- State chemotherapeutic agents that are used to treat fungal infections.
- Describe various characteristics associated with fungi.

7-9 VIRUSES

- Define a virion.
- Describe the steps involved in viral reproduction.
- Discuss aspects of viral structure, reproduction, and infectivity.

7-10 INFECTION CONTROL

- State the causative agent and treatment of choice for patients with acquired immunodeficiency syndrome (AIDS).
- State the causative agent and treatment of choice for patients with respiratory syncytial virus (RSV).
- Describe the procedures known as *universal precautions.*
- Name body fluids that require appropriate barrier protection.
- Discuss Blood and Body Substance Isolation (BSI) procedures.

7-1 CLASSIFICATION OF MICROBES

Understanding infectious disease requires recognition of the relationships between microbes and other living things. There is considerable universality in the basic biochemical processes of life, but often very significant differences in the related structures and functions involved. As such, living things are placed into logical categories based on a systematized arrangement. This science of classifying living things, or *taxonomy,* provides a basis for communicating similarities and differences among species.

Modern taxonomy (Figure 7-1) recognizes five kingdoms for all living things. The two most obvious kingdoms are Plantae and Animalia, more traditionally known as plants and animals. However, it is in the other three kingdoms that many of the agents that may cause infectious disease reside. Bacteria make up the kingdom Procaryotae, fungi the kingdom Fungi, and free-living cells, such as amoebae and other protozoa, the kingdom Protista. It should be recognized that viruses are not placed in any of these kingdoms. Viruses appear to be partial forms of living systems and will be discussed in a separate section.

An especially important characteristic of the kingdom Procaryotae that distinguishes its members from those in the other kingdoms is the lack of a nuclear membrane and other subcellular organelles, such as mitochondria. For this reason, bacteria are referred to as *procaryotes* and are considered to have relatively simple cellular organization compared with those of fungi, protozoa, plants, and animals, which exhibit a true nucleus defined by the

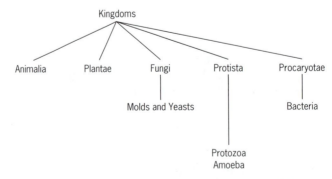

Figure 7-1 *The five kingdoms within the taxonomic classification of living things.*

presence of a nuclear membrane, as well as other subcellular organelles. Because fungi and protozoa have a cellular structure with a defined nucleus, they are referred to as *eucaryotes.*

Recognizing major differences between human cells and procaryotic cells, and similarities between human cells and eucaryotes, is fundamental when considering microbes as infectious agents. Differences between procaryote and human cell structure and metabolism must be taken into account to fully appreciate such concepts as selective toxicity in antimicrobial therapy, cultivating bacteria in the diagnostic laboratory, and techniques for sterilization, disinfection, antisepsis, and infection control.

7-2 BACTERIAL MORPHOLOGY AND STAINING CHARACTERISTICS

Bacteria are the smallest organisms that contain all of the biochemical machinery necessary to sustain life and to allow for reproduction. Bacteria have an average size range of 1 μm to 10 μm. Figure 7-2 compares the relative sizes of a bacterium and eucaryotic cell types (amoeba and hepatocyte).

Bacteria can be grouped on the basis of their morphology as viewed through the light microscope. Cells that are round are called *cocci,* whereas those that are cylindrical or rod-shaped are termed *bacilli.* Some bacteria are oval and are referred to as *coccobacillary.* A few species of bacteria appear comma-shaped and are called *vibrios.* Finally, there are those called *spirochetes,* which are spiral-shaped, similar to coiled springs.

Some genera of bacteria do not separate completely after cell division. As a result, varying spatial arrangements of cells occur depending on the species. Bacteria that divide in a single plane to their axis and develop into chains are called *strep.* For example, cocci that divide in this manner are referred to as *diplococci* if they occur in pairs or *streptococci* if they occur as three or more. Organisms that divide in more than one plane to their axis develop into clusters. An example of organisms that divide in this manner are coccus-shaped bacteria called *staphylococci* (*staph* = grape-like clusters). Figure 7-3 depicts various types and spatial arrangement occurring among bacteria.

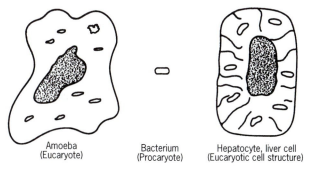

Amoeba
(Eucaryote)

Bacterium
(Procaryote)

Hepatocyte, liver cell
(Eucaryotic cell structure)

Figure 7-2 *Comparison of cell size of a bacterium to an amoeba and a liver cell (hepatocyte).*

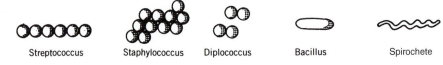

Figure 7-3 *Depiction of various types of spatial arrangements occurring among bacteria.*

In addition to shape and arrangement of bacterial cells, the staining property of various genera is a major means of making initial distinctions between medically important bacteria. The main staining procedures used in this regard are the **Gram stain** and **acid-fast stain.** Both techniques are based on the ability of the organism in question to resist decolorization with an organic solvent after being stained with a basic dye.

In the case of the Gram stain the dye is crystal violet, which stains the organism blue. The decolorizing agent is usually alcohol. After the decolorization step, smears are stained with a counterstain, usually safranin, a red dye. Bacteria that appear blue after the Gram stain procedure are called **gram-positive** bacteria. Those that are decolorized and take up the red counterstain are called **gram-negative.**

The acid-fast stain is reserved mainly for a few microbes that have a high lipid content, for example, the mycobacteria (microbes causing tuberculosis and other diseases). Smears are first stained red with carbol-fuschin. Acid-fast organisms, such as mycobacteria, retain the red stain when treated with a solution of acid-alcohol. Thus, bacteria that appear red after being stained by the acid-fast technique are referred to as *acid-fast.*

Table 7-1 depicts various bacteria with respect to their morphology and staining characteristics.

TABLE 7-1 Morphology and Staining Characteristics of Bacteria that Commonly Cause Respiratory Disease[a]

Bacilli	
Gram-positive	Gram-negative
Corynebacterium diphtheriae	*Klebsiella pneumoniae*
	Hemophilus influenzae
Acid-fast	*Bordetella pertussis*
Mycobacterium tuberculosis	*Pseudomonas aeruginosa*
Mycobacterium species	*Legionella pneumophila*
Nocardia	*Escherichia coli*
Cocci	
Gram-positive	Gram-negative
Streptococcus pyogenes	*Neisseria meningitidis*
Streptococcus pneumoniae	*Neisseria gonorrhea*
Staphylococcus aureus	

[a]*Not all respiratory pathogens are included.*

7-3 BACTERIAL ULTRASTRUCTURE

The overall anatomy of the prototype bacterium can be divided into three distinct regions: the cell envelope, cytoplasm, and appendages. Structures found within these regions are as follows:

1. Cell envelope
    A. Capsule or slime layer
    B. Cell wall
    C. Cell membrane
2. Cytoplasm
    A. Chemical constituents
    B. Nucleoid region (chromosomes)
    C. Plasmids
    D. Ribosomes
    E. Reserve material
3. Appendages
    A. Pilus (fimbriae)
    B. Flagellum

These various structures are depicted in Figure 7-4.

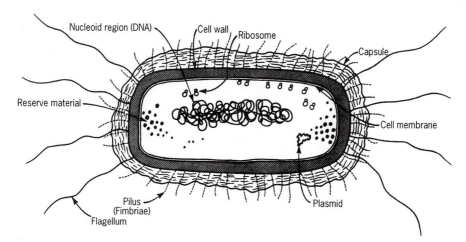

Figure 7-4 *Anatomical features of prototype bacterium showing (1) cell envelope constituents, (2) cytoplasmic components, and (3) appendages.*

Cell Envelope

Most bacteria possess mucilagenous material as a part of their outermost surface layer. If large quantities of this material are clearly detectable, the structure is called a *capsule.* If it is not a distinct structure, it is considered a *slime layer.* The capsule varies widely among bacteria with respect to density, thickness, and chemical composition. Bacterial capsules consist of a **polymer** (a chain of the same type of molecule). For example, the capsule of the organism that causes pneumococcal pneumonia consists of polysaccharides, whereas that of the bacterium that causes streptococcal pharyngitis is a polymer of amino sugars.

Though the capsule is a loose and often a secreted outer material not essential to the survival of a bacterium, in some instances it contributes significantly to the ability of an organism to cause disease by inhibiting the ability of host phagocytic cells to engulf the organism. It should be emphasized, however, that the presence of a capsule does not necessarily mean that the organism will escape **phagocytosis.** There are many disease-causing bacteria whose capsules do not render the organism resistant to phagocytosis. Conversely, with the pneumococcal organism, a capsule is the main factor enabling the organism to establish an infection that can result in disease. The capsules synthesized by many bacteria are antigenic, that is, they induce the synthesis of specific antibodies, which may be used in the serological identification of the organism in the clinical laboratory.

The cell wall is a portion of the procaryotic cell envelope essential for the organism's survival. It is a rigid structure that allows the organism to withstand variations in environmental osmotic pressure. Removal of the cell wall by degradative enzymes or antibiotics leads to the formation of an osmotically sensitive cell called a **protoplast** or **spheroplast.** When such cells are capable of undergoing cell division, they are referred to as **L-forms.** Only the genus *Mycoplasma* does not naturally have a cell wall. As a result, these bacteria are sensitive to **lysis** in a hypotonic environment and require special conditions for their growth in the laboratory.

The rigidity of the cell wall also accounts for the shape of the organism. The numerous antigenic macromolecules on the surface of the cell wall further contribute to serologic identification of many microbes.

The cell wall is unique to bacteria and provides an ideal selective target for antibiotics. Antibiotics that inhibit bacterial cell wall synthesis lead to the death of the organism because osmotic lysis of the protoplast or spheroplast occurs under physiologic conditions.

The biochemical structure of the bacterial cell wall is uniform in that it consists of a single continuous molecule called the **peptidoglycan.** A complete peptidoglycan molecule consists of numerous sugar molecules cross linked to each other creating a fence-like structure that encloses the fragile protoplast (Figure 7-5). However, it should be noted that the gram-negative bacterial cell wall is more complex than the cell wall of a gram-positive bacterium. Gram-negative bacteria have what appears to be a bilayered cell wall. The inner wall component is the same as the peptidoglycan of the gram-positive bacterium. However, the outer component is often referred to as the *outer membrane* because of its structural and chemical resemblance to biological membranes, which are discussed below. The outer membrane of a gram-negative bacterium is composed largely of molecules of lipopolysaccharides (LPS). The LPS material of the gram-negative cell wall has received

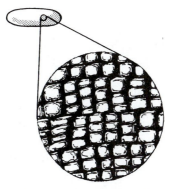

Figure 7-5 *Artistic representation of fence-like structure of peptidoglycan highlighting the cross-linking of constituent sugar molecules.*

considerable attention; it has been shown to have toxic activity responsible in part for many of the symptoms associated with infections by gram-negative species (e.g., vascular collapse, hemorrhage, shock, and leukopenia). Because of these toxic effects, LPS is often referred to as an **endotoxin.**

The cytoplasmic membrane of bacteria is a bilayer of phospholipid molecules interspersed with proteins (Figure 7-6). Unlike the membranes of eucaryotic cells, and with the exception of the *Mycoplasma*, bacterial membranes do not have sterols. Otherwise, as in animal cells, the cytoplasmic membrane of a bacterium functions as a selectively permeable barrier allowing the organism to transport specific nutritional molecules as needed. The function of energy production carried out by mitochondria in eucaryotic cells occurs in the cytoplasmic membrane of the bacterium.

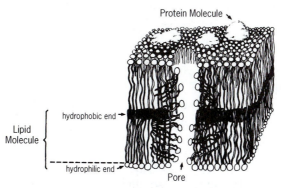

Figure 7-6 *Bacterial cell membrane. Note the phospholipid bilayer and the specific orientation of the hydrophobic and hydrophilic ends of the phsopholipid molecules. Also shown are protein molecules interspersed among the phsopholipids, and a pore allowing for communication between the intra- and extracellular environments.*

Cytoplasm

Approximately 80% of the cytoplasm, which is circumscribed by the cell membrane, is water. The remainder of the cytoplasm consists of proteins, lipids, carbohydrates, nucleic acids, and various electrolytes, such as magnesium and potassium. Enzymes and other molecules involved in metabolism also are located mainly in the cytoplasm. It is important to recognize that the concentration of molecules in the cytoplasm is very high. As a result, there is a substantial osmotic pressure acting on the cell membrane. It is for this reason that if the cell wall is lost the organism will rupture.

The nucleoid region is that region occupied by the bacterial chromosome. Bacteria have only one chromosome, which is a closed, circular, double-stranded DNA molecule. It is about 1,000 times as long as the organism and constitutes the nuclear body by virtue of being densely packed into one region of the organism.

Bacteria often contain various small, autonomously replicating, circular DNA molecules that are distinct from the bacterial chromosome. These pieces of DNA, called **plasmids,** are not necessary for the organism's survival but contain genetic information additional to that of the bacterial chromosome. Genes that confer antibiotic resistance, as well as the ability to produce certain toxins, are often found on plasmids. Bacteria frequently transfer these plasmids to one another by processes called **transduction** and **conjugation.** This transfer may result in serious consequences to drug therapy or to the ability of the recipient microbe to cause disease.

Ribosomes are coarse granular structures that appear in the cytoplasm. As in eucaryotic cells, bacterial ribosomes are prominent in protein synthesis; however, in overall size, bacterial ribosomes are much smaller than eucaryotic cell ribosomes. As a result, antibiotics which prevent protein synthesis have been developed to interact preferentially with bacterial ribosomes. Thus, bacterial protein synthesis, rather than that of the host, is impaired. Taking advantage of this difference between the ultrastructures of bacterial cells and human cells serves as a basis for the development of selectively toxic antimicrobials, which are discussed under the heading "Chemotherapeutic Agents" in Section 7-6.

Depending on the type and amount of nutrients available, bacteria will store molecules as reserves for carbon or energy. Reserve materials include glycogen, lipids, and inorganic polyphosphates, all of which may appear as large granules in stained bacteria.

Appendages

Flagella are long filamentous appendages that extend from the surface of some bacterial cells. The filaments are so fine that they are not visible under the light microscope unless special staining procedures are employed. Flagellum provide motility that results from the propelling force created by undulation of the structure. Some bacteria have flagella distributed over the entire surface of the cell (peritrichous), while others have one (monotrichous) or a few (lopotrichous) found only at one or both ends of the cell. Flagella are antigenic; therefore, flagellar antigens also can be used in the serologic identification of the organism in the clinical laboratory.

Pili, which are much shorter and even thinner than flagella, are appendages on the surface of the cell. They have no role in motility of the cell. However, there are at least two known types. One type of pilus is called a *sex pilus*. It allows one bacterium to attach to another. This attachment facilitates the exchange of genetic information, such as DNA or plasmids, from one cell to another. The second type of pilus is called a *common pilus* or *fimbria*. It is known to assist the organism in attaching to certain types of cells in a given host. For example, the organism that causes gonorrhea establishes infection when the fimbriae attach to the surface of the cells of the urethral tract. Bacterial that cause whooping cough also have fimbriae that enable them to attach readily to epithelial cells of the trachea. There are many other bacteria whose fimbriae-mediated tissue trophism, or selectivity, is suspected to aid in the infectious process by enhancing the organism's ability to colonize the host.

7-4 BACTERIAL GROWTH REQUIREMENTS

Knowing the conditions required for the growth of microorganisms is necessary for understanding the distribution of organisms in nature. Further, it is especially important to understand the growth requirements of microbes in order to cultivate them in the clinical laboratory for identification as possible causative agents of disease.

The vast majority of medically important bacterial species obtain energy and the macromolecular building blocks for growth by utilizing an organic carbon source, such as glucose, and a mixture of inorganic salts. Bacterial growth media of this type are referred to as *minimal synthetic media.* However, most clinically significant microbes need a very complex mixture of organic materials supplemented with inorganic salts. These mixtures are often made from extracts of animal tissues, such as brain or heart. Blood is also a frequent additive. Media preparations of this sort are considered to be *complex media.* In essence, complex media are rich with nutrients of so many different types that they practically cannot be chemically defined.

A few bacterial species have such complex or unusual growth requirements that they can be grown only in living cells, such as tissue culture or embryonated eggs. These bacteria are called **obligate intracellular parasites.** Examples of obligate intracellular parasites are the *Rickettsia,* which cause typhus and Rocky Mountain spotted fever, and the *Chlamydia,* which cause trachoma and other diseases. Chlamydiae and Rickettsiae have all the morphologic characteristics of bacteria but cannot metabolize their necessary energy. Because they need living cells as hosts to support their growth, members of the genera *Chlamydia* and *Rickettsia* are often erroneously classified as nonbacterial.

Finally, a few bacteria can be cultured only in animals. Examples of these microbes are *Treponema pallidum,* which causes syphilis, and *Mycobacterium leprae,* which causes leprosy. However, it is safe to say that the majority of known bacterial pathogens for humans can be cultivated on artificial media (minimal synthetic or complex media).

Endospores

Endospores occur among certain genera of gram-positive bacilli. The medically important genera are *Clostridium* species and *Bacillus anthracis.* The genus *Clostridium* contains species that cause tetanus, botulism, and gas gangrene. *Bacillus anthracis* causes anthrax. These bacteria are triggered to form spores when nutritional needs become depleted or when adverse conditions occur in the environment. During the sporulation process the vegetative form of the bacterium (normal state) undergoes a number of stepwise physiologic changes that result in the formation of a dormant form, that is, the spore, which is resistant to the lethal effects of heat, drying, freezing, various chemicals, antibiotics, and radiation.

Sporulation is not a reproductive process, but a means of cell survival during adverse physical or nutritional conditions. Upon restoration of a favorable environment, the endospore germinates, giving rise to a single vegetative cell, which can resume normal growth and cell division. Endospores are present throughout the environment and serve as a constant source for contamination. In fact, as a result of their resistance to heat, spores are the bane of processes involving sterilization. Figure 7-7 depicts the cycles of sporulation and germination.

Chemical Constituents of Artificial Growth Media

From a basic biochemical standpoint, all bacteria have the same elemental requirements. Analysis of bacterial cytoplasm reveals that bacteria generally contain carbon, nitrogen, sulfur, phosphorus, and trace elements. For bacteria that can be grown on artificial media, these elements can be supplied by various chemical compounds.

Carbon is an element central to the metabolic needs of all cells. It is usually supplied as glucose or some other type of carbohydrate. Carbon provides the backbone necessary for molecules in their role as structural building blocks as well as enzymes and other

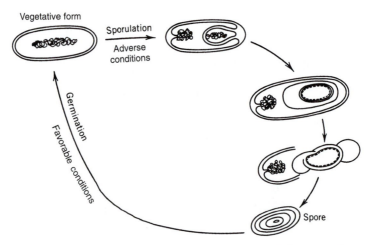

Figure 7-7. *Sporulation and germination cycle characteristic among certain genera of gram-positive bacilli.*

functional molecules. Carbohydrates also can serve as molecules from which the organism derives energy.

Nitrogen is necessary to supply the elemental needs for the synthesis of amino acids and proteins. Nitrogen is often supplied as inorganic nitrates or nitrites or organically by way of protein digests.

Sulfur is essential for the synthesis of certain amino acids, such as cysteine and methionine. Media are often supplemented with sulfate to meet this requirement.

Phosphorus is needed for the synthesis of adenosine triphosphate (ATP) and other nucleotides. It is usually assimilated metabolically by the organism as inorganic phosphate.

Sodium, potassium, and calcium along with the trace metals iron, zinc, magnesium, manganese, and cobalt are required for numerous biochemical functions. They can be included in artificial media as inorganic salts but are usually sufficient in tap water to meet the nutritional requirements of most bacteria.

In addition to these nutritional requirements, some microbes require special supplements known as *growth factors*. Growth factors may include metal chelating agents, vitamins, and various amino acids that the organism can not synthesize on its own from the basic elements just described.

Liquid media are converted into solid media by melting a material derived from seaweed at 100°C. The material is referred to as **agar** and, upon cooling to 47°C, it solidifies as a gelatinous material. The advantage of a solid medium is that bacteria can be observed to grow as distinct colonies. Such colonies are useful in isolating a species in pure culture and using colony morphology as a characteristic for identification.

Environmental Requirements for Bacterial Growth

There are four aspects of the environment that must be taken into consideration when using artificial media to cultivate bacteria. They are hydration, pH, temperature, and aeration.

Water is often called the *universal solvent*. It is essential for the viability of all cells. Although the ability of bacteria to sequester moisture from the environment varies greatly from species to species, the presence of at least a minute amount of water is an absolute requirement for an organism's survival. Of course, when considering that preparation of artificial media includes water as the solvent, hydration is not usually a primary concern for growth of bacteria in the laboratory.

The acidity or alkalinity (pH) of the environment is a key factor to consider when growing microbes in the laboratory. Depending on the species, there are microbes in nature that can grow at a pH as low as that of sulfuric acid, as well as some that can grow at a pH as high as that of sodium hydroxide. However, most medically important microbes tolerate a pH range of about 6.00 to 8.00 with optimal growth conditions being approximately 7.00. As a result of bacterial excretory products changing the pH, artificial media usually contain a buffer that helps to maintain the pH within a narrow range. Still it is important to recognize that the ability of various microbes to produce acid or alkaline byproducts is often used in the systematic identification of organisms. Various pH indicators can be added to a medium that will change color and allow identification of certain microbes based on their ability to change the pH of the medium.

Most bacteria can grow over a wide temperature range but have a narrow range for optimal growth. In nature there are microbes that grow at temperatures near 0°C or as high as 90°C. Microorganisms found in the mammalian body have a temperature optimum of about 37°C. In most cases bacteria cultured in the clinical laboratory are grown at 35°C to 37°C.

The gaseous environment is paramount to the organism. Some species have an absolute requirement for oxygen and are called **obligate aerobes.** Conversely, **obligate anaerobes** are poisoned by the presence of oxygen. Furthermore, there are bacteria that can adapt to the presence or absence of oxygen and adjust their metabolisms accordingly. These microbes are called **facultative.**

Carbon dioxide is another gas that can affect growth. Some organisms have an absolute requirement for the gas because they use it as their sole source of carbon. However, a wide range of clinically important aerobic organisms that utilize carbon-containing compounds also incorporate or "fix" CO_2 into the carbon compounds they synthesize. There are a few organisms, including the bacterial strain causing gonorrhea, that require a greater CO_2 tension than air can supply. In these cases special methods that increase the CO_2 tension must be used to ensure their isolation.

Practical Applications of Artificial Growth Media

The design of media for the growth of bacteria in the clinical laboratory must take into account the specific needs of each organism. There is no single or universal medium that can fulfill all the requirements for all organisms. It is for this reason that complex media are frequently used. Furthermore, by taking advantage of any unique requirements for growth, one may design media and/or conditions of growth that give a particular organism, or groups of organisms, a partial or totally selective advantage. It is often the case in medical bacteriology that diagnosis depends on demonstrating the presence of a disease-producing organism that is a minority group in a sample containing many different kinds of bacteria unrelated to the disease process. Under these conditions, the use of a selective medium that enriches or permits only the growth of the pathogen may be the only way in which isolation and identification of the pathogen can be accomplished. Selection by enrichment can include such methods as incorporating a specific carbon source that only one type of organism can utilize. Conversely, incorporation of compounds inhibitory for most organisms other than the species suspected is a common technique used in diagnostic microbiology for isolation of certain pathogens.

Even when selection is not practical it may be possible to incorporate a reagent into a medium so the organism of interest exhibits its unique properties. A medium that visibly distinguishes one bacterial strain from others during growth is called an *indicator* or **differential medium.** For example, inclusion of lactose and an appropriate pH indicator in an agar medium will permit the visual identification of lactose-fermenting organisms that produce acid and change the color of the indicator. Tests for lactose fermentation are used to detect fecal contamination of water and dairy products, as well as for differentiation of various pathogens that may be present in a clinical specimen.

A medium also commonly used in clinical laboratories for differentiation of some bacterial species, such as streptococci, is blood agar. Various bacteria produce substances that lyse red blood cells to varying degrees. Consequently, the ability of an organism to cause a particular kind of lysis, or hemolysis, on blood agar can be used as a distinguishing factor.

7-5 BACTERIAL GROWTH AND CELL DIVISION

The *viability* of a microorganism is often described as its ability to grow and undergo cell division. Compared with that of animal cells, the rate of growth of most bacteria under optimal conditions is phenomenal. For instance, *Escherichia coli* can optimally divide every 20 minutes. Thus, if a culture of this organism could proliferate indefinitely, it has been estimated that a single cell would give rise to a total mass equal to approximately 4,000 times the earth's mass in about two days! Obviously, such unlimited reproduction of bacterial species does not occur because nutritional limitations and accumulation of toxic products impede their growth. Also, in nature competition among microbes for various ecological niches becomes a factor. Nevertheless, this example illustrates the enormous growth capacity of many bacterial species.

Depending on the availability of nutrients and on environmental conditions, the time required for one bacterium to undergo division to form two is the **generation time.** The minimal generation time varies from species to species. Thus, *Escherichia coli,* which has a 20 minute generation time, will provide a turbid or confluent culture within 12 to 18 hours when a medium is seeded with even a few bacteria. At the other end of the spectrum, most species of mycobacteria, which include the species that causes tuberculosis, have a generation time of about 12 hours. Thus, a specimen from a patient suspected of having tuberculosis would need to be inoculated on an appropriate medium and the culture allowed at least three weeks incubation in order to provide visible growth.

In an ideal liquid culture medium, the growth and division of microbes can be divided into four distinct stages. If a few viable bacteria are inoculated into a fresh medium, they will first begin to sequester nutrients and each individual organism will begin to enlarge. Thus, if one plots the number of viable bacteria present as a function of time, there is no increase in the total number of bacteria during the early stage of incubation, although the mass of each organism increases. This stage is called the *lag phase* (Figure 7-8). During this adjustment period the bacteria are arranging their metabolic priorities to synthesize proteins, lipids, and carbohydrates and are generating a critical mass to support division into two cells. Once the critical mass is reached, the cells begin to divide and "exponential growth" is observed. This stage is the *logarithmic phase* of growth, and the total mass increases proportionally to the total viable cell number. The rate of increase in the total number of viable bacteria is, of course, proportional to the generation time for the particular organism.

As the rapidly increasing number of microbes depletes nutrients in the culture and generates toxic byproducts, the *stationary phase* occurs. During this stage the number of microbes able to divide (i.e., viable) is equal to those that cannot (i.e., nonviable). As a result, there is a plateau in the growth rate. Finally, there is a phase known as the *death phase* during which the number of nonviable microbes begins to exceed the number of microbes that are viable.

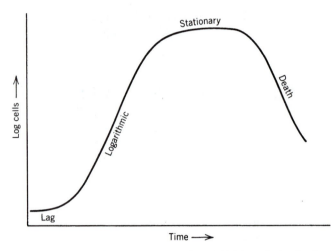

Figure 7-8 *Graphic depiction of the four stages of growth and division of microbes in an ideal liquid culture medium.* Lag phase: *no increase in bacterial number;* logarithmic phase: *exponential growth and increase in viable bacteria;* stationary phase: *equal number of viable and nonviable bacteria;* death phase: *number of nonviable bacteria exceed viable bacteria.*

It is important to be aware that the growth kinetics described above are for microbes grown in a test tube culture. In man and in the environment, this pattern may not apply because factors such as host defenses and competition for nutritional supplies intervene.

7-6 CONTROL OF MICROORGANISM GROWTH

In view of the large number of microbes present throughout the environment, the need for controlling their presence is obvious. This section addresses only sterilization, disinfection, and antimicrobial agents as the primary means by which control of microorganisms can be accomplished; however, it is important to realize that man's natural host defense mechanisms are also exceedingly important in controlling the infectivity of microorganisms and the ultimate outcome of disease processes.

Sterilization

Sterilization is an absolute term that implies complete freedom from all viable forms of all types of microorganisms. In the context of this definition spores are of central concern in the sterilization processes. In fact, various sterilization processes are designed to eliminate spores and often result in overkill for vegetative forms. Sterilization can be accomplished by heat, radiation, or chemical agents.

Moist heat by autoclaving is one of the most common sterilization methods used. Pure saturated steam at 15 psi provides a temperature of 121°C and kills all viable forms of organisms, including spores, within 15 minutes. Higher pressures and higher temperatures are also used for more rapid sterilization, for example, 30 psi and 134°C for 3 minutes.

Autoclaves depend on hydration and coagulation of microbial protein. Heat causes proteins to denature by breaking hydrogen bonds. When water is present, these bonds are more readily broken because hydrogen bonds with water can replace the original intramolecular bonds. Steam must not be superheated because it then behaves as a gas. All air in the autoclave must be replaced by steam; otherwise, sterilizing temperatures might not be attained. Autoclaving is unsuitable for sterilizing the inside of sealed containers or substances such as oils, waxes, some plastics, and sharp metal instruments. Autoclaves are used for sterilizing surgical "packs," instruments, glassware, bacteriological culture media, heavily contaminated materials, and other objects that are not harmed by water or high temperature.

Such items require specific packaging and placement within the autoclave to ensure steam penetration and contact with all item surfaces. Verification of successful autoclaving is rendered by the use of chemical indicator tape. When the tape changes color, sterility of the load is implied.

Dry heat is commonly used to sterilize glassware, certain metals, and hydrophobic substances. Sterilization by this method can be accomplished by heating objects in an oven at 160°C for 2 hours. Higher temperatures than those associated with autoclaving are needed because, as discussed above, proteins are not denatured as readily when water (steam) is absent.

Gamma irradiation is a highly effective means of sterilization. It causes the formation of toxic free radicals in cells. Gamma irradiation is used for sterilizing many disposable plastic articles and syringes because the radiation penetrates prepackaged materials.

Ultraviolet light (radiation) is used for sterilization of surfaces that are completely accessible and have no ultraviolet-absorbing coating. Ultraviolet light causes irreversible damage to the organism's nucleic acids. In practice, ultraviolet light is used to reduce the content of organisms in air under certain limited conditions.

Ethylene oxide (CH_2OCH_2), mixed with inert gases (carbon dioxide, halogenated hydrocarbons, or nitrogen), provides an effective and highly penetrating sterilizing agent that destroys spores. It is used in special chambers under controlled conditions of temperature (50°C to 56°C) and humidity (30% to 70%). Concentrations of ethylene oxide in the chamber can vary from 450 mg/liter to 1,500 mg/liter. It is used to sterilize many plastics or other heat-labile substances and equipment that would be damaged by autoclaving. Items to be sterilized by this method must be washed and thoroughly dried prior to ethylene oxide exposure. Thorough drying must be employed because residual water on the items can react with the ethylene oxide and form the tissue-toxic compound ethylene glycol. Prepackaging of the items with moisture-permeable materials is necessary. Chemical indicator tape is used to verify exposure to ethylene oxide. Once the sterilization process is completed, proper aeration of some items is required for removal of residual amounts of ethylene glycol. Aeration time depends on the nature of the materials sterilized. Metals and glasses are not penetrated by the gas and can be used immediately after sterilization.

Also, it is recommended that items such as polyvinyl chloride products that have been previously gamma irradiated should not be exposed to ethylene oxide. The reason is that polyvinyl chloride and ethylene oxide react to form the tissue-toxic compound ethylene chlorohydrin.

Glutaraldehyde is a chemical compound having bactericidal, tuberculocidal, virucidal, and sporicidal capabilities. It is available in alkaline (Cidex) or acidic (Sonacide) form.

Cidex, which contains 2% glutaraldehyde, has a pH range of 7.50 to 8.50. It is buffered by 0.3% sodium bicarbonate. This solution effectively kills bacteria, mycobacteria, and viruses in 10 minutes; spores are killed in 10 hours.

Sonacide has an active pH range of 2.70 to 3.70. Heating tends to increase its biocidal activity. For example, it is bactericidal and virucidal in 20 minutes at room temperature, but can accomplish the same activities in 5 minutes when heated to 60°C. Furthermore, Sonacide becomes sporicidal after 1 hour at that temperature.

Equipment processed by either solution must be thoroughly rinsed and free of organic residue before immersion. Similarly, equipment must be thoroughly rinsed and dried prior to patient use because glutaraldehyde irritates human tissue.

Maximum potency for both solutions is approximately 28 days depending on the degree of use.

Chemicals cannot generally be guaranteed to bring about complete killing of spores, viruses, or mycobacteria. Formaldehyde plus alcohol, glutaraldehyde, and ethylene oxide are exceptions, but they must have access to all surfaces for a prolonged period. These compounds act as alkylating agents. As such, they interact with the free amine and hydroxyl groups, which are functional groups on proteins and nucleic acids.

Disinfection and Sanitization

Disinfection involves the processes that cause the destruction of most organisms in the vege-tative form. Disinfection is most often accomplished by liquid chemical agents given sufficient time and access. All disinfectants, except some cationic detergents, have varying degrees of toxicity for tissues and are rarely used for treatment of wounds, having been replaced by chemotherapeutic agents. Some disinfectants are used for reducing the microbial flora of skin before surgical procedures, or for the treatment of minor wounds, and are referred to as *antiseptics.* Others are used exclusively for environmental decontamination.

Sanitization is similar in principle to disinfection but involves only reduction of the microbial population and the attainment of an acceptable level of microbial cleanliness for the purpose sought (e.g., surfaces for food preparation).

Pasteurization is the process of heating liquids to 62°C for 30 minutes or to 74°C for 3 to 5 seconds. This process kills most vegetative pathogenic organisms. Immersion of an apparatus such as an anesthetic face mask in water at 70°C to 80°C for 10 to 30 minutes will, likewise, destroy most vegetative bacterial pathogens on accessible surfaces.

Alcohols (ethyl and isopropyl) are widely used as disinfectants for cleaning skin surfaces prior to some invasive procedures. However, alcohols penetrate poorly and are not suitable for use when a large amount of organic matter is present. Because water must be present for the germicidal action of alcohols, a 70% concentration is recommended. Alcohols denature bacterial membranes as a result of their ability to solubilize lipids and denature proteins.

Phenolics (Lysol) are potent antibacterial agents even at low concentrations and act by denaturing proteins and membrane lipids, causing cell lysis. They penetrate well and are not subject to inactivation by organic matter as are alcohols. They are never used as antiseptics because they are highly toxic for tissues.

Quaternary ammonium compounds (cationic detergents) such as benzalkonium chloride have very little toxicity and are highly active against most vegetative bacteria. They have both lipid-soluble and charged water-soluble groups; thus, they concentrate at bacterial cell surfaces, altering membrane permeability. They are inactivated by organic material and ordinary soaps. It is important to be aware that quaternary ammonium compounds have rather poor activity against the genus *Pseudomonas,* whose organisms can grow even in solutions that have lost part of their disinfectant activity. Serious infections have resulted from use of such contaminated solutions.

Iodophors, such as betadine, are combinations of iodine and detergents. They include valuable sanitizers and skin preparation agents. Most iodophors liberate iodine slowly and must not be used on skin if a history of iodine sensitivity exists.

Halogens, such as chlorine or hypochlorite (bleach), are active oxidizing compounds with high antimicrobial activity. Even at high concentrations they are only moderately toxic for tissue. Their main disadvantage is rapid inactivation by organic matter. They are used for disinfection of water and "clean" utensils, for baths, and so on. Tincture of iodine is a highly effective skin antiseptic.

Hexacholorophene is a halogenated phenol incorporated into detergent soaps. It concentrates in the skin and reduces the carriage of pathogenic staphylococci. However, it has little or no activity against most gram-negative organisms. In fact, it may even be conducive to the growth of these organisms. It has been shown that skin absorption of hexachlorophene in premature infants, and from abraded skin in full-term infants, can have toxic effects on the central nervous system. For this reason, hexachlorophene soaps are now a prescription item and, when used in nurseries, are applied for only one or two bathings with special attention to rinsing off after use. They are no longer routinely used with premature babies. Indications for use in nurseries are an increased *Staphylococcus aureus* infection or carrier rate.

Table 7-2 lists some of the common methods employed for sterilization and disinfection.

Chemotherapeutic Agents

Unlike the sterilizing and disinfecting compounds discussed in the previous section, some chemical agents exhibit a high degree of specificity in their action. Thus, these agents affect only a particular step in a metabolic sequence or structural component necessary for the organism's survival. Substances that exhibit this level of specificity for a particular target can be used within the host because the toxic effects on the host tissues are very low or nonexistent. The specificity of a substance in having lethal or inhibitory effects on the microorganism, and little or none on the host, is referred to as **selective toxicity.** Such substances are categorized within a class of chemotherapeutic agents known as *antimicrobials.* Some antimicrobials are chemicals synthesized in the laboratory and thus are called *synthetic drugs.* Others are naturally produced by living organisms such as certain bacteria and fungi. These are the *antibiotics.* Alternatively, some antibiotics are chemically altered in the laboratory to provide pharmacologic advantages and thus offer a wide array of *semisynthetic*

TABLE 7-2   Common Methods of Sterilization or Disinfection[a]

Physical	Radiation	Chemical
Moist heat	Ultraviolet	Antiseptics
Dry heat	Gamma	Iodine
		Merthiolate
		Anionic detergents
		Hexachlorophene
		Alcohol (70%)
		Disinfectants
		Iodophors
		Cresols
		Chlorine
		Cationic detergents
		Phenols
		Sterilization
		Alkylating agents
		Ethylene oxide
		Formaldehyde
		Glutaraldehyde

[a]*Some sterilization or disinfection methods appearing in this table were not discussed in the text because they lack practical application regarding respiratory care equipment. However, they are included here for completeness.*

drugs. Conceptually, the derivations of the numerous antimicrobials are important, but in practice, referring to these distinctions is not common.

The basis for understanding the selective mechanisms of action of antimicrobials rests on a knowledge of structures unique to bacteria and the metabolic pathways that only bacteria employ. For example, in a number of cases the selective toxicity of antibiotics on bacteria has been traced to specific metabolic or structural differences between procaryotic and eucaryotic cells. Specifically, the sulfonamides interfere with a bacterium's ability to convert a metabolic precursor, para-amino benzoic acid (PABA), to the vitamin folic acid. Because humans obtain preformed folic acid in their diet, bacteria that depend on the PABA pathway for folic acid succumb to sulfonamides and human cells remain unaffected. Additional examples of selective toxicity include the action of penicillin on bacterial cell wall synthesis. The fact that the peptidoglycan structure is unique to bacteria has enabled the development of drugs that act specifically on the bacterial cell wall. Antimicrobials that inhibit protein synthesis are selective by virtue of their specificity or by interacting only with procaryotic ribosomes rather than all ribosomes regardless of cell origin.

A number of bacterial metabolic targets with which antimicrobials can interact to inhibit bacterial growth. Table 7-3 depicts the primary sites of action of representative antibiotics.

TABLE 7-3 Classification of Antimicrobial Agents and Their
Corresponding Mechanisms of Action

Inhibitors of Cell Wall Synthesis

Penicillins	Antibacterial
Cephalosporins	Antibacterial
Vancomycin	Antibacterial
Bacitracin	Antibacterial
Ristocetin	Antibacterial
Cycloserine	Antibacterial
Isoniazid	Antibacterial

Disrupters of Membrane Function

Amphotericin B	Antifungal
Nystatin	Antifungal
Clotrimazole	Antifungal
Miconazole	Antifungal
Ketoconazole	Antifungal

Inhibitors of Nucleic Acid Synthesis

Ciprofloxacin (Cipro)	Antibacterial
Rifampin	Antibacterial
Griseofulvin	Antifungal
Flucytosine	Antifungal
Acyclovir	Antiviral
Azidothymidine (AZT)	Antiviral
Pentamidine	Antiprotozoal

Inhibitors of Protein Synthesis

Streptomycin	Antibacterial
Tetracycline	Antibacterial
Chloramphenicol	Antibacterial
Erythromycin	Antibacterial
Gentamycin	Antibacterial
Amikacin	Antibacterial
Tobramycin	Antibacterial
Clindamycin	Antibacterial

Inhibitors of Metabolic Processes

Sulfonamides	Antibacterial
Trimethoprim-sulfamethoxazole (TMP-SMX)	Antibacterial/Antiprotozoal
Ribavirin	Antiviral

It should be noted that amphotericin B is an agent reserved for fungal infections. It disrupts membrane integrity by binding to sterols. Recall from the discussion under the heading "Cell Envelope" in Section 7-3 that, with the exception of *Mycoplasma,* sterols are not present in procaryotic cells. Unfortunately, because sterols are also present in the membranes of mammalian cells, amphotericin B must be administered with caution. Griseofulvin, an inhibitor of nucleic acid synthesis, is likewise used only to treat fungal infections. However, griseofulvin does not have the degree of toxicity associated with amphotericin B.

The selective toxicity of these drugs in binding sterols of fungal membranes as compared with human cells is based on structural differences in the kinds of sterols in each. Human cells have cholesterol as the primary sterol component of membranes and fungal cells have ergosterol. As a result of binding to ergosterol more efficiently than to cholesterol, the selective toxicity effect of clotrimazole, miconazole, ketoconazole, and amphotericin B are more toward the fungus. Though there are some degrees of toxic side effects for the host, ketoconazole and amphotericin B can be administered orally to treat systemic fungal infections, such as in the lungs or central nervous systems. Clotrimazole and miconazole are used topically to treat skin diseases, such as athlete's foot and jock itch.

Another important group of antimicrobics that are now being used effectively are inhibitors of viral nucleic acid synthesis. The drug acyclovir is available to treat various kinds of diseases caused by the herpes viruses. It is available in both topical and oral forms. These diseases include cold sores, genital herpes simplex lesions, chickenpox, and shingles. The most recent antiviral substance to be introduced is azidothymidine (AZT). AZT inhibits the replication of the human immunodeficiency virus (HIV) and is a mainstay in treating HIV infection and acquired immunodeficiency syndrome (AIDS). Although not curative, AZT lengthens the course of survival. Long-term systemic administration of antivirals may have toxic manifestations for the recipient. The target for each is nucleic acid synthesis. However, acyclovir and AZT are not effective until they are activated by enzymes synthesized only in virus-infected cells. It is for this reason that selective toxicity for nucleic acid synthesis is for the virus and not for uninfected cells of the host.

Ribavirin is an antiviral drug used to treat severe respiratory syncytial virus (RSV) infections. The mechanism of action is not fully understood but at least includes inhibition of viral assembly in RSV-infected cells. Ribavirin is administered as an aerosol and licensed for use only in infants not requiring assisted mechanical ventilation.

Pentamidine is an antiprotozoal drug used frequently in combination with trimethoprim-sulfamethoxazole (TMP-SMX) for treatment of pneumonia caused by *Pneumocystis carinii,* an opportunistic protozoan that is a leading cause of death in hospital patients, especially those having AIDS. Pentamidine, which interferes with this organism's RNA and DNA synthesis, is administered as an aerosol.

Resistance to antimicrobial drugs is an ever-increasing problem among all of the various types of infectious agents. A major factor contributing to this situation is indiscriminate use of antimicrobials. A particular problem that has arisen as a result of continuous widespread exposure in hospitals to the antibiotic methicillin is selection of resistant strains of *Staphylococcus aureus.* At one time, methicillin was a mainstay in treating diseases caused by *Staphylococcus aureus,* which is usually resistant to penicillin and most of its other derivatives. Methicillin resistant *Staphylococcus aureus* (MRSA) is now a common cause of hospital acquired infections, especially pneumonia. The organism's antimicrobial resistance pattern makes such infections very difficult to treat. A drug of choice now used to treat MRSA infections is vancomycin. Vancomycin is a rather toxic drug that inhibits cell wall synthesis. Although effective in cases involving MRSA, adverse effects of vancomycin include fever, chills, ototoxicity, and nephrotoxicity.

7-7 NORMAL FLORA AND HOST-PARASITE RELATIONSHIPS

The normal microbial flora are comprised of the microorganisms found in a particular site in normal healthy individuals at most times. For example, in the upper respiratory tract there are streptococci, diphtheroids, neisseria, and numerous other organisms. Establishment of the normal flora begins at birth but changes with respect to physiological conditions, age, and environment.

It is important to be familiar with the concept of normal flora for the following reasons:

1. To know what is normal in particular sites, thereby avoiding the trap of attributing pathological significance to organisms that are usually present in health; for example, alpha hemolytic streptococci in a throat culture do not represent the causative agent of a patient's pharyngitis, but its isolation from a blood culture might be indicative of endocarditis.
2. To be aware that infections are often caused by certain species of normal human flora (e.g., *Escherichia coli* in the urinary tract, actinomycosis of the jaw, and candidiasis in the vagina and/or oral cavity).
3. To understand the protective and beneficial effects of the normal flora.

Normal flora consist of residents and transients. Transients may be found because of temporary contamination or infection without disease. For example, *Streptococcus pneumoniae* (pneumococcus), a common cause of bacterial pneumonia, can be isolated from the respiratory tract and nasopharynx of many healthy individuals, especially during the winter months. The distinction between transient normal flora with the transient carrier state is blurred and largely depends on the epidemiological significance of the organism. For instance, finding *Neisseria meningitidis* (meningococcus) in the nasopharynx of healthy subjects during periods of epidemic meningococcal meningitis is known as "carriage."

Normal Flora of Different Sites

The established normal flora differ greatly at different sites and sometimes change considerably from time to time. The components of the normal flora are determined by physical and chemical conditions of the host, including amount and type of nutrients available and bacterial interactions. Certain members of the normal flora have specific affinity for particular epithelial cells to which they attach and on which they multiply. These phenomena account for normal flora residents. Table 7-4 shows examples of normal flora distributions.

Broad spectrum antibiotics may, through elimination of resident flora, select for a predominance of a particular organism. Once predominant, the organism causes a pathological condition to develop. For example, a severe enterocolitis can occur following intensive antibiotic therapy as a result of selection of *Staphylococcus aureus* as the predominant gastrointestinal tract organism. A generalized fungal infection caused by *Candida* can similarly result when broad spectrum antibiotics eliminate competing flora.

When a member of the normal flora is out of balance with other competing members, or finds its way to a normally sterile site, problems can occur. However, in general the beneficial aspects of the normal flora far outweigh the disadvantages.

Concepts of Pathogenicity

Only a very small percentage of the vast numbers of bacteria with which we share our environment are capable of causing disease in man. Numerous factors must be considered. They include (1) the innate capacity of the microbe to cause disease, (2) the route of entry, (3) the number of bacteria, and (4) the physical condition of the host.

The potential ability of an organism to cause disease is called its **pathogenicity.** Pathogenicity, however, is a relative term. It is well known that there are microbes that take advantage only of altered host defenses to cause infection and disease. Examples of such alterations include immunosuppression resulting from cancer chemotherapy or maintaining organ transplants, circulatory disturbances, alcohol, anesthesia, underlying diseases, such as diabetes, and trauma. An organism that causes disease only in a debilitated host, or does so with increased severity or frequency, is called an **opportunist.** Opportunists include microbes of the normal flora, as well as those of exogenous origin. Often an infection by an opportunistic microbe causes a fatal disease in patients suffering with significant immune suppression (e.g., AIDS). The term **pathogen** is usually reserved for bacteria having the innate capacity to cause disease in a normal host population.

Bacteria that are pathogens are often described in terms of the degree of their pathogenicity, known as **virulence.** In many instances the virulence of an organism can be attributed to specific factors that enable it to be either invasive or toxigenic.

A primary type of virulence due to invasiveness is the ability of an organism to avoid engulfment by phagocytic cells such as various types of leukocytes. This activity is often the result of the presence of capsules surrounding the organisms (e.g., the pneumococcus). Invasiveness also can be attributed to the ability of microbes to survive even after being phagocytized by leukocytes. Such is the case with the mycobacterial species that cause tuberculosis. Microbes that can survive in phagocytes are known as **facultative intracellular parasites.**

Some bacteria are invasive as a result of being able to spread because of the production of a multitude of various extracellular products that destroy tissues. The ability to preferentially attach to certain tissues contributes to invasiveness also.

TABLE 7-4 Microorganisms Found Consistently[a] on Various Integuments of the Human Body

Skin	
Staphylococcus epidermidis	Pityrosporum ovale (scalp and
Corynebacterium acnes	other skin areas)

Conjunctiva	
Corynebacterium species[b]	Hemophilus species

Nose	
Staphylococcus epidermidis	Streptococcus mitis
Corynebacterium species	Streptococcus salivarius
Hemophilus species	Moraxella lacunata

Mouth	
Staphylococcus epidermidis	Anaerobic micrococci
Streptococcus salivarius	Streptococcus mitis
Lactobacillus acidophilus	Anaerobic streptococci
Corynebacterium species	Neisseria species
Actinomyces bifidus	Bacteroides species
Leptotrichia buccalis	Actinomyces israelii
Treponema dentium	Fusobacterium fusiforme
Mycoplasma species	Candida albicans
Spirillum sputigenum	

Pharynx	
Streptococcus salivarius	Streptococcus mitis
Neisseria species	Anaerobic streptococci
Corynebacterium species	Veillonella alcalescens
Fusobacterium fusiforme	Bacteroides species
Treponema dentium	Vibrio sputorum
Klebsiella aerogenes	Actinomyces israelii
Proteus species	Hemophilus species

Lower Intestine	
Streptococcus mitis	Anaerobic micrococci
Streptococcus faecalis	Streptococcus salivarius
Lactobacillus species	Anaerobic streptococci
Escherichia coli	Clostridium species
Pseudomonas aeruginosa	Alcaligenes faecalis
Bacteroides species	Klebsiella aerogenes
Mycoplasma species	Fusobacterium fusiforme
Candida albicans	

(continues)

TABLE 7-4 (continued)

External Genitalia

Staphylococcus epidermidis	Streptococcus species
Streptococcus faecalis	Anaerobic streptococci
Escherichia coli	Spirillum sputigenum
Bacteroides species	Treponema denitum
Mycobacterium smegmatis	Candida albicans
Fusobacterium fusiforme	Mycoplasma species

Vagina

Anaerobic micrococci	Mima vaginicola
Neisseria species	Escherichia coli
Mima polymorpha	Treponema dentium
Hemophilus vaginalis	Mycoplasma species
Streptococcus faecalis	

SOURCE: Myrik, Quentin N., Pearsall, Nancy N., Weiser, Russel S.: Fundamentals of Medical Bacteriology & Mycology, Lea & Febiger, Philadelphia, 1974. Used with permission.
aThis list is not intended to contain all of the organisms of the normal microbial flora.
bMore than one species.

Bacteria that are virulent by virtue of their toxigenic ability excrete products that bring about specific metabolic alterations in various target tissues. These products are gener-ally referred to as **exotoxins.** Depending on the tissue affected, exotoxins are designated *neuro-* for nerve tissue, *entero-* for gastrointestinal, and so forth. Many exo-toxins carry lethal manifestations. Diphtheria is a disease resulting from toxin-produc-ing bacteria, as are whooping cough and tetanus. In fact, the exotoxin that causes tetanus is among the most potent biological toxins known. Estimates are that less than 1.0 µg of tetanus exotoxin is a lethal dose for man. Certain bacterial extracellular enzymes known to be destructive for certain cells (cytotoxic) may also be classified as toxins. Such is the case for enzymes produced by clostridial organisms, which cause gas gangrene.

Certain bacteria are not necessarily either invasive or toxigenic. They may cause disease as a result of having the capacity to be both.

An additional consideration regarding the ability of an organism to cause disease is tis-sue necrosis, which sometimes occurs as a result of what is referred to as *bacterial allergy* or delayed hypersensitivity. Although this response results from the host's immune response to the presence of the organism, localized necrosis can cause detrimental effects. Thus, such "bacterial allergies" may have beneficial and detrimental effects. Pulmonary lesions in cases of tuberculosis involve reactions of this type. For example, when the organism finds its way into the lungs, the immune response is triggered such that lymphocytes infiltrate the infection site. As these cells accumulate, they form granulomatous lesions that may eventually necrose. As these lesions expand, their centers liquify and can serve as reservoirs for a natural culture medium for surviving tubercle bacteria.

7-8 FUNGI

Fungi are assuming an increasingly important role in disease as a result of widespread use of antibiotics and steroids that predispose patients to opportunistic fungal infection. Over 50,000 species of fungi are distributed worldwide; however, only 50 to 70 species are recognized to cause disease in man. Similar to animals and most bacteria, fungi are heterotrophic. As a result of their inability to synthesize carbohydrates from raw carbon sources, they require preformed organic substances as nutrients to form energy. In this respect they either attack organic matter as saprophytes or parasitize man. Thus, fungi are ubiquitous. Ordinarily found as scavengers in the external environment, they grow in soil, vegetation, woods, and nitrogenous wastes, such as excreta of animals or birds. Man is exposed through direct skin penetration, by inhaling the fungal spores, or by becoming an accidental host of the fungal infection from an exogenous source. Because fungal spores are lightweight and become airborne easily, the respiratory tract is a likely portal of entry for exogenous infection. Mild to severe pulmonary involvement is often exhibited. Alternately, some fungi (such as *Candida albicans*) are part of the normal flora of the body. These fungi can produce endogenous fungal infections in the compromised host or as a result of medical intervention, such as the administration of broad-spectrum antibiotics.

Fungi are a diverse group of eucaryotes ranging from mushrooms and toadstools to unicellular forms that cannot be seen with the naked eye. Most fungi can be considered, using colloquial terms, as either *molds* or *yeasts.* Molds grow from spores that germinate to form long tubular projections called **hyphae.** Numerous hyphae intertwine to form a fungal mass called a **mycelium.** This mat is familiar as a velvet-like or a wool-like colony, for example, as mold on cheese or common bread mold.

Yeasts are small, unicellular, oval microorganisms. Too small to be seen without the aid of the light microscope, they range from 3 to 6 microns in size. They are much larger than bacteria and approximate the size of red blood cells.

The vast majority of the fungi are **monomorphic;** that is, they exist as either a mold or a yeast, regardless of their existence in nature, in man, or in a laboratory culture. *Aspergillus* and *Rhizopus* are true molds whether growing on food or in man as an exogenous opportunist in an immunocompromised patient. *Cryptococcus* is a true yeast whether growing in bird excreta or in the cerebral spinal fluid of a patient. Most fungi are saprobes that grow optimally at environmental temperatures. Those that can grow at 37°C may be capable of causing mycotic infections.

A few fungi display thermal dimorphism wherein both mold and yeast phases can be demonstrated in one species depending on the temperature. If the fungus grows as a filamentous mold at room temperature and converts to a yeast form in man or culturally at 37°C, it is considered thermally dimorphic. *Blastomyces* and *Histoplasma* are the agents of blastomycosis and histoplasmosis, respectively. They can cause serious pulmonary and systemic disease. Though the yeast phases of these fungi occur in man, confirmation of these isolates requires cultural conversion between the room temperature mold and 37°C yeast phases. Coccidioidomycosis is a severe systemic mycosis caused by *Coccidioides.* This organism can occur in man either in the yeast form or as mold.

The three systemic fungi, *Blastomyces, Histoplasma,* and *Coccidioides,* are potentially pathogenic to a normal healthy host under appropriate conditions. Although they are not communicable from person to person, they represent a potentially serious hazard to laboratory personnel. Studies to identify and convert the mold-yeast phases should be handled only in specialized microbiology laboratories. Therefore, it is paramount to notify laboratory personnel whenever a systemic mycosis is suspected.

Treatment of serious pulmonary and systemic mycoses presents a problem. Antibacterial drugs that are directed against procaryotic cells are not effective against fungi. Eucaryotic cell walls do not contain peptidoglycans. Hence, penicillin is ineffective in treating fungal infections. Fungal cell walls are composed of chitin, a polysaccharide that is similar to cellulose. Properties of chitin are useful for staining and identification of fungi, but not for therapy. Similarly, the broad spectrum antibiotics that interfere with bacterial protein synthesis do not affect fungal protein synthesis. As a result, the scope of therapy for fungal infections is indeed limited, as was discussed in Section 7-6, "Control of Microorganism Growth," under the subheading "Chemotherapeutic Agents."

Amphotericin B has been effective in treating blastomycosis, histoplasmosis, coccidioidomycosis, and cryptococcosis.

7-9 VIRUSES

The viruses are the leading cause of infectious diseases. The frequency of the common cold alone is enough to emphasize this point. In comparison to other infectious agents, the viruses far outnumber other microbes in causing illnesses. Also important is the fact that viral infections can often predispose an individual to serious infection by bacteria. This point is particularly true with respect to viral infections of the lower respiratory tract such as influenza.

An important question is "What are viruses?" This question can be answered in two ways. One answer is that viruses are the most simple form of microbes known. The other is that they exist somewhere between the "living" and the "nonliving." They are not cells, but particles of protein and nucleic acids occasionally associated with lipids and carbohydrates. The protein forms a coat, or capsid, around a nucleic acid core. The nucleic acid can be either DNA or RNA, but not both. These complex particles of organic biomolecules are known as **virions.** Some virions also have a phospholipid envelope, which is derived from the membrane of a host cell during the infectious process. Viruses range in size from 17 to 300 millimicrons in diameter. Although virions, like bacteria, can have different shapes, a typical icosahedral virion is depicted in Figure 7-9.

Virions reproduce themselves only by penetrating a susceptible cell and taking command of the cell's metabolic machinery. In this regard they are obligate intracellular

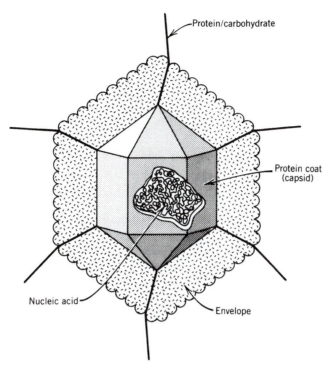

Protein/carbohydrate

Protein coat
(capsid)

Nucleic acid

Envelope

Figure 7-9 *A typical icosahedral virion illustrating the nucleic acid (DNA or RNA) core, surrounded by a capsid (protein coat), which in turn is sometimes enveloped by a phospholipid layer.*

parasites. First the virion attaches to the surface of a susceptible host cell. It subsequently penetrates the cell by invagination of the host cell membrane. The virion loses its protein coat early after penetration. The naked viral nucleic acid then directs synthesis of enzymes, which, in turn, are used to synthesize virus-specific proteins, nucleic acids, or other molecules needed to make up the components of the entire virion. Once synthesized, these individual components are assembled into complete virions and released from the infected cell. These viral progeny infect neighboring cells, resulting in the spread of infection throughout the target tissue. Thus, from this process, one usually thinks of viruses as infectious rather than "living."

The basic steps in virus reproduction can be defined as (1) attachment, (2) penetration, (3) uncoating, (4) production of viral nucleic acids and proteins, (5) assembly of virions, and (6) release. These steps are schematically shown in Figure 7-10.

As previously mentioned, much progress has been made in the development of drugs for treatment of some types of viral infections. Numerous viral diseases can now be prevented by the administration of vaccines. (Table 7-5 lists viral diseases for which vaccines are now available.) Although great advances have been made in understanding viruses and the diseases they cause, treatment still remains largely supportive.

Table 7-6 shows the various infectious agents that cause different types of diseases in the respiratory tract.

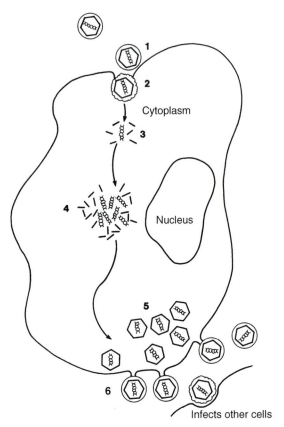

Figure 7-10 *Stages of viral reproduction. (1) attachment to host cell, (2) penetration into host cell, (3) uncoating of virion envelopes, (4) replication of viral nucleic acids and proteins, (5) assembly of virions inside host cell, and (6) release of virions to extracellular environment.*

TABLE 7-5 Vaccines Used in the United States to Prevent Viral Diseases in Humans

Disease	Vaccine
influenza	inactivated virus
measles	attenuated virus
mumps	attenuated virus
rubella	attenuated virus
polio	attenuated or inactivated virus
rabies	inactivated virus
yellow fever	attenuated virus
hepatitis B	component of virus
chicken pox	attenuated virus

TABLE 7-6 Respiratory Disease and Possible Infectious Etiologies

Disease	Possible etiologies	Typical specimens
Common cold	Upper respiratory viruses	Nasopharyngeal swab or nasal washing
Sinusitis	Viruses *Staphylococcus aureus* *Streptococcus pneumoniae*	Puncture of sinus cavity
Pharyngitis	*Streptococcus pyogenes* (Lancefield group A)	Throat or nasopharyngeal swab
Epiglottitis	*Hemophilus influenzae*	Throat swab or blood
Laryngitis	Viruses *Corynebacterium diphtheriae*	Laryngeal swab
Bronchitis (acute)	*Streptococcus pneumoniae* Other streptococci *Hemophilus influenzae* *Mycoplasma pneumoniae* Respiratory viruses, same as upper respiratory viruses *Bordetella pertussis*	Expectorated sputum, tracheal aspirate Bronchial washings, infralaryngeal aspirate Nasopharyngeal swab
Bronchitis (chronic)	*Streptococcus pneumoniae* *Hemophilus influenzae* Enteric gram-negative rods Viruses	Expectorated sputum Bronchial washings, infralaryngeal aspirate
Influenza	Viral	
Pneumonia (bacterial)	*Streptococcus pneumoniae* *Staphylococcus aureus* *Klebsiella pneumoniae* *Hemophilus influenzae* Enteric gram-negative rods *Pseudomonas aeruginosa* Other *Pseudomonas* species *Yersinia pestis* *Francisella tularensis* Anaerobes *Nocardia* species *Actinomyces israelii* *Mycoplasma pneumoniae* *Coxiella burnetii* *Chlamydia psittaci* *Mycobacterium tuberculosis* *Mycobacterium* species *Legionella pneumophila*	Expectorated sputum, tracheal aspirate, transtracheal aspirate, lung biopsy Sputum, nasopharyngeal swab Nasopharyngeal swab, lung biopsy Expectorated sputum, induced sputum, gastric washings Lung biopsy, pleural fluid

(continues)

TABLE 7-6   (continued)

Disease	Possible etiologies	Typical specimens
Pneumonia (viral)	Lower respiratory viruses Influenza viruses	Nasal washings, nasopharyngeal swab
Pneumonia (fungal)	*Blastomyces* *Coccidioides* *Histoplasma* *Aspergillus* *Rhizopus* *Candida* *Cryptococcus*	Expectorated sputum, induced sputum, lung biopsy
Pneumonia (parasitic)	*Pneumocystis carinii* *Paragonimus westermani*	Lung biopsy, bronchial washings Sputum
Lung abscess, empyema	Anaerobes *Klebsiella pneumoniae* *Staphylococcus aureus* *Pseudomonas* species	Transtracheal aspirate Lung tissue, biopsy

7-10 INFECTION CONTROL

In 1981, the first case of AIDS was reported. Because evidence indicates that the causative agent for AIDS, HIV, can be transmitted by contaminated body fluids, concern among health care workers regarding infection control procedures has increased dramatically. However, other blood-borne pathogens also deserve respect. Included among these are hepatitis B and hepatitis C viruses.

In 1982, a vaccine for hepatitis B became commercially available and is recommended for all health care workers who have the potential of being exposed to human blood. It is important that recipients of the vaccine be appropriately tested for seroconversion and reinoculated if negative.

In the absence of a vaccine or cure for AIDS, prevention of contact with HIV remains a paramount consideration. In 1983, the Centers for Disease Control published *Recommendations for Prevention of HIV Transmission in Health Care Settings*. The recommendation was precautions to avoid contact with blood and certain body fluids be taken with all patients regardless of their known infection status. Procedures known as *universal precautions* have now been established by the Office of Occupational Safety and Health Administration under the Department of Labor. Universal precautions protect the health care worker against exposure to blood-borne pathogens through parenteral, mucous membrane, and skin routes of transmission. Under universal precautions, the blood and certain body fluids of all patients are considered to be potentially infectious for HIV, hepatitis B, and other blood-borne pathogens. However, under circumstances in which differentiation between body fluid types is difficult or impossible, all body fluids should be considered potentially infectious materials.

Infection control procedures in contemporary health care settings go beyond standard isolation techniques and proper disposal of contaminated materials and needles. Universal precautions dictate that all blood and certain body fluids should be considered infectious regardless of the patient. A listing of body fluids that fall under requirements for appropriate barrier protection (gloves, gowns, masks, eyewear, etc.) is depicted in Table 7-7.

Be mindful that any body fluids, or other materials, not listed in Table 7-7 but showing visible signs of blood, or suspected to be contaminated with such, require instituting universal precautions. Examples include urine, sputum, and nasal secretions.

Universal precautions are directed toward reducing risk of exposure to blood-borne pathogens. A more global and thorough consideration known as Blood and Body Substance Isolation (BSI) has also been proposed (Gerberding, 1991). BSI procedures require appropriate protection when working with all body substances including moist body surfaces. This system is directed against all nosocomial infectious agents that may be transmitted by contact with skin or mucous membranes, or introduced parenterally. Unlike universal precautions, BSI takes into consideration the degree of contact, and thus is more procedure-specific. This flexibility allows for easier implementation, but should be applied as rigorously and reasonably as possible.

TABLE 7-7   Universal Precautions: Blood and Body Fluids

Apply barrier protection for
Blood
Semen
Vaginal secretions
Amniotic fluid
Cerebrospinal fluid
Synovial fluid
Pleural fluid
Peritoneal fluid
Pericardial fluid
Judgement Required for*
Urine
Sputum
Sweat
Tears
Saliva
Emesis
Feces

*If blood is present, universal precautions must apply.

CHAPTER SUMMARY

Animalia, Plantae, Fungi, Protista, and Procaryotae are the five kingdoms of all living things. Various cellular differences are the basis for this categorization. Bacteria are in the kingdom Procaryote, while viruses (partial forms of living systems) are not included in any of these kingdoms, as viruses are not cells, but particles.

Bacteria are grouped according to their morphology based on light microscopy. Additionally, bacteria are classified according to staining characteristics, i.e., gram-negative, gram-positive, and acid-fast.

Bacteria possess (1) a cell envelope, (2) cytoplasm, and (3) appendages. These three main bacterial components have variable features, leading to numerous forms of bacteria.

Bacteria have different growth requirements, however, medically significant bacteria obtain energy and molecular building blocks for growth using organic carbon sources. Some other bacteria have more complex growth requirements. Others can only be cultured in animals, i.e., *Treponema pallidum*, and *Mycobacterium leprae.*

Certain genera of gram-positive bacilli produce endospores, e.g., *Clostridium* species. Endospores enter a dormant form and can endure harsh conditions until favorable growth conditions prevail.

Despite the variety among bacteria, they all have the same elemental requirements— carbon, nitrogen, sulfur, phosphorus, and trace elements. Environmentally, bacteria have different pH, temperature, and aeration requirements.

Bacterial growth and cell division generally follow a common pathway. The four stages are the lag phase (no increase in bacterial number), logarithmic phase (exponential growth and increase in viable bacteria), stationary phase (equal number of viable and nonviable bacteria), and death phase (number of nonviable bacteria exceeds viable bacteria).

The growth of microorganisms is controlled by a variety of techniques and procedures based on the characteristics of the microbes. Control of growth ranges from sterilization to antiseptic procedures. These techniques and procedures are extremely important for equipment processing.

Chemotherapeutic agents display a high degree of specificity in their action. These agents generally interfere with a particular step in a metabolic pathway or a structural component required for the microbe's survival. Specificity is sought and chemotherapeutic agents, i.e., having lethal or inhibitory effects on the microorganism, and little to none on the host.

Normal flora differs according to location as well as with time. Normal flora is determined by physical and chemical host conditions.

The pathogenecity of microorganisms depends on (1) the innate capacity of the microbe to cause disease, (2) route of entry, (3) number of bacteria, and (4) physical condition of host.

Fungi are a diverse group of eucaryotes. Fungi are considered as either yeasts or molds. Molds grow from spores. Yeasts are small, unicellular, oval microorganisms. A variety of fungal diseases occur in man and are often treated with amphotericin B, nystatin, or ketoconazole.

Viruses exist somewhere between living and nonliving. They contain protein and nucleic acids. The protein forms a coat around the nucleic acid. These microbes enter a susceptible cell and use the cell's metabolic processes for its own growth, development, and reproduction. Some viruses are susceptible to vaccines.

Universal precautions have been established to protect health care workers against blood-borne pathogens. Under these precautions blood and other body fluids of patients are considered potentially infectious for HIV, hepatitis B, and other blood-borne pathogens. These precautions are directed toward reducing risk of exposure to blood-borne pathogens.

REVIEW QUESTIONS

7-1 CLASSIFICATION OF MICROBES

Questions

1. What is the purpose for classifying living things?
2. List the five kingdoms comprising modern taxonomy.
3. List the kingdom under which the following microorganisms are classified: (a) bacteria, (b) fungi, and (c) amoeba.
4. What features of the members of the kingdom Procaryotae distinguish them from members of other kingdoms?
5. Why do bacteria require simple cellular organization compared with that of fungi, protozoa, plants, and animals?
6. Why are fungi and protozoa referred to as eucaryotes?

7-2 BACTERIAL MORPHOLOGY AND STAINING CHARACTERISTICS

Questions

1. Which type of microorganisms contain the necessary biochemistry to sustain life and to allow for reproduction?
2. Based on the light microscope, define the three morphological groups into which bacteria are placed.
3. Describe the manner in which (a) diplococci, (b) streptococci, and (c) staphylococci divide.
4. Describe the Gram stain procedure.
5. What is the significance of (a) blue-stained and (b) red-stained bacteria associated with the Gram stain procedure?
6. State the acid-fast staining procedure.

7-3 BACTERIAL ULTRASTRUCTURE

Questions

1. List the three separate anatomic regions that comprise a typical bacterial cell.
2. Differentiate between a capsule and a slime layer.

3. Describe the disease-causing role of (a) pili, (b) capsule, (c) endotoxin, and (d) plasmids.
4. Define the terms *protoplast* and *spheroplast*.
5. Why are *Mycoplasma* bacteria sensitive to lysis in a hypotonic environment?
6. What bacterial cell component accounts for an organism's shape?
7. Why does inhibition of bacterial cell wall synthesis lead to the microorganism's death?
8. Describe the peptidoglycan molecule.
9. What is the significance of the relationship between lipopolysaccharides and gram-negative organisms?
10. Describe the cytoplasmic membrane of bacteria.
11. Describe the composition of cytoplasm.
12. How many chromosomes are in a bacterial cell, and where is this genetic material located?
13. Define *plasmids*.
14. Describe the process by which bacteria transfer plasmids to one another.
15. State the role of ribosomes in bacterial cells.
16. Describe how antibiotics that inhibit protein synthesis destroy bacteria.
17. Define the terms (a) *flagella*, (b) *peritrichous*, (c) *monotrichous*, and (d) *lopotrichous*.
18. Describe the two types of pili, or fimbriae.

7-4 BACTERIAL GROWTH REQUIREMENTS

Questions

1. Differentiate between *minimal synthetic media* and *complex media*.
2. Describe the media requirements that support the growth of obligate intracellular parasites.
3. Give two examples of obligate intracellular parasites.
4. How do *Chlamydiae* and *Rickettsiae* differ from other bacteria?
5. List two examples of bacteria that can be cultured only in animals.
6. List two genera of gram-positive bacilli that produce endospores.
7. What conditions must prevail to cause these genera to begin forming endospores?
8. From a bacterial survival standpoint, what are the advantages of forming spores?
9. When an endospore germinates, what form or state does the bacterium assume?
10. List the elements that generally constitute bacterial cytoplasm.
11. What element, required for bacterial growth, can usually be supplied by glucose?
12. What element is required for bacteria to synthesize amino acids and proteins?
13. What is the role of sulfur as a constituent of artificial growth media?
14. What constituent of artificial growth media contributes toward the synthesis of adenosine triphosphate?
15. Name the elements that are usually present in sufficient quantity in tap water to meet the nutritional requirements of most bacteria.
16. List the artificial growth media requirements referred to as *growth factors*.
17. Describe how the solid growth medium referred to as *agar* is formed.
18. List the four environmental factors that must be considered when using artificial media to cultivate bacteria.

19. What is the pH range tolerated by medically important microbes?
20. Describe the oxygen requirements for bacteria that are (a) obligate aerobes, (b) obligate anaerobes, and (c) facultative.
21. Describe the circumstances under which a selective medium is used to grow pathogens.
22. Define the term *indicator,* or *differential medium,* as it applies to bacterial growth medium.
23. What two specific constituents must be added to an agar medium to visually identify lactose-fermenting microorganisms?
24. Name the growth medium that supports the growth of the bacterial species *streptococci.*

7-5 BACTERIAL GROWTH AND CELL DIVISION

Questions

1. What term often describes a microorganism's ability to grow and undergo cell division?
2. Define the term *generation time.*
3. What is the impact of bacterial "generation time" on considerations involving growth of an organism in the clinical laboratory?
4. Define the various phases of bacterial growth in an ideal liquid culture medium.
5. What factors may cause the growth kinetics of microbes in a test tube culture to differ in man?

7-6 CONTROL OF MICROORGANISM GROWTH

Questions

1. Define the terms (a) *sterilization,* (b) *disinfection,* and (c) *sanitization.*
2. Describe the process of each of the following sterilization techniques: (a) moist heat (i.e., autoclaving), (b) dry heat, (c) gamma irradiation, (d) ultraviolet light, (e) ethylene oxide, and (f) glutaraldehyde.
3. How do the objectives of sterilization differ from those of disinfection?
4. Describe the process of pasteurization.
5. Describe the use of the following chemicals: (a) alcohols, (b) phenolics, (c) quaternary ammonium compounds, (d) iodophors, and (e) halogens.
6. Identify five classes of chemical agents used as disinfectants.
7. Identify the germicidal mechanism of (a) moist heat, (b) dry heat, (c) irradiation, (d) ethylene oxide, (e) alcohol, and (f) cationic detergents.
8. Discuss the concept of "selective toxicity" with respect to development of antimicrobial agents.
9. Differentiate among the terms (a) *antimicrobials,* (b) *synthetic drugs,* (c) *antibiotics,* and (d) *semisynthetic drugs.*
10. Identify five sites with which antimicrobials can interact to inhibit bacterial growth.
11. What is the mechanism of action of (a) penicillin, (b) cephalosporin, (c) ketocanozole (d) ribavirin, (e) rifampicin, (f) gentamycin, and (g) the sulfonamides?

12. What is the potential problem associated with the use of amphotericin B for the treatment of fungal infections in man?

7-7 NORMAL FLORA AND HOST-PARASITE RELATIONSHIPS

Questions

1. Describe (a) what is meant by the normal microbial flora, (b) when it begins to become established, and (c) what factors contribute to its alteration.
2. Describe the meaning of residents and transients of the normal flora.
3. How can a broad-spectrum antibiotic lead to a predominance of a particular microorganism?
4. What is the significance of the normal flora in determining the causes of infectious diseases?
5. What factors can contribute to a bacterium causing disease in humans?
6. Distinguish between the terms *pathogen* and *opportunist*.
7. Describe bacterial virulence factors that contribute to (a) invasiveness and (b) toxigenicity.
8. Define the term *facultative intracellular parasite*.

7-8 FUNGI

Questions

1. Differentiate between molds and yeasts.
2. List an example of (a) a mold and (b) a yeast.
3. Describe the meaning of *fungal dimorphism*.
4. Name two fungi that are dimorphic.
5. Name the fungi that most often cause disease of the respiratory tract.
6. Why are antibacterial drugs that are directed against procaryotic cells not effective against fungi?
7. Why is penicillin ineffective in treating fungal infections?

7-9 VIRUSES

Questions

1. Why are viruses considered to be "infectious" rather than "living" or "nonliving"?
2. Name the main ultrastructural components of a typical virion.
3. Describe the cycle involved in viral reproduction.
4. List the six steps of viral reproduction.
5. List three viral vaccines that are used to treat viral infections.

7-10 INFECTION CONTROL

Questions

1. In what year was the first case of acquired immunodeficiency syndrome (AIDS) reported?
2. Name the virus responsible for AIDS.
3. Describe the association between contact with body fluids and HIV infection.
4. What is meant by the procedures called *universal precautions*?
5. List the body fluids that require appropriate barrier protection.
6. How do Blood and Body Substance Isolation (BSI) procedures differ from universal precautions?

Bibliography

Barnes, T. *Core Textbook of Respiratory Care Practice.* 2nd ed. St. Louis: Mosby-Year Book, Inc., 1993.

Branson, R. *Respiratory Care Equipment.* 2nd ed., Philadelphia: J.B. Lippincott Company, 1999.

Burton, G., et al. *Respiratory Care: A Guide to Clinical Practice.* 4th ed. Philadelphia: J.B. Lippincott Company, 1997.

Dantzker, D., et al. *Comprehensive Respiratory Care.* Philadelphia: W.B. Saunders Company, 1995.

Federal Register Part II. 1991. *Occupational Exposure to Bloodborne Pathogens*: pp. 64175–64182.

Gerberding, J.L. "Reducing Occupational Risk of HIV Infection." *Hospital Practice* (1991) 26: 103–118.

Scanlan, C., et al. *Egan's Fundamentals of Respiratory Care.* 7th ed. St. Louis: Mosby-Year Book, Inc., 1999.

Stine, G.J. *AIDS Update.* Englewood Cliffs: Prentice Hall, 1995.

Tortora, G.J., Funke, B.R., and Case, C.L. *Microbiology.* 5th ed. New York: Benjamin/Cummings Publishing Company, 1995.

APPENDIX A

SOLUTIONS AND ANSWERS TO PRACTICE PROBLEMS

CHAPTER 1 - MATHEMATICS

1-1 SCIENTIFIC NOTATION AND EXPONENTS

1. $893 \times 10^{-3} = 8.93. \times 10^{-1} = 8.93 \times 10^{-1}$
2. $67.4 \times 10^9 = 6.74 \times 10^{10} = 6.74 \times 10^{10}$
3. $8,562 \times 10^{10} = 8.562. \times 10^{13} = 8.56 \times 10^{13}$
4. $0.0000732 \times 10^8 = 0.00007.32 \times 10^3 = 7.32 \times 10^3$
5. $4,930,000 \times 10^{-7} = 4.930000. \times 10^{-1} = 4.93 \times 10^{-1}$
6. $54,691 \times 10^{-2} = 5.4691. \times 10^2 = 5.47 \times 10^2$
7. 7.03×10^2 (Correct as shown.)
8. $0.000509 \times 10^{-9} = 0.0005.09 \times 10^{-13} = 5.09 \times 10^{-13}$
9. $96.2 \times 10^{-6} = 9.62 \times 10^{-5} = 9.62 \times 10^{-5}$
10. $321.0 \times 10^{-4} = 3.21.0 \times 10^{-2} = 3.21 \times 10^{-2}$
11. *STEP 1:* $\dfrac{9.42}{8.62} = 1.09$

    STEP 2: $\dfrac{10^{-3}}{10^9} = 10^{-3-9} = 10^{-12}$

    STEP 3: 1.09×10^{-12}
12. *STEP 1:* $\dfrac{6.40}{9.81} = 0.652 = 6.52 \times 10^{-1}$

    STEP 2: $\dfrac{10^6}{10^5} = 10^{6-5} = 10^1$

    STEP 3: $6.52 \times 10^{-1} \times 10^1 = 6.52$
13. $14,100.00 \times 10^5$
    $$\underline{- \quad\quad 5.61 \times 10^5}$$
    $14,094.39 \times 10^5$
    $14,094.39 \times 10^5 = 1.41 \times 10^9$

14. *STEP 1:* $\dfrac{8.41}{7.28} = 1.16$

   STEP 2: $\dfrac{10^{-6}}{10^{-7}} = 10^{-6-(-7)} = 10^1$

   STEP 3: 1.16×10^1

15. 7.41×10^{-11}
   $+ 365. \quad \times 10^{-11}$
   $\overline{372.41 \times 10^{-11}} = 3.72 \times 10^{-9}$

   Alternatively,

   0.0741×10^{-9}
   $+ 3.65 \quad \times 10^{-9}$
   $\overline{3.7241 \times 10^{-9}} = 3.72 \times 10^{-9}$

16. $81,500. \quad \times 10^{-10}$
   $- \quad 9.21 \times 10^{-10}$
   $\overline{81,490.79 \times 10^{-10}} = 8.15 \times 10^{-6}$

17. *STEP 1:* $2.40 \times 6.67 = 16.01 = 1.60 \times 10^1$
   STEP 2: $10^{-20} \times 10^{13} = 10^{-20+13} = 10^{-7}$
   STEP 3: $1.60 \times 10^1 \times 10^{-7} = 1.60 \times 10^{-6}$

18. *STEP 1:* $5.89 \times 2.22 = 13.08 = 1.31 \times 10^1$
   STEP 2: $10^{-14} \times 10^{-7} = 10^{-14+(-7)} \times 10^{-21}$
   STEP 3: $1.31 \times 10^1 \times 10^{-21} = 1.31 \times 10^{-20}$

19. *STEP 1:* $\dfrac{3.59}{3.59} = 1.00$

   STEP 2: $\dfrac{10^{-8}}{10^{-9}} = 10^{-8-(-9)} = 10^1$

   STEP 3: 1.00×10^1

20. 0.0111×10^{12}
   $+ 3.12 \quad \times 10^{12}$
   $\overline{3.1311 \times 10^{12}} = 3.13 \times 10^{12}$

   Alternatively,

   1.11×10^{10}
   $+ 312. \quad \times 10^{10}$
   $\overline{313.11 \times 10^{10}} = 3.13 \times 10^{12}$

1-2 SIGNIFICANT DIGITS

21. 2 significant digits
22. 1 significant digit
23. 5 significant digits

24. 3 significant digits
25. 7 significant digits
26. 4 significant digits
27. 3.22 m
  + 3.414 m
  _____
  6.634 m (Round answer to nearest 100th of a meter.)

   Answer: 6.63 m

28. $\dfrac{90.0\ \text{L/min}}{45.000\ \text{L/min}} = 2.0$

29. $\dfrac{63.21\ \text{L}}{10.000\ \text{min}} = 6.32\ \text{L/min}$

30. 10.0 mg
  − 0.00961 mg
  _____
  9.99039 mg (Round answer to nearest 10th of a milligram.)

   Answer: 10.0 mg

31. 3.140 cm
  × 30.6 cm
  _____
  96.084 cm² (Round answer to nearest 10th of a cm².)

   Answer: 96.1 cm²

32.   16.219 kPa
  + 101.33 kPa
  _____
  117.549 kPa (Round answer to nearest 100th of a kPa.)

   Answer: 117.55 kPa

33.   0.9900 ml
  × 0.01   ml
  _____
  0.0099 ml² (Round answer to nearest 10th of a milliliter.)

   Answer: 0.01 ml

34. 12.01 m
  − 7.234 m
  _____
  4.776 m (Round answer to nearest 100th of a meter.)

   Answer: 4.78 m

35.   2.32 cm
  × 20.1   cm
  _____
  46.632 cm² (Round answer to nearest 10th of a cm².)

   Answer: 46.6 cm²

1-3 RATIOS

36. $\dfrac{10\ \text{liters/min airflow}}{10\ \text{liters/min O}_2\ \text{flow}} = \dfrac{1\ \text{air}}{1\ \text{O}_2} = 1:1$

37. $\dfrac{43 \text{ liters/min airflow}}{6 \text{ liters/min O}_2 \text{ flow}} = \dfrac{7 \text{ air}}{1 \text{ O}_2} = 7{:}1$

38. $\dfrac{32 \text{ liters/min total flow}}{8 \text{ liters/min O}_2 \text{ flow}} = \dfrac{4 \text{ total}}{1 \text{ O}_2} = 4{:}1$

39. **For O$_2$ concentrations 35% or greater:**

$\dfrac{\text{air}}{\text{O}_2} = \dfrac{100 - \text{desired O}_2\%}{\text{desired O}_2\% - 20}$

$= \dfrac{100 - 40}{40 - 20}$

$= \dfrac{60}{20}$

$= 3{:}1$

40. $\dfrac{\text{air}}{\text{O}_2} = \dfrac{100 - 100}{100 - 20}$

$= \dfrac{0}{80}$

41. **For O$_2$ concentrations less than 35%:**

$\dfrac{\text{air}}{\text{O}_2} = \dfrac{100 - \text{desired O}_2\%}{\text{desired O}_2\% - 21}$

$= \dfrac{100 - 21}{21 - 21}$

$= \dfrac{79}{0}$

42. $\dfrac{\text{air}}{\text{O}_2} = \dfrac{100 - 29}{29 - 21}$

$= \dfrac{71}{8}$

$= 8.9{:}1$

43. $\dfrac{\text{air}}{\text{O}_2} = \dfrac{100 - 50}{50 - 20}$

$= \dfrac{50}{30}$

$= 1.7{:}1$

44. $\dfrac{3 \text{ sec T}_I}{1.5 \text{ sec T}_E} = \dfrac{2 \text{ T}_I}{1 \text{ T}_E} = 2{:}1$

45. $\dfrac{4.5 \text{ lpm } \dot{V}_A}{5.6 \text{ lpm } \dot{Q}_C} = \dfrac{0.8 \, \dot{V}_A}{1.0 \, \dot{Q}_C} = 0.8{:}1$

46. $\dfrac{225 \text{ ml/min } \dot{V}O_2}{281 \text{ ml/min } \dot{V}CO_2} = \dfrac{0.8 \ \dot{V}O_2}{1.0 \ \dot{V}CO_2} = 0.8{:}1$

47. $\dfrac{1.75 \text{ sec } T_I}{3.50 \text{ sec } T_E} = \dfrac{0.5 \ T_I}{1.0 \ T_E} = 0.5{:}1$

48. 80 cm H_2O and 10 liters/sec cannot be expressed as a true ratio because the units of the two values are not the same.

49. $\dfrac{V_D}{V_T} = \dfrac{PaCO_2 - P\overline{E}CO_2}{PaCO_2} = \dfrac{35 \text{ torr} - 30 \text{ torr}}{35 \text{ torr}} = \dfrac{1}{7} = 1{:}7$

    The V_D/V_T ratio is usually expressed as a decimal; therefore,

    $\dfrac{V_D}{V_T} = \dfrac{1}{7} = 0.14$

50. $\dfrac{V_D}{V_T} = \dfrac{PaCO_2 - P\overline{E}CO_2}{PaCO_2}$

    Because V_D is estimated as 1 cc/lb of ideal body weight (79.5 kg $\times$ 2.2 lb/kg = 175 lbs), 175 cc is inserted in the numerator.

    $$\dfrac{175 \text{ cc}}{565 \text{ cc}} = \dfrac{33 \text{ torr} - P\overline{E}CO_2}{33 \text{ torr}}$$

    $$(0.31)(33 \text{ torr}) = 33 \text{ torr} - P\overline{E}CO_2$$

    $$P\overline{E}CO_2 = 33 \text{ torr} - 10 \text{ torr} = 23 \text{ torr}$$

    or

    $$175 \text{ cc } (33 \text{ torr}) = 565 \text{ cc } (33 \text{ torr}) - 565 \text{ cc } (x)$$

    $$565 \text{ cc } (x) = 18{,}645 \text{ cc·torr} + 5{,}775 \text{ cc·torr}$$

    $$x = \dfrac{24{,}420 \ \cancel{\text{cc}} \cdot \text{torr}}{565 \ \cancel{\text{cc}}} = 23 \text{ torr}$$

51. Before a ratio can be set up with these two factors, one factor must be converted to liters/sec because liters/sec and liters/min cannot be placed in the same ratio, as the units are not the same.

    STEP 1: Convert 80 liters/sec to liters/min

    $$(80 \text{ liters/sec})(60 \text{ sec/min}) = 4{,}800 \text{ liters/min}$$

    STEP 2: Set up the ratio.

    $$\dfrac{4{,}800 \text{ liters/min airflow}}{240 \text{ liters/min } O_2 \text{ flow}} = \dfrac{20}{1} = 20{:}1$$

Alternatively,

STEP 1:   Convert 240 liters/min to liters/sec.

$$\frac{240 \text{ liters/min}}{60 \text{ sec/min}} = 4 \text{ liters/sec}$$

STEP 2:   Set up the ratio.

$$\frac{80 \text{ liters/sec airflow}}{4 \text{ liters/sec O}_2 \text{ flow}} = \frac{20}{1} = 20{:}1$$

52. *STEP 1:* $\dfrac{1{,}034 \text{ cm H}_2\text{O}}{760 \text{ mm Hg}} = 1.36 \text{ cm H}_2\text{O/mm Hg}$

    STEP 2: $\dfrac{1{,}034 \text{ cm H}_2\text{O}}{1.36 \text{ cm H}_2\text{O/mm Hg}} = 760 \text{ mm Hg}$

    STEP 3: $\dfrac{760 \text{ mm Hg}}{760 \text{ mm Hg}} = \dfrac{1}{1} = 1{:}1$

53. $\dfrac{1.8 \text{ sec } T_I}{0.6 \text{ sec } T_E} = \dfrac{3 \ T_I}{1 \ T_E} = 3{:}1$

54. $\dfrac{1.28 \text{ sec } T_I}{3.84 \text{ sec } T_E} = \dfrac{1 \ T_I}{3 \ T_E} = 1{:}3,$ or $\dfrac{0.3 \ T_I}{1 \ T_E} = 0.3{:}1$

55. Use the "Magic Box."

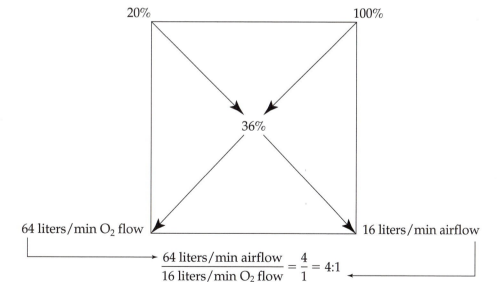

56. Use the "Magic Box."

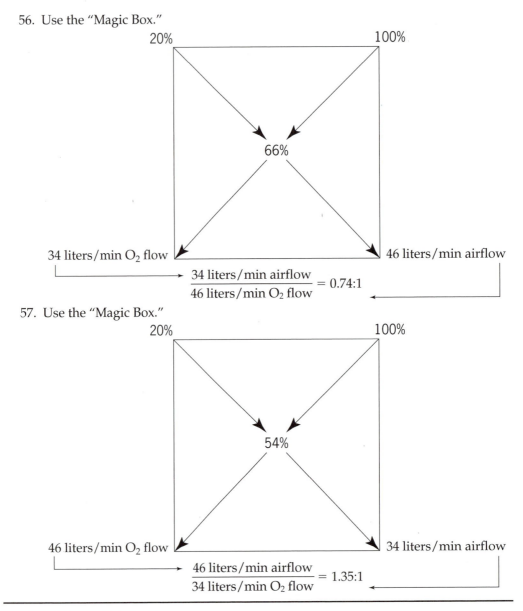

20%   100%

66%

34 liters/min O_2 flow   46 liters/min airflow

$$\frac{34 \text{ liters/min airflow}}{46 \text{ liters/min } O_2 \text{ flow}} = 0.74{:}1$$

57. Use the "Magic Box."

20%   100%

54%

46 liters/min O_2 flow   34 liters/min airflow

$$\frac{46 \text{ liters/min airflow}}{34 \text{ liters/min } O_2 \text{ flow}} = 1.35{:}1$$

1-4 PROPORTIONS

58. 10% W/V Mucomyst = 10 g/100 cc
                     = 10,000 mg/100 cc
                     = 100 mg/cc

$$\frac{4 \text{ cc}}{1 \text{ cc}} = \frac{X}{100 \text{ mg}}$$

$$400 \text{ mg} = X$$

59. 20% W/V Mucomyst = 20 g/100 ml
$$= 20{,}000 \text{ mg}/100 \text{ ml}$$
$$= 200 \text{ mg}/\text{ml}$$

10% W/V Mucomyst = 10 g/100 ml
$$= 10{,}000 \text{ mg}/100 \text{ ml}$$
$$= 100 \text{ mg}/\text{ml}$$

A 20% W/V Mucomyst solution is twice as concentrated as a 10% W/V Mucomyst solution. Therefore, half the volume of the ordered volume of the 10% W/V Mucomyst solution should be given.

$$\frac{2.5 \text{ ml of } 10\% \text{ W/V Mucomyst}}{2} = 1.25 \text{ ml of } 20\% \text{ W/V Mucomyst}$$

60. $$\frac{100 \text{ mg}}{50 \text{ mg}} = \frac{1 \text{ ml}}{X}$$
$$100\,X = 50 \text{ ml}$$
$$X = \frac{50 \text{ ml}}{100} = 0.5 \text{ ml}$$

61. $$\frac{10 \text{ cc}}{X} = \frac{70\%}{40\%}$$
$$400 \text{ cc} = 70\,X$$
$$X = \frac{400 \text{ cc}}{70} = 5.71 \text{ cc}$$

62. $$\frac{6\%}{10\%} = \frac{X}{30 \text{ cc}}$$
$$180 \text{ cc} = 10\,X$$
$$X = \frac{180 \text{ cc}}{10} = 18.0 \text{ cc}$$

63. 20% W/V Mucomyst = 20 g/100 ml
$$= 20{,}000 \text{ mg}/100 \text{ ml}$$
$$= 200 \text{ mg}/\text{ml}$$
$$\frac{200 \text{ mg}}{5 \text{ mg}} = \frac{1 \text{ ml}}{X}$$
$$200\,X = 5 \text{ ml}$$
$$X = \frac{5 \text{ ml}}{200} = 0.025 \text{ ml}$$

64. A $PaCO_2$ of 25 torr signifies hyperventilation. Either the f or V_T needs to be decreased. The patient weighs 180 lbs or 81.8 kg (180 lb ÷ 2.2 lbs/kg). He is receiving a V_T of 11 cc/kg (900 cc ÷ 81.8 kg). Therefore, the V_T is low enough. The f needs to be decreased.

$$\text{desired f} = \frac{(25 \text{ torr})(16 \text{ bpm})}{40 \text{ torr}}$$

$$= \frac{400 \text{ bpm}}{40}$$

$$= 10 \text{ breaths/min}$$

65. A $PaCO_2$ of 30 torr signifies a slight degree of hyperventilation. Either the f or V_T needs to be decreased. The patient weighs 145 lbs, or 65.9 kg (145 lbs ÷ 2.2 lbs/kg). He is receiving a V_T of 15.1 cc/kg (1,000 cc ÷ 65.9 kg). Therefore, the V_T can be lowered because it is too high for the 7–10 cc/kg of IBW tidal volume guideline for COPD patients.

$$\text{desired } V_T = \frac{(30 \text{ torr})(1,000 \text{ cc})}{50 \text{ torr}}$$

$$= 600 \text{ cc}$$

66. A $PaCO_2$ of 60 torr indicates hypoventilation. Either the f or V_T needs to be increased. The patient weighs 80 kg and is receiving 7.5 cc/kg (600 cc ÷ 80 kg) IBW. The V_T may be the setting of choice to change if the patient does not have COPD, status asthmaticus, or ARDS, for which the V_T guideline of 7–10 cc/kg IBW is often used.

$$\text{desired } V_T = \frac{(60 \text{ torr})(600 \text{ cc})}{40 \text{ torr}}$$

$$= 900 \text{ cc}$$

67. A $PaCO_2$ of 50 mm Hg reflects hypoventilation. Either the f or V_T needs to be increased. The patient weighs 165 lbs, or 75 kg (165 pounds ÷ 2.2 lbs/kg) and is receiving a V_T of 12 cc/kg, which is at a reasonable level. The f appears rather low at 8 bpm.

$$\text{desired } f = \frac{(50 \text{ mm Hg})(8 \text{ breaths/min})}{30 \text{ mm Hg}}$$

$$= 13 \text{ breaths/min}$$

1-5 PERCENTS

68. The box contains 100 squares, 21 of which are shaded. Therefore, the shaded squares represent

$$\frac{21}{100} \times 100 = 21\%$$

of the total box. The percent of unshaded squares can be obtained as follows:

$$\begin{array}{l} 100\% \text{ squares} \\ \underline{- 21\% \text{ shaded squares}} \\ 79\% \text{ unshaded squares} \end{array} \qquad \text{or} \qquad \frac{79}{100} \times 100 = 79\%$$

69. $T_I = T_{I\%} \times TCT$

$$= \left(\frac{30}{100}\right)(4 \text{ sec})$$

$$= 1.2 \text{ sec}$$

70. $TCT = \dfrac{T_I}{T_{I\%}} = \dfrac{3 \text{ sec}}{60/100} = \dfrac{3 \text{ sec}}{0.6} = 5.0 \text{ sec}$

71. To achieve saturation implies attaining 100% relative humidity. To achieve 100% saturation at 37°C, air has to contain 43.8 mg of H_2O/L.

   STEP 1:
   $$\begin{array}{r} 43.8 \ \text{mg/L} \\ \times\ 0.75 \\ \hline 32.85 \ \text{mg/L} \ (H_2O \ \text{in air at 75\% RH}) \end{array}$$

   STEP 2:
   $$\begin{array}{r} 43.8 \ \text{mg/L} \ (H_2O \ \text{in air at 100\% RH at 37°C}) \\ -\ 32.85 \ \text{mg/L} \ (H_2O \ \text{in air at 75\% RH}) \\ \hline 10.95 \ \text{mg/L} \ (H_2O \ \text{added to achieve 100\% RH}) \end{array}$$

72. For 1:100 W/V isoproterenol solution,

   $$\frac{1 \ g}{100 \ ml} \times 100 = 1.0\% \ \text{solution (Not a true percent.)}$$

73. *STEP 1:* Calculate the P_AO_2 using the alveolar air equation.

   $$P_AO_2 = F_IO_2 (P_B - P_{H_2O}) - P_ACO_2\left(F_IO_2 + \frac{1 - F_IO_2}{R}\right)$$

   $$= 0.6(760 \ \text{torr} - 47 \ \text{torr}) - 44 \ \text{torr}\left(1 + \frac{1 - 0.6}{0.8}\right)$$

   $$= 0.6(760 \ \text{torr} - 47 \ \text{torr}) - 44 \ \text{torr}(1.5)$$

   $$= 0.6(713 \ \text{torr}) - 66 \ \text{torr}$$

   $$= 362 \ \text{torr}$$

   STEP 2: Calculate the CaO_2.

   $$CaO_2 = ([Hb] \times 1.34 \ ml \ O_2/gHb \times SaO_2) + PaO_2 (0.003 \ \text{vol \%/torr})$$

   $$= (15 \ g\% \times 1.34 \ ml \ O_2/gHb \times \frac{85}{100}) + 70 \ \text{torr} \ (0.003 \ \text{vol \%/to}$$

   $$= 17.1 \ \text{vol\%} + 0.21 \ \text{vol\%}$$

   $$= 17.3 \ \text{vol\%}$$

   STEP 3: Calculate the $C\bar{v}O_2$.

   $$C\bar{v}O_2 = ([Hb] \times 1.34 \ ml \ O_2/gHb \times S\bar{v}O_2) + P\bar{v}O_2 (0.003 \ \text{vol \%/tc}$$

   $$= (15 \ g\% \times 1.34 \ ml \ O_2/gHb \times \frac{60}{100}) + 50 \ \text{torr} \ (0.003 \ \text{vol \%/}$$

   $$= 12.1 \ \text{vol\%} + 0.15 \ \text{vol\%}$$

   $$= 12.3 \ \text{vol\%}$$

   STEP 4: Calculate the $C\acute{c}O_2$.

   $$C\acute{c}O_2 = ([Hb] \times 1.34 \ ml \ O_2/gHb \times 100\%) + P_AO_2 (0.003 \ \text{vol \%/tor}$$

   $$= (15 \ g\% \times 1.34 \ ml \ O_2/gHb \times \frac{100}{100}) + 362 \ \text{torr} \ (0.003 \ \text{vol \%}$$

   $$= 20.1 \ \text{vol\%} + 1.09 \ \text{vol\%}$$

   $$= 21.2 \ \text{vol\%}$$

STEP 5: Insert the calculated values into the shunt equation.

$$\frac{\dot{Q}_S}{\dot{Q}_T} = \frac{C\acute{c}O_2 - CaO_2}{C\acute{c}O_2 - C\bar{v}O_2}$$

$$= \frac{21.2 \text{ vol}\% - 17.3 \text{ vol}\%}{21.2 \text{ vol}\% - 12.2 \text{ vol}\%} \times 100$$

$$= \frac{3.9 \text{ vol}\%}{9.0 \text{ vol}\%} \times 100$$

$$= 43\%$$

74. $\dfrac{\dot{Q}_s}{\dot{Q}_T} = \dfrac{[P(A - a)O_2]0.003}{[P(A - a)O_2]0.003 + (CaO_2 - C\bar{v}O_2)}$

STEP 1: $P_{A}O_2 = F_{IO_2}(P_B - P_{H_2O}) - P_{A}CO_2\left(F_{IO_2} + \dfrac{1 - F_{IO_2}}{R}\right)$

$$= 1.0(760 \text{ torr} - 47 \text{ torr}) - 60 \text{ torr}\left(1.0 + \frac{1 - 1.0}{0.8}\right)$$

$$= 713 \text{ torr} - 60 \text{ torr}$$

$$= 653 \text{ torr}$$

STEP 2: $\dfrac{\dot{Q}_s}{\dot{Q}_T} = \dfrac{(653 \text{ torr} - 515 \text{ torr})0.003}{(653 \text{ torr} - 515 \text{ torr})0.003 + (3.5 \text{ vol}\%)}$

$$= \frac{0.414 \text{ vol}\%}{0.414 \text{ vol}\% + 3.5 \text{ vol}\%}$$

$$= \frac{0.414 \text{ vol}\%}{3.914 \text{ vol}\%} \times 100$$

$$= 10.58\%$$

75. $1{:}1{,}000 = \dfrac{1}{1{,}000} = 0.001(100) = 0.1\%$

76. $\text{actual FEV}_{1\%} = \dfrac{\text{actual FEV}_1}{\text{actual FVC}} \times 100$

$$= \frac{5.19 \text{ L}}{6.38 \text{ L}} \times 100$$

$$= 81.3\%$$

$\text{actual FEV}_{3\%} = \dfrac{\text{actual FEV}_3}{\text{actual FVC}}$

$$= \frac{6.35 \text{ L}}{6.38 \text{ L}} \times 100$$

$$= 99.5\%$$

77. $\text{oxygen content} = [Hb] \times 1.34 \text{ ml } O_2/\text{g Hb} \times S_{O_2}$

$$= (18 \text{ g}\%)(1.34 \text{ ml } O_2/\text{g Hb})\left(\frac{65}{100}\right)$$

$$= 15.68 \text{ vol}\%, \text{ or } 15.68 \text{ ml } O_2/100 \text{ ml plasma}$$

78. $S_{O_2} = \dfrac{\text{oxygen content}}{([\text{Hb}] \times 1.34 \text{ ml } O_2/\text{g Hb})}$

    $= \dfrac{17.5 \text{ ml } O_2/100 \text{ ml plasma}}{(16 \text{ g}/100 \text{ ml bld})(1.34 \text{ ml } O_2/\text{g Hb})} \times 100$

    $= 81.62 \text{ vol}\%$

79. *STEP 1:* $\;CaO_2 = (13 \text{ g}\% \times 1.34 \times 100\%) + (514 \text{ torr} \times 0.003 \text{ vol}\%/\text{torr})$

    $= 17.42 \text{ vol}\% + 1.54 \text{ vol}\%$

    $= 18.96 \text{ vol}\%$

    STEP 2: $\;C\bar{v}O_2 = (13 \text{ g}\% \times 1.34 \times 92\%) + (80 \text{ torr} \times 0.003 \text{ vol}\%/\text{torr})$

    $= 16.03 \text{ vol}\% + 0.24 \text{ vol}\%$

    $= 16.27 \text{ vol}\%$

    STEP 3: $\;P_AO_2 = F_IO_2(P_B - P_{H_2O}) - PaCO_2\left(F_IO_2 + \dfrac{1 - F_IO_2}{R}\right)$

    $= 1.0(760 \text{ torr} - 47 \text{ torr}) - 55 \text{ torr}\left(1.0 + \dfrac{1 - 1.0}{0.08}\right)$

    $= 713 \text{ torr} - 55 \text{ torr}$

    $= 658 \text{ torr}$

    $\dfrac{\dot{Q}_s}{\dot{Q}_T} = \dfrac{[P(A - a)O_2]0.003 \text{ vol}\%/\text{torr}}{[P(A - a)O_2]0.003 \text{ vol}\%/\text{torr} + (CaO_2 - C\bar{v}O_2)} \times 100$

    $\dfrac{\dot{Q}_s}{\dot{Q}_T} = \dfrac{(658 \text{ torr} - 514 \text{ torr})0.003 \text{ vol}\%/\text{torr}}{(658 \text{ torr} - 514 \text{ torr})0.003 + (18.96 \text{ vol}\% - 16.27 \text{ vol}\%)}$

    $= \dfrac{0.432 \text{ vol}\%}{0.432 \text{ vol}\% + 2.69 \text{ vol}\%} \times 100$

    $= \dfrac{0.432 \text{ vol}\%}{3.122 \text{ vol}\%} \times 100$

    $= 13.84\%$

80. $T_{I\%} = \dfrac{T_I}{TCT} \times 100, \text{ or } \dfrac{T_I}{T_I + T_E} \times 100, \text{ or } T_{I\%} = \dfrac{T_I \text{ part}}{TCT \text{ parts}} \times 100$

    $= \dfrac{1}{2.5 + 1} \times 100 = \dfrac{1}{3.5} \times 100 = 0.2857 \,(100)$

    $= 28.57\%$

81. $T_I = T_{I\%} \times TCT$

    $= \left(\dfrac{33}{100}\right)5 \text{ sec}$

    $= 1.65 \text{ sec}$

82. $TCT = \dfrac{T_I}{T_{I\%}} = \dfrac{1.25 \text{ sec}}{25/100} = \dfrac{1.25 \text{ sec}}{0.25} = 5.00 \text{ sec}$

1-6 DIMENSIONAL ANALYSIS

83. $R_{airway} = \dfrac{1,036 \text{ cm H}_2\text{O} - 1,046 \text{ cm H}_2\text{O}}{5 \text{ L/sec}}$

$= \dfrac{10 \text{ cm H}_2\text{O}}{5 \text{ L/sec}}$

$= 2 \text{ cm H}_2\text{O/L/sec}$

84. $O_2 \text{ specific gravity} = \dfrac{1.43 \text{ g/L}}{1.29 \text{ g/L}}$

$= 1.11$

85. $\text{duration of compressed} \atop \text{gas O}_2 \text{ cylinder flow} = \dfrac{2,200 \text{ psig} \times 2.41 \text{ L/psig}}{10 \text{ L/min}}$

$= \dfrac{5,302}{10 \text{ min}}$

$= 530.2 \text{ min}$

86. $\text{C.O.} = \dfrac{250 \text{ ml O}_2/\text{min}}{\left(\dfrac{19.1 \text{ ml O}_2}{100 \text{ ml blood}}\right) - \left(\dfrac{14.1 \text{ ml O}_2}{100 \text{ ml blood}}\right)}$

$= \dfrac{250 \text{ ml O}_2/\text{min}}{0.191 \text{ ml O}_2/\text{ml blood} - 0.141 \text{ ml O}_2/\text{ml blood}}$

$= \dfrac{250 \text{ ml O}_2/\text{min}}{0.05 \text{ ml O}_2/\text{ml blood}}$

$= 5,000 \text{ ml blood/min}$

87. $\text{time constant} = (0.2 \text{ L/cm H}_2\text{O})(2 \text{ cm H}_2\text{O/L/sec})$

$= 0.4 \text{ second}$

88. $\text{pH} = 6.1 + \log\left[\dfrac{24 \text{ mEq/L}}{(40 \text{ torr})(0.03 \text{ mEq/L/torr})}\right]$

$= 6.1 + \log\left[\dfrac{24 \text{ mEq/L}}{1.2 \text{ mEq/L}}\right]$

$= 6.1 + \log 20$

$= 6.1 + 1.30$

$= 7.40$

89. total arterial O_2 content

$= \left[(15 \text{ g Hb/100 ml blood})(1.34 \text{ ml O}_2/\text{g Hb})\left(\dfrac{95.5}{100}\right) + (100 \text{ torr})(0.003 \text{ vol\%/torr})\right]$

$= (19.20 \text{ ml O}_2/100 \text{ ml blood}) + (0.30 \text{ vol\%})$

$= (19.20 \text{ vol\%}) + (0.30 \text{ vol\%})$

$= 19.50 \text{ vol\%}$

90. $\dfrac{r_{CO_2}}{r_{O_2}} = \dfrac{(\sqrt{1.43\ g/L})(0.510\ ml/ml\ plasma/760\ torr)}{(\sqrt{1.96\ g/L})(0.023\ ml/ml\ plasma/760\ torr)}$

$\qquad = \dfrac{(1.20)(0.510)}{(1.40)(0.023)} = \dfrac{0.612}{0.0322}$

$\qquad = \dfrac{19}{1}$

$\quad r_{CO_2} = 19(r_{O_2})$

91. $\bar{P}_{aw} = \left[\dfrac{30\ breaths/min)(0.45\ sec/breath)}{60\ sec/min}\right][(40\ cm\ H_2O - 10\ cm\ H_2O) + 10\ H_2O]$

$\qquad = \left(\dfrac{13.5}{60}\right)[(40\ cm\ H_2O - 10\ cm\ H_2O) + 10\ cm\ H_2O]$

$\qquad = (0.225)[(30\ cm\ H_2O) + 10\ cm\ H_2O]$

$\qquad = 0.225 \times 40\ cm\ H_2O$

$\qquad = 9\ cm\ H_2O$

92. $CI = \dfrac{5\ L/min}{2.5\ m^2} = 2.0\ L/min/m^2$

1-7 UNITS OF MEASUREMENT

93. $1\ Å \times 10^{-8}\ cm/Å = 10^{-8}\ cm$

94. $416\ cm \times 10^1\ mm/cm = 4{,}160\ mm,$ or $4.16 \times 10^3\ mm$

95. $\dfrac{4.96\ g}{1{,}000\ g/kg} = 0.00496\ kg = 4.96 \times 10^{-3}\ kg$

96. $\dfrac{2 \times 10^{-2}\ nm}{10^7\ nm/cm} = 2 \times 10^{-2} \times 10^{-7} = 2 \times 10^{-9}\ cm$

97. $0.00937\ m \times 10^{10}\ Å/m = 0.0094 \times 10^{10}\ Å$

$\qquad\qquad\qquad\qquad\quad = 9.4 \times 10^7\ Å$

98. $\dfrac{609\ mg}{10^6\ mg/kg} = 609 \times 10^{-6}\ kg = 6.09 \times 10^{-4}\ kg$

99. $\dfrac{8.96 \times 10^3\ ml}{10^3\ ml/L} = 8.96 \times 10^3 \times 10^{-3} = 8.96\ L$

100. $19\ L \times 10^3\ ml/L = 19 \times 10^3 = 1.9 \times 10^4\ ml$

101. $0.219\ kg \times 10^6\ mg/kg = 0.219 \times 10^6 = 2.19 \times 10^5\ mg$

102. $\dfrac{0.000006\ \mu m}{10^9\ \mu m/km} = 0.000006 \times 10^{-9} = 6.0 \times 10^{-15}\ kg$

103. $2.125\ lbs\left(\dfrac{16\ oz}{1\ lb}\right)\left(\dfrac{28.35\ g}{1\ oz}\right)\left(\dfrac{1\ kg}{1{,}000\ g}\right) = \dfrac{963.9\ kg}{1{,}000} = 0.96\ kg$

104. $6.2 \times 10^{-2}\ ft\left(\dfrac{12\ in}{1\ g}\right)\left(\dfrac{2.54\ cm}{1\ in.}\right) = 1.89\ cm$

105. $\dfrac{232 \text{ lbs}}{2.2 \text{ lbs/kg}} = 1.05 \times 10^2 \text{ kg}$

106. $693 \text{ m}\left(\dfrac{3.28 \text{ ft}}{1 \text{ m}}\right) = 2273 \text{ ft, or } 2.273 \times 10^3 \text{ ft}$

107. $4.96 \times 10^6 \text{ g}\left(\dfrac{1 \text{ oz}}{28.35 \text{ g}}\right)\left(\dfrac{1 \text{ lb}}{16 \text{ oz}}\right) = 10{,}934.7 \text{ lbs, or } 1.09 \times 10^4 \text{ lbs}$

108. $10^{39} \text{ kg}\left(\dfrac{1{,}000 \text{ g}}{1 \text{ kg}}\right)\left(\dfrac{1 \text{ oz}}{28.35 \text{ g}}\right) = 3.53 \times 10^{40} \text{ oz}$

109. $\dfrac{150 \text{ lbs}}{2.2 \text{ lbs/kg}} = 68.18 \text{ kg}$

110. $1 \text{ ft}\left(\dfrac{12 \text{ in.}}{1 \text{ ft}}\right)\left(\dfrac{2.54 \text{ cm}}{1 \text{ in.}}\right) = 30.48 \text{ cm}$

111. $84 \text{ lbs}\left(\dfrac{1 \text{ kg}}{2.2 \text{ lbs}}\right)\left(\dfrac{1 \text{ g}}{10^3 \text{ kg}}\right) = 3.82 \times 10^{-2} \text{ g}$

112. $325 \text{ ft}\left(\dfrac{1 \text{ m}}{3.28 \text{ ft}}\right) = 9.91 \times 10^1 \text{ m}$

1-8 LOGARITHMS

113. p = base
     r = log, exponent, or power
     t = number

114. 9 = base
     2 = log, exponent, or power
     81 = number

115. $\log_p t = r$

116. $\log_6 216 = 3$

117. $\log_{10} 1 = 0$

118. 0.00003
     $\underbrace{}$
     $1\ 2\ 3\ 4\ ⑤$
     ↓
     $(10 - n) - 10 = \text{characteristic}$
     $(10 - 5) - 10 =$
     $(5) - 10 = 5 - 10, \text{ or } \bar{5}$

119. 987654.3
     ↑ ↑ ↑ ↑ ↑↑
     $1\ 2\ 3\ 4\ 5\ ⑥$
     ↓
     $(x - 1) = \text{characteristic}$
     $6 - 1 = 5$

120. 8 1 4 2
    ↑ ↑ ↑ ↑
    1 2 3 ④

$(x - 1)$ = characteristic

$4 - 1 = 3$

121. $10^{-10} = 0\ .\ 0\ 0\ 0\ 0\ 0\ 0\ 0\ 0\ 0\ 1\ .$
    1 2 3 4 5 6 7 8 9 ⑩

$(10 - n) - 10$ = characteristic

$(10 - 10) - 10 = 0 - 10$, or $\overline{10}$

122. $0.0009 \times 10^{-5} = 0\ .\ 0\ 0\ 0\ 0\ 0\ 0\ 0\ 9$
    1 2 3 4 5 6 7 8 ⑨

$(10 - n) - 10$ = characteristic

$(10 - 9) - 10 = 1 - 10$, or $\overline{9}$

123. 3 8 5 .264
    ↑ ↑ ↑
    1 2 ③

$(x - 1)$ = characteristic

$3 - 1 = 2$

124. 1 0
    ↑ ↑
    1 ②

$(x - 1)$ = characteristic

$2 - 1 = 1$

125. 0 . 0 9 0 0 0 6
    1 ②

$(10 - n) - 10$ = characteristic

$(10 - 2) - 10 = \overline{2}$

126. $3.06 \times 10^{-8} = 0\ .\ 0\ 0\ 0\ 0\ 0\ 0\ 3\ 0\ 6$
    1 2 3 4 5 6 7 ⑧

$(10 - n) - 10$ = characteristic

$(10 - 8) - 10 = 2 - 10$, or $\overline{8}$

127. 5
    ↑
    ①

$(x - 1)$ = characteristic

$1 - 1 = 0$

128. 6.870

characteristic: $1 - 1 = 0$

mantissa: 8370 for 6870

log: 0.8370

129. 0.000979
     characteristic: 6 − 10, or $\overline{4}$
     mantissa: 9908 for 979
     log: −4.0000 (characteristic)
        +0.9908 (mantissa)
        ‾‾‾‾‾‾‾‾‾‾‾‾‾‾‾‾‾‾‾
        $\overline{3}$.0092 (logarithm)

130. $0.0000347 \times 10^6 = 3.47 \times 10^6 \times 10^{-5} = 3.47 \times 10^1 = 34.7$
     characteristic: 2 − 1 = 1
     mantissa: 5403 for 347
     log: 1.5403

131. $55.4 \times 10^{-4} = 0.00554$
     characteristic: 7 − 10, or $\overline{3}$
     mantissa: 7435 for 554
     log: −3.0000 (characteristic)
        +0.7435 (mantissa)
        ‾‾‾‾‾‾‾‾‾‾‾‾‾‾‾‾‾‾‾
        $\overline{2}$.2565 (logarithm)

132. 175.6
     characteristic: 2
     mantissa: 2445 for 1756
     log: 2.2445

133. 1.00
     characteristic: 0
     mantissa: 0 for 1
     log: 0.0000

134. 20
     characteristic: 1
     mantissa: 3010 for 20
     log: 1.3010

135. 0.0000621
     characteristic: 5 − 10, or $\overline{5}$
     mantissa: 7931 for 621
     log: −5.0000 (characteristic)
        +0.7931 (mantissa)
        ‾‾‾‾‾‾‾‾‾‾‾‾‾‾‾‾‾‾‾
        $\overline{4}$.2069 (logarithm)

136. $9.55 \times 10^{-7} = 0.000000955$
     characteristic: 3 − 10, or $\overline{7}$
     mantissa: 9800 for 955
     log: −7.0000 (characteristic)
        + 0.9800 (mantissa)
        ‾‾‾‾‾‾‾‾‾‾‾‾‾‾‾‾‾‾‾
        $\overline{6}$.0200 (logarithm)

137. $0.00452 \times 10^6 = 4,520$
     characteristic: 3
     mantissa: 6551
     log 3.6551

138. $6.00 - 10^{-11} = 0.00000000006$
    characteristic: $\overline{11}$
    mantissa: 7782 for 6
    log: -11.0000 (characteristic)
    $+\quad.7782$ (mantissa)
    $\overline{10}.2218$ (logarithm)

139. log 1.3010
    STEP 1: sequence of digits corresponding to mantissa 3010 = 200
    STEP 2: $x - 1 =$ characteristic
    $\quad x - 1 = 1$
    $\quad\quad x = 2$ digits in number to left of decimal
    STEP 3: 20.0 (number)

140. log 0.9320
    STEP 1: sequence of digits corresponding to mantissa 9320 = 855
    STEP 2: $x - 1 =$ characteristic
    $\quad x - 1 = 0$
    $\quad\quad x = 1$ digit in number to left of decimal
    STEP 3: 8.55 (number)

141. log $\overline{2}.2765$
    STEP 1: $\quad 10.0000$
    $\quad\quad - 2.2765$
    $\quad\quad\quad 7.7235 - 10$
    STEP 2: sequence of digits corresponding to mantissa 7235 = 529
    STEP 3: $7 - 10 = \overline{3}$ (characteristic)
    STEP 4: 0.00529 (number)

142. log $\overline{4}.5670$
    STEP 1: $\quad 10.0000$
    $\quad\quad - 4.5670$
    $\quad\quad\quad 5.4330 - 10$
    STEP 2: sequence of digits corresponding to mantissa 4330 = 271
    STEP 3: $5 - 10 = \overline{5}$ (characteristic)
    STEP 4: 0.0000271 (number)

143. log 3.0043
    STEP 1: sequence of digits corresponding to mantissa 0043 = 101
    STEP 2: $x - 1 =$ characteristic
    $\quad x - 1 = 3$
    $\quad\quad x = 3 + 1$
    $\quad\quad x = 4$ digits in number to left of decimal
    STEP 3: 1,010.0 (number)

144. log $\overline{8}$.1904

    STEP 1:   10.0000
                 − 8.1904
                  1.8096 − 10

    STEP 2: sequence of digits corresponding to mantissa 8096 = 645

    STEP 3: $1 - 10 = \overline{9}$ (characteristic)

    STEP 4: 0.00000000645 (number)

145. log 8.6693

    STEP 1: sequence of digits corresponding to mantissa 6693 = 467

    STEP 2: $x - 1 =$ characteristic
                 $x - 1 = 8$
                    $x = 8 + 1$
                    $x = 9$ digits in number to left of decimal

    STEP 3: 467,000,000.0 (number)

146. log $\overline{3}$.7305

    STEP 1:   10.00000
                 − 3.7305
                  6.2695 − 10

    STEP 2: sequence of digits corresponding to mantissa 2695 = 186

    STEP 3: $6 - 10 = \overline{4}$ (characteristic)

    STEP 4: 0.000186 (number)

147. log $\overline{1}$.6513

    STEP 1:   10.0000
                 − 1.6513
                  8.3487 − 10

    STEP 2:   3502 high mantissa
                − 3483 low mantissa
                   19 high-low mantissa difference

    STEP 3:   2240 high number
                − 2230 low number
                   10 high-low number difference

    STEP 4:   3487 desired mantissa
                − 3483 low mantissa
                    4 desired-low mantissa difference

    STEP 5: $\dfrac{4}{19} = \dfrac{x}{10}$

             $40 = 19x$

                 $x = \dfrac{40}{19} = 2.1$ (desired-low number difference)

STEP 6:   2230 low number
+   2 desired-low number difference
2232 sequence of digits in desired number

STEP 7: $8 - 10 = \overline{2}$ (characteristic)

STEP 8:   0.02232 (number)

148. $\log \overline{5}.8625$

STEP 1:   10.0000
$- 5.8625$
$4.1375 - 10$

STEP 2:   1399 high mantissa
$- 1367$ low mantissa
32 high-low mantissa difference

STEP 3:   1380 high number
$- 1370$ low number
10 high-low number difference

STEP 4:   1375 desired mantissa
$- 1367$ low mantissa
8 desired-low mantissa difference

STEP 5: $\dfrac{8}{32} = \dfrac{x}{10}$

$80 = 32x$

$x = \dfrac{80}{32} = 2.5$ (desired-low number difference)

STEP 6:   1370 low number
+   2 desired-low number difference
1372 sequence of digits in desired number

STEP 7: $4 - 10 = \overline{6}$ (characteristic)

STEP 8:   0.000001372 (number)

149. $\log 6.2399$

STEP 1:   2405 high mantissa
$- 2380$ low mantissa
25 high-low mantissa difference

STEP 2:   1740 high number
$- 1730$ low number
10 high-low number difference

STEP 3:   2399 desired mantissa
$- 2380$ low mantissa
19 desired-low mantissa difference

STEP 4: $\dfrac{19}{25} = \dfrac{x}{10}$

$190 = 25x$

$x = \dfrac{190}{25} = 7.6$

STEP 5:   1730 low number
$\underline{+\quad 7 \text{ desired-low number difference}}$
1737 sequence of digits in desired number

STEP 6: $x - 1 = 6$
$x = 6 + 1 = 7$ (characteristic)

STEP 7:   1,737,000.0 (number)

150. log 4.4444

STEP 1:   4456 high mantissa
$\underline{-\ 4440 \text{ low mantissa}}$
16 high-low mantissa difference

STEP 2:   2790 high number
$\underline{-\ 2780 \text{ low number}}$
10 high-low number difference

STEP 3:   4444 desired mantissa
$\underline{-\ 4440 \text{ low mantissa}}$
4 desired-low mantissa difference

STEP 4: $\dfrac{4}{16} = \dfrac{x}{10}$

$40 = x16$

$x = \dfrac{40}{16} = 2.5$

STEP 5:   2780 low number
$\underline{+\quad 2 \text{ desired-low number difference}}$
2782 sequence of digits in desired number

STEP 6: $x - 1 = 4$
$x = 4 + 1 = 5$ (characteristic)

STEP 7:   27,820.0 (number)

151. log $(0.5241 \div 0.2142)$
log $0.5241 -$ log 0.2142
$-0.2806 - (-0.6692)$
$-0.2806 + 0.6692 = 0.3886$

152. $\log (20 \div 1)$
    $\log 20 - \log 1$
    $1.3010 - 0 = 1.3010$

153. $\log (34 \div 9)$
    $\log 34 - \log 9$
    $1.5315 - 0.9542 = 0.5773$

154. $\log (25 \times 15)$
    $\log 25 + \log 15$
    $1.3979 + 1.1761 = 2.5740$

155. $\log (1532 \times 777)$
    $\log 1532 + \log 777$
    $3.1853 + 2.8904 = 6.0757$

156. $\log (333 \times 0.456)$
    $\log 333 + \log 0.456$
    $2.5224 + (-0.3410)$
    $2.5224 - 0.3410 = 2.1814$

157. $\log \left(\dfrac{24}{1.2}\right)$
    $\log 24 - \log 1.2$
    $1.3802 - 0.0792 = 1.3010$

158. $\log \left(\dfrac{8496}{451}\right) = \log 8496 - \log 451$
    $3.9292 - 2.6542 = 1.2750$

159. $\log (50 \times 100 \times 10^3)$
    $\log 50 + \log 100 + \log 10^3$
    $1.6990 + 2.0000 + 3.0000 = 6.6990$

160. $\log (10^{-2} \times 10^4 \times 36)$
    $\log 10^{-2} + \log 10^4 + \log 36$
    $-2.0000 + 4.0000 + 1.5563 = 3.5563$

1-9 GRAPHS

161. $PIP - P_{plateau}$ = Pressure generated to overcome airway resistance (P_{Raw})
    $45 \text{ cm } H_2O - 20 \text{ cm } H_2O = 25 \text{ cm } H_2O$

162. $PIP - P_{plateau} = P_{Raw}$
    $35 \text{ cm } H_2O - 25 \text{ cm } H_2O = 10 \text{ cm } H_2O$

163. $PIP - P_{plateau} = P_{Raw}$
    $45 \text{ cm } H_2O - 35 \text{ cm } H_2O = 10 \text{ cm } H_2O$

164. Graph UNF App-1:

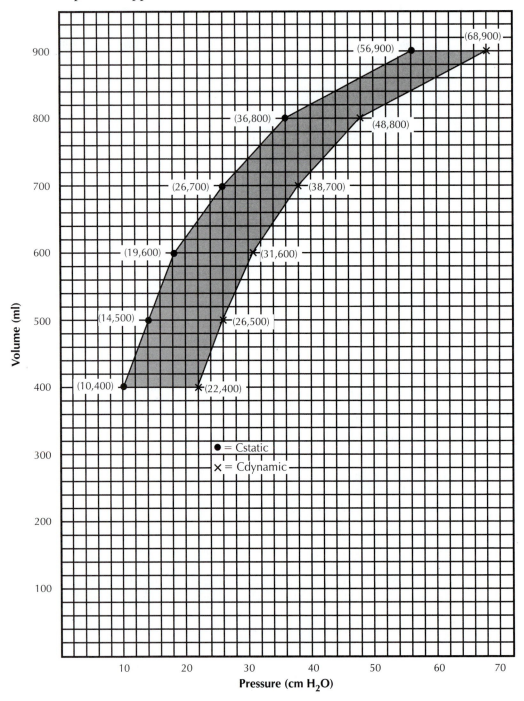

165.

ORDERED PAIR	C_{static}
10, 400	40 ml/cm H_2O
14, 500	36 ml/cm H_2O
19, 600	32 ml/cm H_2O
26, 700	27 ml/cm H_2O
36, 800	22 ml/cm H_2O
56, 900	16 ml/cm H_2O

166.

ORDERED PAIR	$C_{dynamic}$
22, 400	18 ml/cm H_2O
26, 500	19 ml/cm H_2O
31, 600	19 ml/cm H_2O
38, 700	18 ml/cm H_2O
48, 800	17 ml/cm H_2O
68, 900	13 ml/cm H_2O

167.

PIP	–	$P_{plateau}$	=	P_{Raw}
22 cm H_2O		10 cm H_2O		12 cm H_2O
26 cm H_2O		14 cm H_2O		12 cm H_2O
31 cm H_2O		19 cm H_2O		12 cm H_2O
38 cm H_2O		26 cm H_2O		12 cm H_2O
48 cm H_2O		36 cm H_2O		12 cm H_2O
68 cm H_2O		56 cm H_2O		12 cm H_2O

168. Graph UNF App-2:

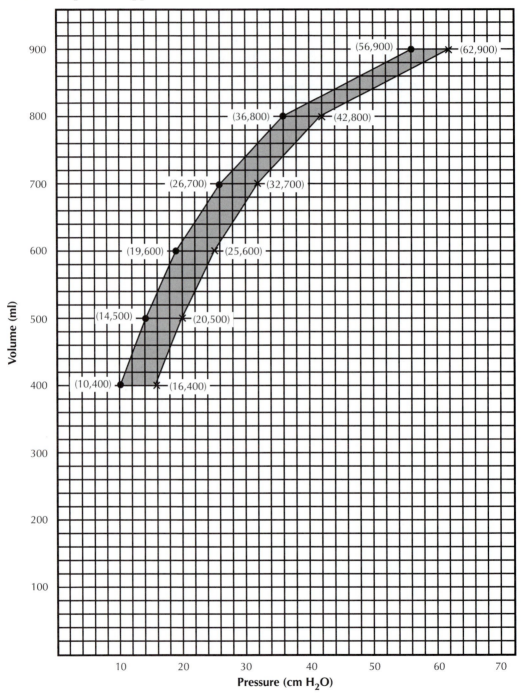

169.

ORDERED PAIR	$C_{dynamic}$
16, 400	25 ml/cm H_2O
20, 500	25 ml/cm H_2O
25, 600	24 ml/cm H_2O
32, 700	22 ml/cm H_2O
42, 800	19 ml/cm H_2O
62, 900	15 ml/cm H_2O

170.

PIP	$-$ $P_{plateau}$	$=$ P_{Raw}
16 cm H_2O	10 cm H_2O	6 cm H_2O
20 cm H_2O	14 cm H_2O	6 cm H_2O
25 cm H_2O	19 cm H_2O	6 cm H_2O
32 cm H_2O	26 cm H_2O	6 cm H_2O
42 cm H_2O	36 cm H_2O	6 cm H_2O
62 cm H_2O	56 cm H_2O	6 cm H_2O

CHAPTER 2 - ALGEBRA

2–1 ALGEBRAIC EXPRESSIONS

1. $6 + x = 6 + 10 = 16$
2. $x + 15 = 10 + 15 = 25$
3. $x + x = 10 + 10 = 20$
4. $\frac{100}{x} = \frac{100}{10} = 10$
5. $x \cdot x = 10 \cdot 10 = 100$
6. $\frac{x}{2} = \frac{10}{2} = 5$
7. $\frac{1}{2}(x) = \frac{1}{2}(10) = 5$
8. $90 - x = 90 - 10 = 80$
9. $x - 5 = 10 - 5 = 5$
10. $0 + x = 0 + 10 = 10$
11. $\frac{xz}{y} = \frac{4 \times 9}{6} = 6$

12. $\dfrac{y}{(x)(z)} = \dfrac{6}{(4)(9)} = \dfrac{1}{6}$

13. $\dfrac{z-3}{y-x} = \dfrac{9-3}{6-4} = \dfrac{6}{2} = 3$

14. $\dfrac{xyz}{8} = \dfrac{4 \times 6 \times 9}{8} = \dfrac{216}{8} = 27$

15. $\dfrac{1}{2}(z+3) = \dfrac{1}{2}(9+3) = \dfrac{12}{2} = 6$

16. $(y+z)\dfrac{1}{3} = (6+9)\dfrac{1}{3} = \dfrac{15}{3} = 5$

17. $7x - y = 7(4) - 6 = 22$

18. $\dfrac{x+y}{10} = \dfrac{4+6}{10} = \dfrac{10}{10} = 1$

19. $2xyz = 2 \times 4 \times 6 \times 9 = 432$

20. $(y+3)\dfrac{1}{3} = (6+9)\dfrac{1}{3} = \dfrac{15}{3} = 5$

21. $\dot{V}_{O_2} = \dot{Q}_T[C(a - \bar{v})O_2]$
    $= (5{,}000 \text{ ml/min})(16.08/100 - 13.5/100)$
    $= (5{,}000 \text{ ml/min})(0.1608 - 0.1350)$
    $= (5{,}000 \text{ ml/min})(0.0258)$
    $= 129 \text{ ml/min}$

22. $\text{time constant} = (R_{aw})(C_L)$
    $(7 \text{ cm } H_2O/L/\text{sec})(0.05 \text{ L/cm } H_2O) = 0.35 \text{ sec}$

23. $E_L = \dfrac{\Delta P}{\Delta V}$

    $= \dfrac{-5 \text{ cm } H_2O - (-9 \text{ cm } H_2O)}{0.8 \text{ L}}$

    $= \dfrac{4 \text{ cm } H_2O}{0.8 \text{ L}}$

    $= 5 \text{ cm } H_2O/L$

24. $C_L = \dfrac{\Delta V}{\Delta P}$

    $= \dfrac{0.8 \text{ L}}{-5 \text{ cm } H_2O - (-9 \text{ cm } H_2O)}$

    $= \dfrac{0.8 \text{ L}}{4 \text{ cm } H_2O}$

    $= 0.2 \text{ L/cm } H_2O$

25. $\dfrac{V_D}{V_T} = \dfrac{PaCO_2 - P\bar{E}CO_2}{PaCO_2}$

$$= \frac{50 \text{ torr} - 35 \text{ torr}}{50 \text{ torr}} = \frac{15 \text{ torr}}{50 \text{ torr}}$$

$$= 0.3$$

26. $P = \dfrac{2ST}{r}$

$$= \frac{2(40 \text{ dynes/cm})}{0.2 \text{ cm}}$$

$$= 400 \text{ dynes/cm}^2$$

27. $T_I = \dfrac{V_T}{\dot{V}_I}$

$$= \frac{0.9 \text{ L}}{1 \text{ L/sec}}$$

$$= 0.9 \text{ second}$$

28. $PSV = \left(\dfrac{PIP - P_{static}}{\dot{V}_{MECH}}\right)\dot{V}_{I_{max}}$

$$= \left(\frac{40 \text{ cm H}_2\text{O} - 25 \text{ cm H}_2\text{O}}{1.5 \text{ L/sec}}\right)0.5 \text{ L/sec}$$

$$= \left(\frac{15 \text{ cm H}_2\text{O}}{1.5 \text{ L/sec}}\right)0.5 \text{ L/sec}$$

$$= (10 \text{ cm H}_2\text{O/L/sec})(0.5 \text{ L/sec})$$

$$= 5 \text{ cm H}_2\text{O}$$

29. $MAP = \dfrac{SP + 2(DP)}{3}$

$$= \frac{120 \text{ mm Hg} + 2(75 \text{ mm Hg})}{3}$$

$$= \frac{270 \text{ mm Hg}}{3} = 90 \text{ mm Hg}$$

30. $G_{aw} = \dfrac{\dot{V}}{PIP - P_{static}}$

$$= \frac{0.5 \text{ L/sec}}{55 \text{ cm H}_2\text{O} - 30 \text{ cm H}_2\text{O}}$$

$$= \frac{0.5 \text{ L/sec}}{25 \text{ cm H}_2\text{O}}$$

$$= 0.02 \text{ L/sec/cm H}_2\text{O}$$

31. $FRC = (TLC - VC) + ERV$

$$FRC = (4{,}000 \text{ ml} - 2{,}500 \text{ ml}) + 800$$

$$FRC = 2{,}300 \text{ ml}$$

32. $VC = (FRC - RV) + IRV + V_T$

    $VC = (2,000 \text{ ml} - 1,000 \text{ ml}) + 2,700 \text{ ml} + 350 \text{ ml}$

    $VC = 4,050 \text{ ml}$

33. $IC = VC - (FRC - RV)$

    $IC = 2,300 \text{ ml} - (1,000 \text{ ml} - 700 \text{ ml})$

    $IC = 2,000 \text{ ml}$

34. $V_T = VC - (ERV + IRV)$

    $V_T = 4,000 \text{ ml} - (1,000 \text{ ml} + 2,700 \text{ ml})$

    $V_T = 300 \text{ ml}$

35. $RV = FRC - [VC - (IRV + V_T)]$

    $\quad = 2,400 \text{ ml} - [4,800 \text{ ml} - (3,100 \text{ ml} + 500 \text{ ml})]$

    $\quad = 2,400 \text{ ml} - [4,800 \text{ ml} - 3,600 \text{ ml}]$

    $\quad = 2,400 \text{ ml} - [1,200 \text{ ml}]$

    $\quad = 1,200 \text{ ml}$

2-2 REAL NUMBERS

36. -10
37. $+5$
38. $+7$
39. $+60$
40. $+19$
41. -10
42. $+64$
43. $+130$
44. -28
45. $+5$
46. -6
47. -2
48. $+4$
49. $+5$
50. -3

2-3 COMPARING NUMBERS

51.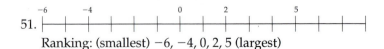

Ranking: (smallest) $-6, -4, 0, 2, 5$ (largest)

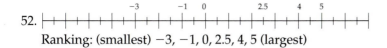

52.

Ranking: (smallest) $-3, -1, 0, 2.5, 4, 5$ (largest)

53.

Ranking: (smallest) $-5, -3.5, -2, 1, 1.5$ (largest)

54.

Ranking: (smallest) $-7, 0, 0.5, 1, 4.5$ (largest)

55.

Ranking: (smallest) $-5.5, -0.5, 2, 3.5, 6.5$ (largest)

56. 8

57. 0.5

58. -4

59. -9

60. -6.5

61. 8.5

62. 2

63. 9

64. 7

65. 0

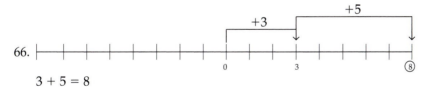

66.

$3 + 5 = 8$

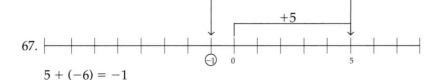

67.

$5 + (-6) = -1$

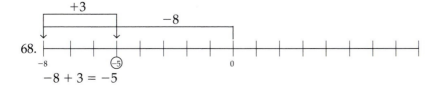

68.

$-8 + 3 = -5$

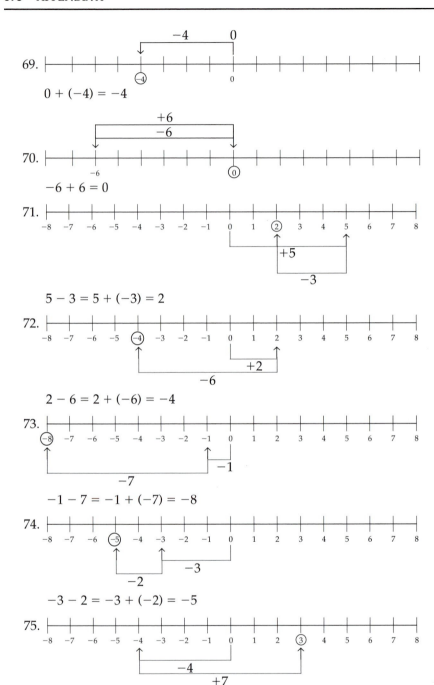

69.

$0 + (-4) = -4$

70.

$-6 + 6 = 0$

71.

$5 - 3 = 5 + (-3) = 2$

72.

$2 - 6 = 2 + (-6) = -4$

73.

$-1 - 7 = -1 + (-7) = -8$

74.

$-3 - 2 = -3 + (-2) = -5$

75.

$-4 - (-7) = -4 + 7 = 3$

76.

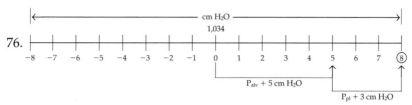

$$P_{trans} = 5 \text{ cm } H_2O - (-3 \text{ cm } H_2O) = 8 \text{ cm } H_2O$$

77.

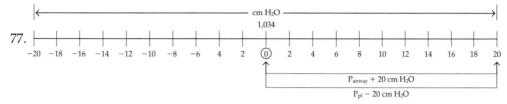

$$P_{transmural} = +20 \text{ cm } H_2O - (+20 \text{ cm } H_2O) = 0 \text{ cm } H_2O$$

78.

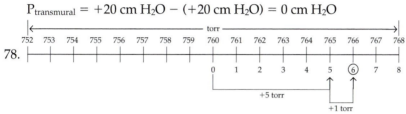

Since 765 torr = 5 torr, then

$$\Delta P = 5 \text{ torr} - (-1 \text{ torr}) = 6 \text{ torr}$$

Alternatively, since -1 torr = 759 torr, then

$$\Delta P = 765 \text{ torr} - 759 \text{ torr} = 6 \text{ torr}$$

79.

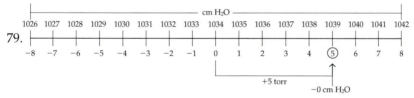

Since 1,034 cm H_2O = 0 cm H_2O, then P_{thorax} = 5 cm H_2O − (0 cm H_2O) = 5 cm H_2O. Alternatively, since 5 cm H_2O = 1,039 cm H_2O, then P_{thorax} = 1,039 cm H_2O − 1,034 cm H_2O = 5 cm H_2O.

80.

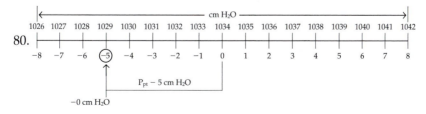

Since 1,034 cm H_2O = 0 cm H_2O, then P_{chest} = −5 cm H_2O − 0 cm H_2O = −5 cm H_2O. Alternatively, since −5 cm H_2O = 1,029 cm H_2O, then P_{chest} = 1,029 cm H_2O − 1,034 cm H_2O = −5 cm H_2O.

2-4 SIMPLIFYING NUMERICAL EXPRESSIONS

81. CaO_2 = [(Hb × 1.34)]SaO_2 + (PaO_2 × 0.003 vol%/torr)

$$= (15 \text{ g}/100 \text{ ml} \times 1.34)\frac{97.5}{100} + (100 \text{ torr} \times 0.003 \text{ vol\%/torr})$$

$$= (20.1 \text{ vol\%})0.975 + 0.3 \text{ vol\%}$$

$$= 19.60 \text{ vol\%} + 0.3 \text{ vol\%} = 19.90 \text{ vol\%}$$

82. $\dot{Q}_T = \dfrac{\dot{V}o_2}{(CaO_2 - C\bar{v}O_2)}$

$$= \frac{250 \text{ ml/min}}{\dfrac{19.1 \text{ ml}}{100 \text{ ml}} - \dfrac{14.1 \text{ ml}}{100 \text{ ml}}} = \frac{250 \text{ ml/min}}{0.191 - 0.141}$$

$$= 5,000 \text{ ml/min}$$

83. $\dfrac{\dot{Q}_s}{\dot{Q}_T} = \dfrac{[P(A - a)O_2]0.003 \text{ vol\%/torr}}{[P(A - a)O_2]0.003 \text{ vol\%/torr} + (CaO_2 - C\bar{v}O_2)}$

$$= \frac{(450 \text{ torr} - 250 \text{ torr})0.003 \text{ vol\%/torr}}{(450 \text{ torr} - 250 \text{ torr})0.003 + (19.85 \text{ vol\%} - 13.95 \text{ vol\%})}$$

$$= \frac{(200 \text{ torr})(0.003 \text{ vol\%/torr})}{(200 \text{ torr})(0.003 \text{ vol\%/torr}) + (5.9 \text{ vol\%})}$$

$$= \frac{0.6 \text{ vol\%}}{0.6 \text{ vol\%} + 5.9 \text{ vol\%}} = \frac{0.6 \text{ vol\%}}{6.5 \text{ vol\%}}$$

$$= 0.092, \text{ or } 0.092 \times 100 = 9.2\%$$

84. (female) IBW = 105 + [5(ht inches − 60)]

$$= 105 + [5(65 \text{ inches} - 60)]$$

$$= 105 + 25 = 130 \text{ lbs}$$

85. $pH = 6.10 + \log\left[\dfrac{HCO_3^-}{(PaCO_2)(0.03)}\right]$

$$= 6.10 + \log\left[\frac{48 \text{ mEq/L}}{(80 \text{ torr})(0.03 \text{ mEq/L/torr})}\right]$$

$$= 6.10 + \log\left(\frac{48}{2.4}\right)$$

$$= 6.10 + \log 20$$

$$= 6.10 + 1.30$$

$$= 7.40$$

2–5 COMBINING LIKE TERMS

86.
$$V_1P_1 = V_2P_2$$
$$(500 \text{ cc})(760 \text{ torr}) = (V_2)(1{,}900)$$
$$V_2 = \frac{380{,}000 \text{ cc-torr}}{1{,}900 \text{ torr}} = 200 \text{ cc}$$

87.
$$C_{static} = \frac{(V_T - V_{lost})}{[P_{plateau} - (PEEP_{applied} + PEEP_{auto})]}$$
$$[P_{plateau} - (PEEP_{applied} + PEEP_{auto})] = \frac{(V_T - V_{lost})}{C_{static}}$$
$$P_{plateau} = X$$
$$X - (10 \text{ cm H}_2O + 7 \text{ cm H}_2O) = \frac{900 \text{ cc} - 100 \text{ cc}}{100 \text{ cc/cm H}_2O}$$
$$X - 17 \text{ cm H}_2O = \frac{800 \text{ cc}}{100 \text{ cc/cm H}_2O}$$
$$X - 17 \text{ cm H}_2O = 8 \text{ cm H}_2O$$
$$X = 25 \text{ cm H}_2O$$
$$P_{plateau} = 25 \text{ cm H}_2O$$

88.
$$\dot{Q}_T = \frac{\dot{V}O_2}{(CaO_2 - C\bar{v}O_2)}$$
$$CaO_2 - C\bar{v}O_2 = \frac{\dot{V}O_2}{\dot{Q}_T}$$
$$C\bar{v}O_2 = X$$
$$\left(\frac{18.50 \text{ ml O}_2}{100}\right) - X = \frac{300 \text{ ml/min}}{6{,}000 \text{ ml/min}}$$
$$0.185 \text{ ml O}_2/\text{ml blood} - X = 0.05$$
$$0.185 \text{ ml O}_2 - 0.05 = X$$
$$X = 0.135 \text{ ml O}_2/\text{ml blood}$$
$$C\bar{v}O_2 = 13.5 \text{ ml O}_2/100 \text{ ml blood, or } 13.50 \text{ vol}\%$$

89.
$$\frac{HR \times SV}{BSA} = CI$$
$$\frac{72 \text{ beats/min } (X)}{1.65 \text{ m}^2} = 3.5 \text{ L/min/m}^2$$
$$72 \text{ beats/min } (X) = (3.5 \text{ L/min/m}^2)(1.65 \text{ m}^2)$$
$$X = \frac{5.78 \text{ L/min}}{72 \text{ beats/min}} = 0.08\text{L, or } 80 \text{ ml}$$
$$SV = 0.08 \text{ L, or } 80 \text{ ml}$$

90.
$$\bar{P}_{aw} = K(PIP - PEEP)(T_I/TCT) + PEEP$$
$$T_I = X$$
$$15 \text{ cm H}_2\text{O} = 1(30 \text{ cm H}_2\text{O} - 10 \text{ cm H}_2\text{O})(X/4 \text{ sec}) + 10 \text{ cm H}_2\text{O}$$
$$15 \text{ cm H}_2\text{O} = (20 \text{ cm H}_2\text{O})(X/4 \text{ sec}) + 10 \text{ cm H}_2\text{O}$$
$$15 \text{ cm H}_2\text{O} - 10 \text{ cm H}_2\text{O} = \frac{20 \text{ cm H}_2\text{O}(X)}{4 \text{ sec}}$$
$$\frac{5 \text{ cm H}_2\text{O} \times 4 \text{ sec}}{20 \text{ cm H}_2\text{O}} = X$$
$$\frac{20 \text{ cm H}_2\text{O-sec}}{20 \text{ cm H}_2\text{O}} = X = 1 \text{ sec}$$
$$T_I = 1 \text{ second}$$

2–6 EVALUATING FORMULAS

91. $CVP = (C.O. \times SVR) - MAP$
$$= (5 \text{ L/min} \times 20 \text{ mm Hg/L/min}) - 90 \text{ mm Hg}$$
$$= 100 \text{ mm Hg} - 90 \text{ mm Hg}$$
$$= 10 \text{ mm Hg}$$

92. $\sqrt{CO_2 \text{ molecular wt}} = \dfrac{(\sqrt{O_2 \text{ molecular wt}})(CO_2 \text{ solubility coefficient})}{(Rco_2 : Ro_2)(O_2 \text{ solubility coefficient})}$
$$= \frac{(\sqrt{32})(0.510)}{(19/1)(0.023)}$$
$$= \frac{(5.66)(0.510)}{(19/1)(0.023)}$$
$$= 6.61$$

Keep in mind that 6.61 is the square root of the molecular weight of carbon dioxide. Squaring 6.61 is 44. The molecular weight of CO_2 is 44 (C = 12 a.m.u., O_2 = 32 a.m.u.).

93. $\dot{V}_I = \dfrac{V_T}{T_I}$
$$= \frac{450 \text{ cc}}{0.75 \text{ sec}}$$
$$= 600 \text{ cc/sec}$$

94. $f(V_T) = f(V_A) + f(V_D)$
$$V_T = \frac{(16 \text{ bpm})(400 \text{ cc}) + (16 \text{ bpm})(200 \text{ cc})}{16 \text{ bpm}}$$
$$= \frac{9,600 \text{ bpm-cc}}{16 \text{ bpm}}$$
$$= 600 \text{ cc}$$
$$f(V_T) = \dot{V}_E = (16 \text{ bpm})(600 \text{ cc}) = 9,600 \text{ cc/min}$$

95. $$[(Hb)1.34]S\bar{v}O_2 = C\bar{v}O_2 - [P\bar{v}O_2(0.003 \text{ vol%/torr})]$$

$$[(Hb)1.34]\frac{65}{100} = 13.75 \text{ vol%} - [35 \text{ torr}(0.003 \text{ vol%/torr})]$$

$$[(Hb)1.34]0.65 = 13.75 \text{ vol%} - 0.105 \text{ vol%}$$

$$(Hb)0.871 \text{ ml } O_2/g \text{ Hb} = 13.65 \text{ vol%}$$

$$Hb = \frac{13.65 \text{ ml } O_2/100 \text{ ml blood}}{0.871 \text{ ml } O_2/g \text{ Hb}}$$

$$= 15.67 \text{ g Hb}/100 \text{ ml blood, or } 15.67 \text{ g%}$$

2–7 RECIPROCALS

96. $7\left(\dfrac{1}{7}\right) = 1$

   The reciprocal of 7 is $\dfrac{1}{7}$.

97. $0.5\left(\dfrac{1}{0.5}\right) = 1$

   The reciprocal of 0.5 is $\dfrac{1}{0.5}$.

98. $4\left(\dfrac{1}{4}\right) = 1$

   The reciprocal of $\dfrac{1}{4}$ is 4.

99. $-6\left(-\dfrac{1}{6}\right) = 1$

   The reciprocal of -6 is $-\dfrac{1}{6}$.

100. $-\dfrac{2}{3}\left(-\dfrac{3}{2}\right) = 1$

   The reciprocal of $-\dfrac{2}{3}$ is $-\dfrac{3}{2}$.

101. $$C_L = \frac{1}{E_L}$$

$$0.4 \text{ ml/cm H}_2O = \frac{1}{E_L}$$

$$E_L = \frac{1}{0.4 \text{ ml/cm H}_2O} = 2.5 \text{ cm H}_2O/ml$$

102. $\dfrac{1}{C_T} = \dfrac{1}{C_L} + \dfrac{1}{C_{cw}}$

$\dfrac{1}{C_{cw}} = \dfrac{1}{C_T} - \dfrac{1}{C_L}$

$= \dfrac{1}{0.15\ ml/cm\ H_2O} - \dfrac{1}{0.30\ ml/cm\ H_2O}$

$= 6.66\ cm\ H_2O/ml - 3.33\ cm\ H_2O/ml$

$\dfrac{1}{C_{cw}} = 3.33\ cm\ H_2O/ml$

$C_{cw} = \dfrac{1}{3.33\ cm\ H_2O/ml} = 0.30\ ml/cm\ H_2O$

103. $E_T = E_L + E_{cw}$

$E_L = E_T - E_{cw}$

$= 5.5\ cm\ H_2O/ml - 3.5\ cm\ H_2O/ml$

$= 2.0\ cm\ H_2O/ml$

$C_L = \dfrac{1}{E_L} = \dfrac{1}{2.0\ cm\ H_2O/ml}$

$= 0.5\ ml/cm\ H_2O$

104. $G_{aw} = \dfrac{1}{R_{aw}}$

$= \dfrac{1}{0.85\ cm\ H_2O/L/sec}$

$= 1.18\ L/sec/cm\ H_2O$

105. $R_{aw} = \dfrac{1}{G_{aw}}$

$= \dfrac{1}{23\ ml/min/mm\ Hg}$

$= 0.043\ mm\ Hg/ml/min$

CHAPTER 3 - CHEMISTRY

3-2 CHEMICAL LAWS

1. $60\ mm\ Hg \times 0.003\ vol\%/mm\ Hg = 0.18\ vol\%$
2. $100\ torr \times 0.003\ vol\%/torr = 0.3\ vol\%$
3. $40\ torr \times 0.003\ vol\%/torr = 0.12\ vol\%$
4. $1,900\ mm\ Hg \times 0.003\ vol\%/mm\ Hg = 5.7\ vol\%$
5. $760\ mm\ Hg \times 0.003\ vol\%/mm\ Hg = 2.28\ vol\%$

6. 40 torr $\times$ 0.067 vol%/torr = 2.68 vol%

7. 75 mm Hg $\times$ 0.067 vol%/mm Hg = 5.03 vol%

8. 25 torr $\times$ 0.067 vol%/torr = 1.68 vol%

9. 63 mm Hg $\times$ 0.067 vol%/mm Hg = 4.22 vol%

10. 760 torr $\times$ 0.067 vol%/torr = 50.92 vol%

11. $\dfrac{2.68\ vol\%}{2.23\ vol\%/mmol/L}$ = 1.20 mmol/L, or 1.20 mEq/L

12. $\dfrac{56.20\ vol\%}{2.23\ vol\%/mmol/L}$ = 25.20 mmol/L, or 25.20 mEq/L

13. $\dfrac{53.52\ vol\%}{2.23\ vol\%/mmol/L}$ = 24 mmol/L, or 24 mEq/L

14. $\dfrac{18.37\ vol\%}{2.23\ vol\%/mmol/L}$ = 8.24 mmol/L, or 8.24 mEq/L

15. $\dfrac{37.81\ vol\%}{2.23\ vol\%/mmol/L}$ = 16.96 mmol/L, or 16.96 mEq/L

16. 40 mm Hg $\times$ 0.03 mmol/L/mm Hg = 1.2 mmol/L, or 1.2 mEq/L

17. 25 mm Hg $\times$ 0.03 mmol/L/mm Hg = 0.75 mmol/L, or 0.75 mEq/L

18. 65 torr $\times$ 0.03 mmol/L/torr = 1.95 mmol/L, or 1.95 mEq/L

19. 90 torr $\times$ 0.03 mmol/L/torr = 2.70 mmol/L, or 2.70 mEq/L

20. 760 torr $\times$ 0.03 mmol/L/torr = 22.8 mmol/L, or 22.8 mEq/L

21. total CO_2 = combined CO_2 + dissolved CO_2

$$combined\ CO_2 = 53.50\ vol\% - (40\ mm\ Hg)(0.067\ vol\%/mm\ Hg)$$
$$= 53.50\ vol\% - 2.68\ vol\%$$
$$= \dfrac{50.82\ vol\%}{2.23\ vol\%/mmol/L}$$
$$= 22.79\ mmol/L$$

22. dissolved CO_2 = total CO_2 - combined CO_2

$$= 35\ mmol/L - \dfrac{75.05\ vol\%}{2.23\ vol\%/mmol/L}$$
$$= 35\ mmol/L - 33.65\ mmol/L$$
$$= \dfrac{1.35\ mmol/L}{0.03\ mmol/L/torr}$$
$$= 45\ torr$$

23. combined CO_2 = total CO_2 - dissolved CO_2

$$= 44\ vol\% - 4.0\ vol\%$$
$$= \dfrac{40\ vol\%}{2.23\ vol\%/mmol/L}$$
$$= 17.94\ mmol/L$$

24. dissolved CO_2 = total CO_2 − combined CO_2

$= 63.6 \text{ vol}\% - (27.1 \text{ mEq/L})(2.23 \text{ vol}\%/\text{mEq/L})$

$= 63.6 \text{ vol}\% - 60.43 \text{ vol}\%$

$= \dfrac{3.17 \text{ vol}\%}{0.067 \text{ vol}\%/\text{torr}}$

$= 47 \text{ torr}$

25. total CO_2 = dissolved CO_2 + combined CO_2

$= 1.7 \text{ mEq/L} + \dfrac{42.37 \text{ vol}\%}{2.23 \text{ vol}\%/\text{mEq/L}}$

$= 1.7 \text{ mEq/L} + 19 \text{ mEq/L}$

$= 20.70 \text{ mEq/L}$

26. $\dfrac{r_{H_2}}{r_{O_2}} = \dfrac{\sqrt{32 \text{ amu}}}{\sqrt{2 \text{ amu}}} = \dfrac{5.66}{1.41} = \dfrac{4}{1}$

$r_{H_2} = 4(r_{O_2})$; H_2 diffuses 4 times faster than O_2.

Alternatively,

$\dfrac{r_{O_2}}{r_{H_2}} = \dfrac{\sqrt{2 \text{ amu}}}{\sqrt{32 \text{ amu}}} = \dfrac{1.41}{5.66} = \dfrac{1}{4} = 0.25$

$r_{O_2} = 0.25 (r_{H_2})$; O_2 diffuses 0.25 times slower than H_2.

27. $\dfrac{r_{CH_4}}{r_{COCl_2}} = \dfrac{\sqrt{99 \text{ amu}}}{\sqrt{16 \text{ amu}}} = \dfrac{9.94}{4.00} = \dfrac{2.49}{1.00}$

$r_{CH_4} = 2.49 (r_{COCl_2})$; CH_4 diffuses 2.49 times faster than $COCl_2$.

Alternatively,

$\dfrac{r_{COCl_2}}{r_{CH_4}} = \dfrac{\sqrt{16 \text{ amu}}}{\sqrt{99 \text{ amu}}} = \dfrac{4.00}{9.94} = \dfrac{1.00}{2.49} = 0.40$

$r_{COCl_2} = 0.40 (r_{CH_4})$; $COCl_2$ diffuses 0.4 times slower than CH_4.

28. $\dfrac{r_{CO_2}}{r_{O_2}} = \dfrac{(\sqrt{32 \text{ amu}})(55.0)}{(\sqrt{44 \text{ amu}})(2.4)} = \dfrac{(5.66)(55.0)}{(6.63)(2.4)} = \dfrac{311.3}{15.9} = \dfrac{19.57}{1}$

$r_{CO_2} = 19.57 (r_{O_2})$; CO_2 diffuses 19.57 times faster than O_2 in water at 38ºC.

Alternatively,

$\dfrac{r_{O_2}}{r_{CO_2}} = \dfrac{(\sqrt{44 \text{ amu}})(2.4)}{(\sqrt{32 \text{ amu}})(55.0)} = \dfrac{(6.63)(2.4)}{(5.66)(55.0)} = \dfrac{1}{19.57} = 0.51$

$r_{O_2} = 0.51 (r_{CO_2})$; O_2 diffuses 0.51 times slower than CO_2 in water at 38ºC.

29. $\dfrac{r_{N_2O}}{r_{C_3H_6}} = \dfrac{(\sqrt{42 \text{ amu}})(0.41)}{(\sqrt{44 \text{ amu}})(0.011)} = \dfrac{(6.48)(0.41)}{(6.63)(0.011)} = \dfrac{2.66}{0.073} = \dfrac{36.44}{1}$

$r_{N_2O} = 36.44 (r_{C_3H_6})$; N_2O diffuses 36.44 times faster than C_3H_6 in water at 38ºC.

Alternatively,

$\dfrac{r_{C_3H_6}}{r_{N_2O}} = \dfrac{(\sqrt{44 \text{ amu}})(0.011)}{(\sqrt{42 \text{ amu}})(0.41)} = \dfrac{(6.63)(0.011)}{(6.48)(0.41)} = \dfrac{0.073}{2.66} = \dfrac{1}{36.44} = 0.027$

$r_{C_3H_6} = 0.027 (r_{N_2O})$; C_3H_6 diffuses 0.027 times slower than N_2O in water at 38ºC.

30. $$\frac{\text{ro}_2}{\text{rco}} = \frac{(\sqrt{28 \text{ amu}})(0.023)}{(\sqrt{32 \text{ amu}})(0.0175)} = \frac{(5.29)(0.023)}{(5.66)(0.0175)} = \frac{0.122}{0.099} = \frac{1.23}{1}$$

ro$_2$ = 1.23 (rco); O$_2$ diffuses 1.23 times faster across the alveolar-capillary membrane than CO.

Alternatively,

$$\frac{\text{rco}}{\text{ro}_2} = \frac{(\sqrt{32 \text{ amu}})(0.0175)}{(\sqrt{28 \text{ amu}})(0.023)} = \frac{(5.66)(0.0175)}{(5.29)(0.023)} = \frac{0.099}{0.122} = \frac{1}{1.23} = 0.81$$

rco = 0.81 (ro$_2$); CO diffuses 0.81 times slower across the alveolar-capillary membrane than O$_2$.

3-3 MOLARITY AND NORMALITY

31. H_3PO_4 = 98 amu molecular weight

$$\frac{98 \text{ g}}{98 \text{ g/mole}} = 1 \text{ mole of } H_3PO_4$$

32. $C_{12}H_{22}O_{11}$ = 342 amu molecular weight

$$\frac{513 \text{ g}}{342 \text{ g/mole}} = 1.5 \text{ moles of } C_{12}H_{22}O_{11}$$

33. C_2H_6O = 46 amu molecular weight

$$\frac{138,000 \text{ mg}}{1,000 \text{ mg/g}} = 138 \text{ g}$$

$$\frac{138 \text{ g}}{46 \text{ g/mole}} = 3 \text{ moles of } C_2H_6O$$

34. $C_3H_8O_3$ = 92 amu molecular weight

$$\frac{68 \text{ g}}{92 \text{ g/mole}} = 0.74 \text{ mole of } C_3H_8O_3$$

35. Hb = 66,700 amu molecular weight

$$\frac{133,400 \text{ g}}{66,700 \text{ g/mole}} = 2 \text{ moles of hemoglobin}$$

36. *STEP 1:* CH_3COOH = 60 amu molecular weight

STEP 2: $\dfrac{60 \text{ g}}{60 \text{ g/mole}} = 1 \text{ mole of } CH_3COOH$

STEP 3: $\dfrac{1,000 \text{ ml}}{1,000 \text{ ml/L}} = 1 \text{ L}$

STEP 4: M = moles/L

$$= \frac{1 \text{ mole}}{1 \text{ L}}$$

$$= 1 \text{ M } CH_3COOH$$

37. *STEP 1:* $C_{12}H_{22}O_{11}$ = 342 amu molecular weight

    STEP 2: $\dfrac{60 \text{ ml}}{1,000 \text{ ml/L}} = 0.06 \text{ L}$

    STEP 3: moles = M × L
    $$= 3 \text{ M} \times 0.06 \text{ L}$$
    $$= 0.18 \text{ mole}$$

    STEP 4: grams = moles × gram–molecular weight
    $$= (0.18 \text{ mole})(342 \text{ g/mole})$$
    $$= 61.56 \text{ g of } C_{12}H_{22}O_{11}$$

38. *STEP 1:* NaOH = 40 amu molecular weight

    STEP 2: $\dfrac{8 \text{ g}}{40 \text{ g/mole}} = 0.2 \text{ mole of NaOH}$

    STEP 3: $L = \dfrac{\text{moles}}{\text{M}}$
    $$= \dfrac{0.2 \text{ mole}}{0.1 \text{ M}}$$
    $$= 2 \text{ L}$$

    STEP 4: 2 L × 1,000 ml/L = 2,000 ml

39. *STEP 1:* KOH = 56 amu molecular weight

    STEP 2: $\dfrac{10 \text{ g}}{56 \text{ g/mole}} = 0.1786 \text{ mole of KOH}$

    STEP 3: $M = \dfrac{\text{moles}}{\text{L}}$
    $$= \dfrac{0.1786 \text{ mole}}{1 \text{ L}}$$
    $$= 0.1786 \text{ M}$$

40. *STEP 1:* H_3PO_4 = 98 amu molecular weight

    STEP 2: moles = M × L
    $$= 0.110 \text{ M} \times 1 \text{ L}$$
    $$= 0.110 \text{ mole of } H_3PO_4$$

    STEP 3: grams = moles × gram–molecular weight
    $$= (0.110 \text{ mole})(98 \text{ g/mole})$$
    $$= 10.78 \text{ g of } H_3PO_4$$

41. *STEP 1:* H_2SO_4 = 98 amu molecular weight

    STEP 2: $H_2SO_4 \rightarrow 2H^+ \times SO_4^{2-}$ (NOTE: 2 positive charges from 2 H^+ ions)

    STEP 3: $\dfrac{98 \text{ g}}{2} = 49 \text{ g}$ (weight of 1 gram equivalent of H_2SO_4)

    STEP 4: $\dfrac{24 \text{ g}}{49 \text{ g/g eq}} = 0.49 \text{ gram equivalent of } H_2SO_4$

42. *STEP 1:* $AlCl_3 = 133.5$ amu molecular weight
    STEP 2: $AlCl_3 \rightarrow Al^{3+} + Cl^{3-}$ (NOTE: 3 positive charges from 1 Al^{3+} ion)
    STEP 3: $\dfrac{133.5 \text{ g}}{3} = 44.5$ g (wt of 1 gram equivalent of $AlCl_3$)
    STEP 4: $\dfrac{28 \text{ g}}{44.5 \text{ g/g eq}} = 0.629$ gram equivalent of $AlCl_3$

43. *STEP 1:* $H_3PO_4 = 98$ amu molecular weight
    STEP 2: $H_3PO_4 \rightarrow 2H^+ + HPO_4^{2-}$ (NOTE: 2 positive charges from 2 H^+ ions)
    STEP 3: $\dfrac{98 \text{ g}}{2} = 49$ g (weight of 1 gram of H_3PO_4)
    STEP 4: $\dfrac{200 \text{ g}}{49 \text{ g/g eq}} = 4.08$ gram equivalents of H_3PO_4

44. *STEP 1:* $Zn(OH)_2 = 99$ amu molecular weight
    STEP 2: $Zn(OH)_2 \rightarrow Zn^{2+} + 2OH^-$ (NOTE: 2 positive charges from 1 Zn^{2+} ion)
    STEP 3: $\dfrac{99 \text{ g}}{2} = 49.5$ g (weight of 1 gram equivalent of $Zn(OH)_2$)
    STEP 4: $\dfrac{100 \text{ g}}{49.5 \text{ g/g eq}} = 2.02$ gram equivalents of $Zn(OH)_2$

45. *STEP 1:* $H_2CO_3 = 62$ amu molecular weight
    STEP 2: $H_2CO_3 \rightarrow 2H^+ + CO_3^{2-}$ (NOTE: 2 positive charges from 2 H^+ ions)
    STEP 3: $\dfrac{62 \text{ g}}{2} = 31$ g (weight of 1 gram equivalent of H_2CO_3)
    STEP 4: $\dfrac{62 \text{ g}}{31 \text{ g/g eq}} = 2$ gram equivalents of H_2CO_3

46. *STEP 1:* $H_2SO_4 = 98$ amu molecular weight
    STEP 2: $H_2SO_4 \rightarrow 2H^+ + SO_4^{2-}$ (NOTE: 2 positive charges from 2 H^+ ions)
    STEP 3: $\dfrac{98 \text{ g}}{2} = 49$ g (weight of 1 gram equivalent of H_2SO_4)
    STEP 4: $\dfrac{2.45 \text{ mg}}{49 \text{ g/g eq}} = 0.05$ gram equivalent of H_2SO_4
    STEP 5: $\dfrac{800 \text{ ml}}{1,000 \text{ ml/L}} = 0.8$ L
    STEP 6: $N = \dfrac{\text{gram equivalents}}{L}$

    $= \dfrac{0.05 \text{ g eq}}{0.8 \text{ L}}$

    $= 0.0625$ N H_2SO_4

47. *STEP 1:* $H_2SO_4 = 98$ amu molecular weight
    STEP 2: $H_2SO_4 \rightarrow 2H^+ + SO_4^{2-}$ (NOTE: 2 positive charges from 2 H^+ ions)

STEP 3: $\dfrac{98\ g}{2} = 49\ g$ (weight of 1 gram equivalent of H_2SO_4)

STEP 4: A 1 M solution of H_2SO_4 contains 98 g of H_2SO_4 per liter. That weight, i.e., 98 g, represents 2 gram equivalents of H_2SO_4. Therefore, 2 gram equivalents of H_2SO_4 in 1 L produces a 2 N solution.

STEP 5: 1 M H_2SO_4 = 2 N H_2SO_4

48. *STEP 1:* NaOH = 40 amu molecular weight

STEP 2: NaOH → Na^+ + OH^- (NOTE: 1 positive charge from 1 Na^+ ion)

STEP 3: $\dfrac{40\ g}{1} = 40\ g$ (weight of 1 gram equivalent of NaOH)

STEP 4: 40 g/L = 1 N NaOH

20 g/L = 0.5 N NaOH

10 g/L = 0.25 N NaOH

STEP 5: Since 2 liters of volume is considered here, twice the number of grams of NaOH will be needed. Therefore, 20 g of NaOH in 2 L will result in a 0.25 N NaOH solution.

49. *STEP 1:* KOH = 56 amu molecular weight

STEP 2: KOH → K^+ + OH^- (NOTE: 1 positive charge from one K^+ ion)

STEP 3: $\dfrac{56\ g}{1} = 56\ g$ (weight of 1 gram equivalent of KOH)

STEP 4: gram equivalents = N × L

= 0.3 N × 1 L

= 0.3 gram equivalent of KOH

STEP 5: gram = (# gram equivalents)(weight of 1 gram equivalent)

= (0.3 gram equivalent)(56 g/g eq)

= 16.8 g KOH

50. *STEP 1:* $Ca(OH)_2$ = 74 amu molecular weight

STEP 2: $Ca(OH)_2$ → Ca^{2+} + 2 OH^- (NOTE: 2 positive charges from 1 Ca^{2+} ion)

STEP 3: $\dfrac{74\ g}{2} = 37\ g$ (weight of 1 gram equivalent of $Ca(OH)_2$)

STEP 4: $\dfrac{50}{1{,}000\ ml/L} = 0.05\ L$

STEP 5: gram equivalents = N × L

= 0.01 N × 0.05 L

= 0.0005 gram equivalent of $Ca(OH)_2$

STEP 6: gram = (# gram equivalents)(weight of 1 gram equivalent)

= (0.0005 gram equivalent)(37 g/g eq)

= 0.0185 g

STEP 7: 0.0185 g × 1,000 mg/g = 18.5 mg of $Ca(OH)_2$

3–4 LAW OF MASS ACTION AND HENDERSON-HASSELBALCH EQUATION

51. $pH = \log\left(\dfrac{1}{10^{-11}}\right)$

$\quad = \log 1 + \log 10^{11}$

$\quad = 0 + 11$

$\quad = 11$

52. $pH = \log\left(\dfrac{1}{2.30 \times 10^{-4}}\right)$

$\quad = -\log (0.00023)$

$\quad = -\log (2.30 \times 10^{-4})$

$\quad = -\log 2.30 + (-\log 10^{-4})$

$\quad = -0.3617 - (-4)$

$\quad = -0.3617 + 4$

$\quad = 3.64$

53. $pH = -\log 4.80 \times 10^{-10}$

$\quad = -\log 4.80 + (-\log 10^{-10})$

$\quad = -0.6812 - (-10)$

$\quad = -0.6812 + 10$

$\quad = 9.32$

54. $pH = -\log 6.30 \times 10^{-1}$

$\quad = -\log 6.30 + (-\log 10^{-1})$

$\quad = -0.7993 - (-1)$

$\quad = 0.7993 + 1$

$\quad = 0.20$

55. $pH = -\log 4.60 \times 10^{-4}$

$\quad = -\log 4.60 + (-\log 10^{-4})$

$\quad = -0.6628 - (-4)$

$\quad = -0.6628 + 4$

$\quad = 3.34$

56. $pH = 9 - \log 33$

$\quad = 9 - 1.52$

$\quad = 7.48$

57. $pH = 9 - \log 34$

$\quad = 9 - 1.53$

$\quad = 7.47$

58. pH = 9 − log 57
    = 9 − 1.756
    = 7.244

59. pH = 9 − log 58
    = 9 − 1.763
    = 7.237

60. pH = 9 − log 100
    = 9 − 2
    = 7.00

61. nanomoles/liter = antilog (9 − 7.49)
    = antilog 1.51
    = 32.36

62. nanomoles/liter = antilog (9 − 7.48)
    = antilog 1.52
    = 33.11

63. nanomoles/liter = antilog (9 − 7.29)
    = antilog 1.71
    = 51.29

64. nanomoles/liter = antilog (9 − 7.35)
    = antilog 1.65
    = 44.67

65. nanomoles/liter = antilog (9 − 7.10)
    = antilog 1.90
    = 79.43

66. nanomoles/liter = antilog (9 − 8.00)
    = antilog 1
    = 10

67. nanomoles/liter = antilog (9 − 8.53)
    = antilog 0.47
    = 2.95

68. nanomoles/liter = antilog (9 − 6.21)
    = antilog 2.79
    = 616.6

69. nanomoles/liter = antilog (9 − 14)
    = antilog −5
    = 1.00×10^{-5}

70. nanomoles/liter = antilog $(9 - 1)$
$$= \text{antilog } 8$$
$$= 1.00 \times 10^8$$

71. $\text{pH} = 6.1 + \log\left[\dfrac{15 \text{ mEq/L}}{(25 \text{ torr})(0.03 \text{ mEq/L/torr})}\right]$
$$= 6.1 + \log 20$$
$$= 7.40$$

72. $\text{P}_{CO_2} = \dfrac{[HCO_3^-]}{[0.03 \text{ mmol/L/torr} \times (\text{antilog pH} - 6.1)]}$

$$= \dfrac{20 \text{ mmol/L}}{[0.03 \text{ mmol/L/torr} \times (\text{antilog } 7.48 - 6.1)]}$$

$$= \dfrac{20 \text{ mmol/L}}{[0.03 \text{ mmol/L/torr} \times (\text{antilog } 1.38)]}$$

$$= \dfrac{20 \text{ mmol/L}}{[(0.03 \text{ mmol/L/torr})(23.99)]}$$

$$= \dfrac{20 \text{ mmol/L}}{0.7196 \text{ mmol/L/torr}}$$

$$= 28 \text{ torr}$$

73. $\text{PaCO}_2 = \dfrac{[HCO_3^-]}{[0.03 \text{ mmol/L/torr}(\text{antilog pH} - 6.1)]}$

$$= \dfrac{26 \text{ mmol/L}}{[0.03 \text{ mmol/L/torr}(\text{antilog } 7.42 - 6.1)]}$$

$$= \dfrac{26 \text{ mmol/L}}{[0.03 \text{ mmol/L/torr}(\text{antilog } 1.32)]}$$

$$= \dfrac{26 \text{ mmol/L}}{0.6268 \text{ mmol/L/torr}}$$

$$= 41 \text{ torr}$$

74. $[HCO_3^-] = (0.03 \text{ mEq/L/torr} \times \text{P}_{CO_2})[\text{antilog}(\text{pH} - 6.1)]$
$$= (0.03 \text{ mEq/L/torr} \times 26 \text{ mm Hg})[\text{antilog}(7.46 - 6.1)]$$
$$= (0.78 \text{ mmol/L})(\text{antilog } 1.36)$$
$$= (0.78 \text{ mmol/L})(22.91)$$
$$= 17.87 \text{ mmol/L, or } 17.87 \text{ mEq/L}$$

75. *STEP 1:* $[HCO_3^-] = (0.03 \text{ mmol/L/torr} \times \text{P}_{CO_2})[\text{antilog}(\text{pH} - 6.1)]$
$$= (0.03 \text{ mmol/L/torr} \times 28 \text{ mm Hg})[\text{antilog}(7.24 - 6.1)]$$
$$= (0.84 \text{ mmol/L})(\text{antilog } 1.14)$$
$$= 11.6 \text{ mmol/L}$$

    STEP 2: total CO_2 = combined CO_2 + dissolved CO_2
$$= 11.6 \text{ mmol/L} + 0.84 \text{ mmol/L}$$
$$= 12.44 \text{ mmol/L}$$

76. $pH = 6.1 + \log\left[\dfrac{36\text{ mEq/L}}{(0.03\text{ mEq/L/torr})(75\text{ torr})}\right]$

$= 6.1 + \log\left(\dfrac{36\text{ mEq/L}}{2.25\text{ mEq/L}}\right)$

$= 6.1 + 1.2$

$= 7.30$

77. $[HCO_3^-] = (0.03\text{ mEq/L/torr} \times P_{CO_2})[\text{antilog}(pH - 6.1)]$

$= (0.03\text{ mEq/L/torr} \times 30\text{ torr})[\text{antilog }(7.48 - 6.1)]$

$= (0.9\text{ mEq/L})(\text{antilog }1.38)$

$= (0.9\text{ mEq/L})(23.9)$

$= 21.6\text{ mEq/L}$

78. $[HCO_3^-] = (0.03\text{ mEq/L/torr} \times P_{CO_2})[\text{antilog}(pH - 6.1)]$

$= (0.03\text{ mEq/L/torr} \times 35\text{ mm Hg})[\text{antilog }(7.33 - 6.1)]$

$= (1.05\text{ mEq/L})\text{antilog }1.23$

$= 1.05\text{ mEq/L} \times 16.98$

$= 17.8\text{ mEq/L}$

79. $pH = 6.1 + \log\left[\dfrac{18\text{ mEq/L}}{(0.03\text{ mEq/L/torr})(55\text{ mmHg})}\right]$

$= 6.1 + \log\left(\dfrac{18\text{ mEq/L}}{1.65\text{ mEq/L}}\right)$

$= 6.1 + \log 10.9$

$= 6.1 + 1.04$

$= 7.14$

80. $[HCO_3^-] = (0.03\text{ mEq/L/torr} \times P_{CO_2})[\text{antilog}(pH - 6.1)]$

$= (0.03\text{ mEq/L/torr} \times 20\text{ torr})[\text{antilog }(7.22 - 6.1)]$

$= (0.6\text{ torr})(\text{antilog }1.12)$

$= 0.6\text{ torr} \times 13.2$

$= 7.92\text{ mEq/L}$

3-5 DENSITY AND SPECIFIC GRAVITY

81. *STEP 1:* $CO_2 = 44$ amu molecular weight

STEP 2: $D = \dfrac{\text{gram–molecular weight}}{\text{ideal gas molar volume at STP}}$

$= \dfrac{44\text{ g}}{22.4\text{ g/L}}$

$= 1.96\text{ g/L}$

82. *STEP 1:* $CO_2 = 44$ amu molecular weight

STEP 2: $D = \dfrac{\text{gram–molecular weight}}{\text{ideal gas molar volume at STP}}$

$= \dfrac{44 \text{ g}}{22.4 \text{ g/L}}$

$= 1.96 \text{ g/L}$

STEP 3: specific gravity $= \dfrac{D_{gas}}{D_{standard}}$

$= \dfrac{1.96 \text{ g/L}}{1.29 \text{ g/L}}$

$= 1.52$

83. *STEP 1:* $N_2O = 44$ amu molecular weight

    STEP 2: $D = \dfrac{\text{gram–molecular weight}}{\text{ideal gas molar volume at STP}}$

$= \dfrac{44 \text{ g}}{22.4 \text{ g/L}}$

$= 1.96 \text{ g/L}$

84. *STEP 1:* volume $= 3.0 \text{ cm} \times 3.0 \text{ cm} \times 3.0 \text{ cm}$

$= 27 \text{ cm}^3, \text{ or } 27 \text{ cc}$

    STEP 2: $D = \dfrac{\text{mass}}{\text{volume}} = \dfrac{90 \text{ g}}{27 \text{ cc}} = 3.33 \text{ g/cc}$

85. *STEP 1:* $CO = 28$ amu molecular weight

    STEP 2: $D = \dfrac{\text{gram–molecular weight}}{\text{ideal gas molar volume at STP}}$

$= \dfrac{28 \text{ g}}{22.4 \text{ g/L}}$

$= 1.25 \text{ g/L}$

    STEP 3: specific gravity $= \dfrac{D_{gas}}{D_{standard}}$

$= \dfrac{1.25 \text{ g/L}}{1.29 \text{ g/L}}$

$= 0.97$

3-6 TEMPERATURE SCALES

86. $°F = 1.8(°C) + 32$

$= 1.8(1°C) + 32$

$= 33.8°F$

87. $°F = 1.8(°C) + 32$
    $= 1.8(89°C) + 32$
    $= 160.2° + 32$
    $= 192.2°F$

88. $°F = 1.8(°C) + 32$
    $= 1.8(-89°C) + 32$
    $= -160.2° + 32$
    $= -128.2°F$

89. $°F = 1.8(°C) + 32$
    $= 1.8(-40°C) + 32$
    $= -72° + 32$
    $= -40°F$

90. $°F = 1.8(°C) + 32$
    $= 1.8(40°C) + 32$
    $= 72° + 32$
    $= 104°F$

91. $°C = (°F - 32)5/9$
    $= (98.6°F - 32)5/9$
    $= (66.6°)5/9$
    $= 37°C$

92. $°C = (°F - 32)5/9$
    $= (-65°F - 32)5/9$
    $= (-97°)5/9$
    $= -53.9°C$

93. $°C = (°F - 32)5/9$
    $= (-459°F - 32)5/9$
    $= (-491°)5/9$
    $= -273°C$

94. $°C = (°F - 32)5/9$
    $= (-32°F - 32)5/9$
    $= (-64°)5/9$
    $= 35.6°C$

95. $°C = (°F - 32)5/9$
    $= (43°F - 32)5/9$
    $= (11°)5/9$
    $= 6.1°C$

96. *STEP 1:* $\degree C = (\degree F - 32)5/9$
$$= (98.6\degree F - 32)5/9$$
$$= (66.6\degree)5/9$$
$$= 37\degree C$$

   STEP 2: $K = \degree C + 273$
$$= 37\degree C + 273$$
$$= 310\ K$$

97. *STEP 1:* $\degree C = (\degree F - 32)5/9$
$$= (-40\degree F - 32)5/9$$
$$= (-72\degree)5/9$$
$$= -40\degree C$$

   STEP 2: $K = \degree C + 273$
$$= -40\degree C + 273$$
$$= 233\ K$$

98. $K = \degree C + 273$
$$= -273\degree C + 273$$
$$= 0\ K$$

99. $K = \degree C + 273$
$$= -118\degree C + 273$$
$$= 155\ K$$

100. $K = \degree C + 273$
$$= 273\degree C + 273$$
$$= 546\ K$$

101. $K = (\degree F - 32)5/9 + 273$
$$= (32\degree F - 32)5/9 + 273$$
$$= 0\degree + 273$$
$$= 273\ K$$

102. $K = (\degree F - 32)5/9 + 273$
$$= (-459\degree F - 32)5/9 + 273$$
$$= (-491\degree)5/9 + 273$$
$$= -273\degree + 273$$
$$= 0\ K$$

103. $K = (\degree F - 32)5/9 + 273$
$$= (-40\degree F - 32)5/9 + 273$$
$$= (-72\degree)5/9 + 273$$
$$= -40\degree + 273$$
$$= 233\ K$$

104. $K = (°F - 32)5/9 + 273$
     $= (72°F - 32)5/9 + 273$
     $= 22° + 273$
     $= 295\ K$
105. $K = °C + 273$
     $= 22° + 273$
     $= 295\ K$

CHAPTER 4 - PHYSICS

4-1 WORK

1. $W = F \times d$
   $= 20\ lbs \times 15\ ft$
   $= 300\ ft\text{-}lbs$

2. $F = \dfrac{W}{d} = \dfrac{240\ J}{2.4\ m} = 100\ N$

3. $F = \dfrac{W}{d} = \dfrac{1.4 \times 10^9\ ergs}{185\ cm} = 7.6 \times 10^6\ dynes$

4. The force applied in this situation is perpendicular to the direction of the motion. Therefore, no work was done, as the equation below shows.
$$W = F \times d$$
$$= 0 \times 460\ cm$$
$$= 0$$

5. *Stairs:* $W = F \times d$ *Ramp:* $W = F \times d$
   $= 180\ lbs \times 15\ ft$ $= 180\ lbs \times 15\ ft$
   $= 2,700\ ft\text{-}lbs$ $= 2,700\ ft\text{-}lbs$

4-4 PRESSURE

6. $\dfrac{760\ mm\ Hg}{9.21 \times 10^6\ mm\ Hg} = \dfrac{1,034\ cm\ H_2O}{X}$
   $X = 1.25 \times 10^7\ cm\ H_2O$

7. $\dfrac{429\ ft\ H_2O}{33\ ft\ H_2O/atm} = 13\ atm$

8. $\dfrac{760\ torr}{380\ torr} = \dfrac{33\ ft\ H_2O}{X}$
   $X = 16.5\ ft\ H_2O$

9. $\dfrac{29.9 \text{ in. Hg}}{80 \text{ in. Hg}} = \dfrac{76 \text{ cm Hg}}{X}$

   $X = 203.34 \text{ cm Hg}$

10. $\dfrac{4.92 \times 10^{-8} \text{ psi}}{14.7 \text{ psi/atm}} = 3.35 \times 10^{-9} \text{ atm}$

11. $\dfrac{760 \text{ mm Hg}}{9.03 \times 10^9 \text{ mm Hg}} = \dfrac{29.9 \text{ in. Hg}}{X}$

    $X = 3.55 \times 10^8 \text{ in. Hg}$

12. $(4.29 \times 10^3 \text{ atm})(760 \text{ torr/atm}) = 3.26 \times 10^6 \text{ torr}$

13. $\dfrac{563 \text{ kPa}}{101.33 \text{ kPa/atm}} = 5.56 \text{ atm}$

14. $\dfrac{101.33 \text{ kPa}}{9.49 \times 10^2 \text{ kPa}} = \dfrac{760 \text{ torr}}{X}$

    $X = 7.12 \times 10^3 \text{ torr}$

15. $\dfrac{1{,}034 \text{ cm H}_2\text{O}}{2.78 \times 10^4 \text{ cm H}_2\text{O}} = \dfrac{101.33 \text{ kPa}}{X}$

    $X = 2.72 \times 10^3 \text{ kPa}$

4-5 GAS LAWS

16. $P_T - P_{H_2O} = P_{T\text{corrected}}$

    $\begin{array}{l} 730 \text{ torr } P_T \\ \underline{-39.9 \text{ torr } P_{H_2O}} \\ 690.1 \text{ torr } P_{T\text{corrected}} \end{array}$

17. $\begin{array}{l} 680 \text{ mm Hg } P_T \\ \underline{-19.8 \text{ mm Hg } P_{H_2O}} \\ 660.2 \text{ mm Hg } P_{T\text{corrected}} \end{array}$

18. $\begin{array}{l} 880 \text{ torr } P_T \\ \underline{-12.8 \text{ torr } P_{H_2O}} \\ 867.2 \text{ torr } P_{T\text{corrected}} \end{array}$

19. $\begin{array}{l} 1{,}000 \text{ torr } P_T \\ \underline{-37.7 \text{ torr } P_{H_2O}} \\ 962.3 \text{ torr } P_{T\text{corrected}} \end{array}$

20. $\begin{array}{l} 740 \text{ mm Hg } P_T \\ \underline{-25.2 \text{ mm Hg } P_{H_2O}} \\ 714.8 \text{ mm Hg } P_{T\text{corrected}} \end{array}$

21. $\dfrac{20.93\% \text{ O}_2}{100} = 0.2093 \ (F_{O_2})$

22. $\dfrac{5\% \text{ CO}_2}{100} = 0.05 \ (F_{CO_2})$

23. *STEP 1:*   550 torr P_T
    -25.2 torr P_{H_2O}
    _____
    524.8 torr $P_{T corrected}$

   STEP 2: $= \dfrac{80\% \text{ He}}{100} = 0.8 \ (F_{He})$

   STEP 3: 0.8×524.8 torr $= 419.8$ torr P_{HE}

24. *STEP 1:* $= \dfrac{26\% \text{ N}_2}{100} = 0.26 \ (F_{N_2})$

   STEP 2: 0.26×600 mm Hg $= 156$ mm Hg P_{N_2}

25. *STEP 1:* $= \dfrac{33\% \text{ CO}}{100} = 0.33 \ F_{co}$

   STEP 2:   980 mm Hg P_T
    -12 mm Hg P_{H_2O}
    _____
    968 mm Hg $P_{T corrected}$

   STEP 3: 0.33×968 mm Hg $= 319.4$ mm Hg P_{co}

26. Gay-Lussac's law.

   STEP 1:   Change the temperatures to K (i.e., K = °C + 273).
    $T_1 = 25°C + 273 = 298$ K
    $T_2 = 45°C + 273 = 318$ K

   STEP 2:   Insert the known values into the formula.

   $$\frac{P_1}{T_1} = \frac{P_2}{T_2}$$

   $$P_2 = \frac{(318 \text{ K})(750 \text{ torr})}{(298 \text{ K})} = 800 \text{ torr}$$

27. Boyle's law.

   $$P_1V_1 = P_2V_2, \text{ or } \frac{P_1}{P_2} = \frac{V_2}{V_1}$$

   $$(900 \text{ torr})(500 \text{ cc}) = (750 \text{ torr})(V_2)$$

   $$V_2 = \frac{(900 \text{ torr})(500 \text{ cc})}{(750 \text{ torr})} = 600 \text{ cc}$$

28. Charles' law.

   STEP 1:   Convert the temperatures from °C to K (i.e., K = °C + 273).
    $T_1 = 30°C + 273 = 303$ K
    $T_2 = 10°C + 273 = 283$ K

   STEP 2:   Insert the known values into the equation.

   $$\frac{V_1}{T_1} = \frac{V_2}{T_2}$$

   $$\frac{100 \text{ ml}}{303 \text{ K}} = \frac{V_2}{283 \text{ K}}$$

   $$V_2 = \frac{(100 \text{ ml})(283 \text{ K})}{303 \text{ K}} = 93.4 \text{ ml}$$

29. Charles' law.

    STEP 1: Change the temperatures from °C to K (i.e., K = °C + 273).

    $T_1 = 30°C + 273 = 303 K$

    $T_2 = -10°C + 273 = 263 K$

    STEP 2: Insert the known values into the equation.

    $$\frac{V_1}{T_1} = \frac{V_2}{T_2}$$

    $$\frac{200 \text{ ml}}{303 \text{ K}} = \frac{V_2}{263 \text{ K}}$$

    $$V_2 = \frac{(200 \text{ ml})(263 \text{ K})}{303 \text{ K}} = 173.6 \text{ ml}$$

30. Boyle's law.

    $$P_1V_1 = P_2V_2$$

    $$(780 \text{ mm Hg})(500 \text{ ml}) = (2,280 \text{ mm Hg})V_2$$

    $$V_2 = \frac{(780 \text{ mm Hg})(500 \text{ ml})}{(2,280 \text{ mm Hg})} = 171 \text{ ml}$$

31. Boyle's law.

    $$P_1V_1 = P_2V_2$$

    $$(101.33 \text{ kPa})(3.0 \text{ L}) = (P_2)(9.0 \text{ L})$$

    $$P_2 = \frac{(101.33 \text{ kPa})(3.0 \text{ L})}{(9.0 \text{ L})} = 33.78 \text{ kPa}$$

32. Combined gas law.

    STEP 1: Convert the temperatures from °C to K (i.e., K = °C + 273).

    $T_1 = 26°C + 273 = 299 K$

    $T_2 = 37°C + 273 = 310 K$

    STEP 2: Correct the pressures at their respective temperatures for the presence of P_{H_2O}. (See Table 4-8.)

    P_1 (corrected): 755 torr at 26°C contains a P_{H_2O} of 25.2 torr.

    P_1 (corrected) = 755 torr − 25.2 torr = 729.8 torr

    P_2 (corrected): 760 torr at 37°C contains a P_{H_2O} of 47 torr.

    P_2 (corrected) = 760 torr − 47 torr = 713 torr

    STEP 3: Insert the known values into the equation.

    $$\frac{P_1V_1}{T_1} = \frac{P_2V_2}{T_2}$$

    $$\frac{(729.8 \text{ torr})(V_1)}{299 \text{ K}} = \frac{(713 \text{ torr})(V_2)}{310 \text{ K}}$$

    $$V_1 = \frac{(299 \text{ K})(713 \text{ torr})V_2}{(729.8 \text{ torr})(310 \text{ K})}$$

$$V_1 = \frac{(213{,}187)V_2}{(226{,}238)}$$

$$V_1 = (0.942)(V_2), \text{ or}$$

$$V_2 = 1.062(V_1)$$

33. Dalton's law of partial pressures.

   STEP 1: Correct the pressure for the presence of P_{H_2O} at 20°C. (See Table 4-8.)

   $P_T(\text{corrected}) = 317 \text{ torr} - 17.5 \text{ torr} = 299.5 \text{ torr}$

   STEP 2: Determine the P_{CO_2}.

   $$P_T = P_{O_2} + P_{N_2} + P_{CO_2}$$

   $$299.5 \text{ torr} = 40 \text{ torr} + 200 \text{ torr} + P_{CO_2}$$

   $$P_{CO_2} = 299.5 \text{ torr} - 40 \text{ torr} - 200 \text{ torr}$$

   $$= 59.5 \text{ torr}$$

   STEP 3: Calculate the percentages of the constitutent gases.

   OXYGEN : $\dfrac{P_{O_2}}{P_T(\text{corrected})} \times 100 = \dfrac{40 \text{ torr}}{299.5 \text{ torr}} \times 100 = 13.3\%$

   NITROGEN : $\dfrac{P_{N_2}}{P_T(\text{corrected})} \times 100 = \dfrac{200 \text{ torr}}{299.5 \text{ torr}} \times 100 = 66.8\%$

   CARBON DIOXIDE : $\dfrac{P_{CO_2}}{P_T(\text{corrected})} \times 100 = \dfrac{59.5 \text{ torr}}{299.5 \text{ torr}} \times 100 = 19.9\%$

34. Ideal gas law.

   STEP 1: Convert the temperature from °C to K (i.e., K = °C + 273).

   $T = 50°C + 273 = 323 \text{ K}$

   STEP 2: Convert kPa to Pa.

   $1 \text{ kPa} = 1.00 \times 10^3 \text{ Pa}$

   $202.66 \text{ kPa} = 202.66 \times 10^3 \text{ Pa}$

   STEP 3: Convert the volume from liters to m³.

   $V = (40.0 \text{ L})(1.00 \times 10^{-3} \text{ m}^3/\text{L}) = 0.040 \text{ m}^3$

   STEP 4: Rearrange the ideal gas equation to solve for n, and insert known values.

   $$n = \frac{PV}{RT}$$

   $$n = \frac{(202.66 \times 10^3 \text{ Pa})(0.040 \text{ m}^3)}{(8.31 \text{ Pa} \cdot \text{m}^3/\text{mole} \cdot \text{K})(323 \text{ K})}$$

   $$= \frac{8106.4}{2{,}684.13 \text{ mole}^{-1}} = 3.0 \text{ moles}$$

35. Combined gas law.

   STEP 1: Convert the temperature from °C to K (i.e., K = °C + 273).

   $T_1 = 0°C + 273 = 273 \text{ K}$

   $T_2 = 37°C + 273 = 310 \text{ K}$

STEP 2: Correct the pressure at BTPS for the presence of P_{H_2O}. (See Table 4-8.)

P_2 (corrected) = 750 torr $-$ 47 torr = 703 torr

STEP 3: Insert the known values into the equation.

$$\frac{P_1 V_1}{T_1} = \frac{P_2 V_2}{T_2}$$

$$\frac{(760 \text{ torr})(V_1)}{273 \text{ K}} = \frac{(703 \text{ torr})(V_2)}{310 \text{ K}}$$

$$V_1 = \frac{(273 \text{ K})(703 \text{ torr})(V_2)}{(760 \text{ torr})(310 \text{ K})}$$

$$V_1 = \frac{(191{,}919)V_2}{(235{,}600)}$$

$$V_1 = (0.8146)(V_2), \text{ or}$$

$$V_2 = 1.2276(V_1)$$

36. Gay-Lussac's law.

STEP 1: Change the temperatures from °C to K (i.e., K = °C + 273).

$T_1 = 22°C + 273 = 295 \text{ K}$

$T_2 = 33°C + 273 = 306 \text{ K}$

STEP 2: Insert the known values into the equation.

$$\frac{P_1}{T_1} = \frac{P_2}{T_2}$$

$$\frac{2{,}200 \text{ psig}}{295 \text{ K}} = \frac{P_2}{306 \text{ K}}$$

$$P_2 = \frac{(2{,}200 \text{ psig})(306 \text{ K})}{(295 \text{ K})} = 2{,}282 \text{ psig}$$

37. Combined gas law.

STEP 1: Convert the temperatures from °C to K (i.e., K = °C + 273).

$T_1 = 27°C + 273 = 300 \text{ K}$

$T_2 = 37°C + 273 = 310 \text{ K}$

STEP 2: Insert the known values into the formula.

$$\frac{P_1 V_1}{T_1} = \frac{P_2 V_2}{T_2}$$

$$\frac{(100.26 \text{ kPa})(V_1)}{300 \text{ K}} = \frac{(101.33 \text{ kPa})(V_2)}{310 \text{ K}}$$

$$V_1 = \frac{(101.33 \text{ kPa})(300 \text{ K})(V_2)}{(100.26 \text{ kPa})(310 \text{ K})}$$

$$V_1 = \frac{(30{,}399)V_2}{(31{,}081)}$$

$$V_1 = (0.9781)(V_2), \text{ or}$$

$$V_2 = 1.0224(V_1)$$

38. Dalton's law of partial pressures and combined gas law.

    STEP 1:   Consult Table 4-8 to obtain the P_{H_2O} at 22°C.

          P_{H_2O} = 19.8 torr at 22°C

    STEP 2:   Convert the P_{H_2O} from mm Hg to cm H_2O.

$$\frac{1{,}034 \text{ cm } H_2O}{760 \text{ mm Hg}} = 1.36 \text{ cm } H_2O/\text{mm Hg}$$

$$P_{H_2O} \text{ (cm } H_2O) = P_{H_2O} \text{ (mm Hg)} \times 1.36 \text{ cm } H_2O/\text{mm Hg}$$
$$= (19.8 \text{ mm Hg})(1.36 \text{ cm } H_2O/\text{mm Hg})$$
$$= 26.9 \text{ cm } H_2O$$

    STEP 3:   Apply Dalton's law.

$$P_T = P_{\text{dry air}} + P_{H_2O}$$
$$P_{\text{dry air}} = P_T - P_{H_2O}$$
$$= 1{,}006 \text{ cm } H_2O - 26.9 \text{ cm } H_2O$$
$$= 979.1 \text{ cm } H_2O$$

    STEP 4:   Insert known values into the combined gas law.

$$\frac{P_1 V_1}{T_1} = \frac{P_2 V_2}{T_2}$$

$$\frac{(979.3 \text{ cm } H_2O)(100 \text{ ml})}{22°C} = \frac{(1{,}006 \text{ cm } H_2O)V_2}{22°C}$$

$$V_2 = \frac{(979.1 \text{ cm } H_2O)(100 \text{ ml})(22°C)}{(1{,}006 \text{ cm } H_2O)(22°C)} = 97.33 \text{ ml}$$

39. Combined gas law.

    STEP 1:   Convert the temperatures from °C to K (i.e., K = °C + 273).

          $T_1 = 37°C + 273 = 310 \text{ K}$

          $T_2 = 24°C + 273 = 297 \text{ K}$

    STEP 2:   Insert known values into the combined gas law.

$$\frac{P_1 V_1}{T_1} = \frac{P_2 V_2}{T_2}$$

$$\frac{(758 \text{ torr})(4.76 \text{ L})}{310 \text{ K}} = \frac{(753 \text{ torr})V_2}{297 \text{ K}}$$

$$V_2 = \frac{(758 \text{ torr})(4.76 \text{ L})(297 \text{ K})}{(753 \text{ torr})(310 \text{ K})} = 4.59 \text{ L}$$

40. Combined gas law.

    STEP 1:   Convert the temperatures from °C to K (i.e., K = °C + 273).

          $T_1 = 28°C + 273 = 301 \text{ K}$

          $T_2 = 0°C + 273 = 273 \text{ K}$

    STEP 2:   Insert known values into the formula.

$$\frac{P_1V_1}{T_1} = \frac{P_2V_2}{T_2}$$

$$\frac{(760 \text{ torr})(3.87 \text{ L})}{301 \text{ K}} = \frac{(760 \text{ torr})V_2}{273 \text{ K}}$$

$$V_2 = \frac{(760 \text{ torr})(3.87 \text{ L})(273 \text{ K})}{(760 \text{ torr})(301 \text{ K})} = 3.51 \text{ L}$$

41. Combined gas law.

STEP 1: Convert the temperatures from °C to K (i.e., K = °C + 273).

$$T_1 = 0°C + 273 = 273 \text{ K}$$

$$T_2 = 37°C + 273 = 310 \text{ K}$$

STEP 2: Insert known values into the combined gas law.

$$\frac{P_1V_1}{T_1} = \frac{P_2V_2}{T_2}$$

$$\frac{(760 \text{ torr})(5.55 \text{ L})}{273 \text{ K}} = \frac{(757 \text{ torr})V_2}{310 \text{ K}}$$

$$V_2 = \frac{(760 \text{ torr})(5.55 \text{ L})(310 \text{ K})}{(757 \text{ torr})(273 \text{ K})} = 6.33 \text{ L}$$

4–6 FLUID DYNAMICS

42. $(\dot{V}_s \times C_s) + (\dot{V}_{ENT} \times C_{ENT}) = (\dot{V}_{DEL} \times C_{DEL})$

Given: $C_{DEL} = 0.70$

$\dot{V}_s = 15 \text{ L/min}$

$C_s = 1.00$

$C_{ENT} = 0.21$

Since $\dot{V}_s + \dot{V}_{ENT} = \dot{V}_{DEL}$, and since $\dot{V}_s = 15 \text{ L/min}$,

$\dot{V}_{ENT} = X - 15 \text{ L/min}$

$\dot{V}_{DEL} = X$

$$(15 \text{ L/min} \times 1.0) + (X \times 0.21) = [(15 \text{ L/min} + X)0.70]$$

$$15 \text{ L/min} + 0.21X = 10.5 \text{ L/min} + 0.7X$$

$$15 \text{ L/min} - 10.5 \text{ L/min} = 0.7X - 0.21X$$

$$4.5 \text{ L/min} = 0.49X$$

$$X = \frac{4.5 \text{ L/min}}{0.49}$$

$$= 9 \text{ L/min}$$

$15 \text{ L/min} + X = \dot{V}_{DEL}$

$15 \text{ L/min} + 9 \text{ L/min} = 24 \text{ L/min}$

Answer: 24 L/min

43. $(4 \text{ L/min} \times 1.0) + (0.21 \times X) = [(4 \text{ L/min} \times X)0.28]$

$$4 \text{ L/min} + 0.21X = 1.12 \text{ L/min} + 0.28X$$

$$2.88 \text{ L/min} = 0.07X$$

$$X = \frac{2.88 \text{ L/min}}{0.07} = 41 \text{ L/min}$$

44. $\dot{V}_{ENT}/\dot{V}_S = $ air:O_2 ratio

$$\frac{41 \text{ L/min}}{4 \text{ L/min}} = 10.2:1$$

45. $[(X - 10 \text{ L/min})1.0] + (10 \text{ L/min} \times 0.21) = (X \times 0.60)$

$$1X - 10 \text{ L/min} + 2.1 \text{ L/min} = 0.6X$$

$$1X - 0.6X = 10 \text{ L/min} - 2.1 \text{ L/min}$$

$$0.4X = 7.9 \text{ L/min}$$

$$X = \frac{7.9 \text{ L/min}}{0.4}$$

$$\approx 20 \text{ L/min}$$

$\dot{V}_{DEL} = X - 10 \text{ L/min}$

$= 20 \text{ L/min} - 10 \text{ L/min}$

$= 10 \text{ L/min}$

Answer: 10 L/min

46. $\dfrac{\dot{V}_{ENT}}{\dot{V}_S} = \dfrac{10 \text{ L/min}}{10 \text{ L/min}} = 1:1$

47. $\dot{V}_S + \dot{V}_{ENT} = \dot{V}_{DEL}$

$$15 \text{ L/min} + 60 \text{ L/min} = 75 \text{ L/min}$$

$$(15 \text{ L/min} \times 1.0) + (60 \text{ L/min} \times 0.21) = X(75 \text{ L/min})$$

$$15 \text{ L/min} + 12.6 \text{ L/min} = 75X \text{ L/min}$$

$$X = \frac{27.6 \text{ L/min}}{75 \text{ L/min}}$$

$$= 0.37$$

Answer: 0.37 F_IO_2

48. $[(X - 60 \text{ L/min})1.0] + (60 \text{ L/min} \times 0.21) = X(0.24)$

$$X - 60 \text{ L/min} + 12.6 \text{ L/min} = 0.24X$$

$$0.76X = 47.4 \text{ L/min}$$

$$X = \frac{47.4 \text{ L/min}}{0.76}$$

$$X \approx 62 \text{ L/min}$$

$$\dot{V}_{DEL} = \dot{V}_S + \dot{V}_{ENT}$$
$$62 \text{ L/min} = X + 60 \text{ L/min}$$
$$X = 62 \text{ L/min} - 60 \text{ L/min}$$
$$X = 2 \text{ L/min}$$

Answer: 2 L/min $\dot{V}_S$; 62 L/min $\dot{V}_{DEL}$

49. $(10 \text{ L/min} \times 1.0) + (X \times 0.21) = [(X + 10 \text{ L/min})0.54]$
$$10 \text{ L/min} + 0.21X = 0.54X + 5.4 \text{ L/min}$$
$$0.33X = 4.6 \text{ L/min}$$
$$X = \frac{4.6 \text{ L/min}}{0.33}$$
$$X \approx 14 \text{ L/min}$$

$$\dot{V}_{DEL} = \dot{V}_S + \dot{V}_{ENT}$$
$$= 10 \text{ L/min} + 14 \text{ L/min}$$
$$= 24 \text{ L/min}$$

Answer: 24 L/min $\dot{V}_{DEL}$

50. $(10 \text{ L/min} \times 1.0) + (30 \text{ L/min} \times 0.21) = (40 \text{ L/min})X$
$$10 \text{ L/min} + 6.3 \text{ L/min} = 40X \text{ L/min}$$
$$X = \frac{16.3 \text{ L/min}}{40 \text{ L/min}}$$
$$X = 0.4$$

Answer: 0.4 F_IO_2

51. $\dfrac{\dot{V}_{ENT}}{\dot{V}_S} = \dfrac{30 \text{ L/min}}{10 \text{ L/min}} = 3{:}1$

52. Series resistances:
$$R_T = R_1 + R_2 + R_3$$

$$R_1 = \frac{4 \text{ torr}}{2 \text{ L/sec}} = 2 \text{ torr/L/sec}$$

$$R_2 = \frac{5 \text{ torr}}{2 \text{ L/sec}} = 2.5 \text{ torr/L/sec}$$

$$R_3 = \frac{6 \text{ torr}}{2 \text{ L/sec}} = 3 \text{ torr/L/sec}$$

$$R_T = 2 \text{ torr/L/sec} + 2.5 \text{ torr/L/sec} + 3 \text{ torr/L/sec}$$
$$= 7.5 \text{ torr/L/sec}$$

Answers: $R_1 = 2$ torr/L/sec; $R_2 = 2.5$ torr/L/sec; $R_3 = 3$ torr/L/sec; $R_T = 7.5$ torr/L/sec

53. Parallel resistances:

$$\frac{1}{R_T} = \frac{1}{R_1} + \frac{1}{R_2} + \frac{1}{R_3}$$

$$R_1 = \frac{9 \text{ cm H}_2\text{O}}{3 \text{ L/min}} = 3 \text{ cm H}_2\text{O/L/min}$$

$$R_2 = \frac{12 \text{ cm H}_2\text{O}}{3 \text{ L/min}} = 4 \text{ cm H}_2\text{O/L/min}$$

$$R_3 = \frac{15 \text{ cm H}_2\text{O}}{3 \text{ L/min}} = 5 \text{ cm H}_2\text{O/L/min}$$

$$\frac{1}{R_T} = \frac{1}{3 \text{ cm H}_2\text{O/L/min}} + \frac{1}{4 \text{ cm H}_2\text{O/L/min}} + \frac{1}{5 \text{ cm H}_2\text{O/L/min}}$$

$$\frac{1}{R_T} = 0.33 \text{ L/min/cm H}_2\text{O} + 0.25 \text{ L/min/cm H}_2\text{O} + 0.2 \text{ L/min/cm H}_2\text{O}$$

$$\frac{1}{R_T} = 0.78 \text{ L/min/cm H}_2\text{O}$$

$$R_T = \frac{1}{0.78 \text{ L/min/cm H}_2\text{O}}$$
$$= 1.28 \text{ cm H}_2\text{O/L/min}$$

Answers: $R_1 = 3$ cm H_2O/L/min; $R_2 = 4$ cm H_2O/L/min; $R_3 = 5$ cm H_2O/L/min; $R_T = 1.28$ cm H_2O/L/min

54. 760 mm Hg = 1,034 cm H_2O

$$R_{aw} = \frac{\Delta P}{V} = \frac{1,034 \text{ cm H}_2\text{O} - 1,029 \text{ cm H}_2\text{O}}{3.5 \text{ L/sec}}$$
$$= 1.4 \text{ cm H}_2\text{O/L/sec}$$

Answer: 1.4 cm H_2O/L/sec, or 1.1 mm Hg/L/sec

55. $\dot{V}_I = \dfrac{\dot{V}_T}{T_I} = \dfrac{0.8 \text{ L}}{2 \text{ sec}} = 0.4$ L/sec

$$R_{aw} = \frac{759 \text{ mm Hg} - 754 \text{ mm Hg}}{\dot{V}_I}$$

$$\frac{5 \text{ mm Hg}}{0.4 \text{ L/sec}} = 12.5 \text{ mm Hg/L/sec}$$

Answer: 12.5 mm Hg/L/sec

56. Series and parallal resistances combination:

$$R_T = R_{T\text{SERIES}} + R_{T\text{PARALLEL}}$$

Series resistances:

$$R_1 = \frac{4 \text{ cm H}_2\text{O}}{2 \text{ L/sec}} = 2 \text{ cm H}_2\text{O/L/sec}$$

$$R_2 = \frac{6 \text{ cm H}_2\text{O}}{2 \text{ L/sec}} = 3 \text{ cm H}_2\text{O/L/sec}$$

$$R_T = 2 \text{ cm } H_2O/L/sec + 3 \text{ cm } H_2O/L/sec$$
$$= 5 \text{ cm } H_2O/L/sec$$

Parallel resistances:

$$R_3 = \frac{10 \text{ cm } H_2O}{2 \text{ L/sec}} = 5 \text{ cm } H_2O/L/sec$$

$$R_4 = \frac{8 \text{ cm } H_2O}{2 \text{ L/sec}} = 4 \text{ cm } H_2O/L/sec$$

$$R_5 = \frac{6 \text{ cm } H_2O}{2 \text{ L/sec}} = 3 \text{ cm } H_2O/L/sec$$

$$R_6 = \frac{4 \text{ cm } H_2O}{2 \text{ L/sec}} = 2 \text{ cm } H_2O/L/sec$$

$$\frac{1}{R_T} = 1/5 \text{ cm } H_2O/L/sec + 1/4 \text{ cm } H_2O/L/sec + 1/3 \text{ cm } H_2O/L/sec$$
$$+ 1/2 \text{ cm } H_2O/L/sec$$

$$\frac{1}{R_T} = 0.2 \text{ L/sec/cm } H_2O + 0.25 \text{ L/sec/cm } H_2O + 0.33 \text{ L/sec/cm } H_2O$$
$$+ 0.5 \text{ L/sec/cm } H_2O$$

$$\frac{1}{R_T} = 1.28 \text{ L/sec/cm } H_2O$$

$$R_T = \frac{1}{1.28 \text{ L/sec/cm } H_2O} = 0.78 \text{ cm } H_2O/L/sec$$

Combination: $R_T = R_{T_{SERIES}} + R_{T_{PARALLEL}}$

$$R_T = 5 \text{ cm } H_2O/L/sec + 0.78 \text{ cm } H_2O/L/sec$$
$$R_T = 5.78 \text{ cm } H_2O/L/sec$$

Answer: 5.78 cm H_2O/L/sec

57.

$$\frac{1}{C_T} = \frac{1}{C_L} + \frac{1}{C_{CW}}$$

$$\frac{1}{0.1 \text{ L/ cm } H_2O} = \frac{1}{0.2 \text{ L/ cm } H_2O} + \frac{1}{C_{CW}}$$

$$\frac{1}{C_{CW}} = \frac{1}{0.1 \text{ L/ cm } H_2O} - \frac{1}{0.2 \text{ L/ cm } H_2O}$$

$$\frac{1}{C_{CW}} = 10 \text{ cm } H_2O/L - 5 \text{ cm } H_2O/L$$

$$\frac{1}{C_{CW}} = 5 \text{ cm } H_2O/L$$

$$C_{CW} = \frac{1}{5 \text{ cm } H_2O/L}$$

$$C_{CW} = 0.2 \text{ L/cm } H_2O$$

Answer: 0.2 L/cm H_2O C_{CW}

58. $C_L = \dfrac{\Delta V}{\Delta P} = \dfrac{0.5 \text{ L}}{2.5 \text{ cm } H_2O} = 0.2 \text{ L/cm } H_2O$

Answer: $C_L = 0.2$ L/cm H_2O, or 200 cc/cm H_2O

59.
$$\frac{1}{C_L} = E_L$$

$$\frac{1}{0.2 \text{ L/cm H}_2\text{O}} = 5 \text{ cm H}_2\text{O/L}$$

Answer: $E_L = 5 \text{ cm H}_2\text{O/L}$, or 0.005 cm H_2O/cc

60. $\dfrac{1}{C_{cw}} = 13.9 \text{ cm H}_2\text{O/L} - \dfrac{1}{0.12 \text{ L/cm H}_2\text{O}}$

$$\frac{1}{C_{cw}} = 13.9 \text{ cm H}_2\text{O/L} - 8.3 \text{ cm H}_2\text{O/L}$$

$$\frac{1}{C_{cw}} = 5.6 \text{ cm H}_2\text{O/L}$$

$$C_{cw} = \frac{1}{5.6 \text{ cm H}_2\text{O/L}} = 0.18 \text{ L/cm H}_2\text{O}$$

Answer: 0.18 L/cm H_2O C_{cw}

61.
$$\frac{1}{C_{cw}} = E_{cw}$$

$$\frac{1}{0.18 \text{ L/cm H}_2\text{O}} = E_{cw}$$

$E_{cw} = 5.6 \text{ cm H}_2\text{O/L}$

Answer: 5.6 cm H_2O/L E_{cw}

62. time constant = $R_{aw} \times 1/E_T$
$= (4 \text{ cm H}_2\text{O/L/sec})(1/1.5 \text{ cm H}_2\text{O/L})$
$= (4 \text{ cm H}_2\text{O/L/sec})(0.67 \text{ L/cm H}_2\text{O})$
$= 2.7 \text{ sec}$

Answer: 2.7 seconds is the length of one time constant

63. a) $1 \times 0.75 \text{ sec} = 0.75 \text{ sec}$ (time of 1 time constant)
b) $2 \times 0.75 \text{ sec} = 1.5 \text{ sec}$ (time of 2 time constants)
c) $3 \times 0.75 \text{ sec} = 2.25 \text{ sec}$ (time of 3 time constants)
Answer: (a) 0.75 sec, (b) 1.5 sec, (c) 2.25 sec

64. *Answer:*   4 time constants

65. Alveolus A: time constant = $(2 \text{ cm H}_2\text{O/L/sec})(0.05 \text{ L/cm H}_2\text{O})$
$= 0.1 \text{ second}$

Alveolus B: time constant = $(4 \text{ cm H}_2\text{O/L/sec})(0.125 \text{ L/cm H}_2\text{O})$
$= 0.5 \text{ second}$

Answers: alveolus A, 0.1 second; alveolus B, 0.5 second

66. Alveolus A: $\dfrac{0.5 \text{ second}}{0.1 \text{ second/time constant}} = 5 \text{ time constants}$

Based on the exponentially increasing alveolar pressure-time constant curve, an alveolus will be 99% filled at 5 time constants, 0.5 second in this case.

Alveolus B: $\dfrac{0.5 \text{ second}}{0.5 \text{ second/time constant}} = 1 \text{ time constant}$

Based on the exponentially increasing alveolar pressure-time constant curve, an alveolus will be 63% filled at 1 time constant, 0.5 second in this case.

Answers: Alveolus A: (a) 5 time constants; (b) 99% filled

Alveolus B: (a) 1 time constant; (b) 63% filled

67. $P = \dfrac{2\,ST}{r}$

STEP 1: Convert the diameter to radius and the units to cm.

$$r = \frac{d}{2} = \frac{2\ mm}{2} = 1\ mm$$

$$1\ mm = 1\ mm \times 0.1\ cm/mm = 0.1\ cm$$

STEP 2: Insert the known values into the law of LaPlace.

$$1.014 \times 10^4\ dynes/cm^2 = \frac{2\,ST}{10^{-1}\ cm}$$

$$ST = 507\ dynes/cm$$

68. $P = \dfrac{2\,ST}{r} = \dfrac{(2)(35\ dynes/cm)}{0.35\ cm} = 200\ dynes/cm^2$

69. *Sphere X*   *Sphere Y*

$P = \dfrac{12\ dynes/cm}{0.005\ cm}$ $P = \dfrac{12\ dynes/cm}{0.0025\ cm}$

$P = 2{,}400\ dynes/cm^2$ $P = 4{,}800\ dynes/cm^2$

Answers: Sphere X = 2,400 dynes/cm²; *Sphere Y* = 4,800 dynes/cm². If the two spheres were in communication with each other, *Sphere Y* would empty into *Sphere X* because *Sphere Y* has the greater pressure. Gas would flow from the high pressure sphere to the low pressure sphere.

4-8 STARLING'S LAW OF THE CAPILLARIES

70. *STEP 1:* Determine the molecular weight of NaCl

$$Na + Cl = NaCl$$

$$23\ amu + 35\ amu = 58\ amu$$

STEP 2: One NaCl molecule ionizes into two ions.

STEP 3: Determine the molarity of 0.45% NaCl.

$$\frac{4.5\ g}{58\ g/mole} = 0.078\ mole\ of\ NaCl$$

$$M = \frac{0.078\ mole}{1\ liter} = 0.078\ M$$

STEP 4: Insert known values into the equation

$$\left(\frac{mole}{liter}\right)\left(\frac{\#\ of\ ionic}{species/molecule}\right)\left(\frac{19{,}304\ torr}{mole/liter}\right) = osmotic\ pressure$$

$$(0.078 \text{ M})(2)\left(\frac{19{,}304 \text{ torr}}{\text{mole/liter}}\right) = 3{,}011 \text{ torr}$$

Answer: 3,011 torr

71. *STEP 1:* H_2SO_4 = 98 amu

$$\boxed{\text{1 component}}$$
$$\downarrow$$

STEP 2: $H_2SO_4 \rightarrow 2H^+ + SO_4^{2-}$
$$\uparrow$$
$$\boxed{\text{2 components}}$$

(3 ionic components/H_2SO_4 molecule)

STEP 3: $\dfrac{196 \text{ g}}{98 \text{ g/mole}} = 2 \text{ moles}$

$$M = \dfrac{2 \text{ moles}}{1 \text{ liter}} = 2 \text{ M}$$

STEP 4: $(2 \text{ M})(3)\left(\dfrac{19{,}304 \text{ torr}}{\text{mole/liter}}\right) = 115{,}824 \text{ torr}$

Answer: 115, 824 torr

72. *STEP 1:* $\dfrac{33 \text{ g}}{100 \text{ g/mole}} = 0.33 \text{ mole}$

STEP 2: $M = \dfrac{0.33 \text{ mole}}{1 \text{ liter}} = 0.33 \text{ M}$

STEP 3: $(0.33 \text{ M})\left(\dfrac{19{,}304 \text{ torr}}{\text{mole/liter}}\right) = 6{,}370 \text{ torr}$

Answer: 6,370 torr

73. $\dfrac{\text{molecular weight}}{\text{\# of ionic species/molecule}} = \text{weight of 1 osmol}$

a. HCl: $\dfrac{36 \text{ g}}{2} = 18 \text{ g/osmol}$

b. H_2SO_4: $\dfrac{98 \text{ g}}{3} = 32.7 \text{ g/osmol}$

c. $Al_2(SO_4)_3$: $\dfrac{342 \text{ g}}{5} = 68.4 \text{ g/osmol}$

d. $NaHCO_3$: $\dfrac{84 \text{ g}}{2} = 42 \text{ g/osmol}$

Answers: a. 18 g/osmol; b. 32.7 g/osmol; c. 68.4 g/osmol; d. 42 g/osmol

74. a. $\dfrac{18 \text{ g/osmol}}{1{,}000 \text{ mosmol/osmol}} = 0.018 \text{ g/mosmol}$

b. $\dfrac{32.7 \text{ g/osmol}}{1,000 \text{ mosmol/osmol}} = 0.033 \text{ g/mosmol}$

c. $\dfrac{68.4 \text{ g/osmol}}{1,000 \text{ mosmol/osmol}} = 0.068 \text{ g/osmol}$

d. $\dfrac{42 \text{ g/osmol}}{1,000 \text{ mosmol/osmol}} = 0.042 \text{ g/mosmol}$

Answers: a. 0.018 g/mosmol; b. 0.033 g/mosmol; c. 0.068 g/mosmol; d. 0.042 g/mosmol

75. $X = \dfrac{B^2}{A + 2B} = \dfrac{(60)^2}{30 + 2(60)} = \dfrac{3,600}{150} = 24$

24 ions (12 cations + 12 anions) migrated from compartment 2 to compartment 1 at equilibrium. The predicted distribution of solutes at equilibrium would be:

Compartment 1	Compartment 2
$[Na^+] = 27$	$[Na^+] = 18$
$[HCO_3^-] = 12$	$[HCO_3^-] = 18$
$[X^-] = 15$	

76. $[Na^+]_1 \times [HCO_3^-]_1 = [Na^+]_2 \times [HCO_3^-]_2$

$27 \times 12 = 18 \times 18$

$324 = 324$

77.

Systemic Capillary

Arterial end of capillary		*Venous end of capillary*	
Interstitium			Interstitium
Capillary endothelium		Capillary endothelium	
CHP	COP	CHP	COP
36 torr	32 torr	30 torr	32 torr
Capillary endothelium		Capillary endothelium	
Interstitium			Interstitium
IHP	IOP	IHP	IOP
5 torr	5 torr	5 torr	5 torr

Arterial end of capillary
1. hydrostatic pressure gradient
   36 torr − 5 torr = 31 torr
2. osmotic pressure gradient
   32 torr − 5 torr = 27 torr
3. filtration pressure
   31 torr − 27 torr = 4 torr

Venous end of capillary
1. hydrostatic pressure gradient
   30 torr − 5 torr = 25 torr
2. osmotic pressure gradient
   32 torr − 5 torr = 27 torr
3. reabsorption pressure
   27 torr − 25 torr = 2 torr

4. filtration-reabsorption pressure gradient
   4 torr − 2 torr = 2 torr

78.   *Arterial end of capillary*   *Venous end of capillary*
1. hydrostatic pressure gradient   1. hydrostatic pressure gradient
40 torr − (−3 torr) = 43 torr   20 torr − (−3 torr) = 23 torr
2. oncotic pressure gradient   2. oncotic pressure gradient
25 torr − 4 torr = 21 torr   30 torr − 4 torr = 26 torr
3. filtration pressure   3. reabsorption gradient
43 torr − 21 torr = 22 torr   26 torr − 23 torr = 3 torr
4. filtration − reabsorption pressure gradient
22 torr − 3 torr = 19 torr

CHAPTER 5 - STATISTICS

5-3 PROBABILITY

1. a. There are three favorable outcomes that result in a sum of 10. The are (5,5), (4,6), and (6,4), and there are a total of 36 possible events, e.g., (1,1), (5,3), (6,1), (6,6), and (4,3). Thus,

$$P(A) = \frac{3}{36} = \frac{1}{12}$$

   b. The number of favorable outcomes for B is 11, as a result of observing any one of the following:

   (1,5), (5,1), (2,4), (4,2), (3,3)

   (3,6), (6,3), (4,5), (5,4)

   (5,6), (6,5)

   Thus, $P(B) = \dfrac{11}{36}$

2. a. A player loses on the first roll if the sum is 2. A 2 results only if the event (1,1) is observed.

   Therefore, chances of losing on the first roll are $\dfrac{1}{36}$.

   b. A player wins on the first roll if the sum is either 7 or 11. A 7 or 11 results if any one of the following 8 favorable outcomes is observed:

   (1,6), (6,1), (2,5), (5,2), (3,4), (4,3), (5,6), (6,5)

   Therefore, chances of winning are $\dfrac{8}{36}$.

   c. If the sum is 3 on the first roll, then the game can end on the second roll if either of the following results is observed:

   (i)   If the sum is 3 on the second roll, the player wins.

   (ii) If the sum is either a 7 or 11 on the second roll, the player loses.

   (iii) If the sum is a 2 on the second roll, the player loses.

The events that are favorable to these three cases are shown below.

(i)   (1,2), (2,1) → 2 events

(ii)   8 events (see (b))

(iii)   (1,1)

Therefore, chances are

$$\frac{2+8+1}{36} = \frac{11}{36}$$

3. Let B_1, B_2, B_3 denote the three blue marbles and R_1 and R_2 denote the two red marbles in the bin. All possible events of drawing two marbles at random are given by:

$$B_1B_2, B_1B_3, B_1R_1, B_1R_2, B_2B_3, B_2R_1, B_2R_2, B_3R_1, B_3R_2, R_1R_2$$

So, there are 10 possible events.

a. Chances that both marbles are blue $= \dfrac{3}{10}$, or 30%.

b. Chances that one is red and the other is blue $= \dfrac{6}{10}$, or 60%.

4. a. 30% + 20% = 50%

   b. 20% + 15% + 15% = 50%

5-4 NORMAL DISTRIBUTION

5. a. *STEP 1:*   Convert 95 beats/min to a z-score.

$$z = \frac{x - \mu}{\sigma} = \frac{95 - 72}{9} = 2.56$$

   STEP 2:   Find the area between 0 and 2.56 by using Table 1, Appendix C. The area is 0.4948.

   STEP 3:   Add 0.5 to 0.4948 to obtain the area below 95 beats/min. Thus, the required percentage is 99.48%.

   b. *STEP 1:*   Convert 54 to a z-score $z = \dfrac{54 - 72}{9} = -2$

   STEP 2:   Find the area between 0 and 2 from Table 1, Appendix C. The area is 0.4772.

   STEP 3:   Subtract 0.4772 from 0.5 to obtain the area below −2 (54 beats/min).

$$\% \text{ below 54 beats/min} = 0.5 - 0.4772 = 2.28\%$$

   c. *STEP 1:*   Convert 54 to a z-score. $z = \dfrac{54 - 72}{9} = -2$

   Convert 90 to a z-score. $z = \dfrac{90 - 72}{9} = 2$

   STEP 2:   Find the area between 0 and 2 from Table 1, Appendix C. This area is 0.4772.

STEP 3: Double the area between 0 and 2 to obtain the area between −2 and 2. Thus, the percent between 54 beats/min and 90 beats/min is 2(0.4772), or 95.44%.

d. STEP 1: Convert 54 to a z-score. $z = \dfrac{90 - 72}{9} = 2$

STEP 2: Find the area between 0 and 2.

STEP 3: Subtract the area between 0 and 2 (which is 0.4772) from 0.5 to obtain the area above 2.

Thus, 0.5 − 0.4772 is 0.0228, or 2.28%.

6. a. Determine the standard score by searching for 0.45 in the body of Table 1, Appendix C, and find the corresponding z-score. The z-score is 1.64 (or 1.65). Thus the 95th percentile heart rate is 1.64 standard deviations above the mean. Therefore, the percentile score is the mean plus 1.64 multiplied by the standard deviation, or

$$\text{percentile score} = 12 + (1.64 \times 3)$$
$$= 16.92$$

b. Determine the standard score by searching for 0.475 in the body of Table 1, Appendix C, and find the corresponding standard score (i.e., z-score). The z-score is 1.96, meaning that the 97.5th percentile score is 1.96 standard deviations above the mean. Therefore, the percentile score is the mean plus 1.96 multiplied by the standard deviation, or

$$\text{percentile score} = 12 + (1.96 \times 3)$$
$$= 17.88$$

5-5 SAMPLING DISTRIBUTION

7. a. Since an n of 36 is large, the sampling distribution of the sample mean ($\bar{x}$) is normally distributed with a mean ($\mu_{\bar{x}}$) of 930 and a standard deviation ($\sigma_{\bar{x}}$) of

$$\frac{\sigma}{\sqrt{n}} = \frac{120}{\sqrt{36}} = 20.$$

b. STEP 1: Convert 910 to a z-score. $z = \dfrac{910 - 930}{20} = -1$

STEP 2: Find the area between 0 and 1 from Table 1, Appendix C. The area is 0.3413.

STEP 3: Subtract 0.3413 from 0.5.

$$0.5 - 0.3413 = 0.1587$$

Thus, the chance that the same mean retardation score is more than 910 is 0.1587, or 15.87%.

c. STEP 1: Convert 950 to a z-score. $z = \dfrac{950 - 930}{20} = 1$

Convert 970 to a z-score. $z = \dfrac{970 - 930}{20} = 2$

STEP 2: Find the area between 0 and 1. The area is 0.3413.

Find the area between 0 and 2. The area is 0.4772 (Table 1, Appendix C).

STEP 3: Subtract 0.3413 from 0.4772 to obtain the area between 1 and 2.

$$0.4772 - 0.3413 = 0.1359$$

Therefore, the chance that the sample mean retardation score is between 950 and 970 is 0.1359, or 13.59%.

5-6 CONFIDENCE INTERVALS FOR THE MEAN

8. *STEP 1:* Since a 95% confidence interval is sought, α equals 5% and $\frac{\alpha}{2}$ equals 2.5%, or 0.025.

STEP 2: Locate the z-score (Table 1, Appendix C) for $z_{0.025}$.

Thus, $z_{0.025} = 1.96$.

STEP 3: Calculate the 95% confidence interval (CI).

$$CI = 12 \pm \left(1.96 \times \frac{2.5}{\sqrt{32}}\right) = (12 - 0.87, 12 + 0.87) = (11.13, 12.87)$$

9. *STEP 1:* Since a 99% confidence interval is sought, α equals 0.01, and $\frac{\alpha}{2}$ equals 0.005.

STEP 2: Locate the z-score (Table 1, Appendix C) for $z_{0.005}$.

Thus, $z_{0.005} = 2.575$.

STEP 3: Calculate the 99% confidence interval.

$$CI = 12 \pm \left(2.575 \times \frac{2.5}{\sqrt{32}}\right) = (12 - 1.14, 12 + 1.14) = (10.86, 13.14)$$

5-7 SAMPLE SIZE DETERMINATION

10. a. Because a 95% confidence interval is sought, α equals 5% and $\frac{\alpha}{2}$ equals 0.025. Therefore, $z_{0.025}$ is 1.96 (Table 1, Appendix C).

Since, the estimate sought needs to be within 2 units, the margin of error (E) is 2. Since σ equals 15, the sample size n is calculated by:

$$n = \left\lceil \frac{z_{0.025} \times \sigma}{E} \right\rceil^2 = \left\lceil \frac{1.96 \times 15}{2} \right\rceil^2 = 216.09 \approx 216$$

Since each observation costs $10, and at least 216 ($n$) observations are needed, $2,160.00 is required. Therefore, insufficient funds exist.

b. Since a 90% confidence interval is required, α equals 10% and $\frac{\alpha}{2}$ equals 0.05. Thus, $z_{0.05}$ is 1.64. E = 2 and $\sigma = 15$ [as in part (a)]. Thus,

$$n = \left\lceil \frac{1.64 \times 15}{2} \right\rceil^2 = 151.29 \approx 151$$

Thus, there are suffcient funds available, as we need at least 151 observations (meaning at least $1,510.00).

5–8 SMALL SAMPLE CONFIDENCE INTERVAL FOR MEAN

11. a. *STEP 1:* Since a 95% confidence interval is sought, α equals 5% and $\frac{\alpha}{2}$ equals 0.025.

    STEP 2: Since the sample size (n) is 16, the d.f. equals 15. Locate $t_{0.025}$ with 15 d.f. in Table 2, Appendix C. Thus, $t_{0.025,15} = 2.131$.

    STEP 3: Calculate the 95% confidence interval (CI).

$$CI = 40.3 \pm \left(2.131 \times \frac{16.0}{\sqrt{15}}\right) = (40.3 - 8.8, 40.3 + 8.8) = (31.5, 49.1)$$

  b. *STEP 1:* $\alpha = 0.01, \frac{\alpha}{2} = 0.005$.

    STEP 2: $n = 16$, d.f. $= 16 - 1 = 15$. Thus, $t_{0.005,15} = 2.947$.

    STEP 3: Calculate the 99% confidence interval.

$$CI = 40.3 \pm \left(2.947 \times \frac{16.0}{\sqrt{15}}\right) = (40.3 - 12.17, 40.3 + 12.17) = (28.13, 52.47)$$

12. a. *STEP 1:* $\alpha = 0.005, \frac{\alpha}{2} = 0.025$.

    STEP 2: Pentobarbitol: $n = 191$, d.f. $= 190$, $t_{0.025,190} \approx z_{0.025} = 1.96$

$$CI = 0.99 \pm \left(1.96 \times \frac{0.235}{\sqrt{191}}\right) = (0.99 - 0.033, 0.99 + 0.033) = (0.957, 1.023)$$

    Urethane: $n = 13$, d.f. $= 12$, $t_{0.025,12} = 2.179$.

$$CI = 1.47 \pm \left(2.179 \times \frac{0.314}{\sqrt{13}}\right) = (1.47 - 0.19, 1.47 + 0.19) = (1.28, 1.66)$$

    Ketamine: $n = 16$, d.f. $= 15$, $t_{0.025,15} = 2.131$.

$$CI = 0.99 \pm \left(2.131 \times \frac{0.164}{\sqrt{16}}\right) = (0.99 - 0.087, 0.99 + 0.087) = (0.903, 1.077)$$

  b. The confidence interval would be much wider. The larger the sample size, the shorter the interval as long as other variables are held constant.

    If n is 13, then d.f. equals 12, and $t_{0.025,12}$ is 2.179.

    Thus, the new CI for Pentobarbitol would be:

$$CI = 0.99 \pm \left(2.179 \times \frac{0.235}{\sqrt{13}}\right) = (0.99 - 0.14, 0.99 + 0.14) = (0.85, 1.13)$$

    Comparing this confidence interval with (0.957, 1.023), the new interval is much wider.

  c. See part (b).

5–10 TESTING OF HYPOTHESIS FOR MEAN

13. a. *STEP 1:* Set up the hypothesis, i.e., $H_o: \mu = 16$, $H_a: \mu > 16$.

    STEP 2: $\alpha = 0.01$

STEP 3: Calculate the test statistic.

$$\frac{\bar{x} - \mu_0}{s/\sqrt{n}} = \frac{18 - 16}{6/\sqrt{40}} = 2.108$$

STEP 4: Define the rejection region. Reject H_o if the test statistic $> z_{0.01} = 2.33$.

STEP 5: Decide whether or not to reject H_o. Since the test statistic 2.108 is not bigger than 2.33, H_o is not rejected.

STEP 6: Conclusion: Based on the data, there is not enough evidence to believe that the average time spent on emergency-related chores is more than 16 person-hours at an α of 0.01.

b. Subtract 0.4826 from 0.5 to obtain the *p*-value. The *p*-value $= 0.5 - 0.4826 = 0.0174$.

14. a. *STEP 1:* $H_o: \mu \geq 3$, $H_a: \mu < 3$.

STEP 2: $\alpha = 0.001$

STEP 3: Calculate the test statistic.

$$\frac{2.1 - 3}{1.5/\sqrt{26}} = -3.06$$

STEP 4: Define the rejection region. Reject H_o if the test statistic $< t_{0.001,25} = -3.45$.

STEP 5: Do not reject H_o.

STEP 6: Not enough evidence exists to conclude that the average stay is less than 3 months at an α of 0.001.

b. Try to locate 3.06 in the row of 25 d.f. in Table 2, Appendix C.

3.06 is located between $t_{0.001,25}$ and $t_{0.005,25}$

Thus, the *p*-value is between 0.001 and 0.005.

15. *STEP 1:* $H_o: \mu = 48.6$, $H_a: \mu \neq 48.6$.

STEP 2: $\alpha = 0.05$

STEP 3: Calculate the test statistic.

$$\frac{44 - 48.6}{8/\sqrt{25}} = -2.875$$

STEP 4: Determine the rejection region. Reject H_o if the test statistic $< -t_{\frac{0.05}{2},24} = -t_{0.025,24} = -2.064$ or if the test statistic > 2.064.

STEP 5: Reject H_o because the test statistic < -2.064.

STEP 6: There is enough evidence to believe that heroin addicts' self-worth assessment mean score is different from the general male population mean score of 48.6.

5-11 COMPARING MEANS OF TWO POPULATIONS (OR GROUPS): INDEPENDENT SAMPLES

16. a. *STEP 1:* Since a 90% confidence interval is sought, $\alpha = 10\%$ and $\frac{\alpha}{2} = 0.05$.

STEP 2: Since n_1 and n_2 are small, use t. d.f. $= n_1 + n_2 - 2 = 8 + 6 - 2 = 12$. Thus, $t_{0.005,12} = 1.782$.

STEP 3: Calculate $s_P^2 = \dfrac{(n_1 - 1)s_1^2 + (n_2 - 1)s_2^2}{n_1 + n_2 - 2}$

Thus,

$$s_P^2 = \frac{(8 - 1) \times 14.80^2 + (6 - 1) \times 13.69^2}{8 + 6 - 2} = 205.86$$

STEP 4: Calculate $\bar{x}_1 - \bar{x}_2 = 70.75 - 77.33 = -6.58$

STEP 5: Calculate the 90% confidence interval (CI).

$$CI = -6.58 \pm 1.782 \sqrt{205.86\left(\frac{1}{8} + \frac{1}{6}\right)}$$

$$= -6.58 \pm 13.8$$

$$= (-6.58 - 13.8, -6.58 + 13.8)$$

$$= (-20.38, 7.22)$$

Since the confidence interval for the difference includes zero, there is no evidence to indicate a statistical difference between the means.

b. *STEP 1:* $H_o: \mu_1 = \mu_2, H_a: \mu_1 \neq \mu_2$.

   STEP 2: $\alpha = 0.1$

   STEP 3: Calculate the test statistic.

$$\frac{(\bar{x}_1 - \bar{x}_2)}{\sqrt{s_P^2\left(\frac{1}{n_1} + \frac{1}{n_2}\right)}} = \frac{-6.58}{\sqrt{205.86\left(\frac{1}{8} + \frac{1}{6}\right)}} = -0.849$$

   STEP 4: Define the rejection region. Reject H_o, if the test statistic $< -t_{0.025,12} = -1.782$ or if the test statistic > 1.782.

   STEP 5: Do not reject H_o because neither of the two conditions in *Step 4* is satisfied.

c. They will always be the same as long as the same α value is used.

17. a. *STEP 1:* $H_o: \mu_1 = \mu_2, \quad H_a: \mu_1 < \mu_2 \qquad \mu_1 =$ mean of treatment group

   STEP 2: $\alpha = 0.05$

   STEP 3: Calculate $s_P^2 = \dfrac{(n_1 - 1)s_1^2 + (n_2 - 1)s_2^2}{n_1 + n_2 - 2}$

$$s_P^2 = \frac{20 \times 7.8^2 + 20 \times 8.3^2}{21 + 21 - 2} = 64.865$$

   STEP 4: Calculate the test statistic.

$$\frac{(\bar{x}_1 - \bar{x}_2)}{\sqrt{s_P^2\left(\frac{1}{n_1} + \frac{1}{n_2}\right)}} = \frac{65.2 - 70.3}{\sqrt{64.865\left(\frac{1}{21} + \frac{1}{21}\right)}} = -2.05$$

   STEP 5: Reject H_o if test statistic $< -t_{\frac{\alpha}{2},n_1+n_2-2} = -t_{0.025,40} = -2.021$, or if test statistic > 2.021.

b. *STEP 1:* Since a 95% confidence interval is needed, $\alpha = 5\%$ and $\frac{\alpha}{2} = 0.025$. d.f. $= n_1 + n_2 - 2 = 21 + 21 - 2 = 40$.

   Thus, $t_{0.025,40} = 2.021$

STEP 2: Construct the 95% confidence interval (CI).

$$CI = (65.2 - 70.3) \pm 2.021 \sqrt{64.865 \left(\frac{1}{21} + \frac{1}{21} \right)}$$

$$= -5.1 \pm 5.023$$

$$= (-10.12, -0.077)$$

18. a. *STEP 1:* $\alpha = 0.05$, $\frac{\alpha}{2} = 0.025$. d.f. $= n_1 + n_2 - 2 = 25 + 25 - 2 = 48$.

Thus, $t_{0.025,48} \approx 2.021$.

STEP 2: Calculate $s_p^2 = \dfrac{24 \times 4.5^2 + 24 \times 5.3^2}{25 + 25 - 2} = 24.17$

STEP 3: Calculate the 95% confidence interval.

$$CI = (25.5 - 24.2) \pm 2.021 \sqrt{24.17 \left(\frac{1}{25} + \frac{1}{25} \right)}$$

$$= 1.3 \pm 2.81$$

$$= (-1.51, 4.11)$$

Since the interval includes zero, there is not enough evidence of significant difference in the means.

b. From the results in part (a) above, it can be concluded that at an α of 0.05, the means do not differ significantly. It can also be concluded that they do not differ at any α smaller than 0.05. Thus, a test at an α of 0.01 does not need to be conducted. It can be concluded, based on part (a) above, that the means do not differ.

5–12 COMPARISON OF MEANS FOR PAIRED (OR DEPENDENT) SAMPLES

19. a. *STEP 1:* Find the paired differences FEV_1 (initial) − FEV_1 (after 2 years) and obtain the mean and standard deviation of the differences.

$$\bar{x}_d = 0.047 \text{ and } s_d = 0.294$$

STEP 2: H_o: $\mu_d = 0$, H_a: $\mu_d > 0$, where $\mu_d = \mu_1 - \mu_2$

STEP 3: $\alpha = 0.05$, d.f. $= n - 1 = 10 - 1 = 9$

Thus, $t_{0.05,9} = 1.833$

STEP 4: Calculate the test statistic.

$$\frac{\bar{x}_d}{s_d/\sqrt{n}} = \frac{0.047}{0.294/\sqrt{10}} = 0.505$$

STEP 5: Define the rejection region: Reject H_o if test statistic > 1.833.

STEP 6: Do not reject H_o because the test statistic is not bigger than 1.833.

b. *STEP 1:* $\alpha = 0.05$, $\frac{\alpha}{2} = 0.025$, d.f. $= n - 1 = 10 - 1 = 9$.

Thus, $t_{0.025,9} = 2.262$

STEP 2: Construct a 95% confidence interval.

$$CI = \bar{x}_d \pm t_{0.025,9} \frac{s_d}{\sqrt{n}}$$

$$= 0.047 \pm 2.262 \times \frac{0.294}{\sqrt{10}}$$

$$= (-0.163, 0.257)$$

20. a. *STEP 1:* Find the paired before and after differences and calculate the mean and standard deviation of the differences.

$$\bar{x}_d = 34.375 \text{ and } s_d = 24.819$$

      STEP 2: H_o: $\mu_d = 0$, H_a: $\mu_d > 0$, $\mu_d =$ mean before $-$ mean after

      STEP 3: $\alpha = 0.01$, d.f. $= n - 1 = 8 - 1 = 7$.

      Thus, $t_{0.01,9} = 2.998$

      STEP 4: Calculate the test statistic.

$$\frac{\bar{x}_d}{s_d/\sqrt{n}} = \frac{34.375}{24.819/\sqrt{8}} = 3.917$$

      STEP 5: Define the rejection region: Reject H_o if test statistic > 2.998.

      STEP 6: Reject H_o because the test statistic is bigger than 2.998.

  b. *STEP 1:* $\alpha = 0.05$, $\frac{\alpha}{2} = 0.025$, d.f. $= n - 1 = 8 - 1 = 7$.

      Thus, $t_{0.025,7} = 2.365$.

      STEP 2: Construct a 95% confidence interval.

$$CI = 34.375 \pm 2.365 \times \frac{24.819}{\sqrt{8}}$$

$$= (13.623, 55.127)$$

5–13 INFERENCES FOR PROPORTIONS OR PERCENTAGES

21. a. *STEP 1:* Calulate $\hat{P} =$ sample recidivism rate.

$$\hat{P} = \frac{29}{62} = 0.47$$

      STEP 2: $\alpha = 0.05$, $\frac{\alpha}{2} = 0.025$. Thus, $z_{0.025} = 1.96$.

      STEP 3: Construct a 95% confidence interval.

$$CI = 0.47 \pm 1.96 \times \sqrt{\frac{0.47(1 - 0.47)}{62}}$$

$$= (0.346, 0.594)$$

  b. *STEP 1:* H_o: $P \geq 0.5$, H_a: $P < 0.5$

      STEP 2: $\alpha = 0.05$.

STEP 3: Calculate the test statistic.

$$\frac{\hat{P} - P_o}{\sqrt{\frac{P_o(1 - P_o)}{n}}} = \frac{0.47 - 0.5}{\sqrt{\frac{0.5(1 - 0.5)}{62}}} = -0.47$$

STEP 4: Reject H_o if test statistic $< -z_\alpha = -z_{0.05} = -1.64$

STEP 5: Do not reject H_o.

22. a. *STEP 1:* Calulate $\hat{P}$ = sample proportion of people surviving 5 years after treatment.

$$\hat{P} = \frac{56}{162} = 0.35$$

STEP 2: H_o: $P \le 0.25$, H_a: $P > 0.25$

STEP 3: $\alpha = 0.001$

STEP 4: Calculate the test statistic.

$$\frac{\hat{P} - P_o}{\sqrt{\frac{P_o(1 - P_o)}{n}}} = \frac{0.35 - 0.25}{\sqrt{\frac{0.25(1 - 0.25)}{162}}} = 2.94$$

STEP 5: Define the rejection region: Reject H_o if the test statistic $> -z_\alpha = -z_{0.001} = 3.08$

STEP 6: Do not reject H_o because the test statistic is less than 3.08.

b. *STEP 1:* Find the area between 0 and 2.94 using Table 1, Appendix C. The area between 0 and 2.94 is 0.4984.

STEP 2: Subtract 0.4984 from 0.5 to obtain the *p*-value.

$$p\text{-value} = 0.5 - 0.4984 = 0.0016$$

5-14 TWO-SAMPLE INFERENCES FOR PROPORTIONS

23. a. *STEP 1:* Calculate $\hat{P}_1$ and $\hat{P}_2$ where

$\hat{P}_1$ = proportion of surgical patients alive.

$\hat{P}_1$ = proportion of medical patients alive.

$$\hat{P}_1 = 0.91 \text{ and } \hat{P}_2 = 0.90$$

STEP 2: Since a 95% confidence interval is sought, $\alpha = 0.05$, $\frac{\alpha}{2} = 0.025$. Thus, $z_{0.025} = 1.96$.

STEP 3: Calculate a 95% confidence interval (CI).

$$CI = (\hat{P}_1 - \hat{P}_2) \pm z_{\frac{\alpha}{2}} \sqrt{\frac{\hat{P}_1(1 - \hat{P}_1)}{n_1} + \frac{\hat{P}_2(1 - \hat{P}_2)}{n_2}}$$

$$= (0.91 - 0.90) \pm 1.96 \sqrt{\frac{0.91(1 - 0.91)}{10,000} + \frac{0.90(1 - 0.90)}{10,000}}$$

$$= (0.01) \pm 0.00813$$

$$= (0.00187, 0.01813)$$

Since the interval does not include zero and is positive, it can be concluded that there is a significant difference in the proportion of patients alive. In fact, it indicates that the proportion of patients alive using the surgical method is significantly (statistically) larger than that using the medical method.

b. Since the α chosen here is the same as that in (a), another test need not be conducted. It can also be concluded that there is a significant difference in the two methods. However, this significance is statistical. In practice, one may not consider the difference to be significant because the percentage of patients surviving using the surgical method is higher than that of those using the medical method by only 0.187% to 1.813%.

5-17 CORRELATION

24. a. *STEP 1:* Calculate Σx, Σx^2, Σy, Σy^2, and Σxy.

Here, $x = $ age, $y = $ BAC

Thus,

$$\Sigma x = 276.6$$
$$\Sigma x^2 = 10680.48$$
$$\Sigma y = 1.664$$
$$\Sigma y^2 = 0.352$$
$$\Sigma xy = 57.192$$

STEP 2: Calculate SS_{xx}, SS_{yy}, and SS_{xy}.

$$SS_{xx} = \Sigma x^2 - \frac{(\Sigma x)^2}{n} = 10680.48 - \frac{(276.6)^2}{8} = 1117.035$$

$$SS_{yy} = \Sigma y^2 - \frac{(\Sigma y)^2}{n} = 0.352 - \frac{(1.664)^2 = 0.005888}{8}$$

$$SS_{xy} = \Sigma xy - \frac{(\Sigma x)(\Sigma y)}{n} = 57.192 - \frac{(276.6)(1.664)}{8} = -0.3408$$

STEP 3: Calculate $\hat{\beta}_1$ and $\hat{\beta}_0$.

$$\hat{\beta}_1 = \frac{SS_{xy}}{SS_{xx}} = \frac{-0.3408}{1117.035} = -0.000305$$

$$\hat{\beta}_0 = \bar{y} - \hat{\beta}_1\bar{x} = 0.208 - (-0.000305)\frac{276.6}{8} = 0.2185$$

STEP 4: Substitute $\hat{\beta}_0$ and $\hat{\beta}_1$ in $\hat{y} = \hat{\beta}_0 + \hat{\beta}_1 x$. Thus, the fitted model is

$$\hat{y} = 0.2185 - 0.000305x$$

b. *STEP 1:* Calculate the mean square error (MSE).

$$\text{MSE} = \frac{SS_{yy} - \hat{\beta}_1 SS_{xy}}{n - 2} = \frac{0.005888 - (-0.000305)(-0.3408)}{8 - 2} = 0.000964$$

STEP 2: Calculate the standard error of $\hat{\beta}_1$.

$$SE(\hat{\beta}_1) = \sqrt{\frac{MSE}{SS_{xx}}} = \sqrt{\frac{0.000964}{1117.035}} = 0.00092898$$

STEP 3: Set up the hypothesis.

$$H_o: \beta_1 = 0, H_a: \beta_1 \neq 0$$

STEP 4: Use $\alpha = 0.05$.

STEP 5: Calculate the test statistic.

$$\frac{\hat{\beta}_1}{SE(\hat{\beta}_1)} = \frac{-0.000305}{0.00092898} = -0.3283$$

STEP 6: Define the rejection region: Reject H_o if the test statistic $< -t_{\frac{\alpha}{2}, n-1} = t_{0.025,7} = -2.365$.

STEP 7: Do not reject H_o. Thus, the model does not seem very useful.

c. *STEP 1:* $\alpha = 0.1, \frac{\alpha}{2} = 0.05, t_{0.05,7} = 1.895$

STEP 2: Construct a 95% confidence interval.

$$CI = \hat{\beta}_1 \pm t_{\frac{\alpha}{2}, n-1} SE(\hat{\beta}_1)$$
$$= -0.000305 \pm 1.895(0.00092898)$$
$$= -0.000305 \pm 0.00176$$
$$= (-0.002065, 0.001455)$$

d. *STEP 1:* Find the point estimate of mean BAC for age $= 20$.

$$\hat{y}_{x=20} = \hat{\beta}_0 + \hat{\beta}_1 \times 20 = 0.2185 + (-0.000305)20 = 0.2124$$

STEP 2: $\alpha = 0.05, \frac{\alpha}{2} = 0.025, t_{0.025,7} = 2.365$

STEP 3: Calculate $\sqrt{MSE\left(\frac{1}{n} + \frac{(x_0 - \bar{x})^2}{SS_{xx}}\right)}$

$$= \sqrt{0.000964\left(\frac{1}{8} + \frac{(20 - 34.575)^2}{1117.035}\right)}$$
$$= 0.01743$$

STEP 4: Calculate the interval.

upper limit $= 0.2124 + 2.365 \times 0.01743 = 0.2536$

lower limit $= 0.2124 - 2.365 \times 0.01743 = 0.1711$

Therefore, the 95% confidence interval is 0.1711 to 0.2536.

APPENDIX B

LOGARITHM TABLES

Common Logarithms of Numbers[a]

N	0	1	2	3	4	5	6	7	8	9
10	0000	0043	0086	0128	0170	0212	0253	0294	0334	0374
11	0414	0453	0492	0531	0569	0607	0645	0682	0719	0755
12	0792	0828	0864	0899	0934	0969	1004	1038	1072	1106
13	1139	1173	1206	1239	1271	1303	1335	1367	1399	1430
14	1461	1492	1523	1553	1584	1614	1644	1673	1703	1732
15	1761	1790	1818	1847	1875	1903	1931	1959	1987	2014
16	2041	2068	2095	2122	2148	2175	2201	2227	2253	2279
17	2304	2330	2335	2380	2405	2430	2455	2480	2504	2529
18	2553	2577	2601	2625	2648	2672	2695	2718	2742	2765
19	2788	2810	2833	2856	2878	2900	2923	2945	2967	2989
20	3010	3032	3054	3075	3096	3118	3139	3160	3181	3201
21	3222	3243	3263	3284	3304	3324	3345	3365	3385	3404
22	3424	3444	3464	3483	3502	3522	3541	3560	3579	3598
23	3617	3636	3655	3674	3692	3711	3729	3747	3766	3784
24	3802	3820	3838	3856	3874	3892	3909	3927	3945	3962
25	3979	3997	4014	4031	4048	4065	4082	4099	4116	4133
26	4150	4166	4183	4200	4216	4232	4249	4265	4281	4298
27	4314	4330	4346	4362	4378	4393	4409	4425	4440	4456
28	4472	4487	4502	4518	4533	4548	4564	4579	4594	4609
29	4624	4639	4654	4669	4683	4698	4713	4728	4742	4757
30	4771	4786	4800	4814	4829	4843	4857	4871	4886	4900
31	4914	4928	4942	4955	4969	4983	4997	5011	5024	5038
32	5051	5065	5079	5092	5105	5119	5132	5145	5159	5172
33	5185	5198	5211	5224	5237	5250	5263	5276	5289	5302
34	5315	5328	5340	5353	5366	5378	5391	5403	5416	5428

Common Logarithms of Numbersª (continued)

N	0	1	2	3	4	5	6	7	8	9
35	5441	5453	5465	5478	5490	5502	5514	5527	5539	5551
36	5563	5575	5587	5599	5611	5623	5635	5647	5658	5670
37	5682	5694	5705	5717	5729	5740	5752	5763	5775	5786
38	5798	5809	5821	5832	5843	5855	5866	5877	5888	5899
39	5911	5922	5933	5944	5955	5966	5977	5988	5999	6010
40	6021	6031	6042	6053	6064	6075	6085	6096	6107	6117
41	6128	6138	6149	6160	6170	6180	6191	6201	6212	6222
42	6232	6243	6253	6263	6274	6284	6294	6304	6314	6325
43	6335	6345	6355	6365	6375	6385	6395	6405	6415	6425
44	6435	6444	6454	6464	6474	6484	6493	6503	6513	6522
45	6532	6542	6551	6561	6571	6580	6590	6599	6609	6618
46	6628	6637	6646	6656	6665	6675	6684	6693	6702	6712
47	6721	6730	6739	6749	6758	6767	6776	6785	6794	6803
48	6812	6821	6830	6839	6848	6857	6866	6875	6884	6893
49	6902	6911	6920	6928	6937	6946	6955	6964	6972	6981
50	6990	6998	7007	7016	7024	7033	7042	7050	7059	7067
51	7076	7084	7093	7101	7110	7118	7126	7135	7143	7152
52	7160	7168	7177	7185	7193	7202	7210	7218	7226	7235
53	7243	7251	7259	7267	7275	7284	7292	7300	7308	7316
54	7324	7332	7340	7348	7356	7364	7372	7380	7388	7396
55	7404	7412	7419	7427	7435	7443	7451	7459	7466	7474
56	7482	7490	7497	7505	7513	7520	7528	7536	7543	7551
57	7559	7566	7574	7582	7589	7597	7604	7612	7619	7627
58	7634	7642	7649	7657	7664	7672	7679	7686	7694	7701
59	7709	7716	7723	7731	7738	7745	7752	7760	7767	7774
60	7782	7789	7796	7803	7810	7818	7825	7832	7839	7846
61	7853	7860	7868	7875	7892	7889	7896	7903	7910	7917
62	7924	7931	7938	7945	7952	7959	7966	7973	7980	7987
63	7993	8000	8007	8014	8021	8028	8035	8041	8048	8055
64	8062	8069	8075	8082	8089	8096	8102	8109	8116	8122
65	8129	8136	8142	8149	8156	8162	8169	8176	8182	8189
66	8195	8202	8209	8215	8222	8228	8235	8241	8248	8254
67	8261	8267	8274	8280	8287	8293	8299	8306	8312	8319
68	8325	8331	8338	8344	8351	8357	8363	8370	8376	8382
69	8388	8395	8401	8407	8414	8420	8426	8432	8439	8445

Common Logarithms of Numbers[a] (continued)

N	0	1	2	3	4	5	6	7	8	9
70	8451	8457	8463	8470	8476	8482	8488	8494	8500	8506
71	8513	8519	8525	8531	8537	8543	8549	8555	8561	8567
72	8573	8579	8585	8591	8597	8603	8609	8615	8621	8627
73	8633	8639	8645	8651	8657	8663	8669	8675	8681	8686
74	8692	8698	8704	8710	8716	8722	8727	8733	8739	8745
75	8751	8756	8762	8768	8774	8779	8785	8791	8797	8802
76	8808	8814	8820	8825	8831	8837	8842	8848	8854	8859
77	8865	8871	8876	8882	8887	8893	8899	8904	8910	8915
78	8921	8927	8932	8938	8943	8949	8954	8960	8965	8971
79	8976	8982	8987	8993	8998	9004	9009	9015	9020	9025
80	9031	9036	9042	9047	9053	9058	9063	9069	9074	9079
81	9085	9090	9096	9101	9106	9112	9117	9122	9128	9133
82	9138	9143	9149	9154	9159	9165	9170	9175	9180	9186
83	9191	9196	9201	9206	9212	9217	9222	9227	9232	9238
84	9243	9248	9253	9258	9263	9269	9274	9279	9284	9289
85	9294	9299	9304	9309	9315	9320	9325	9330	9335	9340
86	9345	9350	9355	9360	9365	9370	9375	9380	9385	9390
87	9395	9400	9405	9410	9415	9420	9425	9430	9435	9440
88	9445	9450	9455	9460	9465	9469	9474	9479	9484	9489
89	9494	9499	9504	9509	9513	9518	9523	9528	9533	9538
90	9542	9547	9552	9557	9562	9566	9571	9576	9581	9586
91	9590	9595	9600	9605	9609	9614	9619	9624	9628	9633
92	9638	9643	9647	9652	9657	9661	9666	9671	9675	9680
93	9685	9689	9694	9699	9703	9708	9713	9717	9722	9727
94	9731	9736	9741	9745	9750	9754	9759	9763	9768	9773
95	9777	9782	9786	9791	9795	9800	9805	9809	9814	9818
96	9823	9827	9832	9836	9841	9845	9850	9854	9859	9863
97	9868	9872	9877	9881	9886	9890	9894	9899	9903	9908
98	9912	9917	9921	9926	9930	9934	9939	9943	9948	9952
99	9956	9961	9965	9969	9974	9978	9983	9987	9991	9996

[a]This table gives the mantissas of numbers with the decimal point omitted in each case. Characteristics are determined by inspection from the numbers.

APPENDIX C

STATISTIC TABLES

Table I   Critical Values of t

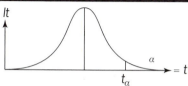

v	$t_{.100}$	$t_{.050}$	$t_{.025}$	$t_{.010}$	$t_{.005}$	$t_{.001}$	$t_{.0005}$
1	3.078	6.314	12.706	31.821	63.657	318.31	636.62
2	1.886	2.920	4.303	6.965	9.925	22.326	31.598
3	1.638	2.353	3.182	4.541	5.841	10.213	12.924
4	1.533	2.132	2.776	3.747	4.604	7.173	8.610
5	1.476	2.015	2.571	3.365	4.032	5.893	6.869
6	1.440	1.943	2.447	3.143	3.707	5.208	5.959
7	1.415	1.895	2.365	2.998	3.499	4.785	5.408
8	1.397	1.860	2.306	2.896	3.355	4.501	5.041
9	1.383	1.833	2.262	2.821	3.250	4.297	4.781
10	1.372	1.812	2.228	2.764	3.169	4.144	4.587
11	1.363	1.796	2.201	2.718	3.106	4.025	4.437
12	1.356	1.782	2.179	2.681	3.055	3.930	4.318
13	1.350	1.771	2.160	2.650	3.012	3.852	4.221
14	1.345	1.761	2.145	2.624	2.977	3.787	4.140
15	1.341	1.753	2.131	2.602	2.947	3.733	4.073
16	1.337	1.746	2.120	2.583	2.921	3.686	4.015
17	1.333	1.740	2.110	2.567	2.898	3.646	3.965
18	1.330	1.734	2.101	2.552	2.878	3.610	3.922
19	1.328	1.729	2.093	2.539	2.861	3.579	3.883
20	1.325	1.725	2.086	2.528	2.845	3.552	3.850
21	1.323	1.721	2.080	2.518	2.831	3.527	3.819
22	1.321	1.717	2.074	2.508	2.819	3.505	3.792
23	1.319	1.714	2.069	2.500	2.807	3.485	3.767
24	1.318	1.711	2.064	2.492	2.797	3.467	3.745
25	1.316	1.708	2.060	2.485	2.787	3.450	3.725
26	1.315	1.706	2.056	2.479	2.779	3.435	3.707
27	1.314	1.703	2.052	2.473	2.771	3.421	3.690
28	1.313	1.701	2.048	2.467	2.763	3.408	3.674
29	1.311	1.699	2.045	2.462	2.756	3.396	3.659
30	1.310	1.697	2.042	2.457	2.750	3.385	3.646
40	1.303	1.684	2.021	2.423	2.704	3.307	3.551
60	1.296	1.671	2.000	2.390	2.660	3.232	3.460
120	1.289	1.658	1.980	2.358	2.617	3.160	3.373
∞	1.282	1.645	1.960	2.326	2.576	3.090	3.291

Table II Normal Curve Areas

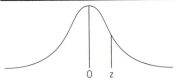

z	.00	.01	.02	.03	.04	.05	.06	.07	.08	.09
.0	.0000	.0040	.0080	.0120	.0160	.0199	.0239	.0279	.0319	.0359
.1	.0398	.0438	.0478	.0517	.0557	.0596	.0636	.0675	.0714	.0753
.2	.0793	.0832	.0871	.0910	.0948	.0987	.1026	.1064	.1103	.1141
.3	.1179	.1217	.1255	.1293	.1331	.1368	.1406	.1443	.1480	.1517
.4	.1554	.1591	.1628	.1664	.1700	.1736	.1772	.1808	.1844	.1879
.5	.1915	.1950	.1985	.2019	.2054	.2088	.2123	.2157	.2190	.2224
.6	.2257	.2291	.2324	.2357	.2389	.2422	.2454	.2486	.2517	.2549
.7	.2580	.2611	.2642	.2673	.2704	.2734	.2764	.2794	.2823	.2852
.8	.2881	.2910	.2939	.2967	.2995	.3023	.3051	.3078	.3106	.3133
.9	.3159	.3186	.3212	.3238	.3264	.3289	.3315	.3340	.3365	.3389
1.0	3.413	.3438	.3461	.3485	.3508	.3531	.3554	.3577	.3599	.3621
1.1	.3643	.3665	.3686	.3708	.3729	.3749	.3770	.3790	.3810	.3830
1.2	.3849	.3869	.3888	.3907	.3925	.3944	.3962	.3980	.3997	.4015
1.3	.4032	.4049	.4066	.4082	.4099	.4115	.4131	.4147	.4162	.4177
1.4	.4192	.4207	.4222	.4236	.4251	.4265	.4279	.4292	.4306	.4319
1.5	.4332	.4345	.4357	.4370	.4382	.4394	.4406	.4418	.4429	.4441
1.6	.4452	.4463	.4474	.4484	.4495	.4505	.4515	.4525	.4535	.4545
1.7	.4554	.4564	.4573	.4582	.4591	.4599	.4608	.4616	.4625	.4633
1.8	.4641	.4649	.4656	.4664	.4671	.4678	.4686	.4693	.4699	.4706
1.9	.4713	.4719	.4726	.4732	.4738	.4744	.4750	.4756	.4761	.4767
2.0	.4772	.4778	.4783	.4788	.4793	.4798	.4803	.4808	.4812	.4817
2.1	.4821	.4826	.4830	.4834	.4838	.4842	.4846	.4850	.4854	.4857
2.2	.4861	.4864	.4868	.4871	.4875	.4878	.4881	.4884	.4887	.4890
2.3	.4893	.4896	.4898	.4901	.4904	.4906	.4909	.4911	.4913	.4916
2.4	.4918	.4920	.4922	.4925	.4927	.4929	.4931	.4932	.4934	.4936
2.5	.4938	.4940	.4941	.4943	.4945	.4946	.4948	.4949	.4951	.4952
2.6	.4953	.4955	.4956	.4957	.4959	.4960	.4961	.4962	.4963	.4964
2.7	.4965	.4966	.4967	.4968	.4969	.4970	.4971	.4972	.4973	.4874
2.8	.4974	.4975	.4976	.4977	.4977	.4978	.4979	.4979	.4980	.4981
2.9	.4981	.4982	.4982	.4983	.4984	.4984	.4985	.4985	.4986	.4986
3.0	.4987	.4987	.4987	.4988	.4988	.4989	.4989	.4898	.4990	.4990

GLOSSARY

abscissa   The horizontal axis (*x*-axis) in a plane Cartesian coordinate system.

absolute scale   A temperature scale with absolute zero ($-273°C$) as the minimum measurement and with calibrations equal in magnitude to those of a Celsius scale.

absolute temperature   Any temperature measured on the absolute scale.

absolute value   The distance a real number is from zero on a number line.

absolute zero   The lowest possible temperature; $-273°C$, or 0 K.

acceleration   The rate of change of velocity; linear distance per time per time (e.g., m/sec^2 or m/sec/sec).

acid   A substance that in aqueous solution increases the hydrogen ion concentration to the extent that the pH value becomes less than 7.00.

acid-fast stain   Bacteriologic staining procedure used to identify bacteria able to retain a carbolfuschin stain when treated with acid alcohol.

active transport   The process of moving molecules or ions across cell membranes against a concentration gradient via the expenditure of energy.

additive inverse   The opposite value of a negative real number, e.g., the additive inverse of -15 is $+15$.

adenine   A purine base found in both DNA and RNA.

adenosine triphosphate (ATP)   A nucleotide that stores energy in phosphate bonds for metabolic use.

adrenergic   1. Of or pertaining to pharmacologic agents that produce epinephrine-like effects; 2. sympathetic nervous system receptors categorized as either β_1, β_2, or α.

agar   A dried substance from seaweed that melts at $100°C$ and solidifies at $48°C$.

agonist   A medication (agent) that stimulates a physiologic or biochemical response at cell receptor sites.

airway generation   Each branching of the conducting airways of the lung with a numerical value assigned to correspond with a specific anatomic location (e.g., trachea = generation 0, alveoli = generation 23).

airway resistance   Results from the interaction between the flowing gas molecules and the walls of the conducting airway and the intermolecular activity among the flowing gas molecules; represented as pressure per flow (e.g., cm H_2O/liter/sec).

alkylating agent   A compound that forms chemical bridges between functional groups on biomolecules.

allosteric interactions Interactions between spatially distinct sites that are transmitted by conformational changes in the protein, e.g., the cooperative binding of oxygen to the hemoglobin molecule, and the effect of H^+ ions, CO_2 and 2-3, DPG on hemoglobin-oxygen affinity.

alpha level (α) The amount of error allowed in making a decision.

alpha receptor An adrenergic receptor that produces vasoconstriction upon stimulation.

alpha tocopherol Vitamin E; a fat-soluble organic compound that functions in all tissues acting as a stabilizer (antioxidant) of cell membrane lipids.

alternative hypothesis (H_a) A statement indicating that the population parameter is some value other than the one specified under the null hypothesis (H_o).

alveolar-arterial oxygen gradient [P(A-a)O_2] The numerical difference between alveolar Po_2 and arterial Po_2, used to assess the diffusibility of oxygen across the alveolar-capillary membrane.

alveolar dead space The volume of gas entering alveoli not being perfused.

alveolar interdependence Phenomenon resulting from the fact that each alveolus relies on adjacent alveoli for its patency.

amino sugar Conjugated molecule consisting of a carbohydrate and one or more amino acids.

ammeter A device for measuring electrical current.

analysis of variance A procedure of comparing means via variances.

anion An ion having more electrons than protons; a negatively charged ion.

anode The electrode of an electrochemical cell where atoms lose electrons (oxidation).

antibiotic A substance produced by one microorganism that inhibits or kills other microorganisms.

antibody A substance produced by the body that inactivates an antigen.

antigen A substance that stimulates the production of antibodies.

antilogarithm The process of determining the logarithm (exponent or power) when the number is known. Opposite process of finding the logarithm.

antioxidant A chemical substance that inhibits the oxidation of other substances.

appendage Structure that extends from the surface of a bacterium.

arachidonic acid An essential fatty acid required for the synthesis of some prostaglandins.

arterial oxygen content (CaO_2) The total amount of oxygen in arterial blood (i.e., amount bound to Hb plus amount dissolved in plasma expressed as volumes percent).

artificial growth medium A preparation of chemical substances that supports the growth of microorganisms.

ascorbic acid Vitamin C.

atmosphere A unit of pressure representing the average pressure exerted on the earth at sea level.

atmospheric pressure Pressure exerted upon the surface of the earth resulting from the molecular movement and the mass of atmospheric gases.

atom The smallest aspect of an element possessing a nucleus (protons and neutrons) and orbiting electrons (number of protons = number of electrons).

atomic mass The arithmetic sum of the number of protons and neutrons inside the nucleus of an atom.

atomic number The number of protons in the nucleus of an atom.

ATPS Ambient temperature and pressure saturated.

augmented diffusion The movement of gas molecules assisted by eddy currents and vortices; the proposed gas movement mechanism in the central and in some peripheral airways during high-frequency ventilation.

A-V difference   The gradient between arterial and venous oxygen content reflecting oxygen consumption at the tissue level.

Avogadro's law   Equal volumes of different gases, at the same temperature and pressure, contain the same number of molecules.

Avogadro's number   The number of molecules in 1 mole of a gas at STP; 6.023×10^{23}.

bacterial envelope   The cell wall, membrane, and capsule of a bacterium.

barometric pressure   Atmospheric pressure as measured on a barometer.

base   A substance that in aqueous solution increases the hydroxyl (OH^-) concentration to the extent that the pH value exceeds 7.00.

Bernoulli principle   Describes the inverse relationship between lateral wall pressure and velocity as a fluid flows through a conducting system.

β_1 receptor   An adrenergic receptor that, when stimulated, increases heart rate and myocardial contractility.

β_2 receptor   An adrenergic receptor that produces bronchodilatation and pulmonary vasodilatation when stimulated.

bias   The influence of variables, other than those accounted for in a study, on the outcome.

binary fission   Division of a single cell to form two equal daughter cells.

blocker   Anything that blocks or prevents passage or activity.

bolus   A volume of fluid or medication rapidly administered intravenously at one time to achieve an immediate response.

bond   A linkage between atoms in a molecule, or in an ion (radical).

Boyle's law   Gas law stating that the volume is inversely proportional to pressure when the mass and absolute temperature of the gas are constant.

Brownian motion   Random movement of molecules or particles in a liquid or gas.

BTPS   Body temperature and pressure saturated.

buffer   Any substance that maintains the relative concentrations of hydrogen and hydroxyl ions in a solution when small amounts of acid or base are added.

carbohydrates   Sugars.

cardiogenic oscillation   Undulations (waviness) occurring on certain physiologic tracings (e.g., SBN_2) caused by cardiac contractions.

carotenoids   Lipid plant products that contribute to animal nutrition as precursors for synthesis of vitamin A.

carriage   The state of harboring a pathogenic microorganism without having clinical signs or symptoms of disease.

Cartesian coordinate system   A two-dimensional coordinate system in which the coordinates are measured from two intersecting perpendicular lines. The plane is divided into four quadrants.

catalase   An enzyme that catalyzes the breakdown of H_2O_2.

catalysis   An increase in the rate of a chemical reaction because of the presence of a catalyst.

catalyst   A compound that accelerates a reaction but is not consumed in the process.

cathode   The electrode of an electrochemical cell where atoms gain electrons (reduction).

cation   An ion having more protons than electrons; a positively charged ion.

cationic detergent   A positively charged molecule that disrupts bacterial membranes by coating the lipid structures, resulting in solubilization.

cell membrane   The outermost bilayer of phospholipids, which envelopes cellular cytoplasm and organelles.

Celsius scale   A temperature scale wherein the freezing point of water is 0°C and its boiling point is 100°C.

centimeter-gram-second (CGS) system   A system of units of measure based on the centimeter, gram, and second.

centrosome   A cytoplasmic body involved in separation of chromosomes during cell division.

characteristic   The integer portion of a logarithm.

Charles' law   Gas law stating that the volume is directly proportional to the absolute temperature when the mass and pressure of the gas are constant.

chemical equilibrium   The state at which the simultaneous forward and reverse chemical reaction rates are equal.

chemotaxis   A mechanism of mobility exhibited by white blood cells and macrophages responsible for the migration of these cells from the bloodstream to an injured area of the body outside the bloodstream. Chemotaxis is initiated by the effect of substances present at the site of injury.

chemotherapeutic agent   Chemical compound used to treat disease.

chloride shift   Refers to the exchange of Cl^- for HCO_3^- across the red blood cell membrane.

cholinergic   1. Of or pertaining to pharmacologic agents that produce acetylcholine-like effects; 2. parasympathetic nervous system receptors.

chromatin   The cell nuclear material consisting of nucleoprotein.

chromosome   A nucleoprotein that contains the genetic information of a cell.

Clark electrode   An electrochemical device used for measuring Po_2.

coefficient   A numerical factor of an elementary algebraic term, as 4 in the term 4X.

coefficient of variation   The standard deviation expressed as a percentage of the mean.

coenzyme   A nonprotein molecule necessary for enzymatic reactions.

colloid   Submicroscopic particles suspended in a continuous medium.

combined CO_2   Carbon dioxide transported in the blood in the form of HCO_3^-.

complement   A system of several serum proteins activated by immune or nonimmune pathways. Complement has a critical role in host protection.

compliance   A measurement representing the degree of elasticity of an expanding or contracting body; unit of volume change per unit of pressure change, (i.e., liter/cm H_2O); the reciprocal of elastance.

complimentary bases   Nitrogen bases of nucleotides in parallel strands of nucleic acids that form hydrogen bonds with each other.

conductance   The reciprocal of resistance (i.e., 1/R represented as the units liter/sec/cm H_2O).

confidence interval   An interval estimate of a parameter. The procedure assures us with a certain high level of confidence about our estimate.

confounders   Variables, other than those considered in a study, affecting the study's outcome.

conjugation   A process of genetic exchange between bacteria involving transfer of chromosomes or plasmids through pili when one bacterium attaches to another.

constant   A quantity that has a fixed numerical value.

continuous variable   A variable that can take on an unlimited number of values, e.g., length, velocity, and weight.

convection   The proposed gas movement mechanism in the central airways and in some peripheral airways during conventional (low-frequency, high tidal volume) ventilation.

cooperativity   Relationship wherein binding of a small-molecular-weight substance to a protein molecule enhances subsequent binding affinity for additional molecules.

corrected barometric pressure   The total barometric pressure minus the water vapor pressure.

correlation   The relationship between two variables.

correlation coefficient   A statistical measure that expresses the degree to which two variables are related.

covalent bond   A combination of atoms resulting from the sharing of electrons.

crista (*pl.*, -ae)   Invagination(s) of the inner membrane of a mitochondrion.

critical velocity   The velocity at which gas flow through a tube converts from a laminar flow pattern to a turbulent one.

crystalloid   A substance that in solution can diffuse through a semipermeable membrane.

current   Electron flow through a conducting medium.

cyclic nucleotide   A nucleotide molecule with two, rather than one, oxygen to phosphate bonds.

cytochrome   A hemoprotein that functions in electron transport; designated as either *a, b, c,* or *d,* depending on the nature of its prosthetic group.

cytochrome oxidase   An enzyme involved in the chain reaction that constitutes cellular oxygen consumption.

cytokines   Hormone-like proteins that act by binding specific receptors on their target cells, e.g., tumor necrosis factor (TNF).

cytoplasm   The internal fluid portion of a cell exclusive of that in the nucleus.

Dalton's law   The total pressure exerted by a mixture of gases is equal to the sum of the partial pressures of the constituent gases.

death phase   The phase of bacterial growth in a closed culture system when there are more bacteria dead than living.

degrees of freedom   The number of values that are free to vary after certain restrictions are placed on the data.

deoxyribose   A five-carbon molecule that is the sugar moiety found in nucleotides of DNA.

denominator   The numeral below the line in a mathematical fraction.

density   Mass per unit volume.

dependent variable   The quantity that changes because of the variation in the independent variable, and plotted on the *y*-axis.

desiccant   A dehumidifying agent.

diamagnetism   The feeble repulsion of a substance with no unpaired electrons by a magnetic field.

diapedesis   The movement of white blood cells out of the blood, through intact vessel walls, into the interstitium.

dichotomous branching   A single branch of a conduction system giving rise to two daughter branches, each of which becomes a parent and branches into two more daughters, and so on.

differential medium   An artificial growth medium containing various indicators that permit visual differentiation of bacterial colonies.

diffusion   The passive movement of molecules, atoms, or ions from an area of high concentration to an area of low concentration.

diluent   A substance used to dilute or reduce the concentration of a solution.

dimension   A unit used to qualify a numerical value (e.g., 760 *mm Hg*).

disaccharide   A sugar molecule consisting of two molecular units of three to six carbon atoms.

discrete variable   A variable that can take on a finite number of values, e.g., the number of white blood cells in one square container.

dispersion   The spread of scores about the measure of central tendency.

disinfection   The process of destroying most pathogenic microorganisms.

dismutase   An enzyme capable of catalyzing a reaction in which two molecules of the same compound are broken down to yield two molecules with different oxidation states, (i.e., $O_2^- \cdot + O_2^- \cdot + 2H^+ \xrightarrow{SOD} H_2O_2 + O_2$).

dissolved CO$_2$ The amount of carbon dioxide dissolved in plasma; P_{CO_2}.

distance   The extent of space between two points.

divalent   Containing two binding sites or degrees of charge.

dividend   The real number located in the numerator. The real number which is divided by the divisor.

divisor   The real number located in the denominator. The real number by which another real number is divided.

DNA   Deoxyribonucleic acid.

driving pressure   A pressure gradient causing a flow of gas or liquid.

dynamic equilibrium   A state of balance in which opposing processes occur at the same rate.

dynes/cm²   A unit of pressure in the CGS system of measurement.

eddy current   The rapid, swirling movement of gas or liquid molecules, atoms, or ions present in turbulent flow.

elastance   The reciprocal of compliance (i.e., 1/C, represented by the units cm H_2O/liter).

elastic recoil   The force which returns a deformed or stretched body to its original shape or position.

elastic limit   The point at which a body will no longer be deformed in proportion to the force applied to it.

elastic resistance   The force opposing ventilation due to the elastic properties of the lung, chest wall, other mediastinal structures, and abdominal viscera.

electrochemical cell   A cell in which spontaneous oxidation-reduction reactions produce an electric current.

electrochemistry   A branch of chemistry concerned with chemical reactions that produce an electric current.

electrode   A conductor through which electric current enters or leaves a conducting medium.

electrolysis   The decomposition of a substance by means of the passage of a galvanic current through it.

electrolyte solution   A solution that conducts electricity.

electron   A negatively charged atomic particle that orbits the nucleus of an atom or ion.

electron orbital   An electron pathway located inside a subshell.

electron spin   A property of an electron that makes it behave as though it were a tiny magnet.

electron transport chain   A biochemical assembly of components located along the inner membrane of mitochondria where oxygen undergoes four univalent reductions to form a molecule of water.

electrostatic   Pertaining to stationary electric charges.

element   A substance whose atoms contain the same atomic number.

endoplasmic reticulum   The network of tubules in the cytoplasm resulting from continuous invaginations of the cytoplasmic membrane.

endospore   A dormant form of bacteria highly resistant to drying, heat, and chemical agents.

endotoxin   The lipopolysaccharide released by gram-negative bacteria when they undergo lysis and cause generalized toxicity.

end-pulmonary capillary oxygen content (CcO₂)   The amount of oxygen in the pulmonary capillary immediately passing the alveoli (expressed in volumes percent).

energy   The ability to do work.

entrain   The addition of another fluid into the flow of the source fluid caused by a reduced lateral wall pressure.

enzyme   A protein molecule that catalyzes metabolic reactions.

equilibrium constant   Represented by K indicating the value of the concentration of the products raised to the power of their respective coefficients in a balanced chemical equation, divided by the product of the concentration of the reactants raised to the power of their respective coefficients in the balanced reaction.

exotoxin   A small molecule excreted by microbes having toxic reactions on specific aspects of cellular metabolism.

exponent   A number of designating the power to which another number is to be raised.

extrapolation   Estimating unknown information by projecting known information.

extreme   The first or last term of a ratio or series.

factor   One of two or more quantities multiplied, thus rendering a specific product.

facultative   Refers to microbes that can grow in either the presence or absence of oxygen.

facultative intracellular parasite   A bacterium that can resist destruction following engulfment by a phagocytic cell.

Fahrenheit scale   A temperature scale having 180 calibrations between the freezing point of water (32°F) and the boiling point (212°F).

F$_IO_2$ Fraction of inspired oxygen represented as a decimal (i.e., 60% O_2 = F$_IO_2$ 0.60).

flagellum   A bacterial appendage that provides the organism motility by undulating in a whiplike motion.

flow rate   A volume of fluid moving across a given point over time; unit of volume per unit of time; liters/min.

fomite   An inanimate vehicle of infection; e.g., eating utensils, hospital equipment, and clothing.

force   A vector that produces or prevents motion.

fractional concentration   The percentage of a gas in the total mixture of gases.

free radical   A highly reactive and potentially destructive biochemical entity carrying an unpaired electron in its outermost shell.

frequency distribution   The values of a variable arranged in the order of their magnitudes showing the number of times each score occurs.

galvanic cell   A cell that generates an electric current by means of chemical reactions.

galvanometer   A device used to sense a voltage difference between two circuits.

gas   A state of matter characterized by low density and low viscosity as compared to those of solids and liquids.

Gay-Lussac's law   Gas law stating that pressure is directly proportional to the absolute temperature when the mass and volume of the gas are constant.

gene   The basic molecular unit of inheritance found on a chromosome.

generation time   The time required for a single cell of a particular microbial species to divide into two progeny cells.

germicidal   Ability to kill microbes.

germination   The process of a spore reverting to a vegetative bacterium.

Gibbs-Donnan rule   States that diffusible ions will cross through a selectively permeable membrane according to specified requirements.

globin   A protein molecule comprising hemoglobin.

Golgi apparatus (body)   A compacted area of endoplasmic reticula involved in cellular-secretory activity.

gradient   A difference in concentration of molecules, atoms, or ions between two points.

Graham's law of diffusion   Gas law stating that the rates of diffusion of two gases are inversely proportional to the square roots of their densities.

gram equivalent weight   Obtained by dividing the molecular weight of a substance of its valence.

gram-negative   Bacterium that does not retain crystal violet when treated with alcohol by the gram procedure.

gram-positive   Designates bacteria that retain crystal violet stain when treated with alcohol by the gram procedure.

grams percent   Expression implying a certain number of grams per 100 ml of blood.

Gram stain   Bacteriologic staining procedure based on the ability of a bacterium to retain crystal violet stain when treated with alcohol.

granule   An insoluble, nonmembranous entity located in cytoplasm.

graph   A pictorial representation of a quantitative relationship.

guanine   A purine nitrogenous base present in nucleotides of both DNA and RNA.

Haldane effect   The influence of CO_2 binding and unbinding on the release and uptake of oxygen, respectively, by the hemoglobin molecule.

half-life   The time required for the concentration of a substance to decrease to one-half its original amount.

half-reaction   The chemical reaction occurring at either electrode of an electrochemical cell.

helix   A curved or coiled structure.

heme   The ring-shaped, iron-containing, nonprotein molecule within hemoglobin responsible for oxygen-binding.

hemoglobin F   The normal hemoglobin of the fetus.

hemoglobin-oxygen dissociation curve   Graph depicting oxygen-hemoglobin affinity based on So_2 and Po_2.

hemoprotein   A conjugated compound comprised of a protein bound to a heme molecule.

Henderson-Hasselbalch equation   An equation demonstrating the relationship of the pH to the logarithmic ratio of base to acid; the general form is pH = pK + log([base]/ [acid]).

Henry's law of solubility   The amount of gas that dissolves in a liquid is directly proportional to the partial pressure of the gas above the surface of the liquid.

histogram   A graph in which data are represented to indicate frequency distribution.

Hooke's law   States that an elastic body will deform proportionally to the force applied to the body until the body's elastic limit is reached.

hydration   The addition of water to a substance.

hydrogen abstraction   The process by which hydrogen is removed as a constituent of a compound.

hydrogen bond   An attraction between hydrogen and oxygen atoms on adjacent molecules.

hydrophilic   Attracted by polar or aqueous environments.

hydrophobic   Repelled by polar or aqueous environments.

hydropholeic   Repulsed by a lipid environment.

hydrostatic pressure   Pressure exerted by a liquid against the walls of the container it occupies; determined by the liquid's density and vertical distance in a column.

hydroxyl radical   An intermediate of oxygen reduction formed from the reaction between superoxide and hydrogen peroxide; symbolized as $OH\cdot$.

hyperbola   A plane curve possessing two branches.

hyperbolic   Pertaining to a hyperbola.

hyphae   Branching, tubular structures that constitute the mycelium of fungi.

hysteresis   The lack of coincidence of two similar or associated phenomena.

ideal gas   A gas whose behavior can be explained by the gas laws.

imidazole   A heterocyclic compound found in the amino acid histidine.

immunoglobulin E (IgE)   An antibody that attaches to mast cell surfaces and causes mast cell degranulation when reacted with a specific antigen.

impedance   The total opposition to flow.

independent variable   The quantity that is intentionally changed and plotted on the x-axis.

inertia   The tendency of a body at rest to remain at rest or the tendency of a body in motion to remain in motion.

inertial resistance   The tendency of the ventilatory system to resist a change in motion.

inorganic chemistry   That branch of chemistry concerned with all the elements and their compounds except for hydrocarbons and hydrocarbon derivatives.

interstitium   The area between the cellular elements of a structure.

integer   A member of the set of positive whole numbers.

interpolation   The process of determining intermediate values within a range of known values.

intraalveolar pressure   The pressure exerted by the volume of air or gas inside the alveoli, expressed as plus or minus atmospheric pressure.

intrapleural pressure   The pressure in the pleural space.

ion   A charged body having an unequal number of protons and electrons.

ionic bond   Combination of atoms from elements resulting from the transfer of electrons.

ionic-covalent bond   A combination of atoms in which electrons are both transferred and shared.

ionization constant   The product of the molar concentrations of the ionized species divided by the molar concentration of the unionized species at a given temperature.

irregular dichotomous branching   An asymmetrical pattern of branching in a conduction system.

isotope   Atom of an element that has the same atomic number but differs in atomic mass.

joule (J)   Work done when a force of 1 newton acts through a distance of 1 meter in the direction of the motion.

Kelvin scale   An absolute scale of temperature whose zero point is $-273°C$, or 0 K.

kinetic energy   The energy caused by the motion of an object, molecule, atom, or ion.

kinetic theory of matter   States that all molecules are in constant motion.

laminae   Cylindrical layers of gas molecules flowing through a tube during laminar flow conditions.

laminar flow   The flow of fluid molecules, atoms, or ions characterized by horizontal layers or laminae.

lateral wall pressure   Pressure exerted against the walls of a conduction system by a flowing fluid.

law of conservation of energy   A law stating that energy gained by a system equals that lost by the system's surroundings.

law of conservation of matter   States that matter can neither be created nor destroyed, only changed from one state to another.

law of continuity   Explains the relationship between total cross-sectional area of a tube and the velocity of the fluid flowing through it.

law of LaPlace   States that the inflation pressure of a sphere is inversely related to the sphere's radius and directly related to the surface tension at the sphere's air-liquid interface.

law of mass action   States that the rate of a chemical reaction is proportional to the concentration of the reactants.

leukotrienes   A group of compounds that produce allergic and inflammatory reactions.

L-form   A bacterium that has lost all or part of its cell wall and is still capable of undergoing cell division.

lipid peroxidation   The process whereby polyunsaturated fatty acid cell membrane components undergo free radical attack.

lipids   Molecules that are constituents of fats.

lipopolysaccharide   A toxic molecule found on the outer surface of all gram-negative bacteria.

liquid   Matter that takes the shape of its container and is uncompressible.

logarithm   The exponent indicating the power to which the base must be raised to give a number.

lysis   Rupturing of a cell.

lysosome   A cytoplasmic organelle containing digestive enzymes.

mantissa   The decimal fraction of a logarithm.

mass   The quantity of matter contained by an object.

mast cell   A perivascular or perilymphatic cell located in connective tissue of all organs.

mean   A statistical term for the sum of values of a variable, or a data set, obtained by dividing the sum of the values by the number of samples in the data set.

mean free path   The average distance traveled by a gas molecule between collisions.

measure of central tendency   An index of central location used in describing frequency distributions.

median   A statistical term for the value in a distribution of scores, above and below which one-half of the frequencies fall; the score of the 50th percentile. The median for an even-numbered data set is obtained by averaging the middle values.

mediator   The chemical agent responsible for the transmission of a nerve impulse across a synapse, also called a *transmitter*.

metabolism   The interactions of biomolecules including synthesis of compounds, degradation of compounds, generation of energy, and associated activities.

metalloporphyrin   A molecule containing a metal ion and a porphyrin (e.g., heme).

metalloprotein   A protein molecule containing a metal ion, (e.g., hemoglobin and myoglobin).

methylene bridge   A chemical bond comprised of the organic radical methylene.

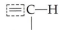

milliequivalent   An expression of concentration of solution obtained by dividing the concentration in milligrams per 100 milliliters by the molecular weight; abbreviated as mEq.

mitochondria   Cytoplasmic organelles of eucaryotic cells that carry out metabolic functions involved in production of energy (ATP).

mitochondrion   A cytoplasmic organelle that contains enzymes necessary for generating ATP.

mitosis   A process involving the stepwise division of the nucleus of a eucaryotic cell into two daughter nuclei each containing the same number of chromosomes as the parent nucleus.

mitotic apparatus   Structures found in the cytoplasm that participate in segregation of chromosomes during cell division.

mode   The statistical term representing the value (score) in a data set that occurs more often than other scores in the same set of data. The mode of the following data set is 8. Data set: 7, 2, 8, 8, 6, 2, 5, 8, 4, 9.

moiety (*pl., -ies*)   A part or portion of indefinite size.

molarity   Moles of solute per liter of solution.

mole   A unit representing the mass of a substance divided by its gram-molecular weight.

molecular diffusion   The movement of gas molecules due to the kinetic energy provided by the ambient temperature.

molecular weight   Sum of the atomic weights of the constituent atoms in a molecule.

momentum   The product of a body's mass and linear velocity.

monomorphic   Refers to fungi having only one shape or appearance.

monosaccharide   A sugar molecule consisting of a single molecular unit of three to six carbon atoms.

monovalent   Containing a single binding site or degree of charge.

monovalent compound   A compound whose gram molecular weight and gram equivalent weight are equal.

multiplicative inverse   Two numbers whose product is one (1), e.g., 1/2 and 2 are multiplicative inverses of each other because $1/2 \times 2 = 1$; also *reciprocal*.

mycelium   Mat of intertwined hyphae comprising a colony of mold.

myoglobin   An oxygen-binding protein located in muscle tissue.

nano-   Greek prefix representing one one-billionth; 0.000000001; 10^{-9}.

nanomole   One one-billionth of a mole; 10^{-9} mole.

neutron   Neutrally charged particle in the nucleus of an atom.

neutropenia   Reduced number of neutrophils in the blood.

neutrophilia   Increased number of neutrophils in the blood.

newton (N)   A force that gives an acceleration of 1 meter/second/second to a 1 kg mass.

Newtonian fluid   A fluid that maintains a constant viscosity at all flow rates.

nominal variable   A variable that is unordered and is assigned a number to identify the class representing that variable; e.g., grouping males and females by assigning the number 1 to represent females and 2 to signify males.

nonelastic resistance   The sum of inertial and airway resistance; also termed nonviscous resistance.

normal curve   A frequency distribution with a bell-shaped curve.

normality   Concentration of a solution expressed in gram equivalent weights per liter of solution.

normal flora   Microbes that are common residents of various bodily tissues and usually do not cause disease.

nuclear membrane   A phospholipid bilayer that partitions the nuclear region of a cell from the cytoplasm.

nucleolus   A region in the nucleus of a eucaryotic cell where RNA is stored.

nucleoprotein   A conjugated protein and nucleic acid that make up a chromosome.

nucleotide   A molecule consisting of a nitrogenous base, a five-carbon sugar, and a phosphate.

nucleotide bases   The nitrogenous ring-structured molecules that when linked together form the molecules deoxyribonucleic acid or ribonucleic acid.

nucleus   The center structure of an atom or ion containing the protons and neutrons, around which the electrons orbit; the intracellular region of a eucaryotic cell that contains the genetic material.

null hypothesis (H_o)   A statement indicating the hypothesized values for one or more of the population parameters. This is usually the status quo or the compliment of the alternative hypothesis.

number line   A line containing real numbers in increasing order from left to right, with positive numbers located to the right of zero (origin) and with negative numbers situated to the left of the origin (zero).

numerator   The numeral above the line in a mathematical fraction.

obligate aerobes   Microbes that require the presence of oxygen for growth.

obligate anaerobes   Microbes for which the presence of oxygen is lethal.

obligate intracellular parasite   An organism that can survive only in the intracellular environment of a cell.

Ohm's law   Electrical law relating resistance, voltage, and current.

opportunist   Microorganism that causes disease when normal host defense mechanisms become altered.

ordered pair   The x and y values signifying the location of a point on a Cartesian coordinate.

ordinal variable   A variable that can be assigned a rank; e.g., the ranking of β_2 agonists in terms of how fast they act or how long their effects persist.

ordinate   The vertical axis (y-axis) in a plane Cartesian coordinate system.

organelle   A subcellular structure found in the cytoplasm and nucleus.

origin   The point of intersection of the ordinate and abscissa on a Cartesian plane.

osmol   A unit of measure used to express the concentration of a solute.

osmosis   The movement of solvent through a semipermeable membrane from a solution of lesser concentration to one of higher concentration.

osmotic pressure   The pressure resulting from the net osmosis of fluid into a solution.

oxidation   The process whereby an atom, ion, or molecule loses one or more electrons.

oxidation potential   Indication of the tendency of a substance to undergo either oxidation or reduction reactions.

oxygen content   Amount of oxygen in blood; expressed in volumes percent.

oxygen saturation   Refers to the percentage of total hemoglobin in blood bound with oxygen; So_2.

parabola   Something cone-shaped.

parallax   The apparent displacement of an object's position caused by the change in an observer's location.

paramagnetic susceptibility   Refers to the magnetic property of atoms or molecules resulting from having one or more unpaired electrons.

parasympathetic   Of or pertaining to that portion of the autonomic nervous system associated with energy conservation.

partial pressure   The pressure exerted by an individual gas in a mixture of gases.

Pascal-second   The units (abbreviated Pas) for viscosity according to International System of Units.

passive transport   The free movement of molecules or ions across cytoplasmic membranes.

pathogen   A parasite capable of causing disease in a significant number of healthy individuals with a normal immune response.

pathogenicity   The disease-producing power of a microbe.

peptidoglycan   The continuous molecular structure making up the bacterial cell wall.

percent   Expressed as a portion of 100.

percentile rank   The number that represents the percent of cases in a comparison group which achieved scores lower than the one cited.

percentiles   Numbers that divide a distribution into 100 equal parts.

permease   An enzyme that facilitates active transport of nutrient molecules across cytoplasmic membranes.

peroxidase   Any of a group of iron-containing porphyrin enzymes that catalyze the oxidation of organic substances in the presence of H_2O_2.

peroxide   The oxide of an element having more oxygen atoms than any of its other components.

pH   A measure of the acidity of a solution.

phagocytes   Cells that envelop and digest microorganisms and cellular debris.

phagocytosis   The process of engulfing bacteria and other particulate matter by cells such as neutrophils and macrophages.

phagolysosome   A digestive compartment in the cytoplasm resulting from fusion of a vacuole and a lysosome.

phenolic group   An aromatic or carbon ring containing one or more hydroxyl (OH^-) groups.

pH indicator   A chemical agent that changes color at specific levels of acidity or alkalinity.

phosphorylation   The biochemical process of incorporating a phosphate group into an organic molecule.

physiologic dead space   The sum of the anatomic dead space and the alveolar dead space.

pili   Appendages extending from the surface of some bacteria and participating in attachment to mammalian tissue or other bacteria during the process of conjugation.

pK   Represents the pH at which maximum buffering capacity can be achieved for a particular reaction.

plasma proteins   Essentially, albumin, fibrinogen, and gamma globulins. These proteins are virtually responsible for the colloid osmotic pressure (oncotic pressure) of the blood.

plasmids   Extrachromosomal pieces of deoxyribonucleic acid (DNA) found in the cytoplasm of bacteria.

plethysmograph   Device used for measuring thoracic gas volume and compliance.

pOH   A measure of the alkalinity of a solution.

point estimate   An estimated value of a parameter.

poise   A unit of measurement of viscosity in the CGS measuring system.

Poiseuille's law of laminar flow   Describes the relationship among a certain number of resistance factors that are encountered as a fluid flows through a conduction system in laminar fashion.

polarographic cell   A device that uses an electrical current to polarize the electrodes for the measurement of oxygen.

polymer   A large molecule consisting of repeating units of a particular smaller molecule.

polymorphonuclear leukocyte   A type of white blood cell containing a multi-lobed, or segmented, nucleus; e.g., a neutrophil, eosinophil, or basophil.

polysaccharide   A sugar molecule consisting of molecular units of three to six carbons in excess of 10.

porphyrin   A metal-containing tetrapyrrole derivative found in cytoplasm; a structural component of hemoglobin.

potential energy   The energy of an object due to its position or configuration.

power   (1) Indicates how many times a number is to be multiplied times itself; an exponent. (2) The rate at which work is done.

precision   The repeatability of a measurement.

pressure   Force per unit area.

primary structure   A protein having an amino acid sequence in a relatively straight (uncoiled) configuration.

principal energy levels   Specific regions wherein electrons are situated and located at varying distances from an atom's or ion's nucleus.

probability   A theory concerned with the possible outcomes of experiments.

product   The number obtained when two factors are multiplied.

proportion   A quantitative relationship equating two ratios.

prosthetic group   The nonprotein portion of a protein molecule.

protein   A molecule consisting of a chain of amino acids.

protein kinase   A protein catalyzing the transfer of a phosphate group from ATP to form a phosphoprotein.

proton   Positively charged particle in the nucleus of an atom.

protoplast   A bacterium that has no cell wall material.

psi   Abbreviation for pounds per square inch; a unit of pressure.

purines   A family of nitrogen-containing, ring-structured molecules with nine atoms.

pyrimidines   Family of nitrogen-containing, ring-structured molecules with six atoms.

pyrrole   The parent compound of the hemoglobin molecule.

quaternary structure   A protein having numerous amino acid (polypeptide) chains linked together forming multichain complexes.

quotient   The quantity resulting from the division of one quantity by another.

radial force   A force developing and extending uniformly around a central axis.

radical   A group of at least two elements having a net charge, e.g., HCO_3^-.

random sampling   Sample selection performed such that each observation has the same probability of being selected.

range   The scale distance between the largest and smallest score.

rate (equilibrium) constant   The numerical value obtained from dividing the product of the molar concentrations of the reactants of a chemical reaction (at equilibrium) by the product of the molar concentrations of the reaction's products (at equilibrium).

ratio   A quantitative relationship between two like entities.

reactant   Substance that chemically interacts with another substance to form an entirely different entity.

reducing agent   A substance that undergoes oxidation and then causes the reduction of some other substance in an oxidation-reduction reaction.

reductase   An enzyme that catalyzes a reduction reaction.

reduction   The process whereby an atom, ion, or molecule gains one or more electrons.

relative humidity   The ratio of the actual amount of water vapor in the air at a specific temperature compared to the maximum capacity of the air for water vapor at that temperature.

respiration   The metabolic reduction of an inorganic molecule, usually oxygen, with the subsequent generation of energy in the form of ATP.

respiratory burst   The release of oxidants (oxidizing agents) from phagocytic cells intended to destroy microorganisms that invade the body.

respiratory quotient   The ratio of carbon dioxide production to oxygen consumption; normal range is 0.8 to 1.0.

Reynold's number   A dimensionless number that reflects the flow pattern present; a value less than 2,000 indicates laminar flow, and one greater than 2,000 indicates turbulent flow.

ribose   Five-carbon molecule that is the sugar moiety found in nucleotides of RNA.

ribosome   A granular cytoplasmic structure involved in the process of protein synthesis.

RNA   Ribonucleic acid.

rule of eight   The natural tendency of all atoms to have eight electrons in their outermost energy level during a chemical reaction.

rules of order of operations   A series of rules which can be applied for the purpose of simplifying a numerical expression.

salt   A neutral ionic compound composed of the cations of a base and the anions of an acid.

sample   A subset of a population.

saprophyte   Organism that usually survives on inert organic matter.

secondary structure   A protein having hydrogen bonds interconnecting a coiled sequence of amino acids.

selectively permeable membrane   A membrane that allows for the passage of solvent and only certain solutes.

selective medium   An artificial growth medium that allows growth of only one or a few members of a desired group of bacteria.

selective toxicity   Refers to antimicrobics that inhibit metabolic systems of bacteria and having little or no effect on metabolism of mammalian cells.

semipermeable membrane   A membrane that allows the passage of some substances (solutes) and prevents the passage of others (solutes and the solvent).

shunt   Blood that does not become arterialized.

shunt effect   Perfusion in excess of ventilation.

sigmoid   S-shaped

significance level   Same as alpha level.

significant digits   The digits (figures) that indicate the precision with which a measurement is made.

singlet oxygen   An oxygen intermediary wherein the two outermost electrons are boosted to a higher electron shell, resulting in one experiencing spin reversal.

solid   A substance of definite shape and volume.

solubility coefficient   The amount of gas that will dissolve in a given liquid at a given temperature at standard pressure.

solute   Substance that is dissolved in a solution.

solution   Homogeneous mixture of molecules, atoms, or ions of two or more substances.

solvent   Substance in which the solute is dissolved when forming a solution.

specific compliance   Indicates the volume at which a compliance measurement is made; expressed as liter/cm H_2O/liter.

specific gravity   The ratio of the density of a solid or liquid to that of water at 4°C; also, the ratio of the density of a gas compared to that of air.

spheroplast   A cell wall-deficient bacterium that retains some of its cell wall material.

sporulation   The process of spore formation from a vegetative bacterium.

standard atmospheric pressure   The total pressure exerted by the ambient air at sea level, often referred to as the downward pressure of air against a unit of area of the earth's surface.

standard deviation   The square root of the sum of the squared deviations of the observations from the mean, divided by the sample size minus 1 ($n-1$); a measure of dispersion.

standard error estimate (SEE)   The standard deviation of scores around a regression line.

standard normal distribution   A frequency distribution with a bell-shaped curve, which has a mean of zero (0), a standard deviation of one (1), and a total area equal to 1.00.

standard score (z-score)   A score representing the deviation from the mean for a specific score.

Starling's law of the capillaries   Explains the direction and magnitude of fluid movement at the capillary level.

static   A condition devoid of motion.

stereochemistry   The area of chemistry dealing with spatial arrangements and relationships among atoms in a compound.

sterilization   The process that results in killing of all viable forms of microorganisms.

sterol   A lipid molecule that contributes to the integrity of cytoplasmic membranes of eucaryotic cells.

STPD   Standard temperature and pressure dry.

subatmospheric pressure   A pressure less than that of the normal atmosphere; also negative pressure.

subshell   A subdivision of an atom's energy level containing the electron orbitals.

sum   The value obtained by adding two or more numbers.

sum of squares   Deviations from the mean squared and summed.

superoxide dismutase (SOD)   An intracellular enzyme (antioxidant) that inactivates the superoxide radical.

superoxide (radical or anion)   An intermediary byproduct of cellular oxygen reduction formed as the oxygen molecule gains one electron; symbolized as $O_2^-\cdot$.

supra-atmospheric pressure   A pressure greater than normal atmospheric pressure; also positive pressure.

surface tension   A property of liquids arising from unbalanced, cohesive molecular forces at an air-liquid interface; expressed as dynes/cm.

surfactant   A surface-active substance that reduces surface tension.

sympathetic   Of or pertaining to that portion of the autonomic nervous system associated with energy expenditure.

t-**distribution**   A symmetrical sampling distribution with a mean of zero (0) and a standard deviation that becomes smaller as the degrees of freedom increase. *t*-distribution will be approximately the same as standard normal distribution for a large sample size.

tertiary structure   A protein having a three-dimensional arrangement as a result of folded amino acid sequences.

tetramer   Having four configurations or shapes.

tetravalent   Containing four binding sites or degrees of charge.

thermal conductivity   The ability of a substance to conduct or dissipate heat.

thoracic gas volume   The total volume of gas in the thoracic cavity.

thymine   A pyrimidine base found only in DNA.

tissue trophism   The property of a parasite that enables it to attach selectivity in tissue.

torque   A rotary force.

torr   Unit of pressure measurement equal to a millimeter of mercury (mm Hg).

total CO$_2$ The sum of combined (HCO$_3^-$) and dissolved carbon dioxide (Pco_2) in the blood.

trace elements   Ionic forms of iron, magnesium, manganese, and cobalt.

tracheobronchial flow   A combination of laminar and turbulent flow as associated with the flow of gas through the tracheobronchial tree.

transairway pressure gradient   The difference between barometric pressure and the intraalveolar pressure; driving pressure of ventilation.

transduction   A process of gene exchange between bacteria involving transfer of chromosomes or plasmids by bacterial viruses.

transpulmonary pressure   The pressure difference (gradient) between intraalveolar pressure and intrapleural pressure.

trivalent   Containing three binding sites or degrees of charge.

turbulent flow   The flow of fluid molecules, atoms, or ions characterized by eddy currents and vortices.

type I error   Rejection of the null hypothesis (H$_o$) when the H$_o$ is actually true.

type II error   Acceptance of the null hypothesis (H$_o$) when the H$_o$ is actually false.

ultrafiltrate   A substance containing small particles that have filtered across a semipermeable membrane.

unit   Qualifies and adds dimension to a quantity.

univalent reduction   The process by which an atom or molecule gains a single electron.

uracil   A pyrimidine nitrogenous base that comprises nucleotide present only in RNA.

vegetative bacterium   The growing and reproducing form of a microbe.

vacuole   A cytoplasmic pocket that forms following phagocytosis of particulate matter.

valence   The combining capacity of an atom.

valence electrons   The electrons in the outermost electron shell, which are either transferred, shared, or both during a chemical reaction.

van der Waals forces   Weak cohesive forces between atoms and nonpolar molecules.

vapor pressure   Pressure exerted by a vapor in equilibrium with its liquid or solid phase.

variance   The sum of the squared deviations of the observations from the mean, divided by the sample size minus 1 ($n-1$); a measure of dispersion.

velocity   A measure of linear distance per time (e.g., m/sec).

velocity profile, asymmetric   The slightly rounded, somewhat flattened configuration of the molecules of a fluid flowing through a tube under turbulent flow conditions.

velocity profile, symmetric   The parabolic configuration of the molecules of a fluid flowing through a tube under laminar flow conditions.

venous oxygen content (C$\bar{v}$O$_2$) The amount of oxygen in venous blood expressed in volumes percent.

Venturi Device used to entrain ambient gas based on Bernoulli's principle.

Venturi principle Phenomenon involving the entrainment of one fluid by another.

Venturi tube A conduit with an architectural configuration within which the inverse relationship between a fluid's velocity of flow and its lateral wall pressure allows for the entrainment of another fluid.

virion The infectious particle that constitutes a virus.

virulence The degree of disease-producing power of a microbe.

viscosity A fluid's resistance to deformity.

volatile The tendency to readily evaporate.

volt The International System unit of electric potential between two points on a conducting wire carrying a current of 1 ampere when the power dissipated between the two points is 1 watt.

voltage Electromotive force or potential.

voltmeter A device that measures voltage.

volumes percent An expression of the number of milliliters of a gas contained in 100 milliliters of blood; abbreviated *vol%*.

vortex A mass of fluid exhibiting a circular motion.

water vapor pressure The pressure exerted in the atmosphere by water vapor.

water vapor Water molecules suspended in the atmosphere in the form of gas.

watt A unit of power that gives rise to the production of energy at a rate of 1 J/second.

weak acid Any acid that does not ionize 100% in solution.

weak alkaline salt Any alkaline salt that does not ionize 100% in solution.

Wheatstone bridge An electronic device used for precise resistance measurements.

work The product of the force exerted on an object and the distance the object is moved.

zwitterion A protein having no net charge. A protein at its isoelectric point has an equal number of positive and negative charges. A protein is a zwitterion at its isoelectric point.

INDEX

Metric Units

Linear Equivalents
  1 km = 1,000 m = 10^3 m
  1 dm =   0.1 m = 10^{-1} m
  1 cm =   0.01 m = 10^{-2} m
  1 mm =   0.001 m = 10^{-3} m
   1 μ =   0.000001 m = 10^{-6} m
  1 μm =   0.000001 m = 10^{-6} m
  1 nm =   0.000000001 m = 10^{-9} m
   1 Å =   0.0000000001 m = 10^{-10} m
Weight Equivalents
  1 kg = 1,000 g = 10^3 g
  1 dg =   0.1 g = 10^{-1} g
  1 cg =   0.01 g = 10^{-2} g
  1 mg =   0.001 g = 10^{-3} g
  1 μg =   0.000001 g = 10^{-6} g
Volume Equivalents
  1 kl = 1,000 liters = 10^3 L
  1 dl =   0.1 liter = 10^{-1} L
  1 cl =   0.01 liter = 10^{-2} L
  1 ml =   0.001 liter = 10^{-3} L
  1 μl =   0.000001 liter = 10^{-6} L

Rules Governing Logarithms (Base 10)

Multiplication
  $\log(A \times B \times C) = \log A + \log B + \log C$
  for example, $\log(100 \times 100 \times 100) = \log(10^2 \times 10^2 \times 10^2) = \log 10^2 + \log 10^2 \times \log 10^2 = 2 + 2 + 2 = 6$
Division
  $\log\left(\dfrac{A}{B}\right) = \log A - \log B$
  for example, $\log\left(\dfrac{100}{100}\right) = \log\left(\dfrac{10^2}{10^2}\right) = \log 10^2 - \log 10^2 = 2 - 2 = 0$

Mathematical Symbols

$=$ is equal to $\approx$ is approximately equal to
$>$ is greater than $\propto$ is proportional to
$<$ is less than $\neq$ is not equal to
$\geq$ is greater than or equal to $\perp$ is perpendicular to
$\leq$ is less than or equal to $//$ is parallel to